Advances in Reproductive Biology

Advances in Reproductive Biology

Editor: Francisco Armstrong

FOSTER ACADEMICS

www.fosteracademics.com

www.fosteracademics.com

FOSTER ACADEMICS

Cataloging-in-Publication Data

Advances in reproductive biology / edited by Francisco Armstrong.
p. cm.
Includes bibliographical references and index.
ISBN 978-1-63242-912-4
1. Reproduction. 2. Biology. 3. Human reproduction. 4. Reproductive technology. I. Armstrong, Francisco.
QH471 .A38 2020
571.8--dc23

Foster Academics,
118-35 Queens Blvd., Suite 400,
Forest Hills, NY 11375, USA

ISBN 978-1-63242-912-4 (Hardback)

Contents

Preface

The human reproductive system is a collection of sex organs operating together in association with hormones, pheromones and other fluids for the purpose of reproduction. The female reproductive system is responsible for the production of egg cells along with the protection and nourishment of offspring till the time of birth. The male reproductive system has one function only- the production and deposition of sperm. Reproductive biology encompasses all aspects of the reproductive system, sexual development, sexual maturity, fertility, endocrinology and reproduction. The field of obstetrics and gynecology is concerned with the clinical aspects of pregnancy, childbirth and the postpartum period, and the health of the female reproductive system. Hormonal dysfunctions, infertility and anatomical reproductive disorders are treated under the sub-field of reproductive endocrinology and infertility. This book unravels the recent studies in the field of reproductive biology. The topics included herein are of utmost significance and bound to provide incredible insights to readers. They would gain knowledge that would broaden their perspective about reproductive biology.

The researches compiled throughout the book are authentic and of high quality, combining several disciplines and from very diverse regions from around the world. Drawing on the contributions of many researchers from diverse countries, the book's objective is to provide the readers with the latest achievements in the area of research. This book will surely be a source of knowledge to all interested and researching the field.

In the end, I would like to express my deep sense of gratitude to all the authors for meeting the set deadlines in completing and submitting their research chapters. I would also like to thank the publisher for the support offered to us throughout the course of the book. Finally, I extend my sincere thanks to my family for being a constant source of inspiration and encouragement.

Editor

1

Uterine Foxl2 regulates the adherence of the Trophectoderm cells to the endometrial epithelium

Michal Elbaz[1], Ron Hadas[2], Louise M. Bilezikjian[3] and Eran Gershon[1*]

Abstract

Background: Forkhead Transcription Factor L2 (FOXL2) is a member of the forkhead family with important roles in reproduction. Recent studies showed that FOXL2 is expressed in human and bovine endometrium and that its levels fluctuate during pregnancy. In this study, we aimed at evaluating the expression and function of FOXL2 in embryo implantation.

Methods: Mouse uteri at different days of pregnancy were isolated and analyzed for the expression and localization of FOXL2. A lentiviral strategy was further employed to either knockdown or overexpress FOXL2 in non-receptive human endometrial AN3-CA cells and in receptive Ishikawa cells, respectively. These genetically modified cells were compared to cells infected with a control lentivirus to determine the function of FOXL2 in trophectoderm cells adherence to Endometrial Epithelium was associated with the expression of genes known to be involved in acquisition of uterine receptivity.

Results: We report that FOXL2 is expressed in both, the luminal epithelium and the myometrium of the mouse uterus and that its expression declines prior to implantation. We found that endometrial cells expressing low FOXL2 levels, either endogenous or genetically manipulated, were associated with a higher attachment rate of mouse blastocysts or human Jeg3 spheroids and mouse blastocysts. In accordance, low-FOXL2 levels were associated with changes in the expression level of components of the *Wnt/Fzd* and apoptotic pathways, both of which are involved in uterine receptivity. Furthermore, FOXL2 expression was inversely correlated with G-protein signaling protein 2 (*Rgs2*) and cytokine expression.

Conclusions: These results suggest that FOXL2 interferes with embryo attachment. Better understanding of the function of FOXL2 in the uterus would possibly suggest novel strategies for treatment of infertility attributed to repeated implantation failure.

Keywords: FOXL2, Uterine receptivity, FOXL2 depletion, FOXL2 overexpression, Embryo attachment, Gene expression, Cell adherence

* Correspondence: eran.gershon1@mail.huji.ac.il
[1]Department of Ruminant Science, Agricultural Research Organization, 50250 Rishon LeZion, Israel
Full list of author information is available at the end of the article

Background

Forkhead transcription factor L2 (FOXL2) is a member of the forkhead family of transcription factors which plays an indispensable role in differentiation of the embryonic gonads into ovaries [1]. Haplo insufficiency of FOXL2 function, resulting from mutations of the *FOXL2* gene has been shown to cause the blepharophimosis–ptosis–epicanthus inversus syndrome (BPES), a genetic disorder characterized by eyelid and mild craniofacial abnormalities, associated with premature ovarian failure in a subset of affected women [2].

The use of DNA chip and quantitative RT-PCR (qRT-PCR) to detect its potential transcriptional targets in granulosa-like cells, revealed that *Foxl2* affects the expression of genes involved in reactive oxygen species (ROS) detoxification, inflammation and apoptosis [3, 4].

Later studies suggest that *Foxl2* regulates granulosa cell proliferation [5] and ovarian G-protein signaling protein 2 (RGS2) [3, 6]. These multi-functional GTPase-accelerating proteins inactivate the alpha-subunit of G proteins and rapidly switch off the G protein-coupled receptor signaling pathways by promoting GTP hydrolysis [7, 8]. Another recent study found that FOXL2 directly modulates estrogen receptor beta (ESR2) expression through a newly identified intronic element [4]. FOXL2 has also been shown to regulate the expression of follistatin and thereby alters activin and SMAD3 signaling, which are key players in the regulation of reproductive functions by their actions in the ovary and the pituitary [9, 10]. In many species activities of the TGFβ super-family members, including activin-like molecules, play a pivotal role in endometrial remodeling, which is essential for placentogenesis during the peri-implantation period [11]. Interestingly, FOXL2 in the murine pregnant uterus, is exclusively expressed in the implantation sites [7].

The expression of FOXL2 has been shown in human myometrium at term [8]. More recently its expression in human endometrium was reported [12] and its downregulation during the pre-receptive to receptive transition has been described [13]. Another paper demonstrated that FOXL2 expression is downregulated in human endometrial cells upon their coculture with trophoblast cells [14]. A recent study demonstrated that FOXL2 is expressed in the mouse neonatal mesenchyme and that expression persists in the stroma and the deep inner myometrial layer during uterine maturation [15]. In the adult mouse, FOXL2 is expressed in the differentiated stromal layer [15]. This study further showed that conditional deletion of *Foxl2* in the postnatal uterus results in infertility, reduced thickness of the stroma layer and a hypertrophic, disorganized inner myometrial layer [15]. Furthermore, the supplementary muscular layer fails to form a coherent layer around uterine arteries in mice with postnatal targeted deletion of *Foxl2* [15].

In the present study, we hypothesized that *Foxl2* might play a role in uterus remodeling, preparing the uterine wall for implantation. To challenge this hypothesis we aimed at evaluating the expression and exploring its specific function in regulating critical processes associated with embryo implantation, such as uterine cell proliferation, genes that are involved in apoptosis, and genes that are involved in embryo-maternal recognition, such as *Rgs2* transcript. Our experiments demonstrated that that FOXL2 expression in the mouse uterus is modified along pregnancy. Its significant decline towards implantation is consistent with our findings that endometrial FOXL2 levels inversely correlate with the rate of embryo attachment. These findings go along with the effects of FOXL2 on the expression of genes implicated in uterine maturation and embryo attachment.

Methods

Animals

To examine FOXL2 expression during pregnancy, sexually mature, cycling female C57BL/6 mice (7–9 wk. old) were purchased from Harlan (Harlan Laboratories, Rehovot, Israel). The females were mated with C57BL/6 male. The next morning, the females were monitored for vaginal plug (indicating day 0.5 of pregnancy). Uteri were isolated at days 3, 4, 6, 12 and 18 of pregnancy and further analyzed.

In all experiments, three independent repeats were performed as follows: for each time point, uteri, implantation sites and placentas from 3 different random animals were collected. Then, the uteri, placenta or implantation sites collected from the 3 animals at each time point were pooled together and the pool was subjected to further analysis. Thus, a total of 9 uteri/implantation sites/placenta from 9 different random animals were used for each lane.

Cells

The AN3-CA cells, non-receptive human endometrial cells (cell line obtained from CLS Cell Line Services GmbH, Eppelheim, Germany), were grown in MEM (Biological Industries, Israel) with 10% fetal bovine serum (FBS, Hyclone, Biological Industries, Israel), Ishikawa cells, receptive human endometrial cells (cell line obtained from ATCC, Manassas, VA), were grown in DMEM (Biological Industries, Israel) with 10% FBS. Both cell lines were grown at 37 °C under 5% CO2.

shRNA-mediated knockdown of FOXL2

The strategy used to achieve siRNA-mediated *Foxl2* knockdown was essentially as described previously [9, 16]. Briefly, lentiviral particles harboring *Foxl2*-targeted shRNA cassettes or scrambled control shRNA in tandem with IRES-controlled GFP cDNA were prepared using HEK293T as described previously [16] and used to infect AN3-CA cells. The cells were expanded under normal growth conditions and monitored for GFP expression. To achieve uniformity of knockdown for functional studies, approximately 10^7 cells expressing either GFP alone, scrambled shRNA as control or *Foxl2* shRNA were subjected to fluorescence-activated cell sorting (FACS) on a FACSVantage SE DiVa (BD Biosciences, San Jose, CA) equipped with a 488-nm argon laser. Initial gating was based on forward scatter and side scatter to maximize recovery of live single cells. According to the fluorescence intensity histogram of each population of infected AN3-CA cells, the top 5% of GFP+ cells were sorted and collected and expanded for further analysis.

Lentivirus mediated method of FOXL2 overexpression

Viral particules harboring *Foxl2* cDNA for overexpression or control vector were prepared using HEK293T as described previously [9]. Briefly, Ishikawa cells were infected with control or FOXL2 overexpressing lentivirus that incorporates IRES-driven GFP as a marker. To achieve uniformity of overexpression for functional studies, the transduced Ishikawa cells were FACS sorted as described above and the top 5% of GFP+ cells were collected and expanded for further analysis.

Establishing a spheroids-endometrial cell attachment assay

The in vitro model for implantation was performed as described previously [17]. Briefly, Jeg3 cells, a human trophoblast cell line, were cultured in a humid atmosphere containing 5% CO_2 at 37 °C on a shaker for 24 h. The resulting spheres were stained using calcein-AM (BD Bioscience, San Jose, CA), and were monitored using G-BOX gel-imager (syngene, Cambridge, UK), in order to test their viability and to count them. Then, labeled Jeg3 spheroids of 50–200 μm in diameter, similar in size to an implanting blastocyst, were transferred to the upper surface of the confluent monolayer of Ishikawa or AN3-CA endometrial cells, with or without *Foxl2* overexpression or knockdown (approximately 50 spheroids/well), and the co-cultures were maintained for 6 h at 37 °C. At the end of incubation, non-adherent spheroids were removed by washing the culture plates and the plates were examined using a G-BOX gel-imager (syngene, Cambridge, UK). The number of tightly attached spheroids in each well was counted using the GeneTools software. The percentage of attached spheroids relative to the total number of spheroids used to initiate the co-incubation experiments (adhesion percent) was calculated.

Embryo attachment assay

Embryo attachment assay was performed as described previously [18]. Briefly, Wild-type ICR females were purchased from Harlan and superovulated by sub-cutaneous injections of 5 units of pregnant mare's serum gonadotropin (PMSG, Chrono-gest Intervest, The Netherlands) followed by 5 units of intraperitoneal injection of human chorionic gonadotropin (hCG, Chrono-gest Intervest, The Netherlands) 48 h later and then mated with wild-type ICR males. Morula and blastocyst stage embryos were collected from the females at 3.5 d after copulation and then incubated in KSOM medium to obtain expanded blastocysts. Embryos were labeled with Vybrant Cell-Labeling Solution (ThermoFisher Scientific, Waltham, MS) before transferring unselectively to confluent Ishikawa (infected with control or *Foxl2* overexpression virus or AN3-CA cells infected with control or *Foxl2* siRNA virus) cell monolayers in a 96-well plate coated with Matrigel (In vitro technologies, Victoria, Australia). Between 3 and 4 blastocysts were transferred per well depending upon the total number recovered. Co-cultures were incubated undisturbed at 37 °C in a 5% CO2 atmosphere for 48 h. The stability of embryo attachment was measured by washing the culture plates and shaking them three times from side to side. Each measurement was performed manually under a microscope (Nikon, Tokyo, Japan), by examining the stability of each mouse embryo upon tapping the stage. The percentage of attached embryos relative to the total number of embryos used to initiate the co-incubation experiments (adhesion percent) was calculated (Additional file 1: Figure S1).

Protein extraction and western blot analysis

Proteins from uteri were extracted at the indicated time points in RIPA buffer using homogenizer, and suspended in Laemmli loading buffer (125 mM Tris, pH 6.8, 4% SDS, 10% glycerol, 0.006% bromphenol blue, and 2% β-mercaptoethanol). The proteins were then separated on a 12% acrylamide gel, followed by their transfer to a nitrocellulose membrane. After blocking with 5% skimmed milk, the membranes were incubated with primary antibodies over-night at 4 °C (rabbit anti-FOXL2 1:1000, Bioss, Woburn, MA; rabbit anti-β-ACTIN 1:2000, Thermo Scientific, Waltham, MS), then with the secondary antibodies for 1 h at room temperature (anti-rabbit 1:5000, Jackson laboratory, Bar Harbor, MI). The immunoreactive bands were detected by ECL (Amersham, England).

RNA extraction and analysis by PCR

Total RNA from uteri and endometrial cell lines was extracted using RNeasy mini columns (Qiagen, Hilden, Germany), according to the manufacturer's guidelines. RNA was converted into cDNA with the High-Capacity cDNA Reverse transcription kit (Applied Biosystems), according to the manufacturer's guidelines using oligo (dT) and Moloney murine leukemia virus reverse transcriptase. The cDNAs were used for PCR amplification with primer sets for *Foxl2* and *Hprt* (Additional file 2: Table S1) in a 25 μl reaction volume, with 10× buffer, 400 μM of each d-NTP and 0.625 units of Taq DNA Polymerase (Fisher Scientific, Waltham, MA). PCR was performed for the indicated number of cycles (initial denaturation at 94 °C for 3 min, then 35 cycles at 94 °C for 1 min, 60 °C for 1 min, 72 °C for 1 min, and a final incubation at 72 °C for 7 min). The reaction mix (10 μl) was run on 1.5% agarose gels, stained with Ethidium Bromide and quantified using UV imaging (Gel Doc 1000, Bio-Rad) and Molecular Analyst software (Bio-Rad, Hercules, Ca.). Experimental replication of each time point was performed in triplicate.

Quantitive RT-PCR

All real-time PCRs were carried out on a step one plus (ThermoFisher Scientific, Waltham, MS), using the Absolute Blue QPCR Master Mix (ThermoFisher Scientific, Waltham, MS) with SYBR Green. The following is the reaction protocol: 15 min at 95 °C for enzyme activation, followed by 40 cycles of: 15 s at 95 °C, 30 s at 60 °C, and 15 s at 72 °C, at the end of which fluorescence was measured with the Rotor-Gene. SYBR Green-I assays also included a melt curve at the end of the cycling protocol, with continuous fluorescence measurement from 65 to 99 °C. All reactions contained the same amount of cDNA, 10 μl Absolute Blue QPCR Master Mix, primers for the indicated genes (Additional file 2: Table S1) and UltraPure PCR-grade water (Biological Industries, Israel) to a final volume of 20 μl. Each real-time PCR included a no-template control, in duplicate. Relative expression levels (ΔΔCt) were calculated by normalizing to hypoxanthine guanine phosphoribosyl transferase (HPRT). Primers were designed using the primer3 website (http://bioinfo.ut.ee/primer3-0.4.0/).

Immunofluorescence staining

FOXL2 immunofluorescence was performed on deparaffinized uterine sections isolated from non-pregnant C57/BL6 females. The sections were washed in PBS (Biological Industries, Israel), followed by antigen retrieval by standard sodium citrate method. Non-specific binding sites were blocked by incubating the sections for 30 min in 20% fetal bovine serum (Biological Industries, Israel), 0.2% Triton X100 (Sigma, Rehovot, Israel) in PBS. Sections were then incubated overnight at 4 °C with anti-FOXL2 antibody (anti-FOXL2 rabbit polyclonal antibody, 1:50, Biosis, Woburn, MA). Sections were washed with PBS and immunoreacted with Cy3-conjugated anti-rabbit IgG in 2% normal horse serum and PBS for 60 min (dilution 1:150, Jackson Laboratories, Bar Harbor, MI). The sections were subsequently washed with PBS and visualized, using fluorescence microscope (Nikon, Tokyo, Japan). All images were taken in identical conditions.

Statistical analysis

For statistical comparisons, replicate experiments were averaged and using Student's 2 tailed unpaired *t*-test and considered statistically different when $P < 0.05$. These statistical analyses were conducted with JMP software (SAS Institute, 2005). All numerical data shown in the figures are from representative experiments expressed as the means −/+S.E.M of replicates.

Results

FOXL2 expression and its localization in the mouse uterus

Our initial experiments were directed at the analysis of the spatio-temporal expression of FOXL2 in the mouse uterus during pregnancy. We found that the FOXL2 protein, which is high upon establishment of pregnancy (days 3 and 4, vaginal plug is day 0.5), significantly decreases prior to implantation (occurring on pregnancy day 4.5 (implantation occurs at day 4.5, vaginal plug is day 0.5, Fig. 1a-b).

In the bovine, FOXL2 has been localized to uterine endometrial, stromal and glandular cells [19]. In agreement, using anti-FOXL2, our immunofluorescence analysis of non-pregnant murine uterine sections showed that FOXL2 localizes to the myometrium, glandular epithelium and the luminal epithelium of (Fig. 2a-b). Analysis of pregnant mouse uterine tissue at embryonic day 4.5 revealed that FOXL2 is expressed by the luminal epithelium as well as by the embryo (Fig. 2c). Interestingly, this

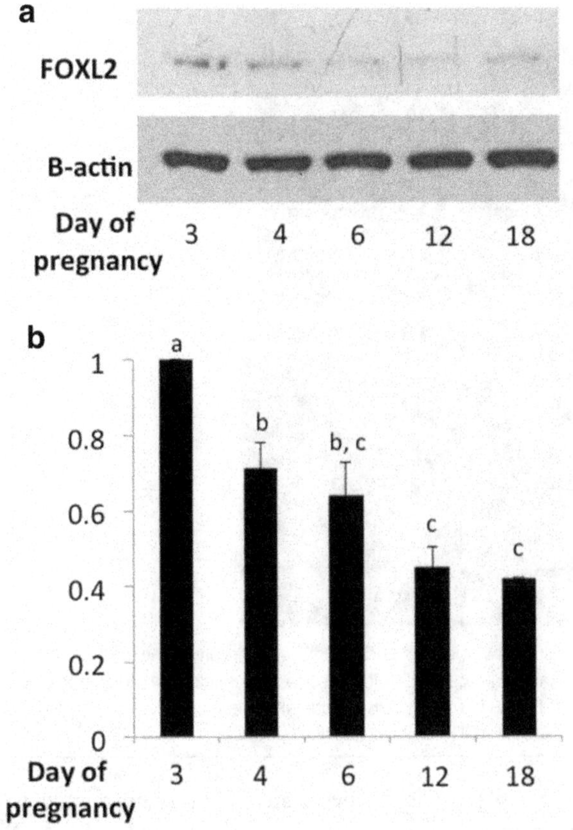

Fig. 1 FOXL2 expression in the murine uterus during pregnancy. **a** FOXL2 protein levels decrease prior to implantation (implantation occurs at pregnancy day 4.5). Western blot analysis of FOXL2 protein using β-actin as a loading control. The results represent one out of 3 independent experiments with similar results. **b** Quantitation of three independent experiments with similar results. Different letters represent significant differences ($p < 0.05$)

experiment showed that FOXL2 could also be detected at the attachment area of the embryo with the luminal epithelium. However, the expression of this protein in luminal epithelial cells surrounding the attached blastocysts is substantially lower than that in the luminal epithelial cells away from the implantation site (Fig. 2c). The specificity of the FOXL2 antibody was confirmed by the absence of signal in sections incubated without the primary anti-FOXL2 antibody (Fig. 2d) The decrease in FOXL2 expression in granulosa cells as folliculogenesis progresses (Additional file 3: Figure S2) confirmed the findings in a previous study [20] and was used as a complementary experiment for specificity demonstration.

Analysis of uterine tissue from healthy women showed that FOXL2 is present in human endometrial tissues [12]. We analyzed two human endometrial cell lines, AN3-CA and Ishikawa cells, and confirmed by RT-PCR that both lines express *FOXL2* mRNA (Additional file 4: Figure S3A).

Establishment of FOXL2 depleted or FOXL2 overexpressing cells

Our next experiments were directed at the validation of human endometrial cell lines models to be employed for further evaluation of the function of FOXL2 in embryo implantation. We used two human endometrial cell lines, AN3-CA and Ishikawa cells that are considered to be representative of non-receptive and receptive endometrium, respectively ([21, 22] and our unpublished data). Interestingly, the two cell lines differ by the level of endogenous FOXL2, with significantly higher levels of *Foxl2* mRNA in AN3-CA non-receptive endometrial cells (Fig. 3 and Additional file 4: Figure S3b). In order to assess the effect of FOXL2 on endometrial functions, we manipulated Foxl2 levels in the two cell lines by knocking down *Foxl2* in AN3-CA cells by shRNA expression using lentiviral particles harboring *Foxl2* -targeted shRNA (shFOXL2) cassettes and, conversely, overexpressing *Foxl2* in Ishikawa cells using lentiviral particles harboring the FOXL2 cDNA. These strategies resulted in a 60–70% reduction of *Foxl2* mRNA levels in AN3-CA cells infected with sh *Foxl2* -encoding lentivirus (Additional file 1: Figure S1A) and as much as a 25-fold increase in *Foxl2* mRNA levels in Ishikawa cells infected with *Foxl2* overexpressing virus, compared to cells infected with a control virus (Additional file 1: Figure S1B). We used these modified and the parent cell lines to examine the effect of *Foxl2* on embryo attachment.

Attachment of murine embryos and Jeg3 spheroids to human endometrial cells with FOXL2 either depletion or overexpression

The effect of changes in *Foxl2* abundance on embryo attachment was assessed by an in vitro adhesion assay (Additional file 5: Figure S4A-C, [18]). We found that the rate of embryo attachment to *Foxl2* -depleted AN3-CA was higher than that to control AN3-CA cells (Fig. 4a). By contrast, overexpression of *Foxl2* in Ishikawa cells led to a reduction in embryo attachment compared to control Ishikawa cells (Fig. 4b). In a complementary experiment we used the in vitro implantation assay to examine Jeg3 human spheroid attachment to the same endometrial cell lines with either high or low FOXL2 protein expression. Similar to our results with mouse embryo attachment, we observed that, Jeg3 spheroid attachment to *Foxl2* -depleted AN3-CA cells was higher than that to control AN3-CA cells (Fig. 4c). Conversely, overexpression of *Foxl2* in Ishikawa cells led to inhibition of spheroid attachment compared to control Ishikawa cells with lower FOXL2 levels (Fig. 4d). These observations support the possibility that the reduced FOXL2 protein expression seen around the time of implantation (Fig. 1b) contribute to the process of implantation by allowing the attachment of the embryo to the endometrial epithelium.

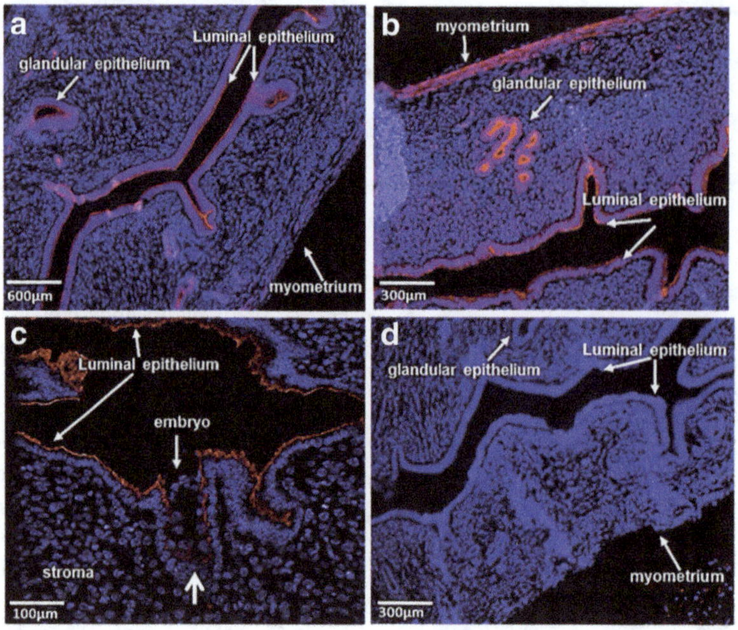

Fig. 2 FOXL2 Localization in the Uterus. **a** FOXL2 is localized to the luminal epithelium, myometrium and glandular epithelium in the non-pregnant uterus of a female mouse. **b** A closer view of FOXL2 localization in the non-pregnant uterus. **c** FOXL2 is localized to the luminal epithelium, and to the embryo on day E4.5 of pregnancy. The thick arrow indicates reduced expression of FOXL2 in uterine cells surrounding the attached embryo. **d** No staining is detected in sections incubated without the primary antibody, anti-FOXL2. Blue = DNA staining (DAPI), RED = FOXL2

FOXL2 effects on the expression of members of the wnt/fzd family

The Wnt/Fzd signaling pathway has been shown to play a role in embryo implantation and stromal cell differentiation [23]. We therefore evaluated the influence of FOXL2 on the expression levels of representative members of the Wnt/Fzd family, *Wnt11* and *Fzd6*, shown to be expressed in the mouse uterus before and around the time of implantation [24]. Using the cellular models described above (Fig. 3 and Additional file 1: Figure S1), we show that *Foxl2* levels are inversely correlated with the expression levels of *Fzd6* and *Wnt11* mRNA. We found that both *Fzd6* and *Wnt11* mRNA are expressed in significantly lower levels in AN3-CA, which contain higher endogenous *Foxl2*, than in Ishikawa cells, which express lower *Foxl2* (Fig. 5a and d). Knockdown of *Foxl2* by siRNAs in AN3-CA cells led to an increase in both, *Fzd6* mRNA (Fig. 5b) and *Wnt11* mRNA (Fig. 5e), while overexpression of *Foxl2* in Ishikawa cells led to a reduction in *Fzd6* mRNA (Fig. 5c) as well as *Wnt11*mRNA (Fig. 5f) expression. We also determined the effect of *Foxl2* levels on the expression of antagonists of this pathway. Indeed, these experiments revealed an opposite effect of FOXL2 on the expression *Kremen2* mRNA, a coreceptor for *Dickkopf 1* and 2, which are Wnt/Fzd signaling antagonists. Cells with lower *Foxl2* expression, either endogenous (Fig. 5g) or genetically manipulated (Fig. 5h), had exhibited lower *Kremen2* mRNA levels (Fig. 5g) whereas FOXL2 overexpression led to induction of *Kremen2* mRNA (Fig. 5i).

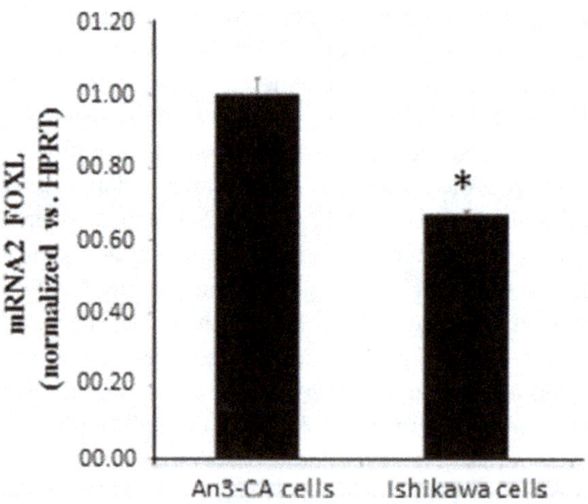

Fig. 3 *Foxl2* expression in uterine cell lines. qRT-PCR of *Foxl2* mRNA expression in AN3-CA and Ishikawa endometrial cell lines. Endogenous expression in Ishikawa cells is significantly lower

FOXL2 regulation of genes involved in cellular stress responses and apoptosis

Uterine cell apoptosis is an important process for normal uterine function [25]. FOXL2 has been implicated in the regulation of processes such as apoptosis, by affecting the expression of relevant genes, including IER3, TNFAIP3 and ATF3 [3]. We evaluated if FOXL2 is also involved in the regulation of these genes in the

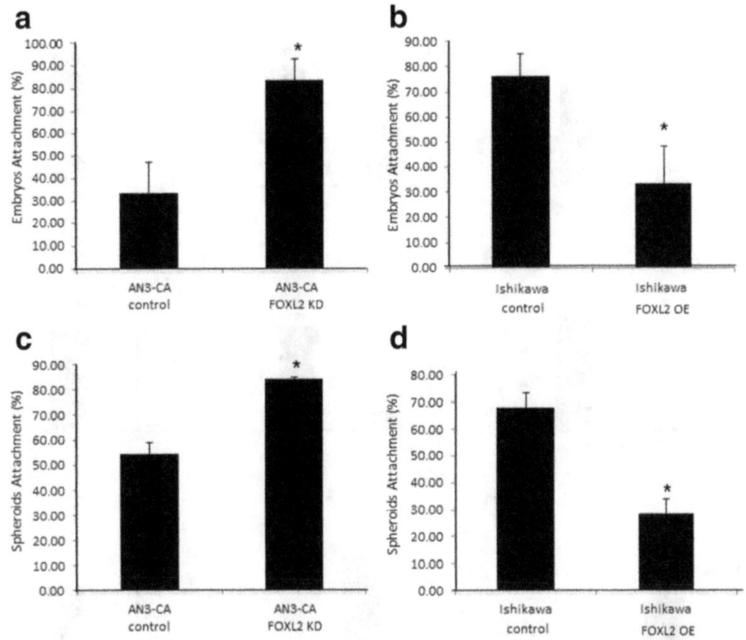

Fig. 4 *Foxl2* effects in an in vitro model of attachment. **a** Mouse embryo attachment is higher after *Foxl2* knockdown in AN3-CA cells. **b** Overexpression of *Foxl2* in Ishikawa cells reduces mouse embryo attachment. **c** Jeg3 spheroid attachment is higher after *Foxl2* knockdown in AN3-CA. **d** Overexpression of *Foxl2* in Ishikawa cells decreases Jeg3 spheroid attachment. * $p < 0.05$

endometrium. We found that *TNFAIP3* mRNA (Fig. 6a and b) and *ATF3* mRNA (Fig. 6d and e) are expressed at higher levels in cells with lower levels FOXL2, namely Ishikawa cells or AN3-CA cells following FOXL2 knockdown. Overexpression of FOXL2 in Ishikawa cells, on the other hand, was associated with a reduction in *TNFAIP3* and *ATF3* mRNA levels (Fig. 6c and f). By contrast, *IER3* mRNA levels were lower in cells with low endogenous FOXL2 (Ishikawa cells) and induced upon FOXL2 overexpression (Fig. 6g and i). AN3-CA cells with FOXL2 depletion, exhibit tendency to express lower levels of *IER3* (Fig. 6h).

FOXL2 effects on genes involved in embryo implantation and uterus receptivity

Uterus receptivity, embryo-maternal recognition and embryo implantation are processes regulated by multiple embryonic and maternal uterine genes. Of these, one of the most intriguing is RGS2, the expression of which in murine pregnant uterus is exclusive to the implantation sites [7]. Another gene that has been demonstrated to play a role in the crosstalk between the embryo and the uterus is the chemokine, CXCl1 [26]. Interestingly, both RGS2 and CXCl1 were reported to be targets of FOXL2 in the ovary [3]. We examined the mRNA expression of both *Rgs2* and *Cxcl1* in our low- and high-FOXL2 expressing cell lines. We found that *Rgs2* mRNA levels are higher in the Ishikawa cells, which express lower levels of FOXL2 and are considered to be representative of a receptive endometrium, as compared to AN3-CA cells, a non-receptive endometrial cell type with higher levels of endogenous FOXL2 (Fig. 7a). Consistent with this trend, *Rgs2* mRNA levels were increased or reduced following FOXL2 knockdown in AN3-CA cells or FOXL2 overexpression in Ishikawa cells, respectively (Fig. 7b and c). Similar to the pattern seen for *Rgs2*, high or low FOXL2 protein expression was inversely associated with low or high *Cxcl1* mRNA expression, respectively (Fig. 7d-f).

Discussion

We demonstrate in this study that FOXL2 is expressed by both human endometrial cells and mouse uteri, and that FOXL2 protein expression in the mouse uterus is pregnancy-stage dependent. We found that FOXL2 is localized to the luminal and glandular epithelium as well as the myometrium of both, non-pregnant and pregnant female mice. FOXL2 expression has been only recently discovered in mouse, human and bovine uteri [12, 15, 27], thus little is known about its role in this tissue. To unveil the functions of FOXL2 in the uterus, we evaluated its influence on the attachment of mouse embryos and spheroids generated from the human trophoblast cell line JEG3 to endometrial cells expressing either low or high FOXL2 levels. Employing complementary experimental models we show an inverse correlation between the abundance of FOXL2 in the endometrial cells and the success rate of trophectoderm cells adherence to Endometrial Epithelium. Our experiments also reveal negative effects of *Foxl2*

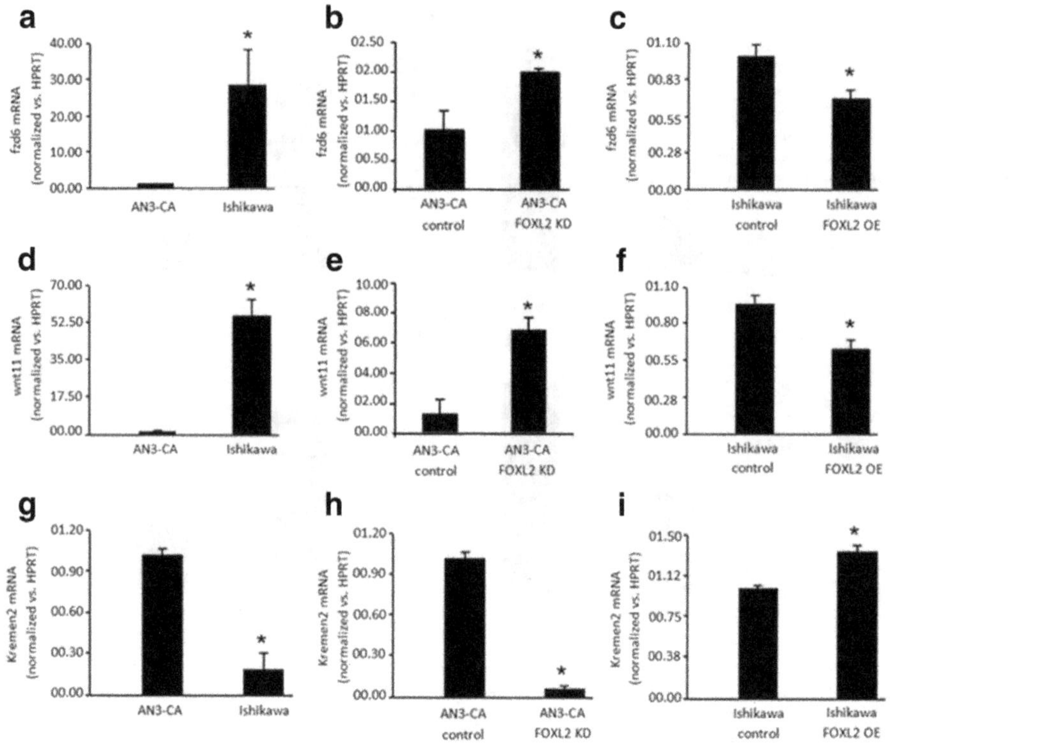

Fig. 5 *Foxl2* effect on the expression of Wnt/Fzd family members. **a**, **d**, **g** The expression of *Fzd6* and *Wnt11* is higher, while the expression of *Kremen2*, a Wnt/Fzd family inhibitor, is lower in receptive endometrial Ishikawa cells, which express low *Foxl2* levels, compared to AN3-CA endometrial non-receptive cells, which express higher levels of *Foxl2*. **b**, **e**, **h** Knockdown of *Foxl2* in AN3-CA leads to an increase in *Fzd6* and *Wnt11* expression and a reduction in *Kremen2* levels. **c**, **f**, **i** Overexpression of *Foxl2* in Ishikawa cells leads to a decrease in *Fzd6* and *Wnt11* levels but elevates *Kremen2* levels. * $p < 0.05$

on the expression of genes known to play crucial roles in uterine function. Altogether our data suggest that, by controlling the expression profile of endometrial genes, *Foxl2* might have an important role in regulating uterus receptivity and embryo implantation. In support to our findings it has been previously reported that *Foxl2* expression decrease during the pre-receptive to receptive transition as well as after co-culturing of human endometrial cells with trophoblast cells [14].

In the current study, we show that FOXL2 localizes to the luminal epithelium and the myometrium. A recent study of neonatal and adult mouse uteri also found FOXL2 protein in the myometrium, but not in the endometrium [15]. The discrepancy between this study and our results might be due to the different methods used. Bellessort et al. used *FOXL2*^{Lacz} mice while we used immunoflorsence staining with FOXL2 specific antibody. Taken altogether, these studies combined with our data suggest that FOXL2 has a key role in uterus remodeling and towards its preparation for implantation. A study of the expression pattern of *Foxl2* in bovine uterus confirmed its presence in the endometrium and showed that *Foxl2* levels are regulated in a hormonal dependent manner [27]. This study showed that both *Foxl2* transcript and FOXL2 protein were expressed from day 5 to day 20 of the estrous cycle, with significant increases during the luteolytic phase followed by a gradual decline corresponding to increased progesterone levels. Consistent with the latter, progesterone supplementation was found to suppress FOXL2 protein levels [27]. These observations are in line with our findings in mouse uteri and human endometrial cells, suggesting that the roles of *Foxl2* in the uterus might be conserved across species, including humans, mice and farm animals. Further studies are needed to examine this possibility. With respect to this, some differences between mice and goats have been found in *Foxl2* effects on gonadal differentiation and function [6, 20, 28–31].

As mentioned above, *Foxl2* expression has been only recently discovered in human, bovine and murine uteri [12, 15, 19, 27]. Thus, little is known about its role in this tissue. In a recent study [15], conditional deletion of *Foxl2* in the postnatal uterus resulted in infertility, severely reduced thickness of the stroma layer and a hypertrophic, disorganized appearance of the myometrium [15]. Moreover, uterine-specific deletion of *Foxl2* in the adult animal resulted in the appearance of a supplementary muscular layer at the stroma/myometrium

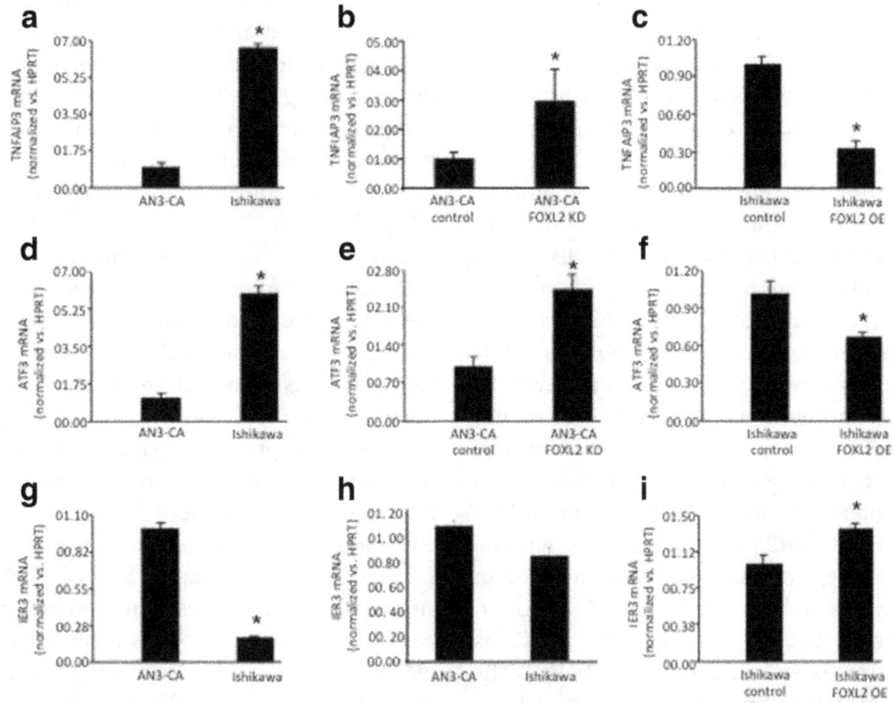

Fig. 6 *Foxl2* effect on the expression of genes involved in apoptosis. **a**, **d**, **g** The expression of *Tnfip3* and *Atf3* is elevated, while the expression of *Ier3* is decreased, in receptive endometrial Ishikawa cells, expressing low *Foxl2* levels as compared to AN3-CA, endometrial non-receptive cells, expressing high levels of *Foxl2*. **b**, **e**, **h** *Tnfip3* and *Atf3* expression is reduced, while the expression of *Ier3* is elevated in AN3-CA after *Foxl2* knockdown. **c**, **f**, **i** Overexpression of *Foxl2* in Ishikawa cells is associated with a decrease in *Tnfip3* and *Atf3* levels and increase in *Ier3* levels. * $p < 0.05$

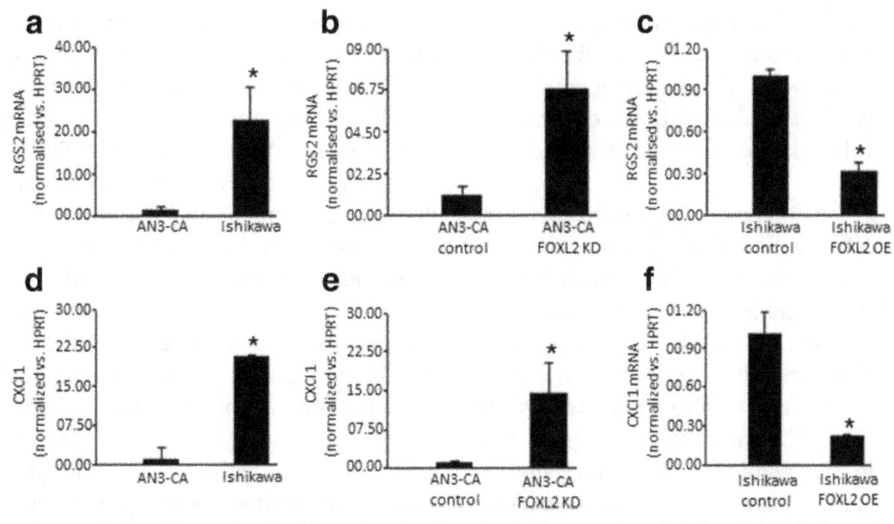

Fig. 7 *Foxl2* effect on the expression of genes involved in embryo implantation. The expression of *Rgs2* and *Cxcl1* is elevated in receptive endometrial Ishikawa cells, expressing low *Foxl2* levels as compared to AN3-CA, endometrial non-receptive cells, expressing high levels of *Foxl2*, (**a**, **d**) as well as in AN3-CA *Foxl2* depleted cells (**b**, **e**). Overexpression of *Foxl2* in Ishikawa cells resulted in a decrease in *Rgs2* and *Cxcl1* levels (**c**, **f**). * $p < 0.05$

border and failure of vascularization of smooth muscle around uterine arteries [15]. In order to expand our understanding of the role of FOXL2 in the human uterus, we utilized two human endometrial cell types to examine the effects of *Foxl2,* either knockdown or overexpression.

In agreement with the findings of Bellassort et al. [15], we observed a reduction in the successful attachment of either mouse blastocysts or Jeg3 trophoblast cells to human Ishikawa receptive endometrial cells with overexpression of *Foxl2,* compared to control Ishikawa cells. Conversely, we found that knockdown of *Foxl2* in AN3-CA non-receptive cells, which express higher levels of endogenous *Foxl2,* improved the attachment of mouse blastocysts and Jeg3 spheroids. Our findings from experiments with human endometrial cells, combined with data from mouse uteri reported by Bellassort et al. [15] support the notion that *Foxl2* plays a negative role in the acquisition uterine receptivity and processes involved in its preparation towards embryo attachment. This notion is further supported by our finding that *Foxl2* is expressed in a lesser extend in uterine epithelial cells surrounding the attached embryo than cells distant from the implantation site.

Additionally, *Wnt* genes were found to be deregulated in this conditional deletion model [15]. Both FOXL2 and the Wnt/Fzd family are necessary for the development of the ovary [32]. In addition, many members of the Wnt/Fzd family are expressed in the uterus [33]. Different Fzd receptors including Fzd6 and Wnt ligands such as Wnt11 were shown to be expressed in the mouse uterus before and around the time of implantation, as well as during stromal cell differentiation [24]. *Wnt11* was detected in the uterus endometrium and epithelial glands in the non-pregnant uterus and its expression was shown to be unregulated by progesterone [24, 34, 35]. *Wnt11* was shown to regulate endometrial gland development [35]. During pregnancy, WNT11 is adjacent to the embryo and FZD6 is localized in the endometrium and stroma during implantation [35].

Our results show an inverse relationship between Wnt/Fzd and *Foxl2* levels. Low *Foxl2* levels are associated with an elevation in *Wnt11* and *Fzd6* and reduction in the levels of Wnt/Fzd inhibitor, *Kremen2,* while the opposite is seen in cells with high *Foxl2* expression levels. Consistent with these findings, conditional deletion of *Foxl2* in the uterus was also found to disrupt *Wnt* gene expression [15]. These results suggest that *Foxl2* has a role in the regulation of normal uterine function, such as uterine glandular generation. Indeed, the decrease in *Foxl2* expression on day 3 of pregnancy might be a crucial mechanism for Wnt/Fzd pathway activation and embryo implantation. Consistent with this notion, the aberrant expression of *Dkk1,* a KREMEN2 receptor, was demonstrated to cause impairment in embryo attachment and implantation [21]. Altogether, these findings provide support for the possibility that conditions that elevate *Foxl2* expression or activity would compromise embryo implantation.

Apoptosis plays an important role in the uterus and is necessary for embryo implantation. *Foxl2* has been implicated in the regulation of both anti- and pro-apoptotic processes in the ovary, based upon microarray data obtained from an ovarian cell line transfected with *Foxl2* [3]. This study reported that *Foxl2* overexpression activated the transcription of several anti-apoptotic genes, such as immediate-early response 3 (*Ier3),* BCL2-related protein A1 (*Bcl2A1*) and tumor necrosis factor alpha-induced protein 3 (*Tnfaip3*) [3], but also increased transcription of pro-apoptotic factors, including activating transcription factor 3 (*Atf3*) [3]. Our results from endometrial cells suggest that, in parallel to the ovary, FOXL2 affects the expression of both, anti-apoptotic and pro-apoptotic genes. This apparently ambivalent behavior of *Foxl2* on apoptosis is likely to reflect the complexity of the pathways that directly, or indirectly regulate apoptosis and the manner in which differential interactions of *Foxl2* might influence or contribute to processes of uterine cell differentiation, proliferation or programmed cell death. The transcriptional regulation of apoptotic proteins is altered in the endometrium of infertile women with chronic endometriosis as compared to healthy women [36]. Estrogen promotes uterine cell apoptosis [37] and estrogen production and actions are influenced by *Foxl2* [4]. Based upon these observations, we predict that altered *Foxl2* expression or activity would compromise uterine cell apoptosis and ultimately lead to impairment of uterine function and the progression of uterine pathology. This prediction requires further investigations although it is consistent with a recent study showing that *Foxl2* levels are elevated in the endometrium of patients with endometriosis [12].

A variety of factors, including *Rgs2* and chemokines, such as *Cxcl1,* are implicated in mediating the crosstalk between the embryo and the uterus [7, 26]. Both factors were reported to be FOXL2 targets in the ovary [3]. Of these, *Rgs2,* exclusively expressed in the implantation sites of the murine pregnant uterus, is of particular interest [3, 7]. RGS's are multi-functional, GTPase-accelerating proteins that promote GTP hydrolysis by the alpha-subunit of G proteins, thereby inactivating G proteins and rapidly switching off G protein-coupled receptor signaling pathways. It is thought that RGS2 regulates implantation and pregnancy by influencing intracellular calcium flux or, alternatively, that it participates in the local immunoregulation of uterine tissues during implantation by activating T cells and interleukin-2 production [38] and attenuating the bioactivity of *Mnsfβ*, a molecule implicated in uterine immune tolerance during pregnancy in mice [39]. Similarly, chemokines, such as *Cxcl1*, are implicated in immunoregulatory and inflammatory processes that play a pivotal role in embryo implantation [26]. Here we show that the expression of both *Rgs2* and *Cxcl1* is sensitive to the level of *Foxl2*, suggesting that *Foxl2* might indirectly regulate processes that are controlled by *Rgs2* and *Cxcl1*. Our results suggest that *Foxl2* depletion just prior to embryo implantation might be necessary for preparing the uterus for successful attachment of the embryo to the uterine wall.

Conclusions

Our data showing a decrease in *Foxl2* levels just before implantation are consistent with the notion that *Foxl2* levels must decline to allow successful embryo attachment, which is an essential prelude for pregnancy progression. This is supported by our observations that *Foxl2* overexpression in endometrial cells reduces embryo and spheroid attachment to receptive cells while attachment is improved by *Foxl2* knockdown in non-receptive cells. Our results further suggest that these effects *Foxl2* are mediated by regulating genes involved in those processes. Further investigations into the contributions of *Foxl2* function to uterus remodeling toward embryo implantation will lead to better understanding of these complex processes. Finding *Foxl2* target genes could also unveil new players in the uterus, both under normal and pathological conditions, and lead to development of new means to improve fertility when implantation fails.

Additional files

Additional file 1: Figure S1. Embryos attachment to endometrial cells. Mouse blastocysts co-incubated with endometrial cell lines for 48 h (A). Attached embryos that stayed on the plate after the plates were washed and shaken (B). Thin arrows indicate attached embryos, thick arrow indicate unattached embryos. (C) The localization of osteopentin, an adhesion molecule, between the embryo and the endometrial cells. Osteopentin-green, DAPI-blue. (TIFF 2025 kb)

Additional file 2: Table S1. PCR primers list. (DOCX 15 kb)

Additional file 3: Figure S2. FOXL2 localization in the ovary. FOXL2 expressed by granulosa cells of early follicles declines at later stages of folliculogenesis. Blue = DNA staining (DAPI), RED = FOXL2. EA-Early antral, GF-Graffian Folicle. (TIFF 2025 kb)

Additional file 4: Figure S3. *Foxl2* expression in human endometrial cell lines. A) Human endometrial cell lines express *Foxl2* mRNA. *Foxl2* mRNA expression in AN3-CA and Ishikawa endometrial cell lines was analyzed by RT-PCR, using *Hprt* mRNA as an internal control. B) *Foxl2* levels are shown as fold mRNA expression, normalized to Hprt. (TIFF 2025 kb)

Additional file 5: Figure S4. Manipulating *Foxl2* expression in human endometrial cell lines. A) *Foxl2* expression is decreased in endometrial non-receptive AN3-CA cells infected with lentivirus expressing *Foxl2* siRNA cassette. B) Ishikawa cells infected with lentivirus overexpress *Foxl2* exhibit higher FOXL2 levels as compared to control. The results of one representative out of a total of 3 independent experiments with similar results is presented. + * $p < 0.05$. (TIFF 2025 kb)

Abbreviations

BPES: Blepharophimosis–ptosis–epicanthus inversus syndrome; FOXL2: Forkhead Transcription Factor L2; hCG: Human chorionic gonadotropin; KD: Knockdown; OE: Overexpression; PMSG: Pregnant mare serum gonadotropin; RGS2: G-protein signaling protein 2

Acknowledgements

We thank Alissa Blackler for her technical contributions to the project.

Funding

This work and L.M.B. were supported in part by Grant 2R01HD046941 awarded by the NICHD. The content is solely the responsibility of the authors and does not necessarily represent the official views of the NICHD or the NIH.

Authors' contributions

ME, RH and EG preformed the experiments, LMB and EG designed the experiments and wrote the manuscript. All authors read and approved the final manuscript.

Competing interests

The authors declare that they have no competing interests.

Author details

[1]Department of Ruminant Science, Agricultural Research Organization, 50250 Rishon LeZion, Israel. [2]Department of Biological Regulation, Weizmann Institute of Science, 76100 Rehovot, Israel. [3]Clayton Foundation Laboratories for Peptide Biology and Laboratory of Neuronal Structure and Function, Salk Institute for Biological Studies, La Jolla, San Diego, CA 92037, USA.

References

1. Carlsson P, Mahlapuu M. Forkhead transcription factors: key players in development and metabolism. Dev Biol. 2002;250:1–23.
2. Zlotogora J, Sagi M, Cohen T. The blepharophimosis, ptosis, and epicanthus inversus syndrome: delineation of two types. Am J Hum Genet. 1983;35:1020–7.
3. Batista F, Vaiman D, Dausset J, Fellous M, Veitia RA. Potential targets of FOXL2, a transcription factor involved in craniofacial and follicular development, identified by transcriptomics. Proc Natl Acad Sci U S A. 2007;104:3330–5.
4. Georges A, L'Hote D, Todeschini AL, Auguste A, Legois B, Zider A, Veitia RA. The transcription factor FOXL2 mobilizes estrogen signaling to maintain the identity of ovarian granulosa cells. elife. 2014;3
5. Caburet S, Georges A, L'Hote D, Todeschini AL, Benayoun BA, Veitia RA. The transcription factor FOXL2: at the crossroads of ovarian physiology and pathology. Mol Cell Endocrinol. 2012;356:55–64.
6. Elzaiat M, Jouneau L, Thepot D, Klopp C, Allais-Bonnet A, Cabau C, Andre M, Chaffaux S, Cribiu EP, Pailhoux E, Pannetier M. High-throughput sequencing analyses of XX genital ridges lacking FOXL2 reveal DMRT1 up-regulation before SOX9 expression during the sex-reversal process in goats. Biol Reprod. 2014;91:153.
7. Huang ZP, Ni H, Yang ZM, Wang J, Tso JK, Shen QX. Expression of regulator of G-protein signalling protein 2 (RGS2) in the mouse uterus at implantation sites. Reproduction. 2003;126:309–16.
8. Ladds G, Zervou S, Vatish M, Thornton S, Davey J. Regulators of G protein signalling proteins in the human myometrium. Eur J Pharmacol. 2009;610:23–8.
9. Blount AL, Schmidt K, Justice NJ, Vale WW, Fischer WH, Bilezikjian LM. FoxL2 and Smad3 coordinately regulate follistatin gene transcription. J Biol Chem. 2009;284:7631–45.

10. McTavish KJ, Nonis D, Hoang YD, Shimasaki S. Granulosa cell tumor mutant FOXL2C134W suppresses GDF-9 and activin A-induced follistatin transcription in primary granulosa cells. Mol Cell Endocrinol. 2013;372:57–64.
11. Sugawara K, Kizaki K, Herath CB, Hasegawa Y, Hashizume K. Transforming growth factor beta family expression at the bovine feto-maternal interface. Reprod Biol Endocrinol. 2010;8:120.
12. Governini L, Carrarelli P, Rocha AL, Leo VD, Luddi A, Arcuri F, Piomboni P, Chapron C, Bilezikjian LM, Petraglia F. FOXL2 in human endometrium: hyperexpressed in endometriosis. Reprod Sci. 2014;21:1249–55.
13. Hu S, Yao G, Wang Y, Xu H, Ji X, He Y, Zhu Q, Chen Z, Sun Y. Transcriptomic changes during the pre-receptive to receptive transition in human endometrium detected by RNA-Seq. *J Clin Endocrinol Metab*. 2014;99(12):E2744–53.
14. Popovici RM, Betzler NK, Krause MS, Luo M, Jauckus J, Germeyer A, Bloethner S, Schlotterer A, Kumar R, Strowitzki T, von Wolff M. Gene expression profiling of human endometrial-trophoblast interaction in a coculture model. Endocrinology. 2006;147:5662–75.
15. Bellessort B, Bachelot A, Heude E, Alfama G, Fontaine A, Le Cardinal M, Treier M, Levi G. Role of Foxl2 in uterine maturation and function. Hum Mol Genet. 2015;
16. Blount AL, Vaughan JM, Vale WW, Bilezikjian LM. A Smad-binding element in intron 1 participates in activin-dependent regulation of the follistatin gene. J Biol Chem. 2008;283:7016–26.
17. Aboussahoud W, Bruce C, Elliott S, Fazeli A. Activation of toll-like receptor 5 decreases the attachment of human trophoblast cells to endometrial cells in vitro. Hum Reprod. 2010;25:2217–28.
18. Kang YJ, Forbes K, Carver J, Aplin JD. The role of the osteopontin-integrin alphavbeta3 interaction at implantation: functional analysis using three different in vitro models. Hum Reprod. 2014;29:739–49.
19. Eozenou C, Mansouri-Attia N, Aubert J, Reinaud P, Giraud-Delville C, Taghouti G, Galio L, Everts RE, Degrelle S, Richard C, et al. Gene expression profiles of bovine caruncular and intercaruncular endometrium at implantation. Physiol Genomics. 2009;39:14–27.
20. Schmidt D, Ovitt CE, Anlag K, Fehsenfeld S, Gredsted L, Treier AC, Treier M. The murine winged-helix transcription factor Foxl2 is required for granulosa cell differentiation and ovary maintenance. Development. 2004;131:933–42.
21. Liu Y, Kodithuwakku SP, Ng PY, Chai J, Ng EH, Yeung WS, Ho PC, Lee KF. Excessive ovarian stimulation up-regulates the Wnt-signaling molecule DKK1 in human endometrium and may affect implantation: an in vitro co-culture study. Hum Reprod. 2010;25:479–90.
22. Rahnama F, Thompson B, Steiner M, Shafiei F, Lobie PE, Mitchell MD. Epigenetic regulation of E-cadherin controls endometrial receptivity. Endocrinology. 2009;150:1466–72.
23. Sonderegger S, Pollheimer J, Knofler M. Wnt signalling in implantation, decidualisation and placental differentiation–review. Placenta. 2010;31:839–47.
24. Hayashi K, Erikson DW, Tilford SA, Bany BM, Maclean JA 2nd, Rucker EB 3rd, Johnson GA, Spencer TE. Wnt genes in the mouse uterus: potential regulation of implantation. Biol Reprod. 2009;80:989–1000.
25. Moumne L, Batista F, Benayoun BA, Nallathambi J, Fellous M, Sundaresan P, Veitia RA. The mutations and potential targets of the forkhead transcription factor FOXL2. Mol Cell Endocrinol. 2008;282:2–11.
26. Hess AP, Hamilton AE, Talbi S, Dosiou C, Nyegaard M, Nayak N, Genbecev-Krtolica O, Mavrogianis P, Ferrer K, Kruessel J, et al. Decidual stromal cell response to paracrine signals from the trophoblast: amplification of immune and angiogenic modulators. Biol Reprod. 2007;76:102–17.
27. Eozenou C, Vitorino Carvalho A, Forde N, Giraud-Delville C, Gall L, Lonergan P, Auguste A, Charpigny G, Richard C, Pannetier M, Sandra O. FOXL2 is regulated during the bovine estrous cycle and its expression in the endometrium is independent of conceptus-derived interferon tau. Biol Reprod. 2012;87:32.
28. Boulanger L, Pannetier M, Gall L, Allais-Bonnet A, Elzaiat M, Le Bourhis D, Daniel N, Richard C, Cotinot C, Ghyselinck NB, Pailhoux E. FOXL2 is a female sex-determining gene in the goat. Curr Biol. 2014;24:404–8.
29. Pailhoux E, Vigier B, Chaffaux S, Servel N, Taourit S, Furet JP, Fellous M, Grosclaude F, Cribiu EP, Cotinot C, Vaiman D. A 11.7-kb deletion triggers intersexuality and polledness in goats. Nat Genet. 2001;29:453–8.
30. Pailhoux E, Vigier B, Vaiman D, Servel N, Chaffaux S, Cribiu EP, Cotinot C. Ontogenesis of female-to-male sex-reversal in XX polled goats. Dev Dyn 2002;224:39–50.
31. Uda M, Ottolenghi C, Crisponi L, Garcia JE, Deiana M, Kimber W, Forabosco A, Cao A, Schlessinger D, Pilia G. Foxl2 disruption causes mouse ovarian failure by pervasive blockage of follicle development. Hum Mol Genet. 2004; 13:1171–81.
32. Richards JS, Pangas SA. The ovary: basic biology and clinical implications. J Clin Invest. 2010;120:963–72.
33. Mohamed OA, Jonnaert M, Labelle-Dumais C, Kuroda K, Clarke HJ, Dufort D. Uterine Wnt/beta-catenin signaling is required for implantation. Proc Natl Acad Sci U S A. 2005;102:8579–84.
34. Hayashi K, Burghardt RC, Bazer FW, Spencer TE. WNTs in the ovine uterus: potential regulation of periimplantation ovine conceptus development. Endocrinology. 2007;148:3496–506.
35. Hayashi K, Yoshioka S, Reardon SN, Rucker EB, 3rd, Spencer TE, DeMayo FJ, Lydon JP, MacLean JA, 2nd: WNTs in the neonatal mouse uterus: potential regulation of endometrial gland development. Biol Reprod 2011, 84:308–319.
36. Di Pietro C, Cicinelli E, Guglielmino MR, Ragusa M, Farina M, Palumbo MA, Cianci A. Altered transcriptional regulation of cytokines, growth factors, and apoptotic proteins in the endometrium of infertile women with chronic endometritis. Am J Reprod Immunol. 2013;69:509–17.
37. Abot A, Fontaine C, Raymond-Letron I, Flouriot G, Adlanmerini M, Buscato M, Otto C, Berges H, Laurell H, Gourdy P, et al. The AF-1 activation function of estrogen receptor alpha is necessary and sufficient for uterine epithelial cell proliferation in vivo. Endocrinology. 2013;154:2222–33.
38. Oliveira-Dos-Santos AJ, Matsumoto G, Snow BE, Bai D, Houston FP, Whishaw IQ, Mariathasan S, Sasaki T, Wakeham A, Ohashi PS, et al. Regulation of T cell activation, anxiety, and male aggression by RGS2. Proc Natl Acad Sci U S A. 2000;97:12272–7.
39. Nie GY, Li Y, Hampton AL, Salamonsen LA, Clements JA, Findlay JK. Identification of monoclonal nonspecific suppressor factor beta (mNSFbeta) as one of the genes differentially expressed at implantation sites compared to interimplantation sites in the mouse uterus. Mol Reprod Dev. 2000;55: 351–63.

2

Associations of sperm DNA fragmentation with lifestyle factors and semen parameters of Saudi men and its impact on ICSI outcome

Basmah Al Omrani[1], Nadia Al Eisa[1], Murid Javed[2*], Maher Al Ghedan[3], Hamoud Al Matrafi[4] and Hamad Al Sufyan[2]

Abstract

Background: Male factor infertility is quite common as 30–50% of infertility cases are due to sperm defects. The high sperm DNA fragmentation is one of the causes of male factor infertility. Many factors cause sperm DNA fragmentation and could be testicular or post-testicular. The purpose of this study was to assess relationships among sperm DNA fragmentation, lifestyle factors and semen values of Saudi men and to determine impact of sperm DNA fragmentation on ICSI cycle outcome.

Methods: The duration of this study was from January 2015 to June 2016. The cases with female factor infertility were excluded. In total 94 couples were selected for investigation. The study parameters were male age, body mass index, smoking, semen values, % sperm DNA fragmentation, fertilization rate and pregnancy outcome. The ICSI procedure was performed in all patients per standard protocol. The semen samples were grouped based on % sperm DNA fragmentation into < 15%, 15–30 and > 30% which corresponded to low, moderate and high sperm DNA fragmentation, respectively.

Results: There was no difference in ICSI outcome in low and moderate sperm DNA fragmentation, however, in high sperm DNA fragmentation no patient achieved pregnancy. In this study, 53.19% Saudi men had low, 32.98% moderate and 13.83% high DFI. Semen volume, sperm morphology and fertilization rate did not show any correlation trend with DNA fragmentation, however, sperm concentration and motility were negatively correlated in all DFI categories. The BMI was positively correlated in moderate DFI category and smoking was positively correlated with low DFI category. The age was positively correlated in moderate and high DFI categories.

Conclusions: The results of this study indicated that 14% Saudi men had high DNA fragmentation. The BMI was positively correlated in moderate DFI category and smoking was positively correlated with low DFI category. The age was positively correlated in moderate and high DFI categories.

Keywords: Sperm DNA fragmentation, Body mass index, ICSI, Infertility, Male factor, Smoking

* Correspondence: murid.javed@gmail.com
[2]Assisted Reproductive Technology Laboratories, Thuriah Medical Center, Riyadh, Saudi Arabia
Full list of author information is available at the end of the article

Background

Infertility is failure to achieve a clinical pregnancy after 12 months or more of regular unprotected sexual intercourse [1]. It is a common problem, with recent publications quoting a 9 to 18% prevalence in the general population [2]. It may be due to male or female factors or unexplained where after an elaborate workup no apparent reason for infertility is found [3]. About 30–50% of infertility cases are attributed to sperm defects [4, 5]. Defective sperm conditions include very low sperm concentration, inadequate sperm motility and morphological abnormalities. The percentage of cells exhibiting fragmented DNA is represented by the DNA fragmentation index (DFI) [6]. The infertile males are found to have a higher percentage of sperm with defective DNA than fertile controls [7–9]. Therefore, DFI is recommended as an appealing fertility predictive element [10–12].

The causes of sperm DNA damage are numerous, of complex nature and could be testicular or post-testicular [13]. These may include defects in spermatogenesis (e.g., genetic or developmental abnormalities) and testicular or post-testicular injury (e.g., gonadotoxins, hyperthermia, oxidants, and endocrine abnormalities). It has been suggested that protamine deficiency (with consequent aberrant chromatin remodeling), reactive oxygen species and abortive apoptosis may be responsible for sperm DNA damage [14].

Lifestyle factors like increased body mass index (BMI) [15], scrotal hyperthermia [16, 17] and smoking [18] increase DFI. An increased risk of cancer in offspring from fathers with increased level of DFI because of smoking has been reported [19].

Intracytoplasmic sperm injection (ICSI) made a paradigm shift of male infertility treatment. It is recommended even in couples with high level of DFI. The Sperm Chromatin Dispersion (SCD) assay is a validated procedure for assessment of DFI [20]. The DFI has been demonstrated to affect naturally induced pregnancy [21, 22] or pregnancy through ART. Furthermore, the high level of DFI (≥ 27%) has been shown to reduce fertility after ART procedure [23]. The objectives of this study were to determine the level of DFI in Saudi men, to see its impact on ICSI outcome and to evaluate its correlations with lifestyle factors (age, body mass index and smoking) and semen parameters.

Methods

We retrospectively conducted a systematic review of data from 94 Saudi men tested for sperm DNA fragmentation by SCD assay before undergoing ICSI from Jan 2015 to June 2016 at an infertility clinic in Riyadh, Saudi Arabia. The cases with female factor infertility were excluded. In total 94 couples were selected for investigation. The study parameters were sperm DFI, semen values, male age, BMI, smoking, fertilization and pregnancy rate. The semen samples were divided into following categories based on DFI: < 15%, 15–30% and > 30, which corresponded to low, moderate and high DFI. Thuriah institutional review board approved this study.

Semen analysis

The patients were instructed to abstain for 3–5 days before providing semen sample by masturbation. After complete liquefaction, semen volume (mL), sperm concentration (10^6/mL), motility (%) and presence of round sperm (10^6/ml) were determined. The percent morphology was assessed from a stained smear under 100× oil immersion objective by analysing 200 spermatozoa. The sample was considered normal if it had 1.5–6 ml volume, ≥ 15 million/mL sperm concentration, ≥40% progressive motility and ≥ 4% normal morphology.

Sperm chromatin dispersion assay

The SCD assay was conducted using Halosperm G2® kit (Halotech®, Spain). At least 300 spermatozoa were scored under an inverted bright-field microscope for each sample. The normal sperm without fragmented DNA showed big or medium size halo and the sperm with fragmented or degraded DNA showed no halo.

Ovarian stimulation, ICSI and embryo culture

Ovarian stimulation in female partner was achieved using agonist or antagonist protocol. Oocytes were collected 36 h post hCG injection. Oocyte denudation and ICSI were performed per standard procedure [24]. On the day of egg collection, the male partner was asked to produce semen sample which was processed for ICSI. The fertilization was checked 16–18 h post-ICSI. Presence of 2 pronuclei and two polar bodies were recognized as normal fertilization. Oocytes without obvious pronuclei were considered unfertilized. Oocytes with a single pronucleus or more than two pronuclei were considered abnormal fertilization and not included in the study. Embryos were cultured in an atmosphere of 6% CO_2 in air. Morphological assessment of each embryo was performed daily based on % cytoplasmic fragmentation. Embryos were graded on a scale of 1 to 5 where 1 was considered the best grade with 10% or less fragmentation. Embryo transfer was performed on day 3. Per our clinic policy; 2 embryos were transferred in patients less than 35 yrs., 3 embryos in patients from 36 to 39 yrs. and 4 embryos in patients 40 yrs. or more. The extra embryos were cryopreserved for subsequent embryo transfers. Biochemical pregnancy rate was calculated based on βhCG test 14 days post oocyte retrieval.

Statistical analysis

The data were analyzed by Statistical Package for Social Sciences (SPSS), Version 23. The main dependent variable in this study was ICSI cycle outcome (successful or unsuccessful). Descriptive statistics were used to calculate mean, medians, maximum and minimum for age, male BMI, semen volume, sperm concentration, sperm motility and morphology. The DFI was categorized into < 15%, 15–30% and > 30, which corresponded to low, moderate and high DFI. The independent t-test was used to detect the difference between two independent groups of ICSI, while Mann-Whitney test was used to assess the significant differences of non-parametric continuous variables (such as semen parameters). Chi-square test was used to assess the significant difference between categorical variables. Pearson's correlation was used to assess the strength and significance of association between parametric variables, while Spearman's correlations were used in non-parametric variables. The degree of association was represented by the correlation coefficient and a statistically significant difference was detected when $P < 0.05$.

Results

From 94 men, 53.19% had low, 32.98% moderate and 13.83% high DFI. The Mean ± SD values for low, moderate and high groups were; 10.46 ± 3.31, 20.80 ± 4.68 and 38.54 ± 10.14%, respectively (Table 1). The distribution of DFI in Saudi sub-fertile men undergoing successful and unsuccessful ICSI treatment is presented in Table 2. The patients in successful group were those who achieved pregnancy in ICSI cycle. The number of embryos transferred in each group were similar. The indication was male factor infertility. There was no significant difference in ICSI outcomes in low ($P = 0.597$) and moderate ($P = 0.235$) DFI categories. In the high DFI category, no patient achieved pregnancy. There were non significant differences between successful and non-successful ICSI groups in regards to the semen parameters. Similarly, there were non significant differences between these two ICSI groups in regards to the age, BMI, and smoking (Table 3).

Table 1 Sperm DNA fragmentation categories in Saudi sub-fertile men undergoing ICSI ($n = 94$)

Category	Number (%)	Mean ± SD	Median	Range
Low DFI (< 15%)	50 (53.19)	10.46 ± 3.31	10.94	2.57–14.90
Moderate DFI (15–30%)	31 (32.98)	20.80 ± 4.68	19.80	15.28–29.73
High DFI (> 30%)	13 (13.83)	38.54 ± 10.14	34.43	31.16–67.75

Values are given as number, Mean ± SD, Median and Range

The correlations between DFI categories, semen parameters and lifestyle factors are given in Table 4. Semen volume, sperm morphology and fertilization rate did not show any correlation trend with DNA fragmentation; however, sperm concentration and motility were negatively correlated in all DFI categories. The BMI was positively correlated in moderate DFI category and smoking was positively correlated with low DFI category. The age was positively correlated in moderate and high DFI categories.

Discussion

In this study, the lowest DFI value was 2.57% and the highest 67.75% in 94 Saudi men tested. In 53% men, the DFI value was 10.46 ± 3.31%. In the moderate and high DFI groups, these values were 20.80 ± 4.68% and 38.54 ± 10.14%, respectively. In the high DFI group no pregnancy was achieved. The DFI has been related to fertility potential [21]. The DFI values are significantly higher in infertile as compared to those in fertile group [25]. A significant inverse correlation was established between DNA fragmentation and sperm concentration, total count, progressive motility (rapid and total) and normal morphology in subfertile and infertile men ($p < 0.05$) as compared to in fertile group [26] Normozoospermic men exhibited lower levels of DNA fragmentation than non-normozoospermic men. Therefore, it was suggested that DNA fragmentation testing and traditional semen analysis should be considered as complementary diagnostic tools in a comprehensive evaluation of male infertility [27].

In our study, the mean DFI value for high DFI group was 38.54% using the SCD assay. The DFI of ≥30% by SCD is considered of poor fertility potential. The other most commonly used techniques to assess sperm DNA integrity are the TUNEL, Comet and Sperm Chromatin Structural Assay (SCSA). A threshold value of 30% DFI was reported for SCSA for IVF/ICSI cases and 20% for the TUNEL assay, although IVF and ICSI term pregnancies have been reported even with semen samples with much higher DFI values [28]. The oocytes and early embryos have the ability to repair sperm DNA damage, with the effect of such damage being dependent on the extent of chromatin damage and the capacity of oocytes to make repairs. This suggests that when sperm has extensively damaged DNA, the capacity of the oocyte to repair damaged DNA might be exceeded and high DFI > 30% may be incompatible with pregnancy [29] in couples with poor oocyte quality.

In the present study, fertilization rate was not different in DFI categories of Saudi men. This finding is in agreement with other studies [30–32]. However, one study found significant association between DFI and fertilization rate [10] which could most likely be due to

Table 2 The distribution of DFI in Saudi sub-fertile men undergoing successful and unsuccessful ICSI treatment (n = 94)

Category	Values in Successful ICSI			Values in Unsuccessful ICSI			*P* Value
	No.	Mean ± SD	Median	No.	Mean ± SD	Median	
DFI < 15%	7	9.83 ± 3.58	10.67	43	10.55 ± 3.29	11.21	0.597
DFI 15–30%	11	19.09 ± 3.78	17.47	20	21.73 ± 4.93	21.75	0.135
DFI > 30%	0	0	0	13	38.54 ± 10.14	34.43	–

Values are given as Mean ± SD and Median. The independent t-test and Chi square were used to compare groups

differences in the oocyte quality because the number of metaphase II oocytes and embryo quality are important factors affecting ICSI outcome. In this study, female age was 33 ± 5.7 yrs. The number of mature oocytes was 10.6 ± 7.5 and oocyte quality was similar in all groups as cases with female factor infertility were excluded.

The sperm DNA fragmentation has been attributed to a variety of intrinsic and extrinsic factors which could be of genetic or environmental origin. Majority of marriages in Saudi population happen in closely related individuals thereby causing some genetic concerns. Among the genetic factors, variations and polymorphisms in genes playing roles in genome integrity have been implicated in an increased risk of sperm DNA fragmentation. The chromosomal structural rearrangements, such as reciprocal translocations are associated with increased DNA damage in infertile men [33]. Analysis of genetic reasons of DNA fragmentation is beyond the scope of this study. A future study addressing this concern is direly needed.

Human sperm DNA is tightly packed. The condensation of nuclear chromatin takes place during the last stages of spermiogenesis and epididymal transport. A few important biochemical changes take place such as the replacement of lysine-rich histones with arginine-rich protamines. At the same time, bisulfidic bonds are formed between cysteine residues. In these ways, the nuclear chromatin is tightly packed to protect it from natural and chemical damaging factors. Abnormalities in sperm chromatin condensation may results in increased sperm DNA fragmentation [34].

This study found that age was significantly positively correlated with moderate and high DFI. This is consistent with an earlier study [35], which aimed to assess the outcomes of ICSI in patients with high DNA fragmentation. It found that male with high and moderate DFI were significantly older than those with the low DFI. This is in disagreement with another study [29] in which there was no significant difference when DFI in males above and below the median age was compared. This non-significant result could be attributed to the life style and young age of included males where maximum age was 48 years, while in the current study the male age reached 55 years.

Among the environmental factors, BMI, smoking and heat to the scrotum are major factors causing DNA fragmentation. In the present study, BMI was significantly correlated with the moderate and total DFI categories. This is in agreement with a study conducted in USA [36], where multiple linear regression detected a significant association between obesity and sperm DNA fragmentation. It found men with BMI higher than 25 to have less DNA integrity, thus, patients should be advised to reduce their body weight in order to achieve maximum possible fertility. This is inconsistent with the

Table 3 The distribution of social and semen characteristics of Saudi sub-fertile men undergoing successful or unsuccessful ICSI treatment

Parameter	Values in Successful ICSI			Values in Unsuccessful ICSI			*P* Value
	No.	Mean ± SD	Range	No.	Mean ± SD	Range	
Male age 23–36 yrs	12	32.75 ± 2.80	28–36	41	32.56 ± 2.67	25–36	0.83
Male age 37–57 yrs	6	42.17 ± 3.19	37–45	35	44.43 ± 5.39	37–55	0.32
BMI = < 30 Kg/m^2	17	22.65 ± 1.93	19.4–26.7	64	23.89 ± 2.61	19–30	0.48
BMI = > 30 Kg/m^2	1	32.0		12	32.44 ± 2.35	30–36	–
Smoker	8			34			0.078
Non-smoker	10			42			
Semen Variables							
Volume (mL)	18	2.72 ± 1.15	0.5–5	79	2.86 ± 1.13	0.2–6	0.154
Conc. (10^6/mL)	18	67.94 ± 74.64	18–350	79	64.13 ± 43.61	15–200	0.628
Prog motility (%)	18	50.16 ± 10.55	40–80	79	49.32 ± 9.19	38–76	0.776
Abn. Morphology (%)	18	94.11 ± 3.32	88–98	79	89.63 ± 11.09	15–98	0.095

Table 4 The correlations between sperm DFI, semen parameters, fertilization rate and lifestyle factors of the sub fertile men

	DFI% (*P* value)		
Characteristics	< 15	15–30	> 30
Semen Volume (mL)	−0.06 (0.68)	0.209 (0.258)	0.18 (0.556)
Sperm Con. (10^6/mL)	−0.02 (0.88)	−0.133 (0.475)	− 0.009 (0.976)
Progressive Motility (%)	−0.36 (0.008)**	− 0.334 (0.06)	−0.334 (0.264)
Sperm Morphology (%)	−0.096 (0.509)	−0.018 (0.925)	0.198 (0.517)
Fertilization Rate (%)	−0.022 (0.878)	0.05 (0.790)	0.497 (0.084)
Age (Yrs.)	−0.273 (0.366)	0.603 (0.001)**	0.548 (0.001)**
BMI	0.21 (0.167)	0.42 (0.041)*	0.561 (0.073)
Smoking	0.292 (0.040)*	0.035 (0.851)	0.340 (0.256)

*$P < 0.05$
*$P < 0.01$

findings of a study conducted in Czech [37], where no significant association between BMI and DFI was reported.

The smoking was significantly correlated with each of the high and total DFI categories. Smoking can affect the sperm by losing their ability to fight off free oxygen radicals in the seminal fluid which make the sperm more sensitive to oxidative stress. Therefore, the increases in the free radicals in the seminal fluid affect DFI, motility and fertilization. [29].

About 15% of infertile Saudi men had normal semen parameters despite high DFI; therefore, testing DFI in addition to other semen parameters is beneficial [38] as the DFI evaluation may reveal a hidden abnormality in apparently normal sperm parameters [39].

Conclusions

In summary, results of this study indicated that 14% Saudi men had high DNA fragmentation. The BMI was positively correlated in moderate DFI category and smoking was positively correlated with low DFI category. The age was positively correlated in moderate and high DFI categories.

Abbreviations

ART: Assisted reproductive technology; BMI: Body mass index; DFI: DNA fragmentation index; DNA: Deoxyribonucleic acid; hCG: Human chorionic gonadotropin; ICSI: Intracytoplasmic sperm injection; SCD: Sperm chromatin dispersion; SPSS: Statistical package for social sciences

Acknowledgements

The authors thank King Saud University and Thuriah Medical Center for assistance in carrying out this study.

Authors' contributions

BO and MJ conceived the idea, analyzed data and drafted the manuscript. NA supervised the study and critically reviewed the manuscript. HM and HS provided data and critically reviewed manuscript. All authors read and approved the final manuscript.

Competing interests

The authors declare that they have no competing interests.

Author details

[1]Zoology Department, King Saud University, Riyadh, Saudi Arabia. [2]Assisted Reproductive Technology Laboratories, Thuriah Medical Center, Riyadh, Saudi Arabia. [3]Genetics Laboratory, Thuriah Medical Center, Riyadh, Saudi Arabia. [4]Urology and Andrology Unit, Thuriah Medical Center, Riyadh, Saudi Arabia.

References

1. Zegers-Hochschild F, Adamson GD, de Mouzon J, Ishihara O, Mansour R, Nygren K, Sullivan E, Vanderpoel S. International Committee for Monitoring Assisted Reproductive Technology (ICMART) and the World Health Organization (WHO) revised glossary of ART terminology. Fertil Steril. 2009;92:1520–4.
2. Hanson B, Johnstone E, Dorais J, Silver B, Peterson CM, Hotaling J. Female infertility, infertility-associated diagnoses, and comorbidities: a review. J Assist Reprod Genet. 2017;34(2):167–77. Published online 2016 Nov 5. https://doi.org/10.1007/s10815-016-0836-8.
3. Lessing JB, Amit A, Barak Y, Kogosowski A, Gruber A, Yovel I, David MP, Peyser MR. The performance of primary and secondary unexplained infertility in an in vitro fertilization-embryo transfer program. Fertil Steril. 1988;50(6):903–5.
4. Oehninger S. Clinical and laboratory management of male infertility: an opinion on its current status. J Androl. 2000;21:814–21.
5. Lamb DJ, Lipshultz LI. Male infertility: recent advances and a look towards the future. Curr Opin Urol. 2000;10:359–62.
6. Speyer BE, Pizzey AR, Abramov B, Saab W, Doshi A, Sarna U, Harper JC, Serhal P. Successful outcomes achieved in assisted reproduction cycles using sperm with high levels of high DNA stainability. Sys biol Reprod Med. 2015;61:293–9.
7. Hammoud AO, Gibson M, Peterson CM, Meikle AW, Carrell DT. Impact of male obesity on infertility: a critical review of the current literature. Fertil Steril. 2008;90:897–904.
8. Saleh RA, Agarwal A, Nada EA, El-tonsy MH, Sharma RK, Meyer A, Nelson DR, Thomas AJ. Negative effects of increased sperm DNA damage in relation to seminal oxidative stress in men with idiopathic and male factor infertility. Fertil Steril. 2003;79:1597–605.
9. Evenson DP, Larson KL, Jost LK. Sperm chromatin structure assay: its clinical use for detecting sperm DNA fragmentation in male infertility and comparisons with other techniques. J Androl. 2002;23:25–43.
10. Benchaib M, Braun V, Lornage J, Hadj S, Salle B, Lejeune H, Guerin JF. Sperm DNA fragmentation decreases the pregnancy rate in an assisted reproductive technique. Hum Reprod. 2003;18:1023–8.
11. Collins JA, Barnhart KT, Schlegel PN. Do sperm DNA integrity tests predict pregnancy with in vitro fertilization? Fertil Steril. 2008;89:823–31.
12. De La Calle JFV, Muller A, Walschaerts M, Clavere JL, Jimenez C, Wittemer C, Thonneau P. Sperm deoxyribonucleic acid fragmentation as assessed by the sperm chromatin dispersion test in assisted reproductive technology programs: results of a large prospective multicenter study. Fertil Steril. 2008;90:1792–9.
13. Henkel RR, Franken DR. Sperm DNA fragmentation: origin and impact on human reproduction. J Reprod Biotech Fertil. 2011;2:88–108.
14. Zini A, Albert O, Robaire B. Assessing sperm chromatin and DNA damage: clinical importance and development of standards. Andrology. 2014;2:322–5.
15. Oliveira JBA, Petersen CG, Mauri AL, Vagnini LD, Renzi A, Petersen B, Franco JG. Association between body mass index and sperm quality and sperm DNA integrity. A large population study. Andrologia. 2017; https://doi.org/10.1111/and.12889.
16. Paul C, Teng S, Saunders PT. A single, mild, transient scrotal heat stress causes hypoxia and oxidative stress in mouse testes, which induces germ cell death. Biol Reprod. 2009;80:913–9.
17. Kanter M, Aktas C, Erboga M. Heat stress decreases testicular germ cell proliferation and increases apoptosis in short term: an immunohistochemical and ultrastructural study. Toxicol Ind Health. 2013;29:99–113.

18. Cui X, Jing X, Wu X, Wang Z, Li Q. Potential effect of smoking on semen quality through DNA damage and the downregulation of Chk1 in sperm. Mol Med Rep. 2016;14:753–6.
19. Rex AS, Aagaard J, Fedder J. DNA fragmentation in spermatozoa: a historical review. Andrology. 2017;5:622–30.
20. Perreault SD, Aitken RJ, Baker HW, Evenson DP, Huszar G, Irvine DS, Morris ID, Morris RA, Robbins WA, Sakkas D, Spano M, Wyrobek AJ. Integrating new tests of sperm genetic integrity into semen analysis: breakout group discussion. Adv Exp Med Biol. 2003;518:253–68.
21. Evenson D, Jost L, Marshall D, Zinaman M, Clegg E, Purvis K, De Angelis P, Claussen O. Utility of the sperm chromatin structure assay as a diagnostic and prognostic tool in the human fertility clinic. Hum Reprod. 1999;14:1039–49.
22. Spano M, Bonde JP, Hjollund HI, Kolstad HA, Cordelli E, Leter G. Sperm chromatin damage impairs human fertility. The Danish first pregnancy planner study team. Fertil Steril. 2000;73:43–50.
23. Larson-Cook KL, Brannian JD, Hansen KA, Kasperson KM, Aamold ET, Evenson DP. Relationship between the outcomes of assisted reproductive techniques and sperm DNA fragmentation as measured by the sperm chromatin structure assay. Fertil Steril. 2003;80:895–902.
24. Larson K, Dejonge C, Barnes A, Jost L, Evenson D. Sperm chromatin structure assay parameters as predictors of failed pregnancy following assisted reproductive techniques. Hum Reprod. 2000;15:1717–22.
25. Wiweko B, Utami P. Predictive value of sperm deoxyribonucleic acid (DNA) fragmentation index in male infertility. Basic Clin Androl. 2017; https://doi.org/10.1186/s12610-016-0046-3.
26. Evgeni E, Lymberopoulos G, Gazouli M, Asimakopoulos B. Conventional semen parameters and DNA fragmentation in relation to fertility status in a Greek population. Eur J Obstet Gynecol Reprod Biol. 2015;188:17–23. https://doi.org/10.1016/j.ejogrb.2015.02.026. Epub 2015 Feb 26
27. Evgeni E, Lymberopoulos G, Touloupidis S, Asimakopoulos B. Sperm nuclear DNA fragmentation and its association with semen quality in Greek men. Andrologia. 2015;47(10):1166–74. https://doi.org/10.1111/and.12398. Epub 2015 Jan 14
28. Sergerie M, Laforest G, Bujan L, Bissonnette F, Bleau G. Sperm DNA fragmentation: threshold value in male fertility. Hum Reprod. 2005;20:3446–51.
29. Nicopoullos JD, Gilling-Smith C, Almeida PA, Homa S, Norman-Taylor JQ, Ramsay JW. Sperm DNA fragmentation in subfertile men: the effect on the outcome of intracytoplasmic sperm injection and correlation with sperm variables. BJU Inter. 2008;101:1553–60.
30. Esbert M, Pacheco A, Vidal F, Florensa M, Riqueros M, Ballesteros A, Garrid N, Calderón G. Impact of sperm DNA fragmentation on the outcome of IVF with own or donated oocytes. RBM Online. 2011;23:704–10.
31. Virro MR, Larson-Cook KL, Evenson DP. Sperm chromatin structure assay (SCSA®) parameters are related to fertilization, blastocyst development, and ongoing pregnancy in in vitro fertilization and intracytoplasmic sperm injection cycles. Fertil Steril. 2004;81:1289–95.
32. Speyer BE, Pizzey AR, Ranieri M, Joshi R, Delhanty JD, Serhal P. Fall in implantation rates following ICSI with sperm with high DNA fragmentation. Hum Reprod. 2010;25:1609–18.
33. Evgeni E, Charalabopoulos K, Asimakopoulos B. Human sperm DNA fragmentation and its correlation with conventional semen parameters. J Reprod Infertil. 2014;15:2–14.
34. Karydis S, Asimakopoulos B, Papadopoulos N, Vakalopoulos I, Al-Hasani S, Nikolettos N. ICSI Outcome is not associated with the incidence of spermatozoa with abnormal chromatin condensation. In Vivo. 2005;19(5):921–5.
35. Dar S, Grover SA, Moskovtsev SI, Swanson S, Baratz A, Librach CL. In vitro fertilization–intracytoplasmic sperm injection outcome in patients with a markedly high DNA fragmentation index (> 50%). Fertil Steril. 2013;100:75–80.
36. Kort HI, Massey JB, Elsner CW, Mitchell-Leef D, Shapiro DB, Witt MA, Roudebush WE. Impact of body mass index values on sperm quantity and quality. J Androl. 2006;27:450–2.
37. Rybar R, Kopecka V, Prinosilova P, Markova P, Rubes J. Male obesity and age in relationship to semen parameters and sperm chromatin integrity. Andrologia. 2011;43:286–91.
38. Al Ghedan MH, Al Matrafi H, Al Sufyan H, Al Tannir M. Sperm DNA fragmentation in Saudi infertile men with normal standard semen parameters. Andrology. 2015;4:126–9.
39. Saleh RA, Agarwal A, Nelson DR, Nada EA, El-Tonsy MH, Alvarez JG, Thomas AJ Jr, Sharma RK. Increased sperm nuclear DNA damage in normozoospermic infertile men: a prospective study. Fertil Steril. 2002; 78:313–8.

3

The in vitro modulation of steroidogenesis by inflammatory cytokines and insulin in TM3 Leydig cells

Kristian Leisegang[1*] and Ralf Henkel[2]

Abstract

Background: Cytokines and hormones, including insulin, are known to modulate the hypothalamic-pituitary-testes axis and steroidogenesis, both centrally and peripherally. In the context of chronic inflammation and hyperinsulinaemia mediating male hypogonadism associated with obesity, metabolic syndrome and type 2 diabetes mellitus, these mechanisms are poorly understood and the impact of cytokines and insulin on Leydig cell steroidogenesis has not been fully elicited. This study aimed to further investigate the in vitro impact of TNFα, IL1ß, IL6, IL8 and insulin on Leydig cell function and steroidogenesis.

Methods: hCG-stimulated TM3 Leydig cells were exposed to various concentrations of TNFα, IL1ß, IL6, IL8 (100 ng/ml, 10 ng/ml, 1 ng/ml and 0.1 ng/ml) and insulin (10 ng/ml, 1 ng/ml, 0.1 ng/ml and 0.01 ng/ml) in optimal cell culture conditions over 48 h. Cell viability (XTT) and testosterone and progesterone concentrations (ELISA) were assessed using standardised laboratory techniques.

Results: TNFα significantly decreased cell viability and progesterone and testosterone concentrations in a dose-dependent relationship. IL1ß and IL6 had a subtle but significant negative effect on cell viability and testosterone concentrations, with a marked significant decrease in progesterone concentration at all concentrations investigated. IL8 showed an increase in cell viability, with no significant effect on testosterone concentrations alongside a significant decrease in progesterone concentrations. Insulin significantly increased cell viability and testosterone concentrations in a dose dependent relationship, but interestingly significantly decreased progesterone concentrations.

Conclusions: The inflammatory cytokines TNFα, IL1β and IL6 cause a dose dependent decline in steroidogenesis in TM3 Leydig cells. These results suggest that chronic inflammation may downregulate steroidogenesis in males via direct modulation of Leydig cell function. However, IL8 may stimulate TM3 Leydig cell growth. Insulin is associated with a dose-dependent increase in testosterone synthesis, with a significant decline in progesterone synthesis. With the phenomenon of insulin resistance, the literature is unclear on the potential role of hyperinsulinaemia in steroidogenesis. Further studies are warranted in order to fully elicit the molecular mechanisms and interactions of these molecules on male steroidogenesis.

Keywords: Steroidogenesis, Testosterone, Progesterone, Leydig cells, Cytokines, TNFα, IL1β, IL6, IL8, Insulin

* Correspondence: kleisegang@uwc.ac.za
[1]School of Natural Medicine, University of the Western Cape, Private Bag X17, Bellville 7535, South Africa
Full list of author information is available at the end of the article

Background

Evidence suggests that immune regulating cytokines, including TNFα [1], IL1 [2] and IL6 [3], and hormones such as insulin [4], modulate the hypothalamic-pituitary-testes (HPT) axis. These effects are mediated centrally via modulating GnRH and LH, and peripherally via direct action on Leydig cells and Sertoli cells [1, 3, 5]. Optimal Leydig cell function within the HPT context is critical for steroidogenesis cascades and primarily testosterone production, a central hormone for male fertility and general male health and well-being [5, 6].

Testosterone is a steroid hormone primarily produced by Leydig cells in the interstitial space of the testes [7]. The role of testosterone in male fertility is well defined, particularly via action on Sertoli cells to promote spermatogenesis [8]. Additional roles for testosterone include muscle formation, body mass composition and fat regulation, bone mineralisation and cognitive functions [7].

Male hypogonadism, characterised by testosterone deficiency and relevant clinical features, affects approximately 6% of males with an increasing incidence and prevalence globally in recent years [5]. Although an uncommon underlying cause of male infertility, serum total and free testosterone concentration should be considered in the assessment of male infertility cases [7]. Clinical features of hypogonadism include sexual dysfunction, reduced muscle strength, increased abdominal adiposity, sleep disturbance and psychological disturbances, and co-morbidities such as dyslipidaemia, hypertension and hyperglycaemia [5]. There are numerous potential causes of male hypogonadism, which can be further classified as testicular failure (primary) or of hypothalamic or pituitary origin (secondary; hypogonadotropic) hypogonadism [7]. Although serious acute and chronic inflammatory pathology is associated with primary gonadal failure [5, 9], obesity and related co-morbidities (e.g. metabolic syndrome and type 2 diabetes mellitus) are considered to be the single most common cause of male hypogonadism, affecting more than 50% of obese males [10, 11].

Traditionally, the steroid hormone progesterone has been viewed as an unimportant precursor hormone in male physiology. However, progesterone is an important modulator of male endocrine and reproductive function [12, 13]. Progesterone in men is synthesised primarily in the adrenal glands, with some production in the testes, and is an essential precursor for all steroid hormones, including testosterone. Progesterone further regulates the hypothalamus and pituitary gland in the synthesis of GnRH and gonadotropins (LH & FSH), respectively, and regulates sexual behaviour in the brain. Evidence also suggests that progesterone has various modulating functions in the central nervous system in males, and therefore affects mood, behaviour and cognitive functions [12].

Although numerous cytokines and insulin are known to modulate the HPT axis, the role of these polypeptides on modulation of male reproduction and steroidogenesis has not been fully elicited and requires further investigation [1, 3]. Inflammatory cytokines are increasingly associated with male hypogonadism, and a direct causal association is postulated [5]. Furthermore, this is relevant in light of the interaction between chronic inflammation, hyperinsulinaemia and male hypogonadism that may mediate obesity, metabolic syndrome and type 2 diabetes mellitus related male reproductive dysfunction and hypogonadism [14–16]. Sex steroids and inflammatory biomarkers are known to be associated with the pathogenesis of various chronic and degenerative diseases in men, although these relationships remain poorly understood [17].

Within this context, the impact and associated mechanisms of action of inflammatory cytokines and insulin on steroidogenesis is required. As testosterone synthesis is predominantly in Leydig cells of males [18], the aim of this study was to investigate the impact of inflammatory cytokines (TNFα, IL1β, IL6 and IL8) and insulin on steroidogenesis using a TM3 mouse Leydig cell line. Results of this study will be of interest to further understand how steroidogenesis may be modulated in chronic inflammatory diseases and obesity related metabolic complications.

Methods

A TM3 Leydig cell culture model was used in order to investigate the effect of insulin and cytokines on cell viability and steroid hormone (testosterone and progesterone) production. TM3 cells are Leydig cell lines derived from 11 – 13d mouse testes (ATCC No CRL – 1714, Manassas, VA, USA). This was an in vitro experimental study comparing various concentrations of experimental exposure to a control group.

In brief, for each set of experiments, cells were seeded and incubated under standard laboratory conditions for 48 h. Following this, the cells were then exposed to various concentrations of TNFα, IL1β, IL6, IL8 (0.1, 1, 10, 100 ng/ml) and insulin (0.01, 0.1, 1, 10 ng/ml) in hCG-enriched (25 mIU/ml) media for a further 48 h. These experiments were done alongside a control group with hCG-enriched (25 mIU/ml) media only. For each set of experiments, all groups were done in duplicate on the same cell line (n = 2). XTT assays were further done in duplicate on the culture plates in order to obtain an average reading for data analysis. Testosterone and progesterone concentrations were quantified via ELISA in duplicate, and the mean of these results were entered for data analysis. Each set of experiments (n = 2) was repeated 6 times, providing n = 12 samples for analysis for each variable investigated. Experimental groups were compared to the control groups for cell viability (%), and testosterone and progesterone concentrations (ng/ml).

Chemicals

Cells were cultured using standard sterile cell culture techniques, maintained using Dulbecco's Modified Eagle Medium F-12 (DMEM/F-12) (Gibco, Johannesburg, South Africa) with 5% Horse Serum (Gibco), 2.5% Fetal Bovine Serum (Gibco) and 1% Penicillin-Streptomycin (Sigma-Aldrich, St. Louis, MO, USA). Cells were cultured in 75 ml culture flasks and incubated at 37 °C with 5% CO_2. When confluent, and ready for experimental preparations, cultured cells were detached using 0.25% Trypsin/EDTA (Gibco).

Recombinant TNFα, IL1β, IL6 and IL8 appropriate for mouse cell culture experiments was obtained from Sigma-Aldrich as a lyophilised powder. As per manufacturer's instructions, powders were reconstituted to achieve a 100 μg/ml solution. This solution was further diluted at 1:10 with culture medium in order to achieve 10 μg/ml stock solutions for each cytokine. Aliquots of this stock solution were frozen at – 20 °C until use. For each experiment, four concentrations of each cytokine were used: 100 ng/ml, 10 ng/ml, 1 ng/ml and 0.1 ng/ml. These were selected based on previous in vitro studies [19–33] and early experimental exposure of the cytokines to TM3 Leydig cells.

Recombinant insulin appropriate for mouse cell culture experiments was obtained from Sigma-Aldrich as a lyophilised powder. As per manufacturer's instructions, the powder was reconstituted in 0.01 M hydrochloric acid (HCl) to achieve a 25 mg/ml solution, which was further serially diluted with culture medium to achieve a stock solution of 20 ng/ml. Aliquots of this stock solution were frozen at – 20 °C until use. For each experiment, four concentrations of insulin were used: 10 ng/ml, 1 ng/ml, 0.1 ng/ml, 0.01 ng/ml. These concentrations are based on previous literature [34–36] and early experimental exposure to TM3 Leydig cells in the laboratory to determine ideal experimental ranges.

Cell culture

For each experiment, approximately 5000 cells per well were seeded in 300 μl medium in sterile 96-well plates and cultured for 48 h. Medium was then removed, and cells further cultured in experimental medium at the experimental concentrations for a further 48 h in the presence of 25 mIU/ml hCG. The respective controls were exposed to culture medium in the presence of 25 mIU/ml hCG only. After 48 h of exposure to the experimental concentrations, the experiments were terminated. Cell viability and steroid hormone (testosterone and progesterone) concentrations were determined for analysis. All experiments were done in duplicate, and repeated six times for data analysis variables (n = 12).

Cell viability and proliferation determination

Cell viability was assessed using the Cell Proliferation Kit II (XTT) (Roche, Illovo, Johannesburg, South Africa). Under sterile conditions, XTT labelling reagent and the electron coupling reagent were thawed at 37 °C, mixed thoroughly, and 1 μl electron coupling reagent was added to 50 μl XTT labelling reagent as per instructions. From this, 50 μl XTT labelling mixture was added to 100 μl experimental medium to achieve a final XTT concentration of 0.3 mg/ml. This was incubated for 6 h in the dark at 37 °C. Following incubation, the plate was read with an ELISA reader (Labtech, East Sussex, UK) at a wavelength of 450 nm. Cell viability was expressed as a percentage of XTT binding as compared to the hCG control group.

Steroid hormone quantifications

Testosterone and progesterone concentrations were determined from experimental cell culture supernatant. The supernatant was removed as cell culture media from each experimental well (300 μl) and stored in Eppendorf vials at – 20 °C until assayed. The testosterone and progesterone ELISA kits (DRG International, Inc., Springfield, New Jersey, USA) were used to determine testosterone and progesterone concentrations as per manufacturer instructions. All assays were carried out in duplicate, with the mean value recorded as the hormone concentration. Final concentration was quantified based on the standard curve determined by the supplied standard concentrations for the assay.

Statistical analysis

Statistical analysis was performed using the MedCalc software (Version 12.0; Mariakerke, Belgium). All experiments were done in duplicate, and repeated six times (n = 12). Data was tested for distribution using the Kolmogorov-Smirnov test. Parametric data (normal distribution) is expressed as mean ± standard deviation in standard bar graphs, and experimental groups compared to the control group using the student T-test. For XTT analysis, the non-parametric Mann-Whitney test for independent samples was used to determine statistical significance of the experimental outcomes compared to the control group. The ANOVA one-way analysis of variance and ANOVA repeated measures analysis of variance were used to determine trends across increasing experimental concentrations on testosterone and progesterone production. A P-value of < 0.05 was considered significant.

Results

Effects of TNFα, IL1β and IL6

Exposure of TM3 Leydig cells to various concentrations of the inflammatory cytokines TNFα (Fig. 1), IL1β (Fig. 2) and IL6 (Fig. 3) resulted in significantly decreased cell viability, testosterone and progesterone concentrations compared to the control experiments. For TNFα and IL6, ANOVA repeated measures analysis and one-way ANOVA were significant ($P < 0.001$) for testosterone and progesterone concentrations, indicating a dose-dependent decline. For IL1β, there was no significant dose-dependent decrease in testosterone concentration observed. However, ANOVA repeated measures analysis and one-way ANOVA were significant ($P < 0.001$) for a dose-dependent decline in progesterone concentrations for IL1β.

Effects of IL8

Exposure of TM3 Leydig cells to the cytokine IL8 resulted in a significant increase in cell viability compared to control for all concentrations (Fig. 4a). There was no effect of IL8 exposure observed on testosterone concentration, nor was there a significant dose-dependent relationship observed for testosterone concentration (Fig. 4b). However, an immediate and significant decrease in progesterone concentration was evident at all concentrations of IL8 investigated (Fig. 4c). Calculated over all IL8 concentrations applied, ANOVA repeated measures analysis ($P = 0.002$) and one-way ANOVA ($P < 0.001$) were significant for progesterone concentration (Fig. 4c).

Effects of insulin

Exposure of TM3 Leydig cells to insulin resulted in a significant increase in cell viability at 0.01 ng/ml ($P = 0.002$), 0.1 ng/ml ($P = 0.029$) and 10 ng/ml ($P = 0.0359$) (Fig. 5a). There was a significant increase in testosterone concentrations at all experimental concentrations tested, and increasing concentrations of insulin resulted in a

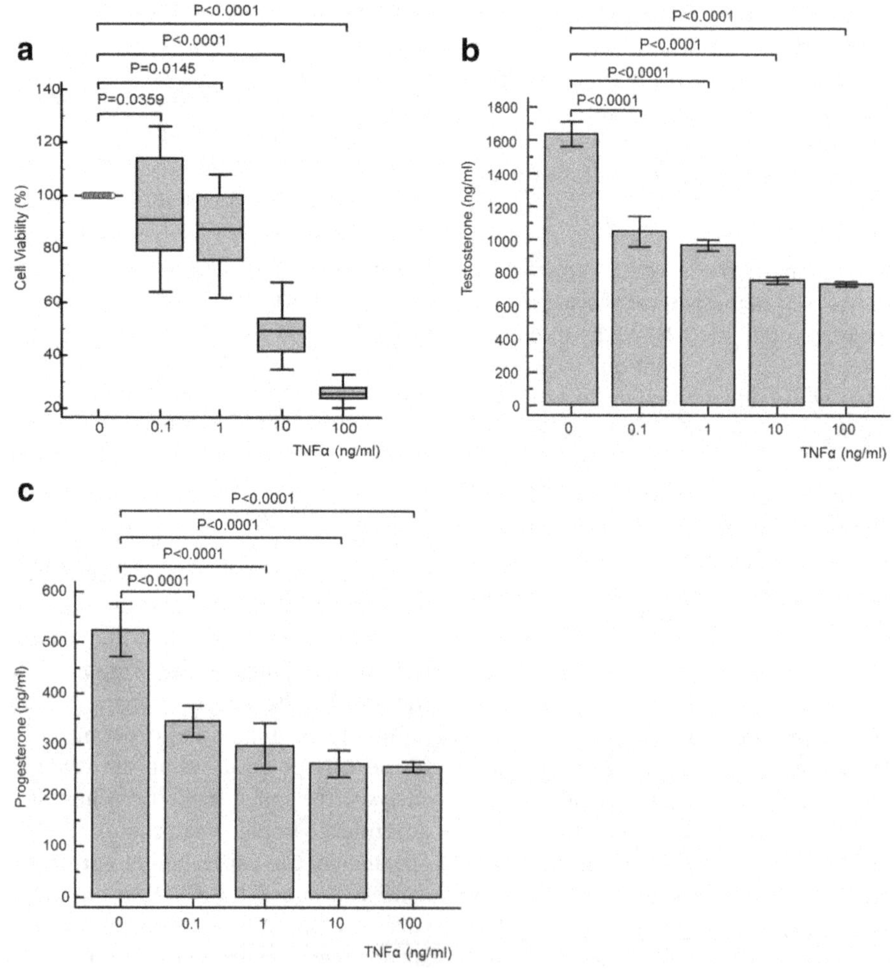

Fig. 1 Cell viability (**a**), testosterone (**b**) and progesterone concentration (**c**) results for TM3 cell exposure to various concentrations of tumour necrosis factor-alpha (TNFα). All tested parameters significantly decreased for all concentrations of TNFα. For testosterone and progesterone results, ANOVA repeated measures analysis of variance was significant ($P < 0.001$), as was the one-way analysis of variance ($P < 0.001$)

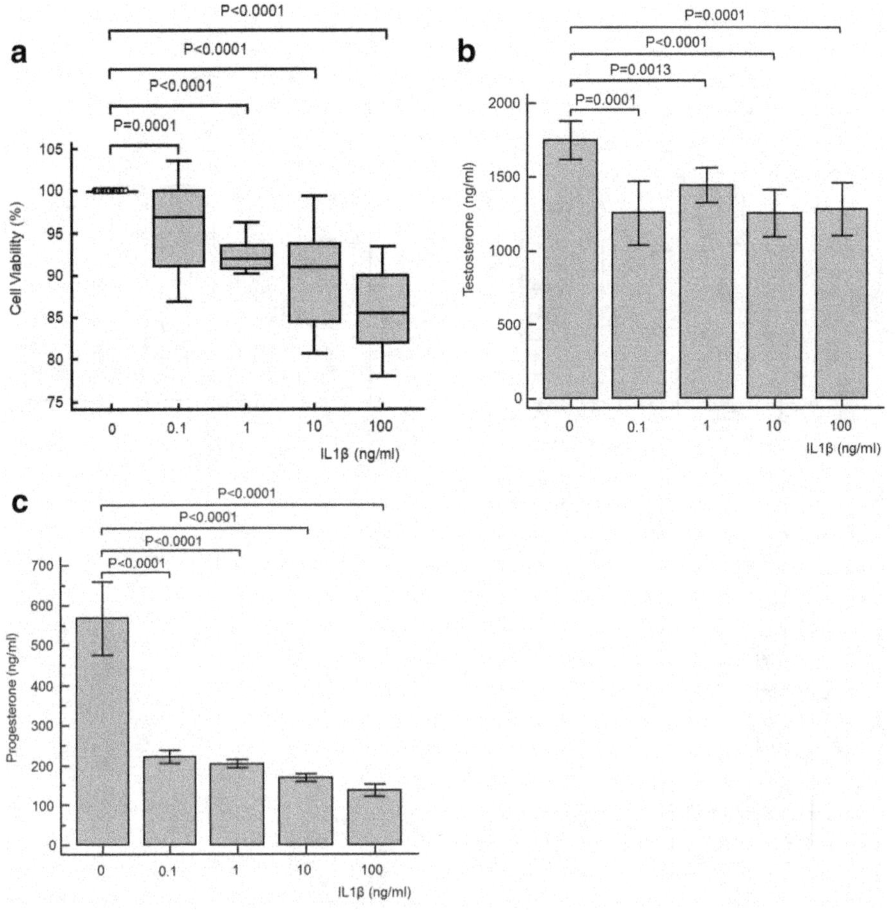

Fig. 2 Cell viability (**a**), testosterone (**b**) and progesterone (**c**) results for TM3 cell exposure to various concentrations of interleukin 1-beta (IL1β). All parameters tested significantly decreased for all concentrations of IL1β. For testosterone, ANOVA repeated measures analysis of variance was not significant ($P = 0.159$), nor was the ANOVA one-way analysis of variance ($P = 0.256$). For progesterone, ANOVA repeated measures analysis of variance was significant ($P < 0.001$), as was the one-way analysis of variance ($P < 0.001$)

dose-dependent and significant increase in testosterone production (ANOVA repeated measures analysis: $P = 0.015$; one-way ANOVA: $P < 0.001$) (Fig. 5b). However, the opposite was discovered for the progesterone production in which a significant decrease was observed at all experimental concentrations. Furthermore, there was a significant and dose-dependent decrease in progesterone concertation (ANOVA repeated measures analysis: $P < 0.001$; one-way ANOVA: $P < 0.001$) (Fig. 5c).

Discussion

Lipophilic steroid hormones are produced via the enzymatic cascade termed steroidogenesis. This process can occur in various tissues (e.g. gonads, adrenal medula and adipose tissue) [13, 16], and testosterone synthesis in males is most prominent in the Leydig cells [16, 18]. Progesterone, although poorly studied, is an important precursor to testosterone and further has regulatory roles on male physiology and pathology [12]. This is mostly investigated on male contraception, the treatment of male hypersexuality and the role of progesterone in fertilisation [12]. In order to further elicit a possible causal relationship between inflammation and hyperinsulinaemia on modulating steroidogenesis, this study suggests that inflammatory cytokines negatively influence steroidogenesis cascades in TM3 Leydig cells, whereas insulin positively modulates testosterone production.

Tumour necrosis factor-alpha

TNFα has been suggested to negatively affect the HPT axis, where in vivo administration is associated with a decrease in serum testosterone [1, 19]. The results of this study agree with previous publications that have assessed the impact of TNFα on Leydig cell function in vitro and in vivo [19–25]. TNFα reduces testosterone production in ranges of 0.1–100 ng/ml, typically in a dose dependant manner, in Leydig cells [20–24]. It is plausible that the enzymes mediating cholesterol uptake into the mitochondria (StAR), conversion to pregnenolone ($P450_{scc}$), pregnenolone conversion to progesterone (3βHSD) and progesterone conversion to 17-

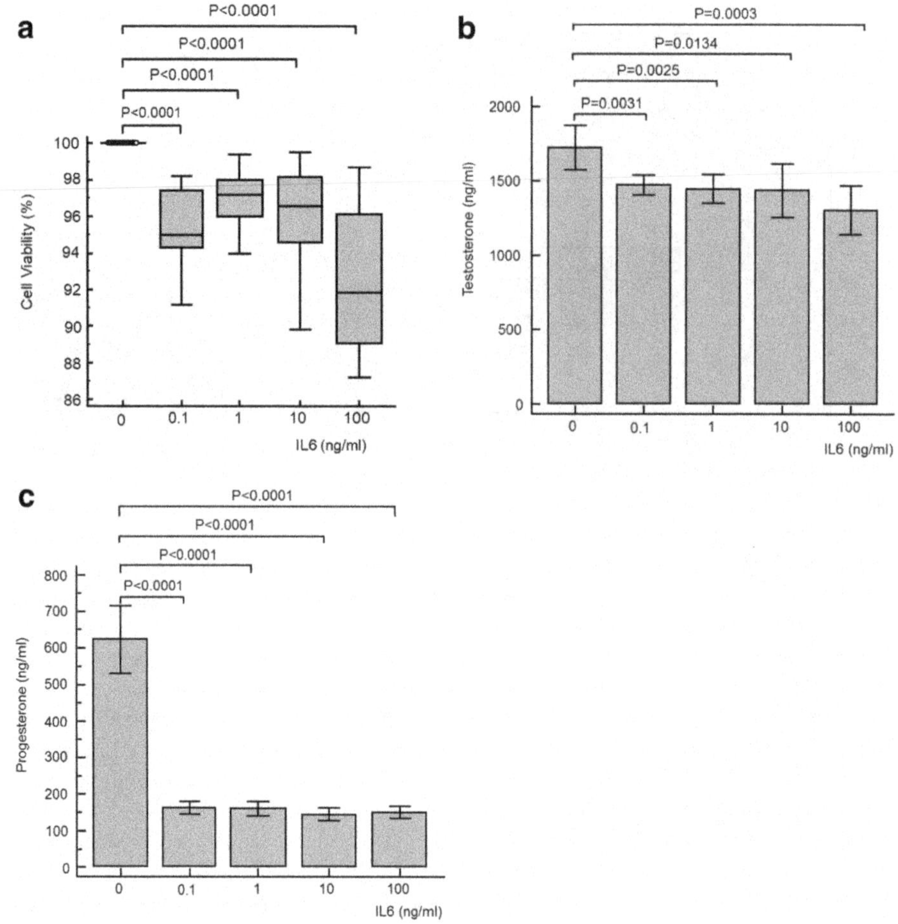

Fig. 3 Cell viability (**a**), testosterone (**b**) and progesterone (**c**) results for TM3 cell exposure to various concentrations of interleukin 6 (IL6). All parameters significantly decreased for all concentrations of IL6. For testosterone and progesterone, ANOVA repeated measures analysis of variance was significant ($P < 0.0001$), as was the one-way analysis of variance ($P < 0.001$)

OH-P (CYP17) are all negatively impacted by increasing TNFα concentrations [20–24]. Furthermore, the significant decrease in cell viability observed in this study would suggest cellular injury at increasing concentrations of TNFα exposure, leading to down-regulation of steroidogenesis enzyme production as a response to cellular injury [23]. TNFα was shown in this study to also decrease progesterone synthesis, agreeing agrees previous studies [20, 25] in Leydig cells. Based on the suggested mechanisms of steroidogenesis down-regulation [20–24], this would be an expected result that has been confirmed in this study.

Interleukin 1-beta

Previous studies on the effect of IL1 on Leydig cell steroid regulation have provided conflicting results. This appears to be due to a variety of different stages of puberty in which primary Leydig cells were obtained from animals [26]. Similar to this study, IL1β has been shown to decrease hCG-stimulated testosterone synthesis in a dose dependant manner using concentrations of 1–100 ng/ml [27, 28]. This may be via a decrease in hCG stimulated cAMP production [27] and reduced $P450_{scc}$ mRNA transcription [28]. In contrast, other studies have shown that IL1β did not significantly alter Leydig cell testosterone synthesis [29], or even increased testosterone synthesis [30].

Similar to this study, IL1 exposure has also previously been associated with a decrease in progesterone levels [25]. However, in contrast to this study, Wu and colleagues reported that a significant decrease in cell viability in TM3 Leydig cells exposed to 0.02 pg/ml IL1β which was interestingly prevented by co-stimulation of Sirt1, associated with cellular protection from inflammatory stress [23].

Interleukin 6

The effect of IL6 on Leydig cell function and steroidogenesis has been less well studied in controlled experiments compared to TNFα and IL1β [3]. However, the available reports generally agree with the results of this study. Human application of subcutaneous single doses

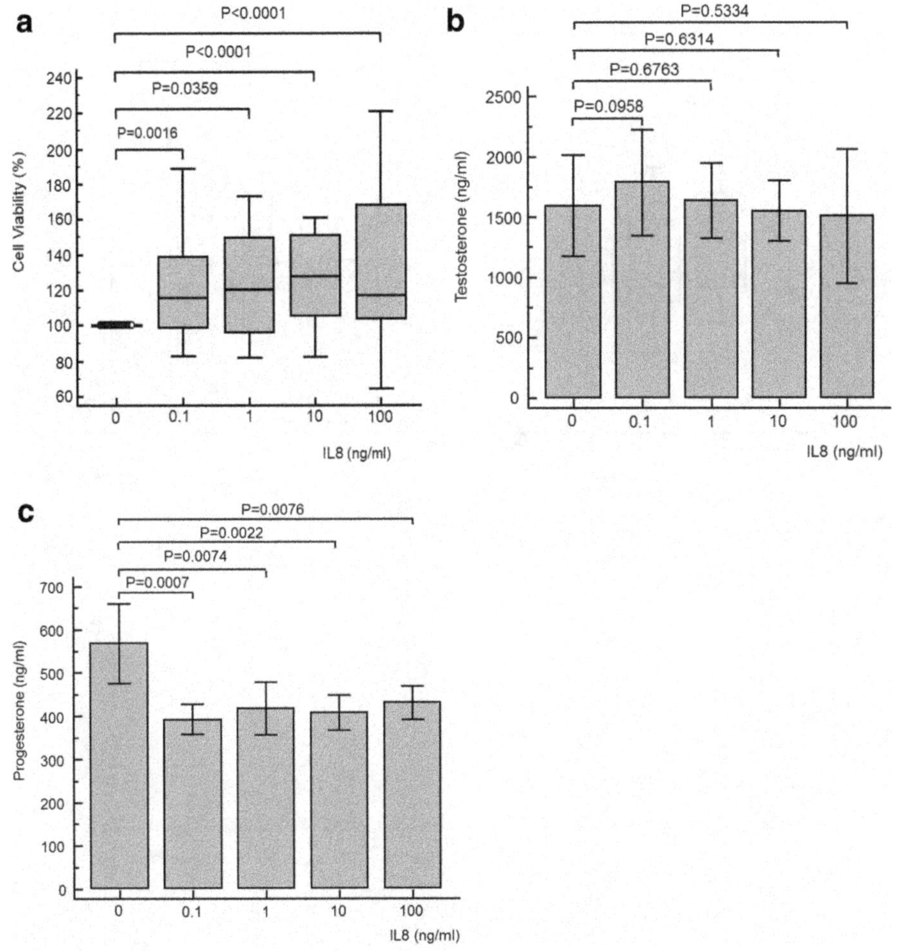

Fig. 4 Cell viability (**a**), testosterone (**b**) and progesterone (**c**) results for TM3 cell exposure to various concentrations of interleukin 8 (IL8). Cell viability was significantly increased for all concentrations, while testosterone concentrations did not significantly change. Contrary, progesterone concentrations declined significantly. For testosterone, ANOVA repeated measures analysis of variance was not significant ($P = 0.052$), nor was the ANOVA one-way analysis of variance ($P = 0.187$). For progesterone, ANOVA repeated measures analysis of variance was significant ($P = 0.002$), as was the one-way analysis of variance ($P < 0.001$)

of IL6 causes significant short term decreases in testosterone levels with increases in LH [31], most marked at 3 μg/Kg [31]. It is also suggested that IL6 compromises cAMP induced expression of CYP17 and, interestingly, 17β-HSD, at concentrations of 100 ng/ml in primary mouse Leydig cells [3], resulting in reduced testosterone synthesis [31, 32]. IL6 also decreases CYP17 and 3βHSD expression [32]. IL6 reportedly reduces Leydig cell viability at 0.02 pg/ml [23] similarly to this study. Interestingly, in adrenal cells from older adult males, IL6 is suggested to increase aldosterone, cortisol and DHEA synthesis [33], up-regulating adrenal steroidogenesis which is predominantly focused on mineralocorticoids and glucocorticoids synthesis [1].

Interleukin 8

Unlike TNFα, IL1β and IL6, there appear to be no published investigations into the possible effects of IL8 on steroidogenesis in Leydig cells. In this study, testosterone concentrations are maintained, but progesterone concentrations significantly decreased. It therefore appears that IL8 may influence progesterone via CYP17 or $P450_{scc}$ or StAR. As testosterone is not different from controls over 48 h, this would imply that the Δ^5-steroid pathway is at least maintained, for which CYP17 or $P450_{scc}$ and StAR are required.

Insulin

The results from this study agrees with reports in which insulin increases testosterone synthesis in the absence of insulin resistance [4, 34–38]. Exposure of primary mouse Leydig cells to 1 μg/ml insulin showed that for one hour prior to addition of LH for a further 3 h increased testosterone production compared to no insulin pretreatment [34]. Lin et al. [36] also demonstrated insulin stimulation of testosterone synthesis in a primary rat

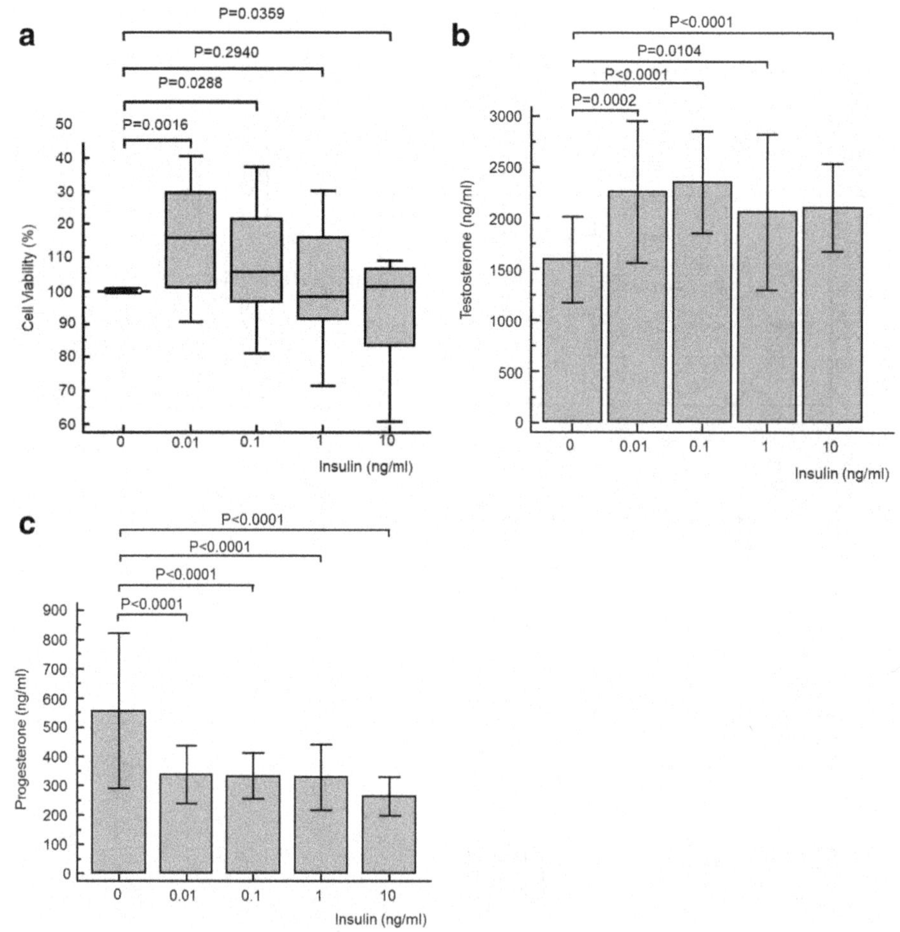

Fig. 5 Cell viability (**a**), testosterone (**b**) and progesterone (**c**) results for TM3 cell exposure to various concentrations of insulin. Cell viability was significantly increased at 0.01, 0.1 and 1 ng/ml insulin. Testosterone concentrations were significantly increased for all concentrations, while progesterone concentrations significantly declined. For testosterone, ANOVA repeated measures analysis of variance was significant ($P = 0.015$), as was the one-way analysis of variance ($P < 0.001$). For progesterone, ANOVA repeated measures analysis of variance was statistically significant ($P < 0.001$), as was the one-way analysis of variance ($P < 0.001$)

Leydig cell culture model. Furthermore, 24-h exposure of primary catfish Leydig cells to 1 ng/ml insulin stimulated testosterone synthesis [39]. However, Ahn and colleagues [40] demonstrated that insulin binds directly to insulin receptors on the Leydig cell membrane, leading to an upregulation of DAX-1 genes expression via the AKT pathway in MA-10 Leydig cells. This in turn resulted in a downregulation of steroidogenesis in these cells [40], which is somewhat contrary to the testosterone results in this study and others [4, 34–38].

Insulin mediates metabolic and mitogenic effects through binding to cell surface insulin receptors, leading to activation of two pathways: the phosphoinositide 3-kinase (PI3K) and the mitogen-activated protein kinase (MAPK) pathways. PI3K results in activation of 3-phosphoinositide-dependent protein kinase 1 (PDK1) and Akt kinase, mediating most of the cellular effects of insulin [41]. The activation of the MAPK pathway generally mediates transcription of factors involved with cell growth. Effects of metabolites in this pathway result in vasoconstriction, increased expression of vascular cell adhesion molecules and growth and mitogenesis of vascular smooth muscle cells [41].

In animals and humans, hyperinsulinaemia and insulin resistance is closely associated with male hypogonadism [37, 42], which also conflicts with these in vivo results. In various cell lines (e.g. hepatocytes, adipocytes, skeletal muscle), the PI3K/Akt intracellular pathway through which insulin exerts its effects breakdown with increasing insulin resistance (hyperinsulinaemia) [41]. The induction of hyperinsulinaemia in mice results in disruption of steroidogenesis cascades via abnormal activation of the oestrogen receptor-alpha pathway, contributing to male hypogonadism pathogenesis [43]. Currently, no significant data exists in which to further postulate on the direct potential impact of hyperinsulinaemia and insulin resistance on Leydig cell function and steroidogenesis molecular mechanisms. Further research is required in order to further elicit these mechanisms.

There are no significant studies identified that investigate the effect of insulin on progesterone synthesis. In stark contrast to testosterone concentrations, progesterone was significantly decreased for all concentrations assessed, in a dose-dependent manner. As progesterone is an essential precursor of testosterone, these results suggest enzymatic activity downstream of progesterone may be upregulated, and not those upstream. Hypothetically, insulin may stimulate an upregulation of testosterone synthesis via the Δ^4-steroid pathway, acting on one or more of these enzymes such as CYP17, CYP17,20 or 17β-HSD. This may also be associated with a down-regulate 3β-HSD, leading to a decrease in the Δ^5-steroid pathway [44]. Further studies on these mechanisms is therefore warranted to further elicit the physiological and pathological mechanisms associated with insulin and Leydig cell steroidogenesis cascades.

Clinical implications

Adequate Leydig cell function with the central purpose of testosterone production via steroidogenesis cascades is critical not only for male reproduction, but in general male health and well-being [6]. Various cytokines, as well as insulin, have been suggested to modulate the HPT axis, and may further regulate steroidogenesis within Leydig cells directly or indirectly [1, 3, 4]. Obesity and related metabolic co-morbidities and complications are closely associated with a low grade, asymptomatic, systemic and chronic inflammatory state and hyperinsulinaemia, amongst other underlying mechanisms [14, 15]. This is also relevant in male ageing and androgen decline in ageing men, which is associated with increasing inflammatory markers and hyperinsulinaemia [45]. Furthermore, increased systemic inflammatory cytokines and insulin have correlated with increased seminal concentrations of cytokines and insulin [14, 15]. As testosterone is critical in male health and well-being [5, 6], the (patho)physiological role of cytokines and insulin is relevant within the context of inflammation in males.

The T_H1-lymphocyte associated inflammatory cytokines, specifically TNFα, IL1β, and IL6, are increasingly associated with male hypogonadism. Although a direct causal association is postulated, this is poorly understood [5, 9]. This is observed in acute inflammatory (infectious) disease associated with gonadal failure [5], and low-grade chronic inflammation associated with obesity and related co-morbidities and complications such as metabolic syndrome and type 2 diabetes mellitus [15]. Testosterone is also inversely correlated to the inflammatory marker C-Reactive Protein (CRP) in males, and males in lower quintiles of serum testosterone concentrations are more likely to have increased inflammatory markers associated with TNFα and IL6 [17]. In addition to having immune (down)regulating functions [17], testosterone therapy reduces inflammatory cytokine production and improves insulin sensitivity in obese and metabolic syndrome males [46].

Although poorly researched in males, reduced serum progesterone is associated with obesity and metabolic syndrome [44, 47, 48]. This study suggests that an associated pro-inflammatory state is associated with reduced progesterone as observed in observational clinical results. However, further research, particularly to understand the mechanisms associated with these results, is required in order to identify potentially novel therapeutic targets in males with chronic inflammation.

Insulin independently stimulates testosterone production and simultaneously inhibits SHBG in normal weight and obese males [4]. Furthermore, insulin resistance is closely associated with low testosterone in males [14, 42]. There is a close relationship between insulin sensitivity and testosterone concentrations in men across a wide range of glucose intolerance, including those with T2DM, and independent of SHBG concentrations [49]. This study is consistent with in vivo evidence from animals and humans that insulin increased testosterone production in insulin sensitive males [49]. However, insulin sensitivity is directly related to testosterone synthesis [34, 36]. Insulin appears to activate the Akt kinase pathway within Leydig cells, which likely mediates the role of this hormone in steroidogenesis [40]. It is further known that this intracellular pathway breaks down with insulin resistance in other cell lines [41]. Numerous studies have shown that TNFα can impair insulin signalling in hepatocytes, adipose tissue and skeletal muscle [50]. It is therefore feasible that induction of insulin resistance may result in the inability of insulin to promote testosterone synthesis in Leydig cells, and further contribute to hypogonadism. Further studies to understand the mechanism of insulin, including the potential induction of insulin resistance, on Leydig cell function and steroidogenesis required.

Strengths and limitations of the study

This in vitro study was done under standard and controlled laboratory conditions. Experiments on each exposure were done in duplicate and assays further done on duplicate to ensure reliability of the results obtained. Experiments were replicated six times, and statistical analysis on the data is appropriate. This study is limited specifically in the number of variables investigated, due to the exploratory nature and aims of the study. Caution should be made in the interpretation of the results within the context of the existing literature, as different in vitro and in vivo models and methods are used in the studies reported. Implications of the results within the broader clinical context, although relevant, require further investigation, and these results are not able to directly prove causation relevant to clinical practice.

Conclusions

The inflammatory cytokines TNFα, IL1β and IL6 cause a dose dependent decline in steroidogenesis in TM3 Leydig cells over 48 h. These results suggest that chronic inflammation may downregulate steroidogenesis in males via direct modulation of Leydig cell function. However, IL8 appears to minimally affect testosterone production in the concentrations observed, with an increase in cell viability and decrease in progesterone concentrations which may suggest inhibition of progesterone synthesis from cholesterol via 17-OH pregnenolone. Insulin was observed to have a dose-dependent increase in testosterone synthesis alongside a significant decline in progesterone synthesis, indicating insulin may directly act on Leydig cells as part of steroid hormone regulation. With the phenomenon of insulin resistance, the literature is unclear on the potential role of hyperinsulinaemia in steroidogenesis. Further studies are warranted in order to fully elicit the molecular mechanisms and interactions of these molecules on male steroidogenesis.

Abbreviations

17β-HSD: 17β-Hydroxysteroid Dehydrogenase; 3β-HSD: 3β-Hydroxysteroid Dehydrogenase; Akt kinase: Protein Kinase B; cAMP: Cyclic Adenosine Monophosphate; CYP17: Cytochrome P450 17α-Hydroxylase; CYP17,20: Cytochrome P450 17,20-Lyase; DHEA: Dehydroepiandrosterone; EDTA: Ethylenediaminetetraacetic acid; FSH: Follicular Stimulating Hormone; GnRH: Gonadotropin releasing hormone; hCG: Human Chorionic Gonadotropin; HPT: Hypothalamic-Pituitary-Testes Axis; IL1β: Interleukin 1-beta; IL6: Interleukin 6; IL8: Interleukin 8; LH: Luteinizing Hormone; NO: Nitric Oxide; $P450_{scc}$: Cholesterol Side-Chain Cleavage Enzyme; SHBG: Sex Hormone Binding Globulin; Sirt1: Sirtuin 1; StAR: Steroidogenic Acute Regulatory Protein; TNFα: Tumour Necrosis Factor-Alpha

Acknowledgements

South African Medical Research Council (MRC) for funding contribution for the experiments.

Funding

Funding was provided by the South African Medical Research Council (MRC), Parow, South Africa. The MRC did not have a role in the study design, data analysis, interpretation of results nor the manuscript drafting;

Authors' contributions

KL conceptualised the study, conducted the laboratory experiments and assays, analysed the data, conducted statistical analysis and drafted the final manuscript. RH critically reviewed the methodology, data analysis and review of manuscript drafts. Both authors read and approved the final manuscript.

Competing interests

The authors declare that they have no competing interests in the study.

Author details

[1]School of Natural Medicine, University of the Western Cape, Private Bag X17, Bellville 7535, South Africa. [2]Department of Medical Biosciences, University of the Western Cape, Private Bag X17, Bellville 7535, South Africa.

References

1. Bornstein SR, Rutkowski H, Vrezas I. Cytokines and steroidogenesis. Mol Cell Endocrinol. 2004;215:135–41.
2. Svechnikov KV, Sultana T, Söder O. Age-dependent stimulation of Leydig cell steroidogenesis by interleukin-1 isoforms. Mol Cell Endocrinol. 2001;182:193–201.
3. Hales DB, Diemer T, Hales KH. Role of cytokines in testicular function. Endocrine. 1999;10:201–17.
4. Pasquali R, Casimirri F, De Iasio R, Mesini P, Boschi S, Chierici R, Flamia R, Biscotti M, Vicennati V. Insulin regulates testosterone and sex hormone-binding globulin concentrations in adult normal weight and obese men. J Clin Endocrinol Metab. 1995;80:654–8.
5. Tremellen K, McPhee N, Pearce K, Benson S, Schedlowski M, Engler H. Endotoxin initiated inflammation reduces testosterone production in men of reproductive age. Am J Physiol Endocrinol Metab. 2017; https://doi.org/10.1152/ajpendo.00279.2017.
6. Walker WH. Testosterone signaling and the regulation of spermatogenesis. Spermatogenesis. 2011;1:116–20.
7. Dohle GR, Smit M, Weber RF. Androgens and male fertility. World J Urol. 2003;21:341–5.
8. Singh J, O'Neill C, Handelsman DJ. Induction of spermatogenesis by androgens in gonadotropin-deficient (hpg) mice. Endocrinology. 1995;136:5311–21.
9. Watson ME, Newman RJ, Payne AM, Abdelrahim M, Francis GL. The effect of macrophage conditioned media on Leydig cell function. Ann Clin Lab Sci. 1994;24(1):84–95.
10. Corona G, Vignozzi L, Sforza A, Mannucci E, Maggi M. Obesity and late-onset 406 hypogonadism. Mol Cell Endocrinol. 2015;418:120–33.
11. Mulligan T, Frick MF, Zuraw QC, Stemhagen A, McWhirter C. Prevalence of hypogonadism 447 in males aged at least 45 years: the HIM study. Int J Clin Pract. 2006;60:762–9.
12. Oettel M, Mukhopadhyay AK. Progesterone: the forgotten hormone in men? Aging Male. 2004;7:236–57.
13. Sherbet DP, Tiosano D, Kwist KM, Hochberg Z, Auchus RJ. CYP17 mutation E305G causes isolated 17,20-lyase deficiency by selectively altering substrate binding. J Biol Chem. 2003;5:48563–9.
14. Leisegang K, Bouic PJ, Menkveld R, Henkel RR. Obesity is associated with increased seminal insulin and leptin alongside reduced fertility parameters in a controlled male cohort. Reprod Biol Endocrinol. 2014;7(12):34.
15. Leisegang K, Bouic PJ, Henkel RR. Metabolic syndrome is associated with increased seminal inflammatory cytokines and reproductive dysfunction in a case-controlled male cohort. Am J Reprod Immunol. 2016;76(2):155–63.
16. Midzak AS, Chen H, Papadopoulos V, Zirkin BR. Leydig cell aging and the mechanisms of reduced testosterone synthesis. Mol Cell Endocrinol. 2009;5:23–31.
17. Tsilidis KK, Rohrmann S, McGlynn KA, Nyante SJ, Lopez DS, Bradwin G, Feinleib M, Joshu CE, et al. Association between endogenous sex steroid hormones and inflammatory biomarkers in US men. Andrology. 2013;1(6):919–28.
18. Miller WL, Auchus RJ. The molecular biology, biochemistry, and physiology of human steroidogenesis and its disorders. Endocr Rev. 2011;32:81–151.
19. van der Poll T, Romijn JA, Endert E, Sauerwein HP. Effects of tumor necrosis factor on the hypothalamic-pituitary-testicular axis in healthy men. Metabolism. 1993;42:303–7.
20. Hong CY, Park JH, Ahn RS, Im SY, Choi HS, Soh J, Mellon SH, Lee K. Molecular mechanism of suppression of testicular steroidogenesis by proinflammatory cytokine tumor necrosis factor alpha. Mol Cell Biol. 2004; 24:2593–604.
21. Mauduit C, Gasnier F, Rey C, Chauvin MA, Stocco DM, Louisot P, Benahmed M. Tumor necrosis factor-alpha inhibits Leydig cell steroidogenesis through a decrease in steroidogenic acute regulatory protein expression. Endocrinology. 1998;139:2863–8.
22. Morales V, Santana P, Díaz R, Tabraue C, Gallardo G, Lopez Blanco F, Hernández I, Fanjul LF, Ruiz de Galarreta CM. Intratesticular delivery of tumor necrosis factor-alpha and ceramide directly abrogates steroidogenic acute regulatory protein expression and Leydig cell steroidogenesis in adult rats. Endocrinology. 2003;144:4763–72.

23. Wu L, Zhang A, Sun Y, Zhu X, Fan W, Lu X, Yang Q, Feng Y. Sirt1 exerts anti-inflammatory effects and promotes steroidogenesis in Leydig cells. Fertil Steril. 2012;98:194–9.
24. Xiong Y, Hales DB. The role of tumor necrosis factor-alpha in the regulation of mouse Leydig cell steroidogenesis. Endocrinology. 1993;132:2568–73.
25. Manna PR, Chandrala SP, Jo Y, Stocco DM. cAMP-independent signaling regulates steroidogenesis in mouse Leydig cells in the absence of StAR phosphorylation. J MolEndocrinol. 2006;37:81–95.
26. Gerendai I, Banczerowski P, Csernus V. Interleukin 1-beta injected into the testis acutely stimulates and later attenuates testicular steroidogenesis of the immature rat. Endocrine. 2005;28:165–70.
27. Calkins JH, Sigel MM, Nankin HR, Lin T. Interleukin-1 inhibits Leydig cell steroidogenesis in primary culture. Endocrinology. 1998;123:1605–10.
28. Lin T, Wang TL, Nagpal ML, Calkins JH, Chang WW, Chi R. Interleukin-1 inhibits cholesterol side-chain cleavage cytochrome P450 expression in primary cultures of Leydig cells. Endocrinology. 1991;129:1305–11.
29. Sun XR, Hedger MP, Risbridger GP. The effect of testicular macrophages and interleukin-1 on testosterone production by purified adult rat Leydig cells cultured under in vitro maintenance conditions. Endocrinology. 1993;132:86–92.
30. Verhoeven G, Cailleau J, Van Damme J, Billiau A. Interleukin-1 stimulates steroidogenesis in cultured rat Leydig cells. Mol Cell Endocrinol. 1998;57:51–60.
31. Tsigos C, Papanicolaou DA, Kyrou I, Raptis SA, Chrousos GP. Dose-dependent effects of recombinant human interleukin-6 on the pituitary-testicular axis. J Interf Cytokine Res. 1999;19:1271–6.
32. Hales DB. Testicular macrophage modulation of Leydig cell steroidogenesis. J Reprod Immunol. 2002;57:3–18.
33. Päth G, Bornstein SR, Ehrhart-Bornstein M, Scherbaum WA. Interleukin-6 and the interleukin-6 receptor in the human adrenal gland: expression and effects on steroidogenesis. J Clin Endocrinol Metab. 1997;82:2343–9.
34. Bebakar WM, Honour JW, Foster D, Liu YL, Jacobs HS. Regulation of testicular function by insulin and transforming growth factor-beta. Steroids. 1990;55:266–70.
35. Benitez A, Perez Diaz J. Effect of streptozotocin-diabetes and insulin treatment on regulation of Leydig cell function in the rat. Horm Metab Res. 1985;17:5–7.
36. Lin T, Haskell J, Vinson N, Terracio L. Characterization of insulin and insulin-like growth factor I receptors of purified Leydig cells and their role in steroidogenesis in primary culture: a comparative study. Endocrinology. 1986;119:1641–7.
37. Pasquali R, Macor C, Vicennati V, Novo F, De Iasio R, Mesini P, Boschi S, Casimirri F, Vettor R. Effects of acute hyperinsulinemia on testosterone serum concentrations in adult obese and normal-weight men. Metabolism. 1997;46:526–9.
38. Pitteloud N, Hardin M, Dwyer AA, Valassi E, Yialamas M, Elahi D, Hayes FJ. Increasing insulin resistance is associated with a decrease in Leydig cell testosterone secretion in men. J Clin Endocrinol Metab. 2005;90:2636–41.
39. Dubey N, Lal B. Paracrine role of macrophage produced-nitric oxide (NO) in Leydig cell steroidogenesis in a teleost, Clarias batrachus: impact of gonadotropin, growth hormone and insulin on NO production by testicular macrophages. Gen Comp Endocrinol. 2009;60:12–8.
40. Ahn SW, Gang GT, Kim YD, Ahn RS, Harris RA, Lee CH, Choi HS. Insulin directly regulates steroidogenesis via induction of the orphan nuclear receptor DAX-1 in testicular Leydig cells. J Biol Chem. 2013;288:15937–46.
41. Huang PL. A comprehensive definition for metabolic syndrome. DMM. 2009;2:231–7.
42. Kasturi SS, Tannir J, Brannigan R. The metabolic syndrome and male infertility. J Androl. 2008;29:251–9.
43. Zhao Y, Li HX, Wang K, Yan BY, Li W. Regulation of testicular steroidogenesis by Foxa3 via transcriptional modulation of ERα signaling in type 2 diabetes mellitus (T2DM). Biochem Biophys Res Commun. 2017;490(3):786–93.
44. Leisegang K, Udodong A, Bouic PJ, Henkel RR. Effect of the metabolic syndrome on male reproductive function: a case-controlled pilot study. Andrologia. 2014;46(2):167–76.
45. Leisegang K, Henkel R, Agarwal A. Redox regulation of fertility in aging male and the role of antioxidants: a savior or stressor. Curr Pharm Des. 2017; 23(30):4438–50.
46. Winter AG, Zhao F, Lee RK. Androgen deficiency and metabolic syndrome in men. Transl Androl Urol. 2014;3(1):50–8.
47. Blanchette S, Marceau P, Biron S, Brochu G, Tchernof A. Circulating progesterone and obesity in men. Horm Metab Res. 2006;38:330–5.
48. Isidori AM, Caprio M, Strollo F, Moretti C, Frajese G, Isidori A, Leptin FA. Androgens in male obesity: evidence for leptin contribution to reduced androgen levels. J Clin Endocrinol Metab. 1999;84:3673–80.
49. Pitteloud N, Mootha VK, Dwyer AA, Hardin M, Lee H, Eriksson KF, Tripathy D, Yialamas M, et al. Relationship between testosterone levels, insulin sensitivity, and mitochondrial function in men. Diabetes Care. 2005;28(7): 1636–42.
50. Galic S, Oakhill JS, Steinberg GR. Adipose tissue as an endocrine organ. Mol Cell Endocrinol. 2010;316(2):129–39.

4

Regulation by FSH of the dynamic expression of *retinol-binding protein 4* in the mouse ovary

Yanwen Jiang[†], Yun Zhao[†], Shuxiong Chen, Lu Chen, Chunjin Li[*] and Xu Zhou[*]

Abstract

Background: Ovarian retinoid homeostasis plays an important role in the physiological function of the ovary. Retinol-binding protein 4 (RBP4) acts as the mediator for the systemic and intercellular transport of retinol and is heavily involved in cellular retinol influx, efflux, and exchange. However, the expression patterns and regulatory mechanisms of *Rbp4* in the ovary remain unclear.

Methods: The expression pattern of ovarian *Rbp4* was examined in immature mice during different developmental stages and in adult mice during different stages of the estrous cycle. The potential regulation and mechanisms of ovarian *Rbp4* expression by estrogen and related gonadotropins in mouse ovaries were also investigated.

Results: The present study demonstrated that the ovarian expression of *Rbp4* remained constant before puberty and increased significantly in the peripubertal period. In adult female mice, the expression of *Rbp4* increased at proestrus and peaked at estrus at both the mRNA and protein levels. The protein distribution of RBP4 was mainly localized in the granulosa cell and theca cell layer in follicles. In addition, the expression of *Rbp4* was significantly induced by follicle-stimulating hormone (FSH) or FSH + luteinizing hormone (LH) in combination in immature mouse (3 weeks old) ovaries in vivo and in granulosa cells cultured in vitro, both at the mRNA and protein levels. In contrast, treatment with LH or 17β-estradiol did not exhibit any observable effects on ovarian *Rbp4* expression. Transcription factors high-mobility group AT-hook 1 (HMGA1), steroidogenic factor 1 (SF-1), and liver receptor homolog 1 (LRH-1) (which have been previously shown to be involved in activation of *Rbp4* transcription), also responded to FSH stimulation. In addition, H-89, an inhibitor of protein kinase A (PKA), and the depletion of HMGA1, SF-1, and LRH-1 by small interfering RNAs (siRNAs), resulted in a dramatic loss of the induction of *Rbp4* expression by FSH at both the mRNA and protein levels.

Conclusions: These data indicate that the dynamic expression of *Rbp4* is mainly regulated by FSH through the cAMP-PKA pathway, involving transcriptional factors HMGA1, SF-1, and LRH-1, in the mouse ovary during different stages of development and the estrous cycle.

Keywords: Follicle-stimulating hormone, Retinol, Ovary, Granulosa cells

* Correspondence: llcjj158@163.com; xzhou65@vip.sina.com
[†]Equal contributors
College of Animal Science, Jilin University, 5333 Xian Road, Changchun, Jilin 130062, China

Summary sentence

Ovarian *Rbp4* expression remains constant before puberty, increases significantly around puberty in immature mice, and peaks at estrus in adult mice, which is mainly regulated by FSH through the cAMP-PKA pathway partly and involves transcriptional factors HMGA1, SF-1, and LRH-1.

Background

Retinol (vitamin A) and its derivatives, collectively known as retinoids, play crucial roles in ovarian development and normal physiological function [1]. Retinol is not biologically active per se, and within cells can be oxidized to retinal and retinoic acid (RA) by dehydrogenases. Most of the cellular actions of retinoids can be accounted for by the transcriptional regulatory activity of RA through their nuclear receptors, known as RA receptors (RARs) and retinoid X receptors (RXRs), which associate with RA response elements (RAREs) within the promoters of retinoid-responsive genes [1]. RA in ovarian antral follicles enhanced FSH-mediated ovarian follicular cell differentiation and female fertility, and vitamin A deficiency inhibited oocyte development and decreased ovulated oocytes in mice [2, 3]. RA also plays a crucial role in both nuclear and cytoplasmic maturation of mouse and bovine oocytes [4, 5] and can also stimulate steroidogenesis, such as testosterone production in human theca cells and estradiol production in mouse granulosa cells [1, 6]. In addition, ovarian retinoid levels vary with the estrous cycle [7], and the concentration of retinol is greater in the follicular fluids of the dominant follicles than that of small follicles [8, 9]. However, the regulatory mechanisms of ovarian retinoid homeostasis have not yet been fully understood.

The data from our laboratory suggest that FSH enhances retinol uptake, accumulation, and metabolism in the mouse ovary (unpublished data), but the mechanisms remain unclear. Retinol-binding protein 4 (RBP4), which acts as the mediator for the systemic and intercellular transport of retinol, plays an important role in cellular retinol influx, efflux, and exchange [10]; and seems to play an important role in retinol intercellular transport and accumulation in follicular fluids of the dominant follicles. Evidence shows that the RBP4 immunostaining was observed in the layers of theca and granulosa cells of antral follicles with the most intense staining noted in the cells of large and healthy follicles. Furthermore, the levels of RBP4 and retinol in the fluids of large follicles were higher than those in the fluids of medium or small follicles [8]. High RBP4 levels are also observed in the serum of women with polycystic ovary syndrome (PCOS) and in the fluids from swine follicular cysts [11, 12]. Based on these data [8–12], the regulation of *Rbp4* expression during follicular development remains an interesting and important point of study and would provide an explanation for the possible mechanisms involved in changing ovarian retinoid levels during follicular development.

The regulatory mechanisms of follicular development and ovarian function are primarily realized through neuroendocrine activities in the hypothalamus–pituitary–ovary (HPO) axial, although early stage occurs independently of the HPO axis. Follicle-stimulating hormone (FSH) or FSH+ luteinizing hormone (LH), which are released by the pituitary gland, principally control follicular development and ovulation by regulating estradiol (E_2) production and the functions of granulosa and theca cells. FSH and LH exert their actions by activating their membrane receptors (namely FSHR and LHR, G-protein coupled receptors) thereby resulting in an increase in intracellular cyclic AMP (cAMP), a second messenger involved in the transduction of hormonal or growth signals that regulate cell functions such as proliferation, differentiation, and metabolism [13, 14]. Elevated cAMP activates protein kinase A (PKA), which phosphorylates certain transcription factors and regulates downstream gene transcription. However, it is not until puberty (at approximately 4 weeks of age in mouse) that gonadotropin pulsatility is sufficient to stimulate fully-grown mature follicles and induce ovulation.

In the adult female mouse (after 6–8 weeks old), under the influence of reproductive hormones (FSH, LH and E_2), ovarian activities (follicular growth, ovulation, and corpus luteum formation and regression) alternate periodically during the estrous cycle (averages 4–5 days: proestrus for 9–18 h, estrus for about 12 h, metestrus for 24–48 h, and diestrus for 48–72 h) [15, 16]. During proestrus, some recruited follicles in the ovary start to grow rapidly under the stimulation of FSH [17]. During the estrus, the dominant follicles mature and ovulate under the influence of FSH, LH, and estradiol [17–19]. After ovulation, the corpus luteum starts to form under the influence of LH and mice enter metestrus [20]; and during diestrus, the mature corpus luteum releases progesterone which inhibits LH and FSH release by the anterior pituitary and inhibits follicular development [17]. Metestrus terminates with the regression of the corpus luteum under the influence of the pulses of prostaglandin ($PG_{F2\alpha}$) released from the uterus [20, 21].

The structural protein high mobility group AT-hook 1 (HMGA1) is important in promoter regulation by uncovering chromatin and facilitating the recruitment of multiple transcription factors [22]. The *cis*-regulatory sequences of the mouse *Rbp4* gene contain several copies of an AT-rich motif, known to be the binding site for HMGA1 proteins. It has also been reported that HMGA1 can bind the *Rbp4* promoter and recruit the transcription factors steroidogenic factor 1 (SF-1) and liver receptor homolog 1 (LRH-1) to form an activation complex and induce *Rbp4* transcription in Hepal mouse hepatoma cells [22].

The present study investigated the expression patterns of *Rbp4* during different stages of development and the estrous cycle. We also explored the potential regulatory mechanisms governing ovarian *Rbp4* expression by estrogen and related gonadotropins in mouse ovaries and examined the involvement of HMGA1, LRH-1, and SF-1. The results of this study are expected to provide mechanistic evidence for the fluctuations in ovarian retinoid levels during follicular development and estrous cycle.

Methods

Animals

Immature (3 weeks old, the same below) and adult (8 weeks old, the same below) BALB/c mice were obtained from the Medical Department of Jilin University (Changchun, China). The mice were raised in an environment with controlled temperature (22–24 °C) and humidity (60–70%) in a 12 h light/dark cycle and provided with food and water ad libitum. Vaginal smear tests were performed on adult female mice (8 weeks old), and ovaries were collected from the mice at various stages of the estrous cycle. Some of the adult female mice (8 weeks old) were mated with male mice, and the ovaries of newborn female mice were collected at different developmental stages (postnatal 1, 2, 3, 4 and 5 weeks). To avoid the effect of endogenous gonadotrophins and E_2, we choose immature female mice (3 weeks old) to investigate hormonal effects on ovarian *Rbp4* expression. They were injected intraperitoneally with a single dose of FSH (10 IU/mouse; Ningbo Second Hormone Factory, Ningbo, China), LH (10 IU/mouse; Ningbo Second Hormone Factory, Ningbo, China), or 17β-estradiol (1 μg/mouse/day in corn oil; Sigma, USA) [23]. Mice were anesthetized with isoflurane and sacrificed via cervical dislocation at 24 or 48 h after injection, and ovarian samples used for RNA isolation were rapidly placed in EZNATM RNA safe stabilizer reagent (Omega, USA) and then stored at − 80 °C. All animal studies were conducted in accordance with the protocol approved by the Animal Care and Use Committee of Jilin University.

Vaginal smear tests

To retrieve ovarian samples from adult mice (8 weeks old) during each of the four stages of the estrous cycle, we performed the vaginal smear tests to identify the specific estrous cycle stages. Briefly, we placed the tip of a plastic pipette filled with 40 μl of phosphate buffered saline after (PBS; Hyclone, USA) into the mouse vagina, and gently flushed the vagina 3–5 times. Vaginal contents (cells and vaginal fluids) from each mouse were collected into a PCR tube and then smeared onto a glass slide. The evaluation of the vaginal smear images was performed under a microscope IX71 system (Olympus, Japan). Proestrus was characterized by the mostly nucleated and some cornified epithelial cells in the smear; estrus by cornified squamous epithelial cells without visible nuclei; metestrus by the predominance of leucocytes and a few nucleated epithelial and/or cornified squamous epithelial cells; and diestrus was characterized by a predominance of leukocytes [24, 25]. The reader is directed to further citations for a full description [24, 25]. Vaginal smear tests were performed at 08:00 and 20:00 each day. When the stages were identified, the mice were sacrificed via cervical dislocation and their ovaries were collected.

Immunohistochemistry

Intact ovaries collected from immature mice (3 weeks old) that were that were untreated controls or treated with FSH for 48 h were fixed in 4% paraformaldehyde (Boster, Wuhan, China) for 12 h at 4 °C. After washed with PBS and dehydrated, these tissues then were embedded in paraffin wax (Thermo, USA); and paraffin-embedded tissue sections (5 μm) were deparaffinized. After washing with PBS, the sections were treated with 10 mM citric acid buffer (pH 6.0) (Boster, Wuhan, China) for antigen activation for 15 min in boiling water. The sections were washed with PBS and blocked by 5% (*v*/v) BSA in PBS (Boster, Wuhan, China). Sections were incubated overnight at 4 °C with mouse monoclonal antibody specific to RBP4 at a 1:200 dilution in PBS (Proteintech, USA). In order to validate the specificity of RBP4 antibody, 5% nonimmune goat serum [26–29] or PBS [30] was used as negative controls instead of RBP4 antibody. After washed by 0.3% (*v*/v) Triton X-100 in PBS, sections were incubated with goat-anti-mouse second antibody (Boster, Wuhan, China) for 1 h at room temperature, stained using ABC kits, and counterstained with hematoxylin.

Follicular granulosa cell isolation and culture in vitro

Primary granulosa cells were isolated from immature female mouse (3 weeks old) ovaries, as described previously [31, 32]. The mice were sacrificed via cervical dislocation after being anesthetized, and the follicles were isolated with no. 5 fine needles. Follicles were then treated with trypsin (Hyclone, USA) for 1 h and filtered using a 100-μm filter (Life Technologies, USA). The isolated granulosa cells were cultured in Dulbecco's Modified Eagle Medium/F12 1:1 (Hyclone, USA) supplemented with 10% fetal bovine serum (Hyclone, USA), 1% insulin–transferrin–selenium (Sigma, USA), and 1% antibiotics (100 IU/ml penicillin and 100 μg/ml streptomycin; Hyclone, USA) at 37 °C in an atmosphere of 5% CO_2 in air. Twenty-four hours later, non-adherent cells were removed and adherent cells were treated with FSH (100 IU/L), LH (100 IU/L), 8-Br-cAMP (500 μM; Sigma, USA), or H-89 (10 μM; PKA inhibitor; Beyotime, Beijing, China).

RNA interference

siRNA oligonucleotides specific for mouse *Hmga1*, *Sf-1*, and *Lrh-1* were designed and synthesized by GenePharma (Shanghai, China). The sequences that provided successful knockdown were *Hmga1* siRNA, 5′-GAGTCAGAAAGAGCCCAGT-3; *Sf-1* siRNA, 5′- GCCTCGATGTGAAATTCCT-3′; and *Lrh-1* siRNA, 5′-GCAGAAGAAAGCCCTCATT-3′. The negative control (NC) siRNA was 5′-TTCTCCGAACGTGTCACGT-3′. Cells were transfected at 50–70% confluency with 50 nM of siRNA duplexes using the FuGENE HD transfection reagent (Roche Applied Science, USA) in accordance with the manufacturer's instructions. FSH was added to the culture medium 24 h after siRNA transfection and cells were treated for an additional 24 h.

Total RNA extraction and real-time quantitative PCR assay

Total RNA from ovarian tissue and granulosa cells cultured in vitro were extracted using an RNAprep pure Micro Kit (Tiangen, Beijing, China) and reverse transcribed into cDNA using a PrimeScript RT reagent kit (Takara, Japan) according to the manufacturer's instructions. Real-time PCR was performed on a sequence detection system (Agilent Technologies, USA) using a SYBR Premix Ex TaqII kit (Takara, Japan). The gene-specific primers (forward and reverse, respectively) that we used for real-time quantitative PCR amplification were as follows: *Rbp4* (NM_011255.3), 5′-AGTCAAGGAGAACTTCGACAAGG-3′, 5′-CAGAAAACTCAGCGATGATGTTG-3′; *Hmga1* (NM_016660.2), 5′-GCAGGAAAAGGATGGGACTG-3′, 5′-AGCAGGGCTTCCAGTCCCAG-3′; *Sf-1* (NM_139051.3), 5′-CCAGACCTTTATCTCCATTGTCG-3′, 5′-AGTGTCATCTGGTCAGCCACCT-3′); *Lrh-1* (NM_030676.3), 5′-TCATGCTGCCCAAAGTGGAGA-3′, 5′-TGGTTTTGGACAGTTCGCTT-3′. The expression level of mouse *β-actin* (NM_007393.3), 5′-TCTGGCACCACACCTTCTA-3′, 5′-AGGCATACAGGGACAGCAC-3′, was used as an internal reference. The relative gene expression levels were calculated using the $2^{-\Delta\Delta Ct}$ method. All primers were obtained from Sangon Biotech (Shanghai, China), all experiments were repeated at least three times.

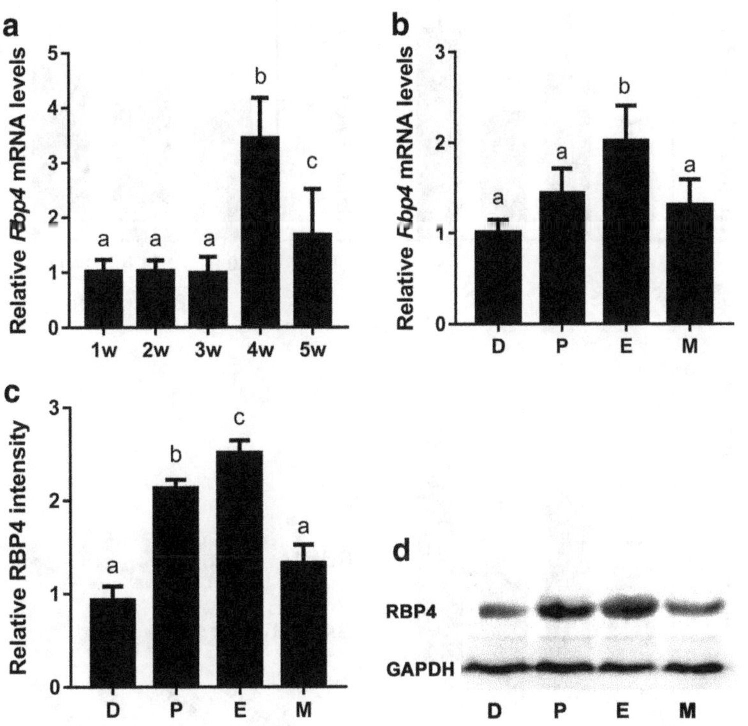

Fig. 1 Dynamic expression of *Rbp4* in mouse ovaries during the different stages of development and the estrous cycle. (A) Real-time qPCR analyses of *Rbp4* mRNA levels in mouse ovaries during different developmental stages. Data are presented as means ± SEM, *n* = 8. (B) Relative *Rbp4* mRNA levels in mouse ovaries during diestrus (D), proestrus (P), estrus (E), and metestrus (M). Data are presented as mean ± SEM, n = 8. RBP4 protein levels in the ovaries of mice during the estrous cycle were determined via Western blot analyses (D), and blots were quantified via densitometry (C). The protein levels were normalized to GAPDH. Data are presented as means ± SEM, *n* = 3. Means with different letters represent a significant difference at the 0.05 level

Western blot analyses

Protein samples were obtained by homogenizing whole ovaries and by lysing granulosa cells in lysate buffer (Beyotime, Beijing, China) with a 10 μg/ml protease and phosphatase inhibitor cocktail (Thermo, USA). Samples were then centrifuged at 13,000 g at 4 °C. Tissue and cell extracts were normalized to the sample protein concentration, as determined by a protein assay kit (Beyotime, Beijing, China). Proteins (40 μg) were separated via sodium dodecyl sulfate polyacrylamide gel (12%) electrophoresis and transferred to polyvinylidene difluoride membranes. The membranes were then blocked in Tris-buffered saline with Tween 20 (TBST) containing 5% non-fat instant milk and incubated overnight at 4 °C with mouse monoclonal antibodies specific to RBP4 or GAPDH (Proteintech, USA); and rabbit monoclonal antibodies specific to HMGA1, SF-1, or LRH-1 (Abcam, USA) each at 1:5000 dilution. After washing with TBST, the membranes were incubated with horseradish peroxidase-conjugated secondary antibody (Proteintech, USA) for 1 h. Enhanced chemiluminescence (ECL) detection was performed using an ECL system according to the specifications of the manufacturer (Beyotime, Beijing, China). Protein levels were normalized to GAPDH and quantified via densitometry using a Tanon gel imaging system (Tanon, Shanghai, China).

Statistical analyses

The statistical analyses of the data were conducted via one-way ANOVA followed by Tukey's multiple-range test. Differences were considered significant at $P < 0.05$. All the statistical analyses were performed using SPSS 22.0 for Windows (StatSoft, USA).

Results

Variable expression of *Rbp4* in mouse ovaries during the different stages of development and the estrous cycle

We first performed experiments to investigate the expression pattern of *Rbp4* in whole mouse ovaries during different developmental stages. *Rbp4* mRNA expression in mouse ovaries remained constant at 1 to 3 weeks postnatally and notably increased at 4 weeks (i.e., peripubertally),

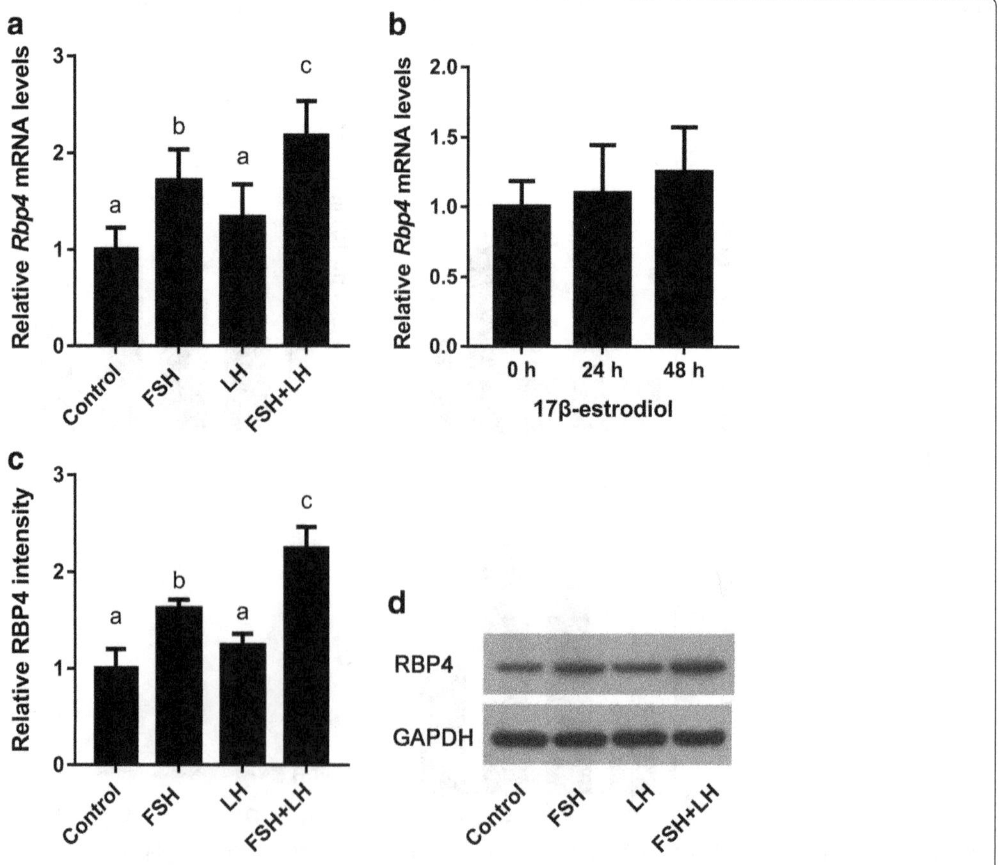

Fig. 2 Effects of gonadotropins and ovarian steroids on the expression of *Rbp4* in the 3-week-old mouse ovary. (A) *Rbp4* mRNA expression levels in the ovaries of mice treated with FSH, LH, or FSH + LH for 48 h. Data are presented as means ± SEM, n = 8. (B) *Rbp4* mRNA expression levels in the ovaries of mice treated with 17β-estradiol for 24 or 48 h. Data are presented as mean ± SEM, n = 8. RBP4 protein levels in the ovaries of mice treated with FSH or LH were determined using Western blot analyses (D), and blots were quantified via densitometry (C). The protein levels were normalized to GAPDH. Data are presented as means ± SEM, $n = 3$. Means with different letters represent a significant difference at the 0.05 level

and dropped at 5 weeks (Fig. 1A). We also investigated the expression patterns of *Rbp4* in whole mouse ovaries during the estrous cycle. The expression of *Rbp4* mRNA in the ovaries of adult mice (8 weeks old) having normal cycles increased at estrus (Fig. 1B), and the levels of RBP4 protein in the ovaries of normally cycling adult mice increased at proestrus and peaked at estrus (Fig. 1C and D). These data imply a potential relationship between *Rbp4* expression and follicular growth [8].

Effects of gonadotropins and ovarian steroids on *Rbp4* expression in mouse ovaries

Follicular growth is mainly controlled by gonadotropins and estrogen. Therefore, we determined the effects of these hormones on *Rbp4* expression in mouse ovaries. First, immature mice (3 weeks old) were treated with FSH, LH, or FSH + LH. The results showed that the expression levels of *Rbp4* in whole ovarian samples increased significantly after treatment with FSH (Fig. 2A) or FSH + LH (Fig. 2A), but not with LH alone (Fig. 2A), and the induction with combined FSH + LH was greater than that with FSH alone (Fig. 2A). The levels of RBP4 protein in the ovaries of mice treated with FSH and/or LH in proportion to the mRNA levels (Fig. 2C and D). 17β-Estradiol showed no evident effect on ovarian *Rbp4* expression (Fig. 2B). Thus, *Rbp4* expression in mouse ovaries appeared to be predominantly regulated by FSH.

Localization of RBP4 protein in mouse ovary

The localization of RBP4 protein in mouse ovaries was analyzed using immunohistochemical staining with specific antibody (Fig. 3). Positive signals for RBP4 were detected in the layers of granulosa and theca cells, and marked staining was also observed in the follicular antrum of large antral follicles in the ovaries of mice treated with FSH for 48 h (Fig. 3).

FSH stimulates the expression of *Rbp4* in mouse granulosa cells

Granulosa cells are one of the two most important types of gonadotropin-sensitive somatic cells in the mammalian ovary. We examined the effect of FSH and FSH + LH on the expression of *Rbp4* using an in vitro culture model of granulosa cells, and our results showed that the expression of *Rbp4* was induced by both FSH and FSH + LH treatments, and that the induction by combined FSH + LH treatment was greater than that by FSH alone (Fig. 4A, B and C).

cAMP-PKA pathway mediates FSH-induced *Rbp4* expression

As previously reported, FSH and LH perform their actions by activating their membrane receptors, the FSH receptor (FSHR) and the LH receptor (LHR), both of which belong to the G-protein coupled receptors [13, 14]. Stimulation of these receptors results in an increase in intracellular cAMP [13, 14], which promotes the rapid activation of

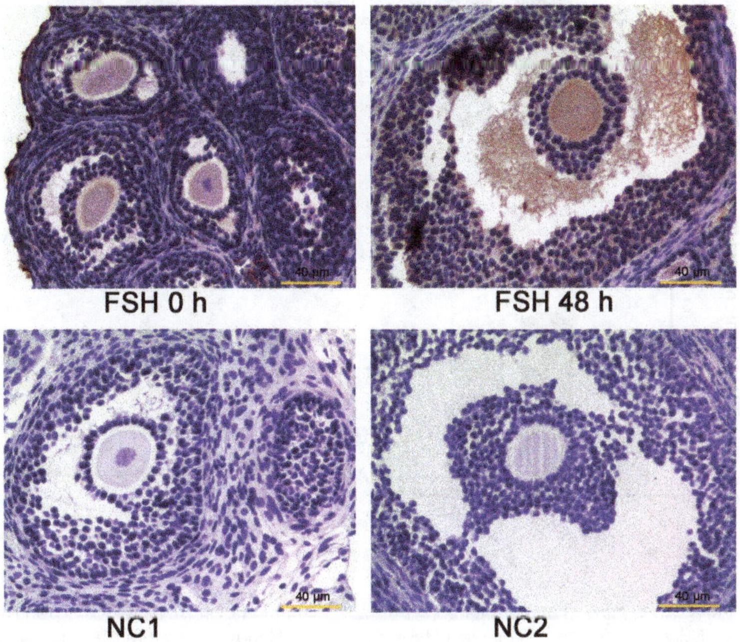

Fig. 3 Localization of RBP4 protein in the ovaries of the immature mice (3 weeks of age) treated with or without FSH for 48 h. Negative controls (NC), which were incubated with 5% goat serum (NC1) or PBS (NC2) instead of the primary antibody, were used to validate the specificity of RBP4 antibody. Positive signals for RBP4 were detected in granulosa and theca cell layers. Bar = 40 μm

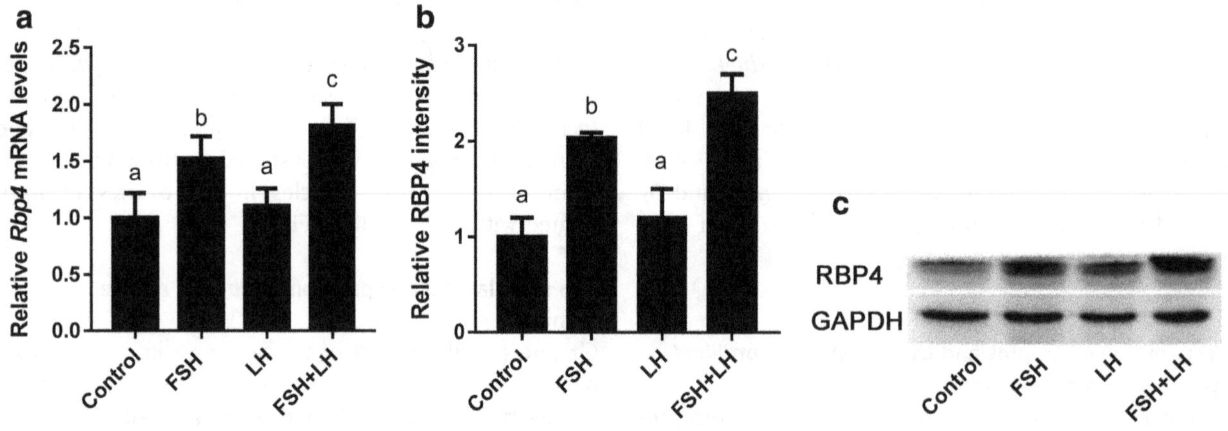

Fig. 4 Effects of gonadotropins on the expression of *Rbp4* in mouse granulosa cells. (A) Relative *Rbp4* mRNA levels in mouse granulosa cells treated with FSH and LH for 24 h. Data are presented as means ± SEM, *n* = 4. RBP4 protein levels in mouse granulosa cells treated with FSH and LH for 24 h were determined using Western blot analyses (C), and blots were quantified via densitometry (B). The protein levels were normalized to GAPDH. Data are presented as means ± SEM, *n* = 3. Means with different letters represent a significant difference at the 0.05 level

protein kinase A (PKA) [33]. To determine whether the cAMP-PKA pathway was involved in FSH-induced *Rbp4* expression in mouse granulosa cells, we first treated the cells in vitro with 500 μM 8-Br-cAMP (a cAMP agonist) or 10 μM H-89 (a PKA inhibitor). If the cAMP-PKA pathway was involved in FSH induction, 8-Br-cAMP would show similar induction effects and H-89 would prevent FSH induction. As expected, the treatment of mouse granulosa cells with 500 μM 8-Br-cAMP for 24 h resulted in a dramatic increase in *Rbp4* expression (Fig. 5A), and

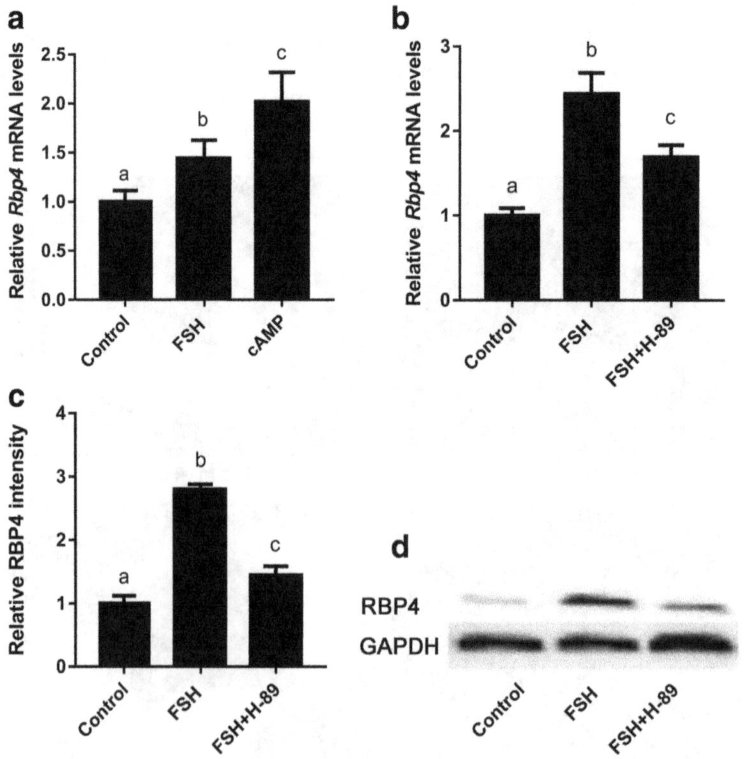

Fig. 5 PKA mediates the FSH induction of *Rbp4* in mouse granulosa cells. (A) Activation of PKA by cAMP and FSH increased *Rbp4* mRNA levels. Data are presented as means ± SEM, n = 4. (B) The PKA inhibitor H-89 abrogated FSH induced *Rbp4* mRNA expression. Granulosa cells were pre-incubated with 10 μM H-89 for 1 h, followed by incubation with 100 IU/L FSH for 24 h. Data are presented as means ± SEM, n = 4. (C) Densitometric quantification of Western blots for RBP4 (D). The protein levels were normalized to GAPDH. Data are presented as means ± SEM, n = 3. Means with different letters represent a significant difference at the 0.05 level

the induction of *Rbp4* by FSH was prevented with 10 μM H-89 (Fig. 5B, C and D). Thus, the cAMP-PKA pathway likely mediates FSH-induced *Rbp4* expression.

HMGA1, SF-1, and LRH-1 mediate FSH stimulation of *Rbp4*

HMGA1 can bind to the promoter of *Rbp4* and recruit SF-1 and LRH-1 to regulate the transcriptional activity of *Rbp4* [22]. The present study examined the effects of FSH on the expression of these transcription factors, and the results showed that FSH significantly stimulated the expression of these genes in granulosa cells. Moreover, the PKA inhibitor H-89 significantly inhibited FSH induction of these genes (Fig. 6A, B, and C). These data suggest that FSH stimulated the expressions of HMGA1, SF-1, and LRH-1 via PKA. To determine whether HMGA1, SFI, and LRH-1 mediated the FSH induction of *Rbp4*, we sought to knock down the corresponding genes using specific siRNAs. As expected, the expressions of these genes at the mRNA and protein levels were diminished to approximately 50% in cells transfected with 50 nM siRNA compared with controls (Fig. 7A, B, C, D, E, and F). After 24 h of transfection, the cells were treated with FSH for an additional 24 h. The cells were harvested and *Rbp4* mRNA and protein levels were examined. *Rbp4* expression was significantly reduced in cells transfected with *Hmga1* siRNA (Fig. 7G and H); while, knockdown of *Lrh-1* or *Sf-1* also prevented FSH induction of *Rbp4* (Fig. 7G, I, and J). Thus, the transcription factors HMGA1, SF-1, and LRH-1 are likely to be involved in the induction of *Rbp4* expression by FSH.

Discussion

Firstly, the present study presented the dynamic expression patterns for *Rbp4* in mouse ovaries during different stages of development and the estrous cycle. The expression of ovarian *Rbp4* remained constant at 1 to 3 weeks postnatally, notably increased at 4 weeks (i.e., peripubertally), and dropped at 5 weeks. Numerous studies have supported the concept that the gonadotropin-releasing hormone (GnRH) neuronal network generates pulse and surge modes of gonadotropin secretion that are critical for puberty [34], and stimulate the secretion of a mass of local ovarian factors and follicular growth in females. This modulation in *Rbp4* expression may be related to the pituitary gonadotropin wave at the onset of puberty. After puberty, some follicles in ovary start to grow and ovulate irregularly under the influence of serum gonadotropins, and at 5 weeks of age, some mice may be in the follicular-growth phase and some in the post ovulatory period. The different levels of gonadotrophins in these mice may constitute a possible explanation for the drop in *Rbp4* expression at 5 weeks. Furthermore, the expression of *Rbp4* in the ovaries of adult mice (8 weeks old) having normal cycles was found to increase at proestrus and peaked at estrus, the phase with higher serum levels

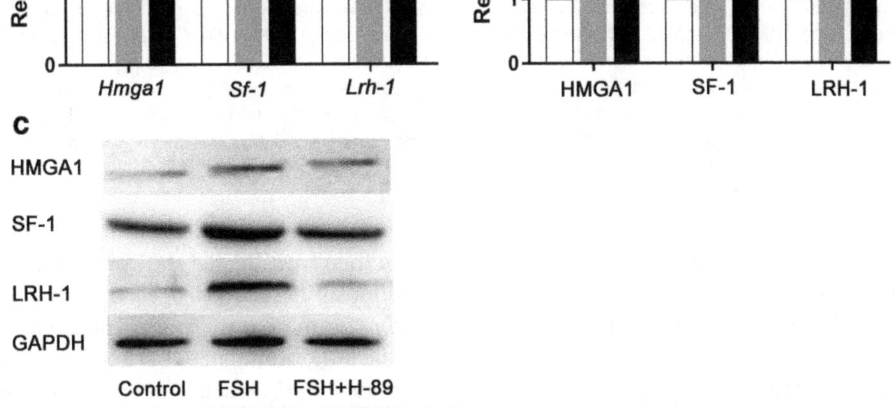

Fig. 6 FSH upregulates HMGA1, SF-1, and LRH-1 via PKA. (A) Relative mRNA levels of *Hmga1*, *Sf-1*, and *Lrh-1* in mouse granulosa cells incubated with FSH and H-89 for 24 h. Data are presented as means ± SEM, n = 4. SF-1 and LRH-1 protein levels were determined using Western blot analyses (C), and blots were quantified via densitometry (B). The protein levels were normalized to GAPDH. Data are presented as means ± SEM, n = 3. $^*p < 0.05$, $^{**}p < 0.01$

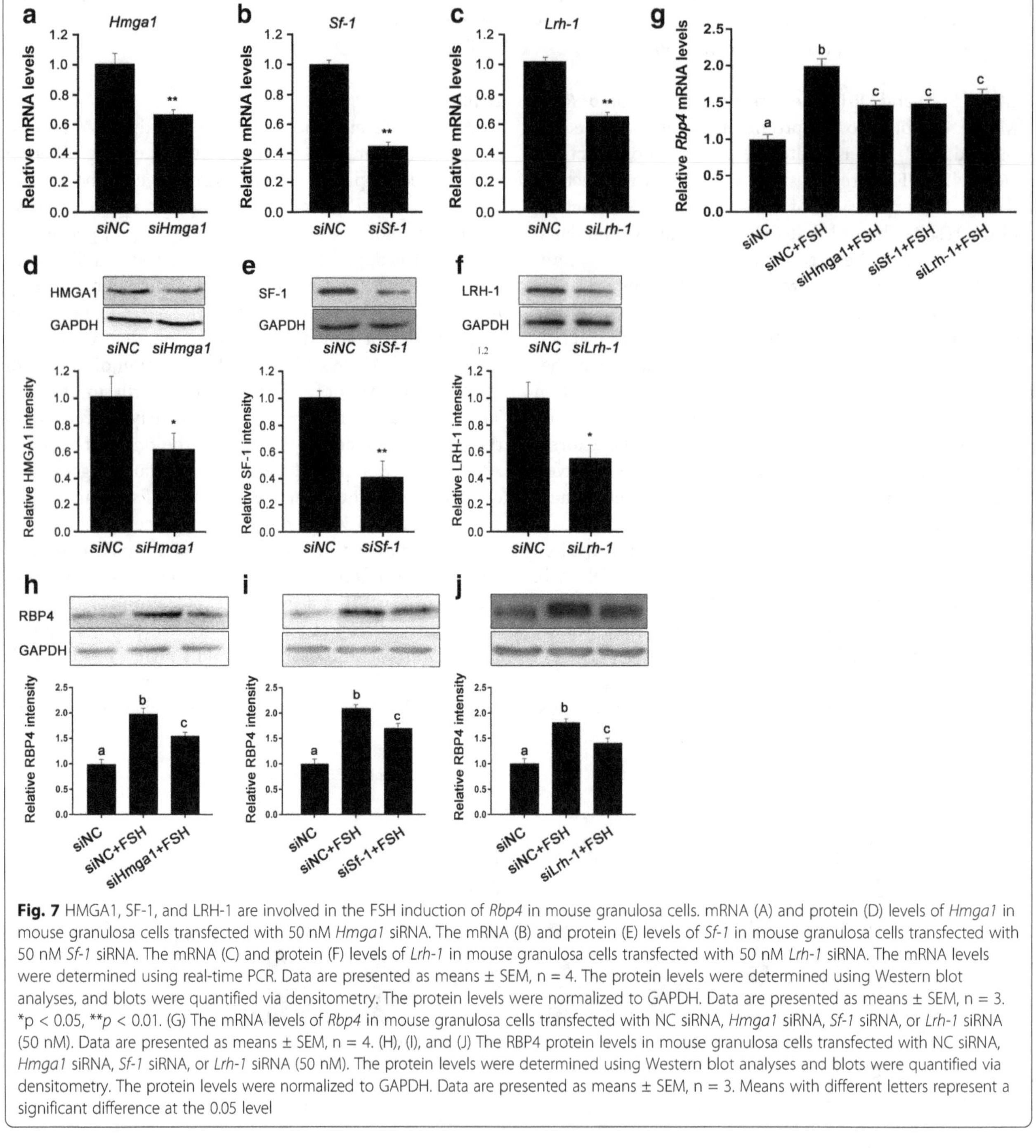

Fig. 7 HMGA1, SF-1, and LRH-1 are involved in the FSH induction of *Rbp4* in mouse granulosa cells. mRNA (A) and protein (D) levels of *Hmga1* in mouse granulosa cells transfected with 50 nM *Hmga1* siRNA. The mRNA (B) and protein (E) levels of *Sf-1* in mouse granulosa cells transfected with 50 nM *Sf-1* siRNA. The mRNA (C) and protein (F) levels of *Lrh-1* in mouse granulosa cells transfected with 50 nM *Lrh-1* siRNA. The mRNA levels were determined using real-time PCR. Data are presented as means ± SEM, n = 4. The protein levels were determined using Western blot analyses, and blots were quantified via densitometry. The protein levels were normalized to GAPDH. Data are presented as means ± SEM, n = 3. *$p < 0.05$, **$p < 0.01$. (G) The mRNA levels of *Rbp4* in mouse granulosa cells transfected with NC siRNA, *Hmga1* siRNA, *Sf-1* siRNA, or *Lrh-1* siRNA (50 nM). Data are presented as means ± SEM, n = 4. (H), (I), and (J) The RBP4 protein levels in mouse granulosa cells transfected with NC siRNA, *Hmga1* siRNA, *Sf-1* siRNA, or *Lrh-1* siRNA (50 nM). The protein levels were determined using Western blot analyses and blots were quantified via densitometry. The protein levels were normalized to GAPDH. Data are presented as means ± SEM, n = 3. Means with different letters represent a significant difference at the 0.05 level

of FSH and LH. In a previous study, higher RBP4 protein concentrations were observed in the follicular fluids of dominant follicles relative to small follicles [8, 9]. The dynamic expression patterns of *Rbp4* in mouse ovaries during different stages of development and the estrous cycle motivated us to pose an alternative hypothesis: that the expression of ovarian RBP4 is affected by gonadotropins and gonadal steroids and is related to follicular growth.

We then investigated the potential regulatory effects of gonadotropins and estrogen on the dynamic expression of *Rbp4* in the mouse ovary. The expression of *Rbp4* was significantly stimulated by administration of FSH and combined FSH + LH, but unaffected by administration of LH or 17β-estradiol. In addition, intense immunostaining was observed in granulosa cell layers of large antral follicles in the ovaries of mice treated with FSH. To determine whether the induction of *Rbp4* by FSH and FSH + LH occurred due to increased expression of *Rbp4* in granulosa cells, we examined primary granulosa cells cultured in vitro. Our results showed that the expression of *Rbp4* was induced by FSH and combined FSH + LH treatments, and that the induction by combined FSH + LH treatment was stronger than that by FSH alone. The administration of LH alone did not exert an effect. Because the primary granulosa cells were isolated from the immature female mouse (3 weeks old) ovaries without FSH or equine chorionic gonadotropin (eCG) pretreatment and with no or low LHR expression, the cells were mainly immature granulosa cells without LHR expression [35]. This may be the reason as to why LH alone manifested no obvious effects on granulosa cells and immature ovaries in the present study. However, LHR in granulosa cells can be induced by FSH [35], and during late maturation of granulosa cells in antral follicles, LH exerts a relatively more notable effect than FSH on cAMP formation [14, 36, 37], suggesting that LHR density was relatively greater than FSHR density or that LHR was more effectively coupled to cAMP generation. These findings may explain the stronger induction of *Rbp4* expression by FSH + LH than by FSH alone, and the higher levels of RBP4 in the follicular fluids of the large antral follicles [8].

To determine whether the induction of *Rbp4* by FSH was mediated by the cAMP-PKA pathway, we examined the effects of the cAMP analog 8-Br-cAMP and the PKA inhibitor H-89 on the induction of *Rbp4* in granulosa cells. The treatment of cells with 500 μM 8-Br-cAMP showed a dramatic increase in *Rbp4* expression, whereas 10 μM H-89 significantly prevented the induction of *Rbp4* by FSH. Thus, the cAMP-PKA pathway likely participates in the induction of *Rbp4* by FSH.

The cis-regulatory sequences of the mouse *Rbp4* gene contain a bipartite promoter, i.e., a proximal region necessary for basal expression and a distal segment that contains several binding sites for the structural HMGA1 proteins that are structural components of chromatin [22, 38]. HMGA1 binds to the adenine thymine (AT)-rich regions of DNA, changes the structure of DNA and recruit transcription factors to the promoter, and facilitates gene transcription [39]. There are several AT-rich motifs homologous to the binding sites of HMGA1 in the promoter region of mouse *Rbp4*, and HMGA1 proteins can bind upstream sequences of the *Rbp4* promoter. In the present study, *Hmga1* was sensitive to FSH and this response was prevented by the PKA inhibitor H-89; whereas the knockdown of *Hmga1* with siRNA resulted in a dramatic loss of FSH-induced *Rbp4* expression. In addition, HMGA1 can interact with SF-1 and LRH-1 and recruit them to the complex [22]. In the present study, the depletion of SF-1 and LRH-1 resulted in a dramatic loss of FSH-induced *Rbp4* expression. SF-1 was shown to be expressed at higher levels in theca cells, and also found in granulosa cells; whereas LRH-1 expression was found to be abundant and highly restricted to the granulosa cells of developing follicles [40, 41]. Consistent with our data, the two transcription factors were shown to be induced in granulosa cells by FSH/cAMP through the activation of PKA [40, 41], as cAMP signals are mediated largely via PKA [33] and can be elevated in granulosa cells by FSH [42, 43] or LH [44]. Thus, the expression of ovarian *Rbp4* was likely regulated by FSH via the cAMP-PKA pathway, involving HMGA1, SF-1, and LRH-1.

Conclusion

In conclusion, the present study showed a dynamic expression pattern of *Rbp4* in the mouse ovary during different stages of development and the estrous cycle, which was predominantly regulated by FSH. Furthermore, the cAMP-PKA pathway and transcription factors HMGA1, SF-1, and LRH-1 were likely involved in the induction of *Rbp4* by FSH (Fig. 8). This work expands

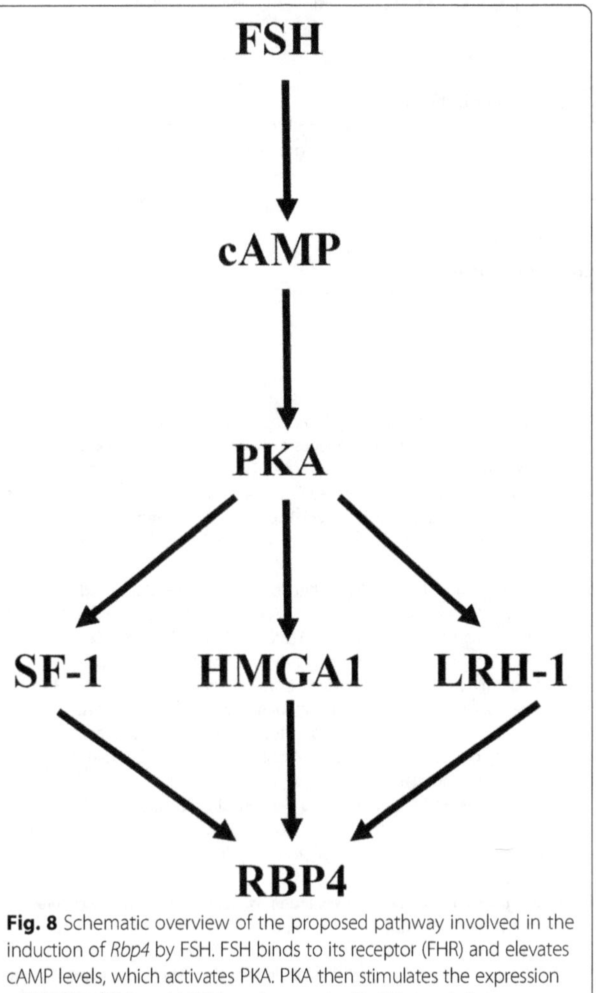

Fig. 8 Schematic overview of the proposed pathway involved in the induction of *Rbp4* by FSH. FSH binds to its receptor (FHR) and elevates cAMP levels, which activates PKA. PKA then stimulates the expression of HMGA1, SF-1, and LRH-1, and promotes *Rbp4* transcription

our understanding of the mechanisms underlying the regulation of *Rbp4* expression patterns in the ovary during different stages of development and the estrous cycle. Although further research needs to be conducted in this area, our data are important for the understanding of the molecular regulation of retinol transport and accumulation in the follicular fluids during ovarian follicular growth.

Abbreviations

8-Br-cAMP: 8-Bromoadenosine 3',5'-cyclic monophosphate; FSH: Follicle-stimulating hormone; GAPDH: Glyceraldehyde 3-phosphate dehydrogenase; HMGA1: High-mobility group AT-hook 1; LH: Luteinizing hormone; LRH-1: Liver receptor homolog 1; PKA: Protein kinase A; RBP4: Retinol-binding protein 4; SF-1: Steroidogenic factor 1

Acknowledgments

We would like to thank LetPub (www.letpub.com) for providing linguistic assistance during the preparation of this manuscript.

Funding

This work was supported by the National Natural Science Foundation of China (grants numbers 31372308, 31672417 and 31301969).

Authors' contributions

YJ, CL, and XZ conceived and designed the study; YJ performed the experiments; YJ and YZ analyzed the data; YJ, SC, and LC wrote the manuscript. All authors read and approved the final manuscript.

Competing interests

The authors declare that they have no competing interests.

References

1. Jiang YW, Li CJ, Chen L, Wang FG, Zhou X. Potential role of retinoids in ovarian physiology and pathogenesis of polycystic ovary syndrome. Clin Chim Acta. 2017;469:87–93.
2. Kipp JL, Golebiowski A, Rodriguez G, Demczuk M, Kilen SM, Mayo KE. Gene expression profiling reveals Cyp26b1 to be an activin regulated gene involved in ovarian granulosa cell proliferation. Endocrinology. 2011;152: 303–12.
3. Kawai T, Yanaka N, Richards JS, Shimada M. De novo-synthesized retinoic acid in ovarian antral follicles enhances FSH-mediated ovarian follicular cell differentiation and female fertility. Endocrinology. 2016;157:2160–72.
4. Ikeda S, Kitagawa M, Imai H, Yamada M. The roles of vitamin a for cytoplasmic maturation of bovine oocytes. J Reprod Dev. 2005;51:23–35.
5. Tahaei LS, Eimani H, Yazdi PE, Ebrahimi B, Fathi R. Effects of retinoic acid on maturation of immature mouse oocytes in the presence and absence of a granulosa cell co-culture system. J Assist Reprod Genet. 2011;28:553–8.
6. Wickenheisser JK, Nelson-DeGrave VL, Hendricks KL, Legro RS, Strauss JF, McAllister JM. Retinoids and retinol differentially regulate steroid biosynthesis in ovarian theca cells isolated from normal cycling women and women with polycystic ovary syndrome. J Clin Endocrinol Metab. 2005;90: 4858–65.
7. Haliloglu S, Baspinar N, Serpek B, Erdem H, Bulut Z. Vitamin a and beta-carotene levels in plasma, corpus luteum and follicular fluid of cyclic and pregnant cattle. Reprod Domest Anim. 2002;37:96–9.
8. Brown JA, Eberhardt DM, Schrick FN, Roberts MP, Godkin JD. Expression of retinol-binding protein and cellular retinol-binding protein in the bovine ovary. Mol Reprod Dev. 2003;64:261–9.
9. Schweigert FJ, Zucker H. Concentrations of vitamin a, beta-carotene and vitamin E in individual bovine follicles of different quality. J Reprod Fertil. 1988;82:575–9.
10. Kawaguchi R, Zhong M, Kassai M, Ter-Stepanian M, Sun H. Vitamin a transport mechanism of the Multitransmembrane cell-surface receptor STRA6. Membranes (Basel). 2015;5:425–53.
11. Jia J, Bai J, Liu Y, Yin JN, Yang P, Yu SQ, et al. Association between retinol-binding protein 4 and polycystic ovary syndrome: a meta-analysis. Endocr J. 2014;61:995–1002.
12. Sun YL, Ping ZG, Li CJ, Sun YF, Yi KL, Chen L, et al. Comparative proteomic analysis of follicular fluids from normal and cystic follicles in sows. Reprod Domest Anim. 2011;46:889–95.
13. Richards JS. Hormonal control of gene expression in the ovary. Endocr Rev. 1994;15:725–51.
14. Richards JS, Russell DL, Robker RL, Dajee M, Alliston TN. Molecular mechanisms of ovulation and luteinization. Mol Cell Endocrinol. 1998;145: 47–54.
15. McLean AC, Valenzuela N, Fai S, Bennett SA. Performing vaginal lavage, crystal violet staining, and vaginal cytological evaluation for mouse estrous cycle staging identification. J Vis Exp. 2012;67:e4389.
16. Cora MC, Kooistra L, Travlos G. Vaginal cytology of the laboratory rat and mouse: review and criteria for the staging of the estrous cycle using stained vaginal smears. Toxicol Pathol. 2015;43:776–93.
17. Parkening TA, Collins TJ, Smith ER. Plasma and pituitary concentrations of LH, FSH, and prolactin in aging C57BL/6 mice at various times of the estrous cycle. Neurobiol Aging. 1982;3:31–5.
18. Kumar TR, Wang Y, Lu N, Matzuk MM. Follicle stimulating hormone is required for ovarian follicle maturation but not male fertility. Nat Genet. 1997;15:201.
19. Montgomery V, Loutradis D, Tulchinsky D, Kiessling A. FSH-induced ovulation in intact and hypophysectomized mice. J Reprod Fertil. 1988;84:1–6.
20. McCracken JA, Custer EE, Lamsa JC. Luteolysis: a neuroendocrine-mediated event. Physiol Rev. 1999;79:263–323.
21. Stocco C, Telleria C, Gibori G. The molecular control of corpus luteum formation, function, and regression. Endocr Rev. 2007;28:117–49.
22. Bianconcini A, Lupo A, Capone S, Quadro L, Monti M, Zurlo D, et al. Transcriptional activity of the murine retinol-binding protein gene is regulated by a multiprotein complex containing HMGA1, p54(nrb)/NonO, protein-associated splicing factor (PSF) and steroidogenic factor 1 (SF1)/liver receptor homologue 1 (LRH-1). Int J Biochem Cell Biol. 2009;41:2189–203.
23. Wang C, Dehghani B, Li YX, Kaler LJ, Proctor T, Vandenbark AA, et al. Membrane estrogen receptor regulates experimental autoimmune encephalomyelitis through up-regulation of programmed death 1. J Immunol. 2009;182:3294–303.
24. Byers SL, Wiles MV, Dunn SL, Taft RA. Mouse estrous cycle identification tool and images. PLoS One. 2012;7:e35538.
25. Caligioni CS. Assessing reproductive status/stages in mice. Curr Protoc Neurosci. 2009; Appendix 4:Appendix 4I
26. Mankhey RW, Bhatti F, Maric C. 17beta-estradiol replacement improves renal function and pathology associated with diabetic nephropathy. Am J Physiol Renal Physiol. 2005;288:F399–405.
27. Chen H, Guan R, Lei Y, Chen J, Ge Q, Zhang X, et al. Lymphangiogenesis in gastric cancer regulated through Akt/mTOR-VEGF-C/VEGF-D axis. BMC Cancer. 2015;15:103.
28. Mhawech-Fauceglia P, Wang D, Samrao D, Godoy H, Pejovic T, Liu S, et al. Pair-box (PAX8) protein-positive expression is associated with poor disease outcome in women with endometrial cancer. Br J Cancer. 2012;107:370–4.
29. Di Somma S, Marotta M, Salvatore G, Cudemo G, Cuda G, De Vivo F, et al. Changes in myocardial cytoskeletal intermediate filaments and myocyte contractile dysfunction in dilated cardiomyopathy: an in vivo study in humans. Heart. 2000;84:659–67.
30. Ronkainen H, Soini Y, Vaarala MH, Kauppila S, Hirvikoski P. Evaluation of neuroendocrine markers in renal cell carcinoma. Diagn Pathol. 2010;5:28.
31. Liang N, Xu YL, Yin YM, Yao GD, Tian H, Wang GS, et al. Steroidogenic Factor-1 is required for TGF-beta 3-mediated 17 beta-estradiol synthesis in mouse ovarian granulosa cells. Endocrinology. 2011;152:3213–25.
32. Yao GD, Yin MM, Lian J, Tian H, Liu L, Li X, et al. MicroRNA-224 is involved in transforming growth factor-beta-mediated mouse granulosa cell proliferation and granulosa cell function by targeting Smad4. Mol Endocrinol. 2010;24:540–51.

33. Hunzicker-Dunn M, Maizels ET. FSH signaling pathways in immature granulosa cells that regulate target gene expression: branching out from protein kinase a. Cell Signal. 2006;18:1351–9.
34. Herbison AE. Control of puberty onset and fertility by gonadotropin-releasing hormone neurons. Nat Rev Endocrinol. 2016;12:452–66.
35. Camp TA, Rahal JO, Mayo KE. Cellular localization and hormonal regulation of follicle-stimulating hormone and luteinizing hormone receptor messenger RNAs in the rat ovary. Mol Endocrinol. 1991;5:1405–17.
36. Yong EL, Baird DT, Hillier SG. Mediation of gonadotrophin-stimulated growth and differentiation of human granulosa cells by adenosine-3′,5′-monophosphate: one molecule, two messages. Clin Endocrinol. 1992;37:51–8.
37. Yong EL, Baird DT, Yates R, Reichert LE Jr, Hillier SG. Hormonal regulation of the growth and steroidogenic function of human granulosa cells. J Clin Endocrinol Metab. 1992;74:842–9.
38. Jessen KA, Satre MA. Induction of mouse retinol binding protein gene expression by cyclic AMP in Hepa 1-6 cells. Arch Biochem Biophys. 1998; 357:126–30.
39. Bustin M, Reeves R. High-mobility-group chromosomal proteins: architectural components that facilitate chromatin function. Prog Nucleic Acid Res Mol Biol. 1996;54:35–100.
40. Falender AE, Lanz R, Malenfant D, Belanger L, Richards JS. Differential expression of steroidogenic factor-1 and FTF/LRH-1 in the rodent ovary. Endocrinology. 2003;144:3598–610.
41. Hinshelwood MM, Repa JJ, Shelton JM, Richardson JA, Mangelsdorf DJ, Mendelson CR. Expression of LRH-1 and SF-1 in the mouse ovary: localization in different cell types correlates with differing function. Mol Cell Endocrinol. 2003;207:39–45.
42. Mukherjee A, Park-Sarge OK, Mayo KE. Gonadotropins induce rapid phosphorylation of the 3′,5′-cyclic adenosine monophosphate response element binding protein in ovarian granulosa cells. Endocrinology. 1996;137: 3234–45.
43. Salvador LM, Park Y, Cottom J, Maizels ET, Jones JC, Schillace RV, et al. Follicle-stimulating hormone stimulates protein kinase A-mediated histone H3 phosphorylation and acetylation leading to select gene activation in ovarian granulosa cells. J Biol Chem. 2001;276:40146–55.
44. Wang YK, Hao XQ, Yang J, Li J, Zhang MJ. CREB activity is required for luteinizing hormone-induced the expression of EGF-like factors. Mol Reprod Dev. 2016;83:1116–27.

5

Parental genetic material and oxygen concentration affect hatch dynamics of mouse embryo in vitro

Shaoquan Zhan[1†], Shanbo Cao[1,2†], Hongzi Du[1], Yuan Sun[1], Li Li[1], Chenhui Ding[3], Haiyan Zheng[1*] and Junjiu Huang[1,3*]

Abstract

Background: Hatching is crucial for mammalian embryo implantation, since difficulties during this process can lead to implantation failure, ectopic pregnancy and consequent infertility. Despite years of intensive researches, how internal and external factors affecting embryo hatch are still largely unclear.

Methods: The effects of parental genetic material and oxygen concentration on hatch process were examined. Fertilized and parthenogenetic mouse preimplantation embryos were cultured in vitro under 5 and 20% oxygen for 120 h. Zona pellucida drilling by Peizo micromanipulation were performed to resemble the breach by sperm penetration.

Results: Firstly, parthenogenetic embryos had similarly high blastocyst developmental efficiency as fertilized embryos, but significantly higher hatch ratio than fertilized embryos in both O_2 concentrations. 5% O_2 reduced the hatch rate of fertilized embryos from 58.2 to 23.8%, but increased that of parthenogenetic embryos from 81.2 to 90.8% significantly. Analogously, 5% O_2 decreased the ratio of *Oct4*-positive cells in fertilized blastocysts, whereas increased that in parthenogenetic blastocysts. Additionally, 5% O_2 increased the total embryonic cell number in both fertilized and parthegenetic embryos, when compared to 20% O_2, and the total cell number of fertilized embryos was also higher than that of parthegenetic embryos, despite O_2 concentration. Real-time PCR revealed that the expression of key genes involving in MAPK pathway and superoxide dismutase family might contribute to preimplantation development and consequent blastocyst hatch in vitro. Finally, we showed that fertilized and parthenogenetic embryos have diverse hatch dynamics in vitro, although the zona pellucida integrity is not the main reason for their mechanistic differences.

Conclusion: Both parental genetic material and O_2 concentration, as the representative of intrinsic and extrinsic factors respectively, have significant impacts on mouse preimplantation development and subsequent hatch dynamics, probably by regulating the gene expression involving in MAPK pathway and superoxide dismutase family to control embryonic cell proliferation and allocation of ICM cells.

Keywords: Hatch, Fertilized embryo, Parthenogenetic embryo, Oxygen, Zona pellucida

* Correspondence: ceozhy_1985@126.com; hjunjiu@mail.sysu.edu.cn
†Equal contributors
[1]Center for Reproductive Medicine, Key Laboratory for Reproductive Medicine of Guangdong Province, Key Laboratory for Major Obstetric Diseases of Guangdong Province, and Key Laboratory for Reproduction and Genetics of Guangdong Higher Education Institutes, the Third Affiliated Hospital of Guangzhou Medical University, Guangzhou 510150, China
Full list of author information is available at the end of the article

Background

Hatching is a process essential for mammalian embryo implantation, in which the embryo at blastocyst stage escapes from its zona pellucida (ZP), an outer shell which is composed of glycoproteins and is responsible for the preventation of polyspermy and ectopic pregnancy [1–3]. The mechanism regulating the preimplantation embryos when and where to hatch is very critical for implanting in uterus exactly and successfully, since difficulties during this process can lead to implantation failure, ectopic pregnancy and consequent infertility [4, 5].

Many factors have been proved to function in embryo implantation in the past few decades, including embryonic cell number, trypsin-like proteinases, progranulin, prostanoid pathways, uterine function and the leukaemia inhibitory factor, zygote genomic expression and epigenetic changes, such as DNA methylation and histone deacetylation [6–14]. However, none of them has been identified as the determinant factor for embryo hatching. Additionally, the external culture environment is regarded as a key factor for preimplantation embryo growth in vitro, one of which is the oxygen (O_2) concentration [15]. O_2 plays an important role in the regulation of embryonic gene expression, allocation of cells to inner cell mass (ICM) and trophectoderm (TE) lineages and subsequent fetal development [16, 17]. Recent studies have showed that low O_2 (5%) can promote embroyonic cell proliferation and reduce apoptosis, whereas it inhibit trophoblast cell invasion [17–25]. Conversely, other studies argued that there are no beneficial effects of 5% O_2 culture on embryo subsequent development, such as implantation rate, pregnancy rate and fetal weight, when compared with atmospheric O_2 culture [19, 26, 27]. It is also still controversial whether low O_2 concentrations can be adopted as the standard for human embryo culture, at least for blastocyst formation. Thus, one of aims in our current study is to find out the relationship between O_2 concentration and embryo hatching ability in vitro.

Furthermore, many oxygen-regulated genes have been proved to function in embryonic development and metabolish [9, 28], whereas it remains poorly understood whether there are any oxygen-regulated imprinted genes, connecting with the process of blastocyst hatch. Parthenogenetic embryos produced in vitro enable us to study the effect of maternally expressed genes in preimplantation embryos, since it is still unknown how parental genetic background influence embryo hatching [29, 30].

Besides that, sperm's penetration through the ZP during fertilization, triggers the exocytosis of cortical granules in oocytes and biochemically alters the structure of ZP, thus making it impermeable to additional sperm, to prevent polyspermy [31–34]. So the integrity of ZP structure in normally in vivo fertilized embryos, is distinctly different from that in parthenogenetic embryos activated by chemicals in vitro, which is intact and completely hermetical. This provides us a powerful tool to study the effects of physical structural changes of ZP on embryo hatching process.

Therefore, this study aims to determine the effects of oxygen concentrations, parental genetic material, and integrity of ZP structure on blastocyst hatch, and tries to find out the molecular mechanisms regulating the blastocyst hatch, by utilizing fertilizated and parthenogenetic mouse embryos collected and cultured in vitro.

Methods

Unless otherwise specified, all reagents were obtained from Sigma Chemical Co. (St. Louis, MO).

Animal care and ethics statement

B6C3F1 mice were maintained in an environmentally controlled room at 22 ± 1 °C, under a light cycle of 14 h light/10 h dark, with free access to food and water in animal facility of specific pathogen-free (SPF) in Sun Yat-sen University. All experimental protocols involving the handling of mice were approved by the Institutional Animal Care and Use Committee of Sun Yat-sen University (Approval No. IACUC-2014-0102), People's Republic of China.

Collection of mouse oocytes and zygotes

Collection and culture of zygotes were performed as previously described [35–37]. B6C3F1 female mice aged at 5–8 weeks (weighed 16–19 g) were superovulated with 5 IU pregnant mare serum gonadotropin by intraperitoneal injection (PMSG, Calbiochem, La Jolla, CA), followed by 5 IU human chorionic gonadotrophin (hCG) 46–48 h later. Female mice were mated individually with B6C3F1 males of proven fertility, and successfully mated females indicated by a vaginal plug in the next morning, were used for collecting zygotes (day 0.5) at 20–21 h after hCG injection. Oocytes enclosed in cumulus masses were collected from oviduct ampullae 14 h after hCG injection. Cumulus cells were removed by pipetting after brief incubation in 0.03% hyaluronidase prepared in potassium simplex optimized medium (KSOM) containing 14 mM Hepes and 4 mM sodium bicarbonate (HKSOM). After removal of cumulus cells, zygotes and oocytes were then washed and incubated in 50 μL droplets of pre-equilibrated KSOM supplemented with non-essential and essential amino acids and 2.5 mM hepes ($KSOM_{AA}$) and then covered with mineral oil pending further treatments. Zygotes and Oocytes culture and all subsequent embryonic culture experiments were carried out at 37 °C in a humidified atmosphere of 6.0% CO_2 in air. All manipulations in vitro were performed at 36–37 °C on heated stages or in incubators. Embryos normally cleaved to two-cells at day 1–1.5, and formed morulae at day 2.5 (48 h in culture). Early blastocysts were formed at day 3.5 (72 h in culture), and late expanded blastocysts at day 4.5 (96 h in culture). Hatched blastocysts appeared at day5.5 (120 h in culture).

Parthenogenetic activation of oocytes

Freshly ovulated metaphase II oocytes were collected from the ampullae 14 h after hCG injection, and cumulus cells were removed as described above. Diploid parthenogenetic embryos were produced by activation of oocytes with $SrCl_2$ and cytochalasin D in 20% O_2, as described before [30].

Embryo culture in vitro

Both zygotes and parthenogenetic embryos were cultured in groups of 20–30 embryos per 50 μL droplet of $KSOM_{AA}$ overlaid with embryo-tested mineral oil. Embryos were cultured in humidified atmospheres (Thermo) with 5% or 20% O_2. Culture plates (35-mm petri dish; Corning Inc., Corning, NY) were prepared and equilibrated in the incubator 1 h before embryos collection. All control groups were made in the same day and the same treatment groups were cultured in the same dish with distinct makers. In all experiments, embryos were cultured for 5 days in vitro, and observed respectively at 24, 72, 96 and 120 h in vitro and graded for the stage of development including blastula formation and hatch.

Embryo hypotonicity

The embryos culured for 48 h were transferred into a 20 μL droplet of pure water under mineral oil in 35 mm Petri dish directly, and immediately observed under Zeiss inverted microscope for live image.

Zona pellucida drilling by Peizo micromanipulation

Ovulated metaphase II oocytes were collected at 14 h after hCG, and transferred into HKSOM microwell. A tiny breach (about 1 μm) on ZP was drilled with a pronuclear injection pipette or a 5 μm blunt-end pipette by Piezo micromanipulator.

Live image with embryo

Each 4 un-hatched blastocysts cultured for nearly 96 or 120 h in vitro were transferred into 2 μL HKSOM medium covered with mineral oil in a 35 mm coated glass bottom microwell dish (MatTek corporation). The dish was put on a heating plate controlled by a temperature controller (Medical systems corp. Model: TC-202A) to keep 37 °C. Zeiss inverted microscope and AxionVision LE software were used to make live image.

Immunofluorescence (IF) staining

Embryos were washed twice in phosphate buffered saline containing 0.1% polyvinyl pyrrolidone (PBS-PVP), then fixed in freshly prepared 3.7% paraformaldehyde in PBS-PVP (pH 7.4) for 15 min at 4 °C, permeablized in 0.1% Triton X-100 in blocking solution (3% goat serum in PBS-PVP) for 30 min, washed three times, and then left in blocking solution for 1 h. Embryos were incubated at 4 °C overnight with anti-*Oct4* mouse monoclonal antibody (sc5279, santa cruz) diluted 1:50 in blocking solution, washed, and then incubated for 1 h with secondary antibodies conjugated to Alexa Fluor 568 (Molecular Probes) diluted 1:100 in blocking solution. Embryos were washed, and mounted onto a slide under a coverslip in the Vectashield with 0.2 μg/mL Hoechst 33342 mounting medium. Alexa Fluor-labeled *Oct4* and Hoechst-labeled nuclei were observed with a Leica inverted fluorescence microscope.

Detection of apoptosis by TUNEL assay

Embryos were collected, washed three times in PBS-PVP, and fixed in 3.7% paraformaldehyde overnight at 4 °C. Nuclear DNA fragmentation was detected by the TUNEL method using the In Situ Cell Death Detection Kit (Fluorescein, Roche Applied Science) according to the manufacturer's instructions, and nuclei were counterstained with propidium iodide (PI, 50 μg/mL, Sigma). Fluorescence was detected using a Leica inverted fluorescence microscope.

Real-time PCR relative quantitation of gene expression

Thirty blastocysts from both fertilized and parthenogenetic groups cultured in 5% or 20% O_2 for 96 h in vitro were collected and used for mRNA extraction with RNeasy micro Kit (Qiagen, 74004). Total mRNA was subjected to cDNA synthesis using Reverse Transcription System (Toyobo). Primers for amplification of all the selected genes were designed using GeneTool Lite 1. 0 (BioTools) (see Additional file 1). Polymerase chain reaction (PCR) was performed with ABI Prism 7900 Sequence Detection System (Applied Biosystems) using SYBR Green Real-time PCR Master Mix (Toyobo, QPK-201). Gene expression levels were analyzed and normalized to housekeeping gene β-actin as the reference gene.

Statistical analysis

Percentages were transformed using arcsin transformation. Unless otherwise indicated, percentage transformed data, cell number, embryo hatch time and real-time PCR data were analyzed by one-way analysis of variance (ANOVA) and means were compared by Fisher's protected least-significant difference (PLSD) using the StatView software from SAS Institute Inc. (Cary, NC). Significant difference was defined as $P < 0.05$.

Results

Both the oxygen concentration and genetic material affect the blastocyst hatch process in vitro

To assess the effects of oxygen concentration and genetic material on embryo development and hatch process, we carried out four combinatorial treatments in a two-factor design by using the in vitro model of embryo culture, in which both fertilized zygotes from naturally mated female mice and parthenogenetic embryos from chemically activated MII oocytes were cultured for 120 h in 5 and 20% O_2 respectively.

No detectable differences were observed in the blastocyst rates (around 97%) and morphology, among these four groups cultured for 96 h (Table 1 and Fig. 1a). However, the hatch rates among these groups showed significant differences after culture for 120 h (Table 1 and Fig. 1b). About 58.2% of fertilized embryos in 20% O_2 hatched, which was notably higher than those in 5% O_2 (23.8%, Table 1 and Fig. 1b). Conversely, the percentage of hatched parthenogenetic blastocysts in 5% O_2 (90.8%) was significantly increased, compared with that in 20% O_2 (81.2%, Table 1 and Fig. 1b). These results demonstrate that the oxygen concentration does not affect the development of either fertilized or parthenogenetic embryos to blastocyst (day 3), but influences the blastocyst hatch following blastulation (days 5). Interestingly, 5% O_2 reduced the hatch ratio of fertilized embryos, but increased that in parthenogentic embryos, suggesting that there are distinct mechanistic differences between fertilized and parthenogentic embryos in regulating the effects of oxygen on blastocyst hatch. Moreover, the hatch ratio of parthenogenetic embryos was markedly higher than that of fertilized embryos, regardless of oxygen concentration (Table 1), implying a significant influence of parental genetic background on blastocyst hatch.

The allocation of ICM cells is affected diversely in fertilized and parthenogenetic blastocysts in vitro

To better understand the mechanism regulating embryo hatch, immunostaining for *Oct4* protein, a crucial marker for ICM and embryonic stem cells (ESCs), and TUNEL assay were performed to check the cell allocation, apoptosis, and total embryonic cell number in these blastocysts among groups after culture for 120 h. There were no overt differences for the number of *Oct4*-positive cells in either fertilized or parthegenetic groups, when embryos cultured in 20% O_2 was compared with those in 5% (Table 2 and Fig. 2a). Likewise, we found no any change for the number of apoptotic cells among groups, with less than two apoptotic cells observed in all groups of blastocysts by TUNEL assay (Table 2 and Fig. 2b). Congruently, when they were cultured for 96 h, that is, prior to hatching, embryos among groups had a comparable mRNA expression level of both *Oct4* and apoptosis-associated genes, *Bcl2* and *Bax*, confirmed by real-time PCR analysis (Fig. 2c).

However, the ratio of *Oct4*-positive cells in each embryo after culture for 120 h varied considerably among these groups, due to a marked difference in the total embryonic cell number (Table 2). When compared with 20% O_2, obviously, 5% O_2 decreased the ratio of *Oct4*-positive cells in fertilized blastocysts, whereas increased that in pharthenogenetic blastocysts. This result resembles the data on hatch ratio (Table 1), and thus suggests a possible regulatory role for the allocation of ICM cells in blastocyst hatch. Furthermore, we found that the total cell number of fertilized embryos was higher than that of parthegenetic embryos in both 5% and 20% O_2 (Table 2), and that 5% O_2 increased the total cell number in both fertilized and parthenogenetic embryos, comparing to 20% O_2 (Table 2). These data unambiguously illustrates the importance of both the parental genetic material and oxygen concentration on preimplantation development, and thus subsequent embryo hatch.

Oxygen concentration affects the gene expression in fertilized and parthenogenetic blastocysts before hatching

To find the key genes involved in the control of embryo hatch, several important genes involving in different cellular events were analyzed by real-time PCR, using fertilized and parthenogenetic blastocysts cultured in vitro for 96 h under 5% or 20% O_2. Firstly, the expression patterns of three common imprinted genes in these

Table 1 Development potential of fertilized and parthenogenetic embryos cultured in 5 and 20% oxygen in vitro

Groups	Oxygen concentration %	Replicates No.	Total embryos No.	96 h No. (%) Blastocysts+	120 h No. (%) Hatched Blastocysts
FE	20	7	324	312 (96.2 ± 1.4)	179 (58.2 ± 4.2)[a]
	5	7	350	337 (97.3 ± 1.1)	83 (23.8 ± 2.6)[b]
PA	20	9	346	336 (97.6 ± 0.8)	278 (81.2 ± 2.7)[c]
	5	9	346	335 (96.8 ± 1.0)	306 (90.8 ± 1.8)[d]

FE fertilized embryos, *PA* parthenogenetically activated embryos
+Mean ± SEM
[a] vs. [b], $p < 0.001$; [a] vs. [c], $p < 0.01$; [c] vs. [d], $p < 0.05$; [b] vs. [d], $p < 0.001$

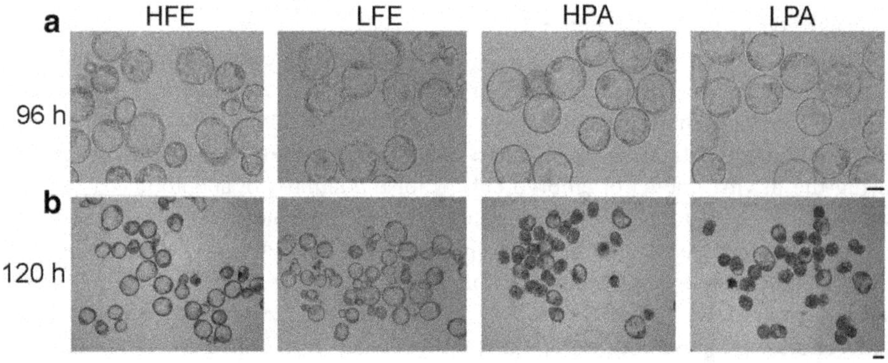

Fig. 1 Morphology and hatch process of embryos cultured in vitro. **a** Morphology of fertilized and parthenogenetic embryos cultured in vitro for 96 h in 20% or 5% O_2. Bar = 50 μm. **b** Morphology of fertilized and parthenogenetic embryos cultured in vitro for 120 h in 20% or 5% O_2. Bar = 50 μm. HFE and LFE, fertilized embryos cultured in 20% and 5% O_2 respectively; HPA and LPA, parthenogenetic embryos cultured in 20% and 5% O_2 respectively

four groups differed greatly as following: the expression of maternally-expressed *H19* was significantly increased but paternally-expressed Snrpn notablely reduced in both parthenogenetic embryo groups, when compared with fertilized embryo groups, and the expression of *Igf2r* was not changed among groups (Fig. 3a), indicating that their expressions are influenced only by the parental genetic background, rather than oxygen concentration. Secondly, the proteinase genes, *Pitrm1, Prnt3, Psmc4* and *Psmd11,* which were reported to function in regulating the hatch process [7, 38], demonstrated a similar expression level in all groups (Fig. 3b). Given that the mitogen-activated protein kinase (MAPK) signal pathway plays a key role in embryonic cell division [39], then, the expressions of three important regulating genes in this pathway were confirmed including *Erk1, Erk2* and *Gab1,* since we have found a significant change in the total cell number among groups (Table 2). As expected, the expression of all three genes in fertilized embryo groups were significantly increased in 5% O_2 group (Fig. 3c). Similarly, in parthenogenetic embryo groups, *Erk1* expression significantly rised and *Erk2* and *Gab1* slightly increased in 5% O_2 group (Fig. 3c). What's more, *Gab1* expression was significantly reduced in parthenogenetic embryos in both 5 and 20% O_2, when compared to paralleled fertilized embryos (Fig. 3c), showing a expression pattern similar to imprinted gene *Snrpn.* Finally, we checked the expression of *Sod1* and *Sod2,* two menbers from superoxide dismutases (SODs) family, which is the first and most important line of antioxidant enzyme defense systems against reactive oxygen species (ROS) and can thus help embryo developing well in vitro [40, 41]. While there was no difference found among all groups for *Sod2* expression, slightly higher expression level of *Sod1* was observed in parhtenogenetic embryos, when compared with fertilitzed embryos (Fig. 3d). There results clearly illuminate that oxygen concentration affects the gene expression in fertilized and parthenogenetic embryos, suggesting a potential role of MAPK in regulation of the preimplantation development and consequent blastocyst hatch in vitro.

Sperm-drilling breach is not the main reason for different hatch dynamics between fertilized and parthenogenetic embryos

To furthur elucidate how the embryo hatch was affected in both fertilized and parthenogenetic embryos, we monitored the embryo hatch process by living imaging and found that fertilized embryos spend about 42 h completing the hatch process, while parthenogenetic embryos spend only 6 h (see Additional files 2 and 3, Table 3). In detail, we found that fertilized embryos started hatching

Table 2 Cell allocation and apoptosis in fertilized and parthenogenetic embryo cultured in vitro for 120 h

Groups	No. embryos	120 h Blastocysts$^+$			No. embryos	120 h Blastocysts
		No. total cells	No. *Oct4* positive cells	*Oct4* positive cells/ Total cells (%)		No. apoptosis cells
HFE	37	116.0 ± 3.2^a	25.2 ± 1.2	21.7 ± 0.8^e	14	1.9 ± 0.6
LFE	39	129.4 ± 4.4^b	24.5 ± 1.2	18.8 ± 0.6^f	13	1.2 ± 0.6
HPA	49	105.7 ± 2.6^c	23.2 ± 1.0	21.9 ± 0.7^e	11	1.4 ± 0.4
LPA	60	112.6 ± 2.7^{acd}	27.6 ± 0.9	24.7 ± 0.6^g	12	1.3 ± 0.4

HFE and LFE fertilized embryos cultured in 20 and 5% oxygen, *HPA and LPA* parthenogentic embryos cultured in 20 and 5% oxygen
$^+$Mean ± SEM
^{a} vs. ^{b}, $p < 0.01$; ^{a} vs. ^{c}, $p < 0.05$; ^{b} vs. ^{c}, $p < 0.0001$; ^{b} vs. ^{d}, $p < 0.001$; ^{c} vs. ^{d}, $p < 0.05$; ^{e} vs. ^{f}, ^{g} $P < 0.01$; ^{f} vs. ^{g}, $P < 0.01$

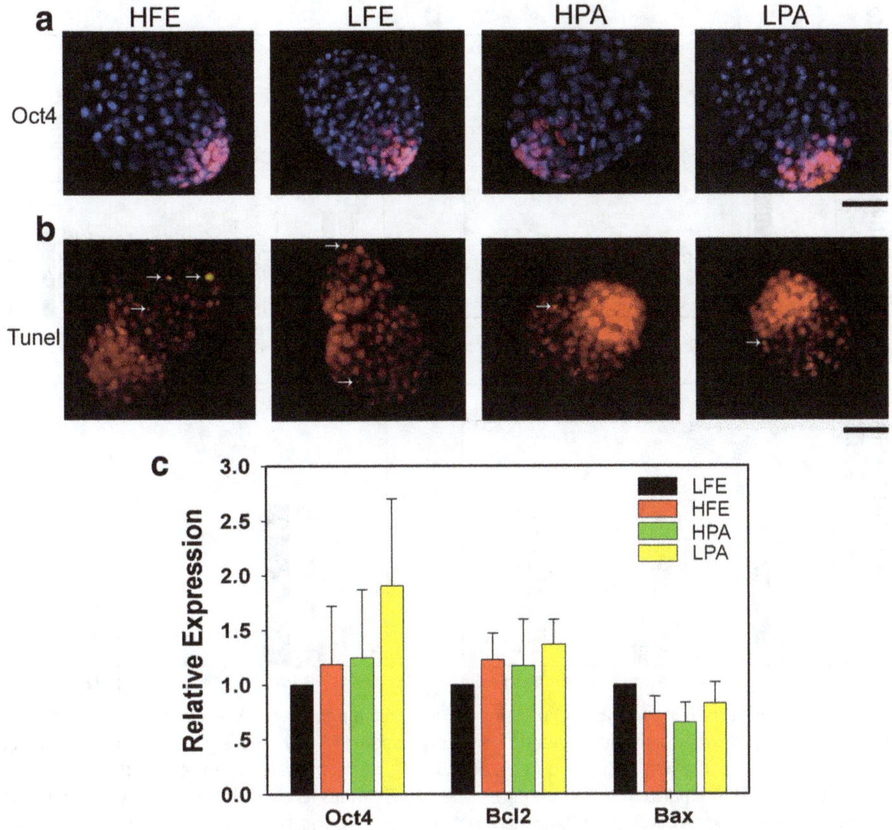

Fig. 2 Embryonic cell differentiation and apoptosis in blastocysts cultured in vitro. **a** Immunofluorescent images showing *Oct4*-positive cells in fertilized and parthenogenetic blastocysts cultured for 120 h in 5% or 20%, indicative of inner cell mass (pink), with nuclei stained with Hoechst (blue). Bar = 50 μm. **b** Representative merged images showing apoptotic cells (yellow, white arrows) in fertilized and parthenogenetic blastocysts cultured for 120 h in 5% or 20% by TUNEL assay, with nuclei stained with PI (red). Bar = 50 μm. **c** Quantification of *Oct4* and apoptotic genes, including *Bcl2* and *Bax*, in fertilized and parthenogenetic embryos cultured for 96 h. Relative mRNA expression levels are determined by real-time PCR and normalized to β-actin as internal reference, with the average value of LFE groups as control set to one and compared across groups. Data are presented as mean ± SEM. LFE and HFE, fertilized embryos cultured in 5% and 20% O_2 respectively; LPA and HPA, parthenogenetic embryos cultured in 5% and 20% O_2 respectively

at 72 h and about 43% completed hatching at 120 h in 20% O_2 (Fig. 4a and Table 3). Nevertheless, none of the 71% parthonegenetic embryos started to hatch until 120 h, without any signs observed at 72 or even at 96 h (Fig. 4a and Table 3), indicating a significant difference in the hatch dynamics between fertilized blastocysts and parthonegenetic blastocysts.

Since sperm penetration through the oocyte ZP makes the resultant fertilized embryos different from parthenogenetic embryos in the physical structure of ZP, we wondered whether this divergence could also lead to marked differences in hatch process. To answer this question, we performed the hypotonic experiment using embryos cultured for 48 h. Significantly, the cytoplasm permeated out through a breach on ZP from all fertilized embryos after transferred into pure water, while no cytoplasm leaked out in parthenogenetic embryos (Fig. 4b, Additional files 4 and 5), indicating that the breach generating from sperm's penetration may be the reason leading to two different hatched mechanisms.

In order to verify this possiblibity, a tiny breach (about 1 μm) was artificially made on the mature oocyte ZP using pronuclear injection method. After the oocytes were parthenogenetically activated and then cultured for 48 h, we found that no cytoplasm permeated out from the ZP-drilled parthenogenetic embryos in hypotonic experiment, and no hatching embryo was observed before 96 h, and 80% embryos (8/10, Table 3) hatched in 120 h, indicating the same hatch pattern as normal parthenogenetic embryos. One of the potential reasons for the above results is that the breach drilled by pronuclear injection pipette was much smaller than that generated by sperm penetration in fertilized embryo, which would block the cytoplasm outflowing in hypotonic experiment. Thus, a wider injection pipette (approximate 5 μm in blunt-end) was used to make a larger breach on

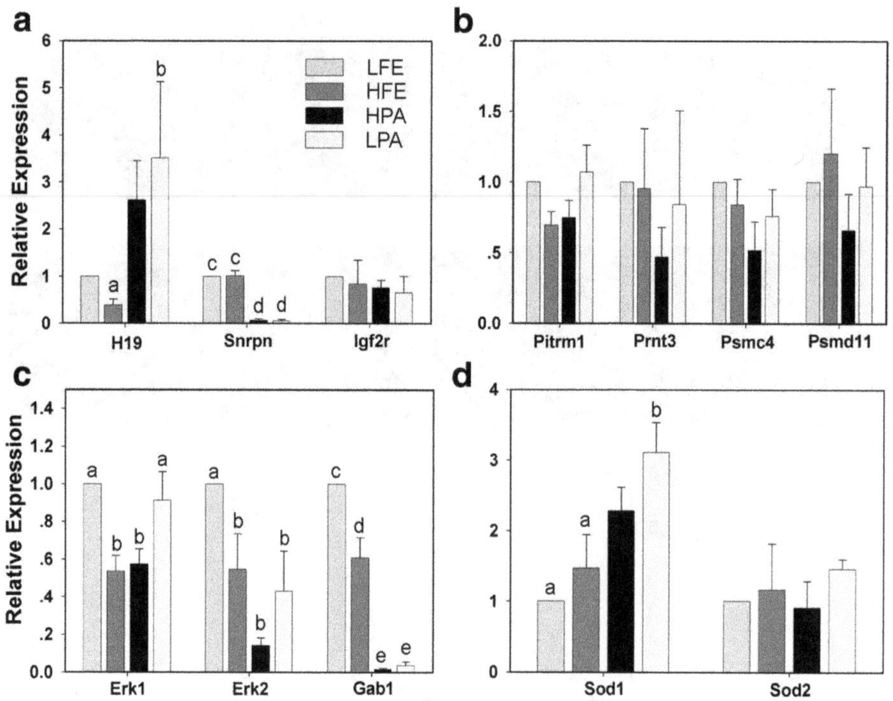

Fig. 3 Quantification of key genes expression in embryos cultured in vitro for 96 h. **a** Imprinted genes expression. **b** Proteinase genes expression. **c** MAPK signal pathway genes expression. **d** Superoxide dismutase genes expression. LFE and HFE, fertilized embryos cultured in 5% and 20% O_2 respectively; LPA and HPA, parthenogenetic embryos cultured in 5% and 20% O_2 respectively. Gene-expression data are determined by real-time PCR and normalized to the levels of β-actin mRNA, with the average value of LFE groups as controls set to one and compared across groups. Data are presented as mean ± SEM, with letters indicating differences between groups, a vs. b, $p < 0.05$; c vs. d, $p < 0.001$; c vs. e, $p < 0.0001$; d vs. e, $p < 0.0001$

oocyte ZP at similar size as sperm penetration in fertilized embryos. After hypotonic treatment at 48 h, the cytoplasm permeated out from ZP-drilled parthenogenetic embryos (Fig. 4b, Additional file 6). Furthermore, ZP-drilled parthenogenetic embryos started to hatch at 96 h, and 75% embryos (15/20) completed hatching in 120 h, which were similar to normal parthenogenetic embryos but significantly higher than fertilized embryos (Fig. 4a and Table 3). However, we found that the blastocysts did not come out from the aritificial breach on ZP, but kept expanding and then hatched out from another place of ZP suddenly and quickly, although some trophoderm cells had already came out through the sperm-like breach at 96 h (see Additional file 7). These results indicate that the sperm-like breach on ZP was not the main reason for the mechanistic difference of hatch between parthenogenetic and fertilized embryos.

Discussion

Uterus interacts with embryos and secretes lots of lytic factors to help embryo hatch and implant [42, 43]. Whereas, uterus is not the determinant issue for embryo hatch, since the embyos are able to hatch by themselves in vitro, through a way different from that developed in vivo [13, 44]. Assisted hatching (AH), an invasive technique aiming to facilitate embryo implantation by artificially manipulating zona pellucida in vitro, has been widely used, although its clinical efficacy remains controversial [4, 45–47]. Understanding molecular mechanisms involving in embryo hatching will enable the

Table 3 Hatched percentage and time of different types of embryo

Embryo types	Diameter of hole on ZP	No. embryos	96 h Blastocysts	120 h Hatched Blastocysts (%)	Total Hatched time (repeats)
FE	Sperm-size	23	23	10 (43)^a	41.7 ± 5.1^c (9)
PA	None	24	24	17 (71)^b	6.0 ± 1.8^d (10)
PA-ZPI	~ 1 μm	10	10	8 (80)^b	
PA-ZPI	~ 5 μm	20	20	15 (75)^b	

^{a} vs. ^{b}, $p < 0.05$; ^{c} vs. ^{d}, $p < 0.0001$

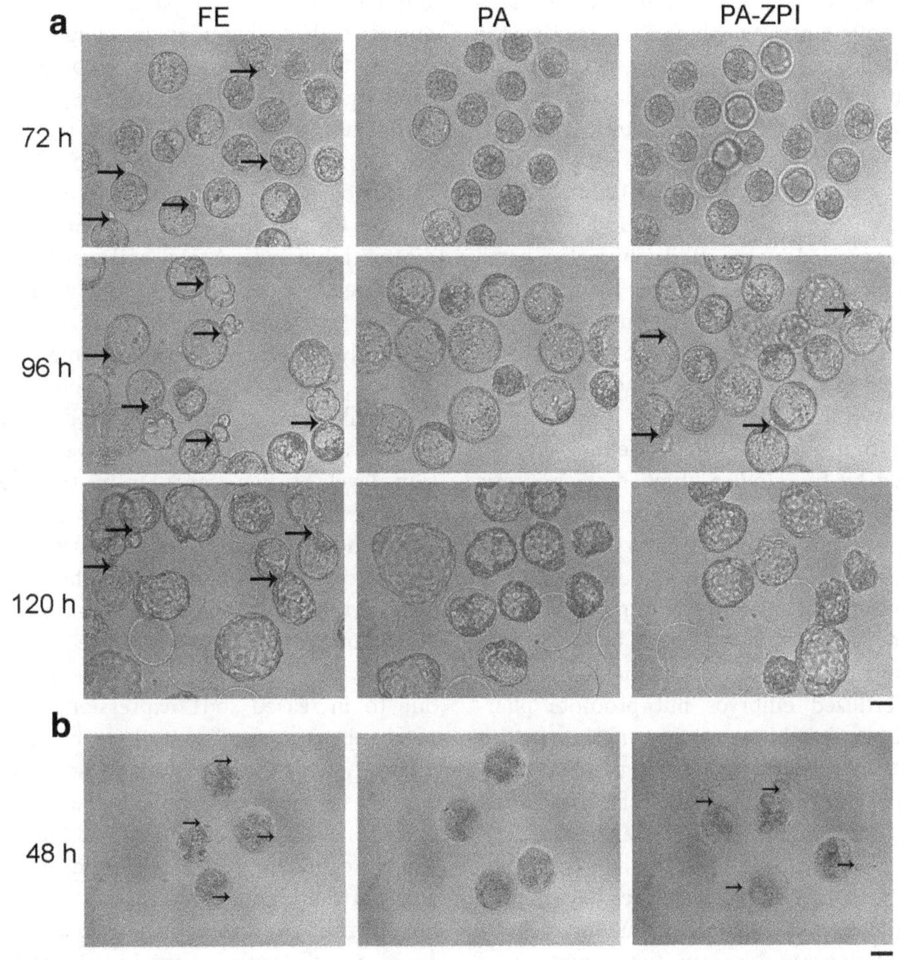

Fig. 4 Different hatch patterns between fertilized and parthenogenetic embryos cultured in vitro. **a** Morphology of fertilized, normal and ZP-drilled parthenogenetic embryos cultured in vitro for 72, 96 and 120 h. Thick and black arrows indicated the place where embryos began to hatch. **b** Hypotonicity treatments with embryos cultured for 48 h. Thin and black arrows indicated the place where cytoplasm permeated out. FE, fertilized embryos cultured in 20% O_2; PA, normal parthenogenetic embryos cultured in 20% O_2; PA-ZPI, parthenogenetic embryos with a breach about 5 μm on ZP, drilled by a way like pronuclear injection with Piezo micromanipulator and cultured in 20% O_2. Bar = 50 μm

development of new interventions for embryo implantation and thus improve the human reproductive outcomes. Here, our results indicate that the mechanism of mouse embryo hatch is regulated by both intrinsic and extrinsic factors in vitro.

Both oxygen concentration and parental genetic material affect preimplantation development and subsequent blastocyst hatching

Oxygen concentration is one of the most important extrinsic factors for embryo culture in vitro [15–17]. In our present study, we found that both fertilized and parthenogenetic embryos developed to blastocyst stage well in 5% and 20% O_2 at 96 h, which means that oxygen concentration does not affect embryo developmental morphology, as reported in bovine [17], mouse [19], and human [26, 27]. However, after culture for 120 h, that is, after blastocyst formation, we found that 5% O_2 increased the total cell number in both fertilized and parthenogenetic embryos, comparing to 20% O_2. This result is accordant with a previous conclusion that 5% O_2 is better for mouse embryo development [19, 22, 48, 49]. Moreover, in both 5% and 20% O_2, the total cell number of fertilized embryos was significantly higher than that of parthegenetic embryos. These data indicate that both oxygen concentration and parental genetic background can regulate embryonic cell proliferation after blastulation, and thus affect the subsequent hatch process in vitro.

As for the effects of oxygen concentration on hatch, we found that 5% O_2 reduced the hatch rate of fertilized embryos, which is consistent with Fischer's report that bovine fertilized embryos have notablely higher hatched rate cultured under 20% O_2 in KSOM medium [17]. On the contrary, we found that 5% O_2 increased the hatch rate in parthenogentic embryos, which suggests that the mechanism regulating the effects of oxygen concentration on hatch process in parthenogentic embryos is distinctly different from that in fertilized embryos. Moreover, the hatch ratio of blastocysts showed significant differences among groups after culture for 120 h, and implied a significant effect of maternal genetic background on embryo hatch, revealed by the markedly higher hatch ratio observed in parthenogenetic embryos than fertilized embryos, regardless of oxygen concentration.

We suppose that 5% O_2 increased the total embryonic cell number in both fertilized and parthenogenetic blastocysts, mainly by stimulating TE cells proliferation, since we did not find any difference in either embryo qualities, indicated by the similar number of apoptotic cells and camparable expression level of apoptosis related genes in all embryo groups, or embryonic cell differentiation, indicated by no changes for the expression level of pluripotent gene *Oct4* and the number of *Oct4*-positive cells that are considered as ICM cells [50]. Nevertheless, comparing with 20% O_2, the reason why 5% O_2 inhibit fertilized embryos but promote pharthenogenetic embryos hatching remains unclear. In this study, we amazedly found that 5% O_2 significantly decreased the ratio of *Oct4*-positive cells in fertilized blastocysts, whereas increased that in pharthenogenetic blastocysts. That is to say, both fertilized and parthenogenetic embryos with higher hatched rate, have higher ratio of *Oct4*-positive cells accordingly, thus indicating a potential close relationship between the allocation of ICM cells and subsequent blastocyst hatch. We speculate that embryos with higher ICM ratio likely secrete more factors, which may be benefiticial for embryo hatch [42, 43].

Taking into account that oxygen can regulate the expression of embryonic genes, and that low oxygen can affect the expression of oxygen-regulated genes in mouse and bovine embryos [9, 16, 28], we performed real-time PCR to analyze the expression levels of key genes that may be involved in the control of embryo hatch, by using fertilized and parthenogenetic blastocysts cultured in 5% and 20% O_2 for 96 h, when the mRNA transcript expression level would be changed at this stage, if any of these genes is functioned in regulating embryo hatch. Since we found that the expression level of three common imprinted genes including *H19*, *Snrpn*, and *Igfr2*, are influenced only by the parental genetic background, as previously reported [16], further studies are required to better characterize whether there are any aother imprinted genes involving in the blastocyst hatch process. Also, our results showed no changes for all the four proteinase genes including *Pitrm1*, *Prtn3* and *Psmd11* as well as *Psmc*, indicating that these proteinase genes might not be impacted by oxygen concentration during embryo hatching, although they were demonstrated to be important for embrygenesis and embryo hatching in previous studies [7, 38].

However, we found that 5% O_2 significantly indeed increased *Erk1* and *Erk2* expression in both fertilized and parthenogenetic embryos, which is one of the reasons why 5% O_2 can promote embryonic cell proliferation, indicated by increased total embryonic cell number, when compared with 20% O_2. Simultaneously, the expression level of *Gab1*, another gene in MAPK pathway, was significantly increased in fertilized embryos in both 5% and 20% O_2, which accounts for their significantly higher total cell number, when compared to paralleled parthegenetic embryos. Furthermore, we analyzed the expression level of two genes from superoxide dismutases (SODs) family, and found no change for *Sod2* expression, whereas slight higher expression level of Sod1 was observed in parhtenogenetic embryos, when compared with fertilitzed embryos. Given that superoxide dismutases can protect against reactive oxygen species (ROS) [40, 41], we hence presume that reduced oxidative stress, due to increased sod1 expression, may be one of the mechanisms to faciliate embryo hatch, indicated by the higher hatch rate in parhtenogenetic embryos. But, this hypothesis might not be suitable for normal fertilized embryos, because of the distinct differences in mechanisms regulating the hatch process between fertilized and parthonegenetic blastocysts. Therefore, it will be meaningful to further explore whether antioxidants, such as N-Acety-L-Cysteine (NAC) or resveratrol [37, 51], can increase the hatch rate of human embryos and thereby improve the clinic outcomes, since the relationship between the oxidative stress and embryo hatch remains largely unknown.

Sperm-like breach induces embryo hatch and genetic background determines the hatch mechanism

In our present study, markedly higher hatch rate observed in parthenogenetic embryos than fertilized embryos, regardless of oxygen concentration, resembled the result as previous reported [12]. Furthermore, when we use living imaging to monitor the hatch process in vitro, we amazedly found that fertilized embryos showed a hatch pattern different from parthenogenetic embryos. Fertilized embryos usually started hatching earlier and spent about 42 h to complete hatching, which was nearly seven times longer than parthenogenetic embryos that initiate hatching after 96 h. This result indicated that these two types of embryos had totally different mechanisms to regulate hatch, which might be caused by the genetic background and ZP structure.

On the one hand, Parental genetic background difference can affect TE cells function and make parthenogenetic embryo have much more rapid expansion ability [12], which thus lead to such a short time hatched. On the other hand, there is at least one breach on the ZP of fertilized embryos due to sperm penetration, making them different that of parthenogenetic embryos. The hypotonic experiment result showed that the fertilized embryos prefer to start hatching from sperm-driling gaps at about 72 h by plumping TE cells, thinning ZP and then breaking ZP, after which they continue to widen the ZP gap with "zona breaker" cells and the TE cells emerg to form dumb-bell shap like human embryos, and finally the whole embryo come out gradually [52, 53]. Unlike fertilized embryos, parthenogenetic embryos have hermetical and intact ZP, and they usually keep plumping TE cells and thinning ZP till 96 h or later, and then suddenly break ZP and come out quickly.

To identify whether it is caused by the change of ZP integrity, we tried to make a breach on parthegenetic embryo's ZP artificially by Peizo micromanipulation [54]. No change happened when a tiny breach was made, whereas ZP-drilled parthenogenetic embryos started hatching at 96 h with a small mass of zona breaker cells when the breach size reached to 5 μm which is as large as sperm penetration. Unexpectedly, instead of keeping emerging as fertilized embryos, these cells stoped and the whole embryo hatched suddently and quickly from another place of ZP after long-term expansion, just like normal parthenogenetic embryos. These results indicate that the divergence in ZP structure is not the main reason for the different hatching patterns between fertilized and parthenogenetic embryos. These data suggest that the sperm-drilling breach just induces embryo hatching but embryo itself knows how to continue this process by an unknown mechanism that requires further investigation.

Conclusion

In conclusion, the mechanism of mouse embryo hatch is regulated by both intrinsic and extrinsic factors in vitro. This result has significant clinical implications for the patients who requires AH during IVF treatment, meaning that, in addition to patients' clinical indications, the embryo culture condition should be taken into consideration, when this technique is used to facilitate embryo implantation. O_2 concentration had different influences on the expression of key genes involving in MAPK pathway and superoxide dismutase family between fertilized and pharthenogenetic blastocysts. The regulation of gene expression might control embryonic cell proliferation and the allocation of ICM cells, indicated by the total embryonic cell number and ratio of *Oct4*-positive cells, and thus leads to diverse blastocyst hatch dynamics in different parental genetic background. Therefore, human embryos awaiting AH should be cultured under the atmospheric O_2 (20%) after fertilization, aiming to promote hatching and improve the reproductive outcomes, if the result of mouse study can be applied to humans. However, more animal and human clinical studies are required to clarify the mechanism underlying embryo hatching.

Additional files

Additional file 1: Real time PCR primers for genes expression analysis of 96 h blastocysts. (DOC 41 kb)

Additional file 2: Hatch process of fertilized embryos in vitro. Fertilized embryos started hatching in 72 h and then spent about 42 h emerging from it gradually and slowly until completely hatched in 120 h. (MP4 1099 kb)

Additional file 3: Hatch process of parthenogenetic embryos in vitro. Parthenogenetic embryos kept expansion until broken out suddenly and quickly within approximately 6 h after culture for 96 h. (MP4 283 kb)

Additional file 4: Hypotonicity of 48 h fertilized embryo in vitro. Cytoplasm came out from sperm-breach quickly after transferred into pure water. (MP4 333 kb)

Additional file 5: Hypotonicity of parthenogenetic embryo in vitro. No cytoplasm came out from parthenogenetic embryos after transferred into pure water. (MP4 341 kb)

Additional file 6: Hypotonicity of parthenogenetic embryo with 5 μm breach drilled on zona pellucid in vitro. Cytoplasm came out from artificial breach quickly as same as fertilized embryos after transferred into pure water. (MP4 330 kb)

Additional file 7: Hatch process of parthenogenetic embryo with 5 μm breach drilled on zona pellucid in vitro. Parthenogenetic embryos started hatching slightly from artificial breach in 96 h, but embryonic cells did not keep emerge from it. They kept expansion and broke out from another place on zona pellucid in a short time as normal parthenogenetic embryos did. (MP4 580 kb)

Abbreviations

AH: Assisted hatching; ANOVA: One-way analysis of variance; ESCs: Embryonic stem cells; hCG: Human chorionic gonadotrophin; HKSOM: KSOM containing 14 mM Hepes and 4 mM sodium bicarbonate; ICM: Inner cell mass; IF: Immunofluorescence; KSOM: Potassium simplex optimized medium; $KSOM_{AA}$: KSOM supplemented with nonessential and essential amino acids and 2.5 mM hepes; MAPK: Mitogen-activated protein kinase; NAC: N-Acety-L-Cysteine; O_2: Oxygen; PBS-PVP: Phosphate buffered saline containing 0.1% polyvinyl pyrrolidone; PCR: Polymerase chain reaction; PLSD: Fisher's protected least-significant difference; ROS: Reactive oxygen species; SODs: Superoxide dismutases; SPF: Specific pathogen-free; TE: Trophectoderm; ZP: Zona pellucida

Funding

This work was supported by the National Key R&D Program of China (2017YFC1001901 and 2017YFA0102801); National Natural Science Foundation of China (31671540, 81771579 and 81501327); Guangdong Science and Technology Department Planning Project (2015B020228002); and Science and Technology Planning Project of Guangdong Province (Grant No. 2014A020213017).

Authors' contributions

JH conceived the study. JH and HZ designed the overall experimental scheme. SZ, SC, YS, LL, CD, and HD executed the experiments. SZ, CS, HZ and JH analyzed the data. SZ, HZ and JH wrote the paper. All authors read and approved the final manuscript.

Competing interests
The authors declare that they have no competing interests.

Author details
[1]Center for Reproductive Medicine, Key Laboratory for Reproductive Medicine of Guangdong Province, Key Laboratory for Major Obstetric Diseases of Guangdong Province, and Key Laboratory for Reproduction and Genetics of Guangdong Higher Education Institutes, the Third Affiliated Hospital of Guangzhou Medical University, Guangzhou 510150, China. [2]Beijing Acorndx Biotechnology Co. Ltd, Beijing 100176, China. [3]Key Laboratory of Reproductive Medicine of Guangdong Province, School of Life Sciences and the First Affiliated Hospital, Sun Yat-sen University, Guangzhou 510275, China.

References

1. Soupart P, Strong PA. Ultrastructural observations on polyspermic penetration of zona pellucida-free human oocytes inseminated in vitro. Fertil Steril. 1975;26:523–37.
2. O'Sullivan CM, Rancourt SL, Liu SY, Rancourt DE. A novel murine tryptase involved in blastocyst hatching and outgrowth. Reproduction. 2001;122:61–71.
3. Wassarman PM, Litscher ES. Mammalian fertilization: the egg's multifunctional zona pellucida. Int J Dev Biol. 2008;52:665–76.
4. Cohen J, Elsner C, Kort H, Malter H, Massey J, Mayer MP, et al. Impairment of the hatching process following IVF in the human and improvement of implantation by assisting hatching using micromanipulation. Hum Reprod. 1990;5:7–13.
5. McLaren A. Can mouse blastocysts stimulate a uterine response before losing the zona pellucida? J Reprod Fertil. 1969;19:199–201.
6. Carlone DL, Skalnik DG. CpG binding protein is crucial for early embryonic development. Mol Cell Biol. 2001;21:7601–6.
7. Chen HW, Chen JJ, Yu SL, Li HN, Yang PC, Su CM, et al. Transcriptome analysis in blastocyst hatching by cDNA microarray. Hum Reprod. 2005;20:2492–501.
8. Gwatkin RB, Williams DT, Hartmann JF, Kniazuk M. The zona reaction of hamster and mouse eggs: production in vitro by a trypsin-like protease from cortical granules. J Reprod Fertil. 1973;32:259–65.
9. Harvey AJ, Kind KL, Pantaleon M, Armstrong DT, Thompson JG. Oxygen-regulated gene expression in bovine blastocysts. Biol Reprod. 2004;71:1108–19.
10. Huang JC, Wun WS, Goldsby JS, Wun IC, Falconi SM, Wu KK. Prostacyclin enhances embryo hatching but not sperm motility. Hum Reprod. 2003;18:2582–9.
11. Kelleher AM, Peng W, Pru JK, Pru CA, DeMayo FJ, Spencer TE. Forkhead box a2 (FOXA2) is essential for uterine function and fertility. Proc Natl Acad Sci U S A. 2017;114:E1018–E26.
12. Latham KE, Kutyna K, Wang Q. Genetic variation in trophectoderm function in parthenogenetic mouse embryos. Dev Genet. 1999;24:329–35.
13. Montag M, Koll B, Holmes P, van der V. Significance of the number of embryonic cells and the state of the zona pellucida for hatching of mouse blastocysts in vitro versus in vivo. Biol Reprod. 2000;62:1738–44.
14. Qin J, Diaz-Cueto L, Schwarze JE, Takahashi Y, Imai M, Isuzugawa K, et al. Effects of progranulin on blastocyst hatching and subsequent adhesion and outgrowth in the mouse. Biol Reprod. 2005;73:434–42.
15. Pool TB. An update on embryo culture for human assisted reproductive technology: media, performance, and safety. Semin Reprod Med. 2005;23:309–18.
16. Feil D, Lane M, Roberts CT, Kelley RL, Edwards LJ, Thompson JG, et al. Effect of culturing mouse embryos under different oxygen concentrations on subsequent fetal and placental development. J Physiol. 2006;572:87–96.
17. Fischer-Brown A, Monson R, Parrish J, Rutledge J. Cell allocation in bovine embryos cultured in two media under two oxygen concentrations. Zygote. 2002;10:341–8.
18. Harlow GM, Quinn P. Foetal and placental growth in the mouse after pre-implantation development in vitro under oxygen concentrations of 5 and 20%. Aust J Biol Sci. 1979;32:363–9.
19. Karagenc L, Sertkaya Z, Ciray N, Ulug U, Bahceci M. Impact of oxygen concentration on embryonic development of mouse zygotes. Reprod BioMed Online. 2004;9:409–17.
20. Karja NW, Wongsrikeao P, Murakami M, Agung B, Fahrudin M, Nagai T, et al. Effects of oxygen tension on the development and quality of porcine in vitro fertilized embryos. Theriogenology. 2004;62:1585–95.
21. Lash GE, Otun HA, Innes BA, Bulmer JN, Searle RF, Robson SC. Low oxygen concentrations inhibit trophoblast cell invasion from early gestation placental explants via alterations in levels of the urokinase plasminogen activator system. Biol Reprod. 2006;74:403–9.
22. Quinn P, Harlow GM. The effect of oxygen on the development of preimplantation mouse embryos in vitro. J Exp Zool. 1978;206:73–80.
23. Rho GJ, Kim DS, Son WJ, Cho SR, Kim JG, et al. Influence of in vitro oxygen concentrations on preimplantation embryo development, gene expression and production of Hanwoo calves following embryo transfer. Mol Reprod Dev. 2007;74:486–96.
24. Umaoka Y, Noda Y, Narimoto K, Mori T. Effects of oxygen toxicity on early development of mouse embryos. Mol Reprod Dev. 1992;31:28–33.
25. Yuan YQ, Van Soom A, Coopman FO, Mintiens K, Boerjan ML, Van Zeveren A, et al. Influence of oxygen tension on apoptosis and hatching in bovine embryos cultured in vitro. Theriogenology. 2003;59:1585–96.
26. Dumoulin JC, Vanvuchelen RC, Land JA, Pieters MH, Geraedts JP, Evers JL. Effect of oxygen concentration on in vitro fertilization and embryo culture in the human and the mouse. Fertil Steril. 1995;63:115–9.
27. Dumoulin JC, Meijers CJ, Bras M, Coonen E, Geraedts JP, Evers JL. Effect of oxygen concentration on human in-vitro fertilization and embryo culture. Hum Reprod. 1999;14:465–9.
28. Kind KL, Collett RA, Harvey AJ, Thompson JG. Oxygen-regulated expression of GLUT-1, GLUT-3, and VEGF in the mouse blastocyst. Mol Reprod Dev. 2005;70:37–44.
29. Liu L, Ju JC, Yang X. Parthenogenetic development and protein patterns of newly matured bovine oocytes after chemical activation. Mol Reprod Dev. 1998;49:298–307.
30. Liu L, Trimarchi JR, Keefe DL. Haploidy but not parthenogenetic activation leads to increased incidence of apoptosis in mouse embryos. Biol Reprod. 2002;66:204–10.
31. Cheeseman LP, Boulanger J, Bond LM, Schuh M. Two pathways regulate cortical granule translocation to prevent polyspermy in mouse oocytes. Nat Commun. 2016;7:13726.
32. Bianchi E, Wright GJ. Sperm meets egg: the genetics of mammalian fertilization. Annu Rev Genet. 2016;50:93–111.
33. Okabe M. The cell biology of mammalian fertilization. Development. 2013;140:4471–9.
34. Wassarman P, Chen J, Cohen N, Litscher E, Liu C, Qi H, et al. Structure and function of the mammalian egg zona pellucida. J Exp Zool. 1999;285:251–8.
35. Huang J, Okuka M, McLean M, Keefe DL, Liu L. Telomere susceptibility to cigarette smoke-induced oxidative damage and chromosomal instability of mouse embryos in vitro. Free Radic Biol Med. 2010;48:1663–76.
36. Huang J, Okuka M, McLean M, Keefe DL, Liu L. Effects of cigarette smoke on fertilization and embryo development in vivo. Fertil Steril. 2009;92:1456–65.
37. Liu J, Liu M, Ye X, Liu K, Huang J, Wang L, et al. Delay in oocyte aging in mice by the antioxidant N-acetyl-L-cysteine (NAC). Hum Reprod. 2012;27:1411–20.
38. Sakao Y, Kawai T, Takeuchi O, Copeland NG, Gilbert DJ, Jenkins NA, et al. Mouse proteasomal ATPases Psmc3 and Psmc4: genomic organization and gene targeting. Genomics. 2000;67:1–7.
39. Maekawa M, Yamamoto T, Kohno M, Takeichi M, Nishida E. Requirement for ERK MAP kinase in mouse preimplantation development. Development. 2007;134:2751–9.
40. Goto Y, Noda Y, Narimoto K, Umaoka Y, Mori T. Oxidative stress on mouse embryo development in vitro. Free Radic Biol Med. 1992;13:47–53.
41. Orsi NM, Leese HJ. Protection against reactive oxygen species during mouse preimplantation embryo development: role of EDTA, oxygen tension, catalase, superoxide dismutase and pyruvate. Mol Reprod Dev. 2001;59:44–53.
42. Genbacev OD, Prakobphol A, Foulk RA, Krtolica AR, Ilic D, Singer MS, et al. Trophoblast L-selectin-mediated adhesion at the maternal-fetal interface. Science. 2003;299:405–8.
43. Thouas GA, Dominguez F, Green MP, Vilella F, Simon C, Gardner DK. Soluble ligands and their receptors in human embryo development and implantation. Endocr Rev. 2015;36:92–130.
44. Gonzales DS, Bavister BD. Zona pellucida escape by hamster blastocysts in vitro is delayed and morphologically different compared with zona escape in vivo. Biol Reprod. 1995;52:470–80.

45. Schimmel T, Cohen J, Saunders H, Alikani M. Laser-assisted zona pellucida thinning does not facilitate hatching and may disrupt the in vitro hatching process: a morphokinetic study in the mouse. Hum Reprod. 2014;29:2670–9.
46. Park SB, Kim HJ, Choi YB, Ahn KH, Lee KH, Yang JB, et al. The effect of various assisted hatching techniques on the mouse early embryo development. Clin Exp Reprod Med. 2014;41:68–74.
47. Martins WP, Rocha IA, Ferriani RA, Nastri CO. Assisted hatching of human embryos: a systematic review and meta-analysis of randomized controlled trials. Hum Reprod Update. 2011;17:438–53.
48. Bavister B. Oxygen concentration and preimplantation development. Reprod BioMed Online. 2004;9:484–6.
49. Harvey AJ. The role of oxygen in ruminant preimplantation embryo development and metabolism. Anim Reprod Sci. 2007;98:113–28.
50. Liu L, Czerwiec E, Keefe DL. Effect of ploidy and parental genome composition on expression of Oct-4 protein in mouse embryos. Gene Expr Patterns. 2004;4:433–41.
51. Liu M, Yin Y, Ye X, Zeng M, Zhao Q, Keefe DL, et al. Resveratrol protects against age-associated infertility in mice. Hum Reprod. 2013;28:707–17.
52. Cohen J, Feldberg D. Effects of the size and number of zona pellucida openings on hatching and trophoblast outgrowth in the mouse embryo. Mol Reprod Dev. 1991;30:70–8.
53. Sathananthan H, Menezes J, Gunasheela S. Mechanics of human blastocyst hatching in vitro. Reprod BioMed Online. 2003;7:228–34.
54. Huang J, Deng K, Wu H, Liu Z, Chen Z, Cao S, et al. Efficient production of mice from embryonic stem cells injected into four- or eight-cell embryos by piezo micromanipulation. Stem Cells. 2008;26:1883–90.

6

Is Afamin a novel biomarker for gestational diabetes mellitus?

Angela Köninger[1], Annette Mathan[1,2], Pawel Mach[1], Mirjam Frank[3], Boerge Schmidt[3], Ekkehard Schleussner[4], Rainer Kimmig[1], Alexandra Gellhaus[1] and Hans Dieplinger[5,6*]

Abstract

Background: In search of potential early biomarkers for timely prediction of gestational diabetes mellitus (GDM), we focused on afamin, a vitamin E–binding protein in human plasma.. Afamin plays a role in anti-apoptotic cellular processes related to oxidative stress and is associated with insulin resistance and other features of metabolic syndrome. During uncomplicated pregnancy its serum concentrations increase linearly. The aim of this study was to investigate the suitability of afamin as early marker for predicting GDM.

Methods: In a first-trimester cohort from a prospective observational study of adverse pregnancy outcomes we secondarily analyzed afamin concentrations in 59 patients diagnosed with GDM and 51 controls. Additionally, afamin concentrations were cross-sectionally examined in a mid-trimester cohort of 105 women and compared with results from a simultaneously performed oral glucose tolerance test (OGTT). Subgroup analysis comparing patients treated with either insulin (iGDM) or dietary intervention (dGDM) was performed in both cohorts. Patients were recruited at the University Hospital Essen, Germany, between 2003 and 2016.

Results: Results were adjusted for body-mass-index (BMI) and gestational age. First and mid-trimester cohorts yielded significantly elevated afamin concentrations in patients with pathological OGTT compared to patients without GDM (first trimester cohort: mean, 113.4 mg/l; 95% CI, 106.4–120.5 mg/l and 87.2 mg/l; 95% CI, 79.7–94.7 mg/l; mid-trimester cohort: mean, 182.9 mg/l; 95% CI, 169.6–196.2 mg/l and 157.3 mg/l; 95% CI, 149.1–165.4 mg/l, respectively). In the first-trimester cohort, patients developing iGDM later in pregnancy presented with significantly higher afamin concentrations compared to patients developing dGDM and compared to patients without GDM. In the mid-trimester cohort, mean concentrations of afamin differed significantly between patients with dGDM compared to controls and between patients with iGDM and controls. Patients with iGDM showed only slightly higher afamin levels compared to patients with dGDM.

Conclusion: Afamin may serve as a new early biomarker for pathological glucose metabolism during pregnancy. Further research is needed to determine afamin's concentrations during pregnancy, its predictive value for early detection of pregnancies at high risk to develop GDM and its diagnostic role during the second trimester.

Keywords: Afamin, Pregnancy, Insulin resistance, Gestational diabetes mellitus, Oral glucose tolerance test

* Correspondence: hans.dieplinger@i-med.ac.at
[5]Division of Genetic Epidemiology, Department of Medical Genetics, Molecular and Clinical Pharmacology, Medical University of Innsbruck, Schöpfstrasse 41, 6020 Innsbruck, Austria
[6]Vitateq Biotechnology GmbH, 6020 Innsbruck, Austria
Full list of author information is available at the end of the article

Background

Gestational diabetes mellitus (GDM) is a common disorder that occurs in approximately 7% to 14% of pregnancies [1]. GDM is defined as "any degree of glucose intolerance with onset or first recognition during pregnancy" [2].

The prevalence of GDM depends strongly on ethnicity and the diagnostic criteria used [3]. The absence of a worldwide standard concerning the best criteria for diagnosing GDM results in unequal management concepts, variances in incidence rates, and a lack of scientific evidence of the consequences for the mother and the baby. As shown by the Hyperglycemia and Adverse Pregnancy Outcome (HAPO) trial, pathological findings from the 75-g oral glucose tolerance test (OGTT) are strongly associated with adverse pregnancy outcome [4, 5]. Some studies have demonstrated a benefit for the mother and the baby if diabetes is screened, diagnosed, and treated during pregnancy [6, 7]. As shown by Crowther et al. [7], the number of patients who need to be treated to prevent one serious event, such as shoulder dystocia, a high-grade birth injury such as nerve palsy, bone fracture, or neonatal death, is approximately 34. An important finding in Landon's [6] interventional trial involving patients with mild GDM was a reduction in the risk of cesarean section and of preeclampsia if GDM was screened, diagnosed, and treated. In summary, the exact and timely diagnosis of GDM allows successful interventions and improves pregnancy outcomes.

The 75-g OGTT is currently considered to be the gold standard for diagnosing GDM [8]. However, the test presents some problems in performance and pre-analytic requirements, such as the need for patients to be in a fasting state, the need to avoid glycolysis of the samples, and the need to perform laboratory analysis in accordance with highly standardized analysis procedures and low inter-assay variations. Some countries recommend screening tests for determining which pregnant women may be at high risk of GDM; these tests include the 50-g OGTT, which was performed in the two interventional studies reported thus far [6, 7, 9]. However, this test has limitations in terms of sensitivity, specificity, and reproducibility [10, 11]. For these reasons, the consensus statement of the *International Association of the Diabetes and Pregnancy Study Groups* (IADPSG) [8] recommends that "in future clinical practice, simpler and more cost-effective strategies that do not require performing an OGTT on most pregnant women may be developed".

In the current study, our search for potential new and early biomarkers that can offer timely prediction of GDM focused on afamin, a previously described vitamin E–binding protein found in human plasma [12]. Vitamin E is an important antioxidant that protects against oxidative stress. Afamin is a member of the albumin gene family [13] that seems to play a role in anti-apoptotic cellular processes related to oxidative stress [14]. Plasma concentrations of afamin are independent of fasting status, age, and sex [15, 16] and increase linearly approximately 2-fold during an uncomplicated pregnancy [17]. Afamin concentrations are strongly correlated with clinical and laboratory parameters of the metabolic syndrome, such as elevations in body mass index (BMI) and plasma glucose concentrations, dyslipidemia, and hypertension [18]. It was subsequently shown in a very recent population-based study in more than 20,000 individuals that afamin concentrations are also associated with the prevalence and incidence of type 2 diabetes mellitus as well as insulin resistance (IR) [19].

As we have previously shown, afamin concentrations are also associated with the presence of IR among patients with polycystic ovary syndrome (PCOS) [20]. IR can be determined by the Homeostasis-Model Assessment (HOMA) [21]. Physiologically, IR increases during pregnancy with the aim of adequate maternofetal glucose transfer. Increased IR at the beginning of pregnancy is strongly associated with the development of GDM [22]. Additionally, insulin concentrations regulate the expression of sex hormone–binding protein (SHBG) in the liver [23] and low concentrations of SHBG during the first trimester of pregnancy may indicate the development of GDM [24]. However, no reliable method of screening for diabetes during the first trimester currently exists.

The aim of this study was to explore the predictive and diagnostic value of afamin concentrations regarding GDM, in the first and second trimester, respectively. In a secondary analysis of samples which were taken from a prospective observational study with the aim to predict adverse pregnancy outcomes, we examined the association between serum afamin concentrations during the first trimester and the subsequent development of GDM during the ongoing pregnancy. In a mid-trimester cross-sectional analysis we also examined serum afamin concentrations in serum samples from women with and without a pathological 75-g OGTT in median gestational age of 26th week of pregnancy.

Methods

Subjects characteristics

First-trimester cohort

Frozen serum samples from 110 women with singleton pregnancies in the first trimester of pregnancy were secondarily analyzed. We included all patients who gave birth at the Department of Obstetrics and Gynecology of the University Hospital of Essen between 2003 and 2014 with either a GDM diagnosis at the time of delivery or an uncomplicated pregnancy and from whom frozen blood samples collected during the first trimester were available. 59/110 developed GDM in the second trimester and 51/110 did not develop GDM and served as controls. Patients were 19 to 44 years old (median, 34 years; interquartile range [IQR], 31–37 years) and presented between gestational day 43 and 98 (median 89 days of pregnancy [IQR 85–92]). 8 patients from the cohort, all with GDM, had confirmed polycystic ovarian syndrome (PCOS) corresponding to the prevalence of PCOS in the general population [25].

Information about GDM was available from our medical records or from patient interviews. GDM was diagnosed by the women's gynecologists according to the current guidelines for obstetric care in Germany [9]. GDM is diagnosed if at least one value of the 75 g-OGTT was elevated. Before 2011, the following definition was used: fasting glucose: 95 mg/dl, glucose after 1 h: 180 mg/dl, glucose after 2 h: 155 mg/dl [9, 26]. The values are based on maternal life-time risk for diabetes [26]. Since 2011, the following definition is used in Germany to diagnose GDM: fasting glucose: 92 mg/dl, glucose after 1 h: 180 mg/dl, glucose after 2 h: 153 mg/dl [4, 9, 26]. These values are based on adverse pregnancy outcomes (HAPO trial 2008). 36 patients with GDM presented before 2011 and 23 after 2011.

According to current guidelines, only patients at elevated risk for GDM e.g. obesity, family history with diabetes or macrosomia in a pregnancy before or patients with a pathological 50 g-OGTT got a 75 g-OGTT before 2013. Since 2013 to the end of the study period, the performance of a 50 g-OGTT as a screening tool for GDM was a standard procedure in Germany. Patients with either glucose levels ≥135 mg/dl in the 50 g-OGTT or patients with risk factors got a 75 g-OGTT [9]. Consequently, not all pregnant women in Germany got a 75 g-OGTT. Since we performed a secondary analysis using data from clinical routine, a 75 g-OGTT was not available from all patients of the control group because they were screened according to current guidelines and after screening OGTT was not indicated for all of the controls.

Mid-trimester cohort

We also performed a cross-sectional analysis involving 105 pregnant women with singleton pregnancies aged 20 to 43 years (median, 32 years; IQR, 28–36 years). Between 2014 and 2016, women were enrolled in the study as they presented to the University Hospital of Essen Department of Obstetrics and Gynecology for antenatal care in high-risk pregnancies. 5/107 suffered from PCOS. Patients underwent a 75-g OGTT for GDM screening between gestational day 44 and 272 (median 184; IQR 162–209). Simultaneously with the test, blood samples were collected for afamin determination. Patients in whom the test was performed before 24 weeks and with no pathological results in the OGTT, received another OGTT after reaching the 24th week of pregnancy. If both results differed from each other, they were excluded from the study. OGTT was performed according to the practice guideline of the German Diabetes Association (DDG) and the German Association for Gynecology and Obstetrics (DGGG) [9]. To avoid glycolysis, we transported venous blood samples to the laboratory of the University Hospital Essen within 15 min after sampling. Fasting insulin concentrations were determined at presentation (0 h), after 1 h, and after 2 h. Insulin resistance was defined according to HOMA [20]. Serum collected while patients were fasting was also used to determine afamin concentrations. All women of both cohorts provided written informed consent, and the study was approved by the local research ethics committee (number 125212-BO).

Blood sampling

First trimester cohort: 9 ml of blood was drawn with the S-Monovette Blood Collection System (Sarstedt AG and Co., Nürnbrecht, Germany) for freezing and later determination of parameters of interest. Samples were stored immediately at 4 °C and processed within 4 h to avoid cell lysis. Blood fractionation was carried out by centrifugation at 2500×g for 10 min, and 3 to 4 ml of the supernatant constituting blood serum was removed and stored at – 80 °C. For afamin analysis, all samples were thawed to divide them into aliquots and restored at – 80 °C. Frozen aliquots were sent to the Medical University of Innsbruck, Division of Genetic Epidemiology in 2016 for determination of afamin concentrations.

Mid-trimester cohort: 2.7 ml blood were collected into 2.7-ml fluoride/EDTA monovettes for analyzing glucose concentrations. The S-Monovette Blood Collection System (Sarstedt AG and Co., Nürnbrecht, Germany) was used to collect 9 ml blood for insulin determination. Glucose and insulin concentrations were immediately determined in the central laboratories of the University Hospital Essen. 9 ml of blood was also drawn with the S-Monovette Blood Collection System (Sarstedt AG and Co., Nürnbrecht, Germany) for determination of afamin. These samples were stored at 4 °C immediately and processed within 4 h to avoid cell lysis. Blood fractionation was carried out by centrifugation at 2500×g for 10 min, and 3 to 4 ml of the supernatant constituting blood serum was removed and stored at – 80 °C. For afamin analysis all samples were thawed to divide them into aliquots and restored at – 80 °C. Frozen samples were sent to the Medical University of Innsbruck, Division of Genetic Epidemiology in 2016 for determination of afamin concentrations.

Laboratory parameters

Afamin concentrations were measured with a commercially available sandwich enzyme-linked immunosorbent assay (ELISA; BioVendor, Brno, Czech Republic) using two different monoclonal antibodies against human afamin as modified from a previously described protocol

[15]. Recombinantly expressed and purified human afamin served as the assay standard. According to the manufacturer's manual, within-run and run-to-run coefficients of variation were 3.6% and 3.4%, respectively, at a mean afamin concentration of 80 mg/l.

Glucose concentrations were determined photometrically (ADVIA Centaur CP Immunoassay System; Siemens Healthcare Diagnostics, Eschborn, Germany). Analyses were performed according to the guidelines of the German Medical Association (www.bundesaerztekammer.de). Automated chemiluminescence immunoassay systems (Immulite 2000 XPi; Siemens Healthcare Diagnostics) were used to determine insulin concentrations. Intra-assay variations were ≤1.1% for glucose and ≤5.5% for insulin; inter-assay variations were ≤1.8% for glucose and ≤7.3% for insulin.

Statistical analysis

Characteristics of both study populations were presented as mean with standard deviations (SD) as well as medians with interquartile ranges (IQR). Mann-Whitney-U-Test or t-test were used to analyse group differences in maternal age, gestational age, BMI, newborn weight, gestational age at birth, afamin, glucose and insulin concentrations and HOMA-IR. In both cohorts, differences in afamin concentrations between subgroups were analyzed using linear regression models including gestational age and BMI at the time of blood sampling as covariate and status of iGDM or dGDM as categorical independent variables to estimate gestational age- and BMI -adjusted least-squares means with 95% confidence intervals (CIs) as marginal averages. The alpha level was set at 0.05 to determine statistical significance. All analyses were performed with the R statistical package, version 3.0.2 [27].

Results

First-trimester study population

Patient characteristics (n = 110) are shown in Table 1. Of the 59 participants who had GDM diagnosis later in their pregnancy, 25 were treated with dietary intervention (dGDM) and 34 were treated with insulin (iGDM). Patient characteristics of the subgroups are shown in Table 2.

Since afamin levels depend on BMI and gestational age, the subsequent results comparing afamin levels between controls, iGDM and dGDM patients, were adjusted for BMI and gestational age:

Serum afamin concentrations measured during the first trimester were significantly higher among patients with GDM (mean, 113.4 mg/l; 95% CI, 106.4–120.5 mg/l) than among patients without GDM diagnosis later in their pregnancy (mean, 87.2 mg/l; 95% CI, 79.7–94.7 mg/l; $P = < 0.0001$).

Patients which developed iGDM (mean, 132.8 mg/l; 95% CI, 124.6–141.0 mg/l) presented with significantly higher afamin concentrations than patients which developed dGDM (mean, 91.2 mg/l; 95% CI, 82.4–100.0 mg/l; $P < 0.0001$) and than patients without GDM in their ongoing pregnancy (mean, 84.7 mg/l; 95% CI, 78.4–91.1 mg/l; $P < 0.0001$). No significant difference was seen between afamin concentrations of patients with dGDM in their later pregnancy and controls ($p = 0.23$) (Fig. 1).

Table 1 Patients' characteristics and afamin concentrations in the first-trimester cohort study

Parameter	Controls n = 51	Gestational diabetes mellitus (GDM) n = 59	p-value
Maternal age (years)			
Mean (± standard deviation, SD)	32.65 (4.79)	34.36 (5.26)	0.05
Median (Interquartile range, IQR)	33.00 (29.25–36.00)	36.00 (32.00–38.00)	
Body-mass-index (kg/m^2)			
Mean (± SD)	24.76 (5.00)	30.05 (8.02)	< 0.001
Median (IQR)	24.00 (21.80–26.85)	28.85 (24.40–34.30)	
Afamin (mg/l)			
Mean (± SD)	84.59 (17.75)	115.46 (31.72)	< 0.001
Median (IQR)	82.18 (68.68–100.57)	117.13 (86.27–146.99)	
Newborn weight (gram)			
Mean (± SD)	3517 (453)	3148 (730)	0.03
Median (IQR)	3490 (3270–3865)	3320 (2868–3568)	
Gestational age at parturition (days)			
Mean (± SD)	276 (8)	266 (21)	0.02
Median (IQR)	278 (272–282)	273 (262–280)	

Table 2 Patients' characteristics and afamin concentrations in the first-trimester cohort study of patients with diagnosis of gestational diabetes mellitus (GDM) later in pregnancy

Parameter	Gestational diabetes mellitus treated with dietary intervention (dGDM) n = 25	Gestational diabetes mellitus treated with insulin (iGDM) n = 34	*p*-value
Maternal age (years)			
Mean (± standard deviation, SD)	33.60 (6.37)	34.91 (4.29)	0.50
Median (Interquartile range, IQR)	36.00 (28.50–37.25)	36.00 (32.00–39.00)	
Body-mass-index (kg/m^2)			
Mean (± SD)	26.19 (5.98)	32.78 (8.23)	0.002
Median (IQR)	24.85 (22.10–30.80)	29.50 (27.90–37.40)	
Afamin (mg/l)			
Mean (± SD)	91.33 (21.43)	133.20 (25.87)	< 0.001
Median (IQR)	86.99 (75.88–100.94)	140.18 (118.20–154.70)	
Newborn weight (gram)			
Mean (± SD)	3376 (709)	2985 (711)	0.008
Median (IQR)	3510 (3165–3680)	3105 (2768–3453)	
Gestational age at parturition (days)			
Mean (± SD)	269 (20)	264 (21)	0.25
Median (IQR)	277 (266–281)	272 (251–280)	

Mid-trimester cohort

Patient characteristics are shown in Table 3. Of the 105 patients, 29 exhibited abnormal OGTT results and 76 exhibited normal OGTT results. Of the 29 patients with GDM, 12 were treated with insulin (iGDM) and 17 with dietary intervention (dGDM). Patient characteristics of the two subgroups are shown in Table 4.

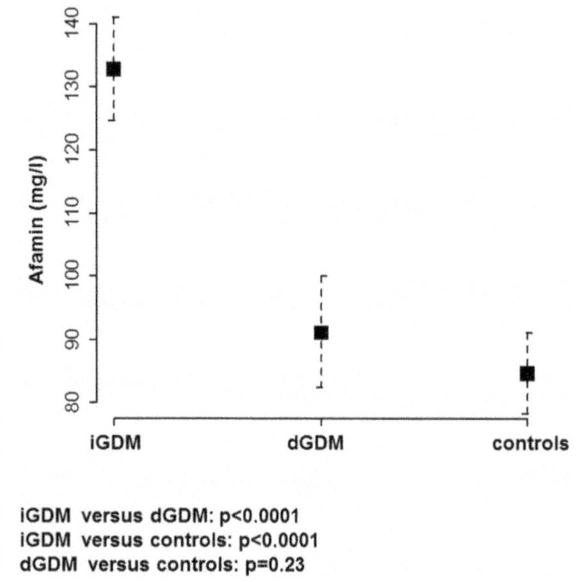

Fig. 1 Afamin concentrations in the first trimester cohort (between gestational day 8 and 98). Serum concentrations of afamin among patients with gestational diabetes mellitus (GDM) treated with insulin (iGDM; *n* = 34), treated with dietary intervention (dGDM; *n* = 25) and control subjects (*n* = 51) adjusted for gestational age and body-mass-index (BMI)

When the analysis was adjusted for gestational age and BMI, the differences in afamin concentrations were significant between GDM patients (mean, 182.9 mg/l; 95% CI, 169.6–196.2 mg/l) and control subjects (mean, 157.3 mg/l; 95% CI, 149.1–165.4 mg/l; $P = 0.002$).

Mean concentrations of afamin differed significantly between control subjects (mean, 157.2 mg/l; 95% CI, 149.0–165.4 mg/l) and dGDM patients (mean, 179.5 mg/l; 95% CI, 162.5–196.5 mg/l; $P = 0.02$) as well as patients with iGDM (mean, 188.2 mg/l; 95% CI, 166.8–209.7 mg/l; $P = 0.01$). Patients with iGDM showed only slightly higher afamin levels compared to patients with dGDM ($P = 0.53$) (Fig. 2).

HOMA-IR was significantly higher in patients with iGDM (median 2.90, IQR 1.78–5.75) compared to controls (median 1.50; IQR 0.77–2.48; $P = 0.001$) and compared to patients with dGDM (median 1.80; IQR 0.95–3.05; $P = 0.04$). The difference between HOMA-IR of patients with dGDM and controls was not significant ($P = 0.34$).

Discussion

The aim of this pilot study was to evaluate new screening or diagnostic tools for GDM. Currently, no screening tool exists that can be used during the first trimester of pregnancy to determine which patients will experience GDM during the course of pregnancy. The gold standard for diagnosing GDM during the second trimester is the 75-g OGTT [4, 5]. The corresponding trial showed that an increase in each of the measured values (fasting

Table 3 Patients´ characteristics and laboratory parameters in the mid-trimester cohort study

Parameter	Normal 75 g-oral glucose-tolerance-test (OGTT) n = 76	Pathological 75 g-oral glucose-tolerance-test (OGTT) *n* = 29	*p*-value
Gestational age at 75 g-oral glucose-tolerance-test (OGTT) performance (days)			
Mean (± standard deviation, SD)	189 (40)	168 (43)	0.06
Median (Interquartile range, IQR)	189 (165–221)	176 (151.25–200.00)	
Maternal age (years)			
Mean (± SD)	30.59 (5.08)	35.00 (5.01)	< 0.001
Median (IQR)	30.50 (27.50–34.00)	37.00 (31.50–39.00)	
Body-mass-index (kg/m^2)			
Mean (± SD)	28.35 (7.13)	31.15 (8.56)	0.08
Median (IQR)	26.80 (23.40–32.00)	29.30 (25.60–34.65)	
Fasting Insulin (μIU/ml)			
Mean (± SD)	9.68 (7.53)	12.68 (7.94)	0.02
Median (IQR)	7.90 (4.40–12.25)	10.00 (7.63–14.90)	
1 h Insulin (μIU/ml)			
Mean (± SD)	90.26 (54.17)	110.45 (57.89)	0.07
Median (IQR)	76.30 (52.35–121.00)	102.00 (68.23–123.50)	
2 h Insulin (μIU/ml)			
Mean (± SD)	69.76 (46.40)	121.16 (54.21)	< 0.001
Median (IQR)	58.15 (42.90–85.10)	120.00 (84.63–148.25)	
Fasting glucose (mg/dl)			
Mean (± SD)	77.70 (5.68)	83.79 (11.93)	0.03
Median (IQR)	77.00 (74.00–81.50)	81.00 (73.75–93.25)	
1 h glucose (mg/dl)			
Mean (± SD)	135.25 (24.86)	179.00 (25.97)	< 0.001
Median (IQR)	136.50 (119–156.50)	175.00 (161.00–189.25)	
2 h glucose (mg/dl)			
Mean (± SD)	103.04 (21.02)	152.69 (26.02)	< 0.001
Median (IQR)	101.50 (87.00–121.00)	156.00 (148.25–170.25)	
HOMA-IR			
Mean (± SD)	1.90 (1.52)	2.72 (1.96)	0.01
Median (IQR)	1.50 (0.80–2.45)	2.20 (1.53–3.33)	
Afamin (mg/l)			
Mean (± SD)	157.90 (36.32)	180.83 (41.21)	0.003
Median (IQR)	160.49 (142.63–177.33)	180.20 (158.68–211.94)	
Gestational age at parturition (days)			
Mean (± SD)	259 (21)	256 (22)	0.38
Median (IQR)	266 (249–273)	263 (249–269)	
Newborn weight (gram)			
Mean (± SD)	2851 (786)	2916 (821)	0.71
Median (IQR)	3075 (2465–3385)	3170 (2496–3473)	

glucose concentrations at baseline and glucose concentrations after 1 and 2 h) was positively correlated with the risk of adverse outcome. These findings highlight the importance of a carefully performed 75-g OGTT. However, the 75-g OGTT requires high quality in pre-analytic steps, analysis, performance and requires patients to be in a fasting state. For these reasons, the 75-g OGTT cannot be offered to all pregnant women. In addition, the 50-g OGTT,

Table 4 Gestational diabetes mellitus (GDM) patients´ characteristics and laboratory parameters in the mid-trimester cohort study

Parameter	Gestational diabetes mellitus treated with dietary intervention (dGDM) n = 17	Gestational diabetes mellitus treated with insulin (iGDM) n = 12	*p*-value
Gestational age at 75 g-oral glucose-tolerance-test (OGTT) performance (days)			
Mean (± standard deviation, SD)	174 (32)	158 (55)	0.32
Median (Interquartile range, IQR)	183 (157–200)	167 (120–199)	
Maternal age (years)			
Mean (± SD)	34.59 (4.64)	35.58 (5.85)	0.40
Median (IQR)	36 (32.25–38.00)	37.50 (30.00–39.50)	
Body-mass-index (kg/m^2)			
Mean (± SD)	28.05 (5.28)	35.53 (10.49)	0.02
Median (IQR)	26.60 (24.55–31.33)	30.50 (29.70–38.90)	
Fasting Insulin (μIU/ml)			
Mean (± SD)	9.95 (5.04)	16.53 (9.79)	0.06
Median (IQR)	9.90 (5.48–14.30)	13.40 (9.35–20.35)	
1 h Insulin (μIU/ml)			
Mean (± SD)	82.04 (24.47)	150.69 (68.15)	0.003
Median (IQR)	75.50 (63.98–103.25)	125.00 (111.50–213.00)	
2 h Insulin (μIU/ml)			
Mean (± SD)	101.59 (40.58)	148.88 (60.45)	0.02
Median (IQR)	102.00 (71.80–123.50)	141.00 (107.50–187.50)	
Fasting glucose (mg/dl)			
Mean (± SD)	79.47 (9.27)	89.92 (12.93)	0.02
Median (IQR)	77.00 (73.00–89.25)	93.50 (82.00–98.00)	
1 h glucose (mg/dl)			
Mean (± SD)	171.53 (16.90)	189.58 (33.07)	0.14
Median (IQR)	171.00 (160.25–187.50)	183.50 (171.50–202.50)	
2 h glucose (mg/dl)			
Mean (± SD)	155.35 (20.34)	148.92 (33.08)	0.81
Median (IQR)	155.00 (151.25–172.00)	157.00 (135.00–169.00)	
HOMA-IR			
Mean (± SD)	2.00 (1.07)	3.75 (2.47)	0.04
Median (IQR)	1.80 (0.98–2.98)	2.90 (1.90–4.90)	
Afamin (mg/l)			
Mean (± SD)	176.40 (48.33)	187.10 (29.19)	0.50
Median (IQR)	175.80 (158.68–206.39)	184.72 (160.23–214.95)	
Gestational age at parturition (days)			
Mean (± SD)	257 (26)	256 (14)	0.33
Median (IQR)	266 (252–270)	260 (243–267)	
Newborn weight (gram)			
Mean (± SD)	2935 (945)	2889 (644)	0.89
Median (IQR)	3170 (2570–3505)	2915 (2303–3448)	

an established screening method for determining which women are at risk of GDM, lacks sensitivity and specificity [10, 11]. Therefore, new and effective screening and diagnostic tools for GDM are recommended [8].

In the current study, we analysed serum concentrations of afamin in samples collected from 215 pregnant women. Because afamin concentrations are known to increase during the course of pregnancy [17] and depend

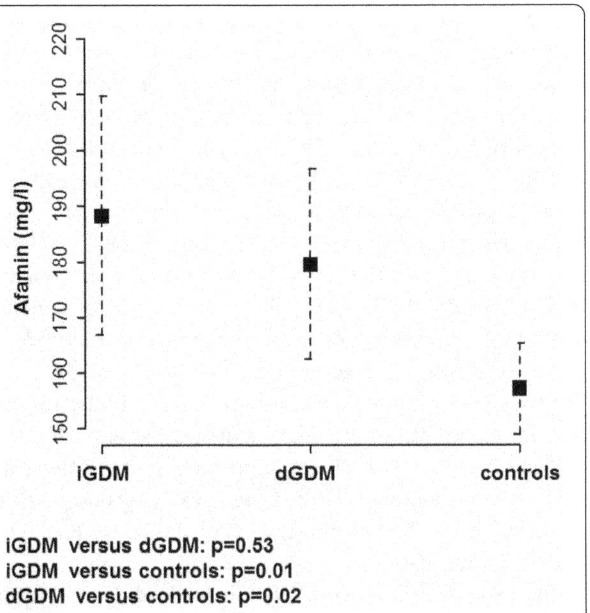

Fig. 2 Afamin concentrations in the mid-trimester cohort (between gestational day 44 and 272). Serum concentrations of afamin among patients with gestational diabetes mellitus (GDM) treated with insulin (iGDM; $n = 12$), treated with dietary intervention (dGDM; $n = 17$) and control subjects ($n = 76$) adjusted for gestational age and body-mass-index (BMI)

on BMI [18], we adjusted the analysis for gestational age and BMI. Women which developed GDM presented with significantly higher afamin concentrations during the first trimester than patients without GDM in their ongoing pregnancy.

Women with subsequent iGDM presented higher serum afamin concentrations during the first trimester than women with subsequent dGDM or women free of GDM. Women which developed dGDM showed only slightly higher afamin levels in the first trimester compared to women free of GDM. Since in the first trimester cohort the blood samples were secondarily collected in a prospective observational study between 2003 and 2014, not all of the participants received a 75 g-OGTT because in Germany, 75 g-OGTT was only recommended in pregnant women at elevated risk for GDM or with a pathological 50 g-OGTT until 2017. Therefore, patients with undiagnosed GDM may be part of the control cohort. This may explain the comparable results in the control and the dGDM group. In the cohort of GDM patients who had confirmed GDM, however, a significant difference in afamin concentrations was found between patients with iGDM and patients who did not need insulin therapy.

In a mid-trimester cohort we evaluated cross-sectionally the ability of serum afamin concentrations to predict pathological results from a 75-g OGTT. We analyzed serum afamin concentrations among 105 patients undergoing 75-g OGTT with a median gestational age of 26th weeks of pregnancy. We found that serum afamin concentrations were significantly higher among patients with pathological findings by OGTT than among control subjects.

Additionally, serum afamin concentrations, determined when the 75 g-OGTT was performed, were higher among iGDM than among dGDM patients without reaching statistical significance. This is in contrast to the results from the first trimester group, but may be due to the smaller subgroups. We also determined HOMA-IR in the subgroups since afamin levels are known to correlate with HOMA-IR [18, 20]. The HOMA-IR was also significantly higher among patients with pathological OGTT. HOMA-IR differed significantly between iGDM patients and controls and between iGDM patients and dGDM patients, but no difference was observed between patients with dGDM compared to controls. This is in contrast to the result of a significant difference in afamin values between dGDM patients and controls. However, the study design was not suitable to compare the diagnostic accuracy of HOMA-IR and afamin values to predict insulin dependence. Further research with a larger sample size is recommended to explore the role of afamin concentrations, the HOMA-IR or the combination of both parameters in the prediction of iGDM or dGDM in the second trimester.

Because afamin concentrations increase during the course of uncomplicated pregnancies [17] and because OGTT is a test routinely performed between 24 and 28 weeks of gestation, our study design could not determine a cut-off value indicating pathological conditions that exactly corresponded with gestational age.

In all investigated subgroups, including individuals with uncomplicated pregnancies, we found surprisingly high concentrations of afamin, considerably higher than those measured in the general population and pregnant women from other ethnic origins [15, 17]. The ethnic background seems to play a (not yet widely investigated) role in determining afamin concentrations since a previous study from individuals from the same regional origin had also markedly higher average afamin concentrations compared to previously published work analyzing afamin concentrations from different regions [20].

Afamin is known as an indicator of oxidative stress [18]. Oxidative stress itself is strongly associated with IR and with obesity [28, 29]. Previous studies have shown that higher serum concentrations of afamin are associated with IR and with elevated glucose concentrations [18–20]. During pregnancy, the severity of IR increases with ongoing gestational age [30]. The physiological role of the decrease in insulin sensitivity appears to be the appropriate materno-fetal transfer of glucose. Interestingly, IR increases similarly in every woman independent of preconception IR or obesity [22]. As a consequence, women with elevated IR concentrations before conception experience pathologic glucose metabolism during pregnancy, and this condition results in pathologic materno-fetal glucose transfer followed by adverse pregnancy outcomes. Mediators of the increasing severity of IR are produced by the placenta [31]. As shown by Kirwan et al. [32], tumor necrosis factor alpha (TNF-α) plays the most important role in physiologic IR. Adipose tissue produces a cytokine pattern nearly identical to that of the placenta [33]. This condition explains the fact that obese women are at higher risk of GDM. However, concentrations of mediators of IR, such as TNF-α, are also known to be increased during conditions of oxidative stress [34]. TNF-α itself inhibits insulin activity [35]. A well-known condition of IR associated with the presence of mediators of oxidative stress is PCOS [34, 36]. With regard to the association between oxidative stress and glucose metabolism, afamin concentrations seem to indicate the presence of IR among PCOS patients, as we have previously shown [20].

The present study showed that afamin concentrations are significantly higher among pregnant patients with pathological findings of 75-g OGTT. Increased afamin concentrations during the first trimester also indicated the development of iGDM. Afamin seems to be able to early predict a pathologic glucose metabolism during pregnancy. In accordance with the pathomechanisms of GDM, serum afamin concentrations probably reflect situations in which increased IR and oxidative stress result in GDM. The finding that afamin concentrations are higher among iGDM patients than among dGDM patients indicates that high afamin concentrations are also associated with increased severity of IR.

Because tests for serum afamin concentrations do not require the patient to be in a fasting state, these concentrations are very suitable as a biomarker of GDM [15, 16]. Until 2017, the 50-g OGTT was established as a screening method for GDM [6, 9]. In addition to limitations in the accuracy of results from this test, the test also requires a high level of personal and standardized procedures. This may be one reason why this method was not routinely integrated into maternal care in Germany before 2013 [8].

In accordance with the recommendations of the IADPSG in searching for "simpler and more cost-effective strategies that do not require performing an OGTT," serum afamin concentrations may be a very suitable and easily applicable biomarker that can be used to diagnose patients for GDM during the second trimester of pregnancy or even to screen patients in high risk to develop GDM as early as possible during the first trimester.

However, the use of serum afamin concentrations has also limitations. Because high afamin concentrations indicate IR, the results may be non-specific in detecting GDM. Other conditions, such as preeclampsia [17] or preterm labor, are also associated with IR [37, 38]. Furthermore, the first trimester part of the current study may also have limitations: screening for GDM with a 50 g- or 75 g-OGTT was not a standard procedure in Germany before 2013. Therefore, the control group in our first-trimester cohort consisted of patients without GDM diagnosis at birth according to currently available guidelines, but undiagnosed GDM cannot be completely excluded. In 2005, the prevalence of GDM was 2.5% and in 2015, it was 13.2% [39]. This increased prevalence is most likely a consequence of the changed methods of GDM screening and reflects the situation in Germany. For these reasons, we did not determine a first-trimester afamin cut-off value that distinguishes patients developing GDM or not in their ongoing pregnancy in this pilot study. Additionally, we performed no subgroup analysis to the slightly differing thresholds of the 75 g-OGTT before and after 2011.

The cross-sectional part of our study did not require administration of the OGTT at the identical gestational age for every patient. Our analysis of afamin concentrations was adjusted for gestational age because afamin concentrations increase during the course of pregnancy, but our study design did not allow us to determine cut-off values for each gestational week. The mean gestational age at parturition was 36 weeks indicating the high-risk group. However, this is a pilot study presenting first data of afamin concentrations in correlation with pathological 75 g OGTT.

Conclusion

This study demonstrates a statistically significant difference between afamin serum concentrations in pregnant women with pathologic OGTT results and those with normal 75-g OGTT in the second trimester. Patients with GDM requiring insulin showed slightly higher afamin serum concentrations as patients treated with diet. These findings were also observed in blood samples collected in the first trimester of women developing GDM during their ongoing pregnancy. Patients with subsequent iGDM in their later pregnancy exhibited higher afamin concentrations during the first trimester than women free of GDM or women with later GDM not requirering insulin therapy.

Afamin indicates IR, the pathophysiological key mechanism underlying GDM, which is linked to oxidative stress. The results of this pilot study indicate a promising role of a novel biomarker for pathological glucose metabolism in pregnancy.

Further research is recommended for determining afamin concentrations prospectively during the first trimester of pregnancy and correlating them with the results of 75-g OGTT during the second trimester. Additionally, studies involving larger populations are recommended for determining whether afamin concentrations are superior to the 50-g OGTT as a screening test that can determine which women are at high risk of GDM. An interesting question that remains unanswered is whether elevated mid-trimester serum concentrations of afamin are associated with adverse pregnancy outcomes. Future research is warranted in this area and may have an impact on how we manage pregnancies at risk to develop GDM.

Abbreviations

CI: Confidence interval; DDG: Deutsche Diabetesgesellschaft; dGDM: Gestational diabetes mellitus treated with diet; DGGG: Deutsche Gesellschaft für Gynäkologie und Geburtshilfe; GDM: Gestational diabetes mellitus; HOMA: Homeostasis-Model Assessment; IADPSG: International Association of the Diabetes and Pregnancy Study Groups; iGDM: Insulin dependent gestational diabetes mellitus; IQR: Interquartile range; IR: Insulin resistance; OGTT: Oral glucose tolerance test; PCOS: Polycystic ovary syndrome; SHBG: Sexual hormone binding protein; TNF: Tumor-necrosis-factor

Acknowledgments

We thank the laboratory staff members Sieglinde Arndt, Ute Kirsch, Claudine Kühn, Jens Rasch, Gabriele Sehn and our nurses for technical assistance and data documentation. We are grateful to Dr. Florence Witte for English editing and critical reading of the manuscript.

Funding

Provided by the University of Duisburg-Essen to A.K. and the Austrian Research Fund (P19969-B11) to H.D.

Authors' contributions

AK, AM and HD substantially contributed to the study's conception and design, to acquisition and interpretation of data, drafting the manuscript and final approval of the version to be published. RK and AG substantially contributed to acquisition of data, revising the manuscript critically for important intellectual content and final approval of the version to be published. PM, MF, BS and FS substantially contributed to the analysis and interpretation of data, drafting the manuscript, revising it critically for important intellectual content and final approval of the version to be published.

Competing interests

Dr. Dieplinger is owner and shareholder of Vitateq Biotechnology GmbH, a spin-off company of the Medical University of Innsbruck, holding several patents related to research described in this article. All other authors disclose no conflicts of interest.

Author details

[1]Department of Gynecology and Obstetrics, University of Duisburg-Essen, Hufelandstrasse 55, 45122 Essen, Germany. [2]Department of Gynecology and Obstetrics, Klinikum Würzburg Mitte, Salvatorstrasse 7, 97074 Würzburg, Germany. [3]Institute for Medical Informatics, Biometry and Epidemiology (IMIBE), University of Duisburg-Essen, Hufelandstrasse 55, 45122 Essen, Germany. [4]Department of Obstetrics, Jena University Hospital, Am Klinikum 1, 07747 Jena, Germany. [5]Division of Genetic Epidemiology, Department of Medical Genetics, Molecular and Clinical Pharmacology, Medical University of Innsbruck, Schöpfstrasse 41, 6020 Innsbruck, Austria. [6]Vitateq Biotechnology GmbH, 6020 Innsbruck, Austria.

Germany. [4]Department of Obstetrics, Jena University Hospital, Am Klinikum 1, 07747 Jena, Germany. [5]Division of Genetic Epidemiology, Department of Medical Genetics, Molecular and Clinical Pharmacology, Medical University of Innsbruck, Schöpfstrasse 41, 6020 Innsbruck, Austria. [6]Vitateq Biotechnology GmbH, 6020 Innsbruck, Austria.

References

1. Hunt KJ, Schuller KL. The increasing prevalence of diabetes in pregnancy. Obstet Gynecol Clin N Am. 2007;34(2):173–99. vii
2. American Diabetes Association. Diagnosis and classification of diabetes mellitus. Diabetes Care. 2009;32(Suppl 1):S62–7.
3. Koning SH, Hoogenberg K, Lutgers HL, van den Berg PP, Wolffenbuttel BH. Gestational diabetes mellitus: current knowledge and unmet needs. J Diabetes. 2016;8(6):770–81.
4. HAPO Study Cooperative Research Group, Metzger BE, Lowe LP, Dyer AR, Trimble ER, Chaovarindr U, Coustan DR, Hadden DR, McCance DR, Hod M, McIntyre HD, Oats JJ, Persson B, Rogers MS, Sacks DA. Hyperglycemia and adverse pregnancy outcomes. N Engl J Med. 2008;358(19):1991–2002.
5. Waters TP, Dyer AR, Scholtens DM, Dooley SL, Herer E, Lowe LP, Oats JJ, Persson B, Sacks DA, Metzger BE, Catalano PM. HAPO cooperative study research group. Maternal and neonatal morbidity for women who would be added to the diagnosis of GDM using IADPSG criteria: a secondary analysis of the hyperglycemia and adverse pregnancy outcome study. Diabetes Care. 2016;39(12):2204–10.
6. Landon MB, Spong CY, Thom E, Carpenter MW, Ramin SM, Casey B, Wapner RJ, Varner MW, Rouse DJ, Thorp JM Jr, Sciscione a, Catalano P, harper M, Saade G, lain KY, Sorokin Y, Peaceman AM, Tolosa JE, Anderson GB. Eunice Kennedy Shriver National Institute of Child Health and Human Development maternal-fetal medicine units network. A multicenter, randomized trial of treatment for mild gestational diabetes. N Engl J Med. 2009;361(14):1339–48.
7. Crowther CA, Hiller JE, Moss JR, McPhee AJ, Jeffries WS, Robinson JS. Australian carbohydrate intolerance study in pregnant women (ACHOIS) trial group. Effect of treatment of gestational diabetes mellitus on pregnancy outcomes. N Engl J Med. 2005;352(24):2477–86.
8. International Association of Diabetes and Pregnancy Study Groups Consensus Panel, Metzger BE, Gabbe SG, Persson B, Buchanan TA, Catalano PA, Damm P, dyer AR, Leiva a, Hod M, Kitzmiler JL, Lowe LP, McIntyre HD, oats JJ, Omori Y, Schmidt MI. International association of diabetes and pregnancy study groups recommendations on the diagnosis and classification of hyperglycemia in pregnancy. Diabetes Care. 2010;33(3):676–82.
9. Kleinwechter H, Schäfer-Graf U, Bührer C, Hoesli I, Kainer F, Kautzky-Willer A, Pawlowski B, Schunck K, Somville T, Sorger M. German diabetes association; German Association for Gynaecology and Obstetrics. Gestational diabetes mellitus (GDM) diagnosis, therapy and follow-up care: practice guideline of the German diabetes association (DDG) and the German Association for Gynaecology and Obstetrics (DGGG). Exp Clin Endocrinol Diabetes. 2014;122(7):395–405.
10. Lewis GF, McNally C, Blackman JD, Polonsky KS, Barron WM. Prior feeding alters the response to the 50-g glucose challenge test in pregnancy. The Staub-Traugott effect revisited. Diabetes Care. 1993;16:1551–6.
11. Sacks DA, Abu-Fadil S, Greenspoon JS, Fotheringham N. How reliable is the fifty-gram, one-hour glucose screening test? Am J Obstet Gynecol. 1989;161(3):642–5.
12. Voegele AF, Jerković L, Wellenzohn B, Eller P, Kronenberg F, Liedl KR, Dieplinger H. Characterization of the vitamin E-binding properties of human plasma afamin. Biochemistry. 2002;41:14532–8.
13. Lichenstein HS, Lyons DE, Wurfel MM, Johnson DA, McGinley MD, Leidli JC, Trollinger DB, Mayer JP, Wright SD, Zukowski MM. Afamin is a new member of the albumin, alpha-fetoprotein, and vitamin D-binding protein gene family. J Biol Chem. 1994;269(27):18149–54.
14. Heiser M, Hutter-Paier B, Jerkovic L, Pfragner R, Windisch M, Becker-André M, Dieplinger H. Vitamin E binding protein afamin protects neuronal cells in vitro. J Neural Transm Suppl. 2002;62:337–45.
15. Dieplinger B, Egger M, Gabriel C, Poelz W, Morandell E, Seeber B, Kronenberg F, Haltmayer M, Mueller T, Dieplinger H. Analytical characterization and clinical evaluation of an enzyme-linked immunosorbent assay for measurement of afamin in human plasma. Clin Chim Acta. 2013;425:236–41.
16. Dieplinger H, Dieplinger B. Afamin–a pleiotropic glycoprotein involved in various disease states. Clin Chim Acta. 2015;446:105–10.
17. Hubalek M, Buchner H, Mörtl MG, Schlembach D, Huppertz B, Firulovic B, Köhler W, Hafner E, Dieplinger B, Wildt L, Dieplinger H. The vitamin E-binding protein afamin increases in maternal serum during pregnancy. Clin Chim Acta. 2014;434:41–7.
18. Kronenberg F, Kollerits B, Kiechl S, Lamina C, Kedenko L, Meisinger C, Willeit J, Huth C, Wietzorrek G, Altmann ME, Thorand B, Melmer A, Dähnhardt D, Santer P, Rathmann W, Paulweber B, Koenig W, Peters A, Adham IM, Dieplinger H. Plasma concentrations of afamin are associated with the prevalence and development of metabolic syndrome. Circ Cardiovasc Genet. 2014;7(6):822–9.

19. Kollerits B, Lamina C, Huth C, Marques-Vidal P, Kiechl S, Seppälä I, Cooper J, Hunt SC, Meisinger C, Herder C, Kedenko L, Willeit J, Thorand B, Dähnhardt D, Stöckl D, Willeit K, Roden M, Rathmann W, Paulweber B, Peters A, Kähönen M, Lehtimäki T, Raitakari OT, Humphries SE, Vollenweider P, Dieplinger H, Kronenberg F. Plasma concentrations of afamin are associated with prevalent and incident type 2 diabetes: a pooled analysis in more than 20,000 individuals. Diabetes Care. 2017;40(10):1386–93.
20. Köninger A, Edimiris P, Koch L, Enekwe A, Lamina C, Kasimir-Bauer S, Kimmig R, Dieplinger H. Serum concentrations of afamin are elevated in patients with polycystic ovary syndrome. Endocr Connect. 2014;3(3):120–6.
21. Matthews DR, Hosker JP, Rudenski AS, Naylor BA, Treacher DF, Turner RC. Homeostasis model assessment: insulin resistance and beta-cell function from fasting plasma glucose and insulin concentrations in man. Diabetologia. 1985;28(7):412–9.
22. Catalano PM, Huston L, Amini SB, Kalhan SC. Longitudinal changes in glucose metabolism during pregnancy in obese women with normal glucose tolerance and gestational diagetes mellitus. Am J Obstet Gynecol. 1999;180(4):903–16.
23. Plymate SR, Matej LA, Jones RE, Friedl KE. Inhibition of sex hormone-binding globulin production in the human hepatoma (Hep G2) cell line by insulin and prolactin. J Clin Endocrinol Metab. 1988;67(3):460–4.
24. Thériault S, Giguère Y, Massé J, Girouard J, Forest JC. Early prediction of gestational diabetes: a practical model combining clinical and biochemical markers. Clin Chem Lab Med. 2016;54(3):509–18.
25. Azziz R, Woods KS, Reyna R, Key TJ, Knochenhauer ES, Yildiz BO. The prevalence and features of the polycystic ovary syndrome in an unselected population. J Clin Endocrinol Metab. 2004;89:2745–9.
26. Carpenter MW, Coustan DR. Criteria for screening tests for gestational diabetes. Am J Obstet Gynecol. 1982;144(7):768–73.
27. R Core Team. R: A language and environment for statistical computing. R Foundation for Statistical Computing, Vienna, Austria; 2014. http://www.R-project.org/. Last accessed 30 Nov 2016.
28. González F, Rote NS, Minium J, Kirwan JP. Increased activation of nuclear factor kappaB triggers inflammation and insulin resistance in polycystic ovary syndrome. J Clin Endocrinol Metab. 2006;91:1508–12.
29. González F, Rote NS, Minium J, Kirwan JP. Reactive oxygen species-induced oxidative stress in the development of insulin resistance and hyperandrogenism in polycystic ovary syndrome. J Clin Endocrinol Metab. 2006;91:336–40.
30. Catalano PM, Tyzbir ED, Wolfe RR, Calles J, Roman NM, Amini SB, Sims EA. Carbohydrate metabolism during pregnancy in control subjects and women with gestational diabetes. Am J Phys. 1993;264(1 Pt 1):E60–7.
31. Yamashita H, Shao J, Friedman JE. Physiologic and molecular alterations in carbohydrate metabolism during pregnancy and gestational diabetes mellitus. Clin Obstet Gynecol. 2000;43(1):87–98.
32. Kirwan JP, Hauguel-De Mouzon S, Lepercq J, Challier JC, Huston-Presley L, Friedman JE, Kalhan SC, Catalano PM. TNF-alpha is a predictor of insulin resistance in human pregnancy. Diabetes. 2002;51(7):2207–13.
33. Hauguel-de Mouzon S, Guerre-Millo M. The placenta cytokine network and inflammatory signals. Placenta. 2006;27(8):794–8.
34. González F, Sia CL, Shepard MK, Rote NS, Minium J. Inflammation in response to glucose ingestion is independent of excess abdominal adiposity in normal-weight women with polycystic ovary syndrome. J Clin Endocrinol Metab. 2012;97(11):4071–9. 31
35. Hotamisligil GS, Murray DL, Choy LN, Spiegelman BM. Tumor necrosis factor alpha inhibits signaling from the insulin receptor. Proc Natl Acad Sci U S A. 1994;91(11):4854–8.
36. Diamanti-Kandarakis E, Piouka A, Livadas S, Piperi C, Katsikis I, Papavassiliou AG, Panidis D. Anti-mullerian hormone is associated with advanced glycosylated end products in lean women with polycystic ovary syndrome. Eur J Endocrinol. 2009;160:847–53.
37. Anim-Nyame N, Sooranna SR, Jones J, Alaghband-Zadeh J, Steer PJ, Johnson MR. Insulin resistance and pre-eclampsia: a role for tumor necrosis factor-alpha? Gynecol Endocrinol. 2004;18(3):117–23.
38. Abhari FR, Ghanbari Andarieh M, Farokhfar A, Ahmady S. Estimating rate of insulin resistance in patients with preeclampsia using HOMA-IR index and comparison with nonpreeclampsia pregnant women. Biomed Res Int. 2014;2014:140851.
39. Melchior H, Kurch-Bek D, Mund M. The prevalence of gestational diabetes: a population-based analysis of a Nationwide screening program. A population-based analysis of a nationwide screening program. Dtsch Arztebl Int. 2017;114(24):412–8.

7

Progestin-primed milder stimulation with clomiphene citrate yields fewer oocytes and suboptimal pregnancy outcomes compared with the standard progestin-primed ovarian stimulation in infertile women with polycystic ovarian syndrome

Hongjuan Ye[1*], Hui Tian[1], Wen He[2], Qifeng Lyu[2], Yanping Kuang[2], Qiuju Chen[2*] and Lihua Sun[1*]

Abstract

Background: Oral progestin has recently been used to prevent premature LH surges in ovarian stimulation, and this progestin-primed ovarian stimulation (PPOS) is effective and safe in patients with different ovarian reserves. The current data are lacking regarding how to individualize the gonadotropin dose and regimen for women with polycystic ovarian syndrome (PCOS). A retrospective cohort trial was performed to evaluate the efficacy of progestin-primed milder stimulation with clomiphene citrate (CC) compared to the standard progestin-primed ovarian stimulation (PPOS) protocol for infertile women with PCOS.

Methods: A total of 220 PCOS women were collected and classified into the study group (HMG 150 IU/d + CC 50 mg/d + MPA 10 mg/d) and control group (HMG 225 IU/d + MPA 10 mg/d). Ovulation was triggered by GnRH agonist 0.1 mg and hCG 1000 IU when dominant follicles matured. Viable embryos were cryopreserved for later transfer. The primary endpoint was the ongoing pregnancy rate. Secondary outcomes included the cycle characteristics and the live birth rate.

Result(s): The study group consumed less HMG (1470.0 ± 360.1 IU vs 1943.8 ± 372.0 IU, $P < 0.001$) and harvested fewer oocytes than the control group (12.2 ± 7.4 vs 18.2 ± 9.7, $P < 0.001$). The study group showed a higher mid-follicular LH concentration (4.49 ± 2.49 mIU/ml vs 2.52 ± 2.09 mIU/ml, $P < 0.05$) but no endogenous LH surge. No between-group difference was found in the incidence of ovarian hyperstimulation syndrome (OHSS) (0.91% vs 0.91%, $P > 0.05$). The cumulative ongoing pregnancy rate and live birth rate per patient were lower but did not reach significance compared with the control group (71.8% vs 81.8 and 64.5% vs 75.5%, respectively, both $P > 0.05$).

(Continued on next page)

* Correspondence: yehongjuan7777@163.com; chenqj75@126.com; lihua-sun@163.com
[1]Centre of assisted reproduction, Shanghai East Hospital, Tongji University, Shanghai, People's Republic of China
[2]Department of Assisted Reproduction, Shanghai Ninth People's Hospital, Shanghai Jiaotong University School of Medicine, Shanghai, People's Republic of China

(Continued from previous page)
Conclusion(s): The milder PPOS with CC in PCOS women led to lower oocyte yields and suboptimal pregnancy outcomes compared to the standard PPOS treatment. The two regimens both achieved a low incidence of OHSS. The results from the CC combination regimen provide a new insight for developing a more patient-friendly protocol for PCOS women.

Keywords: Polycystic ovarian syndrome, Progestin-primed ovarian stimulation, Clomiphene citrate, In vitro fertilization, Freeze-only

Background

Polycystic ovarian syndrome (PCOS) is an endocrine disorder affecting 5–10% of reproductive-age women worldwide [1]. Approximately 74% of women with PCOS seeks pregnancy assistance, including induced ovulation, insemination or in vitro fertilization (IVF) [2]. However, PCOS women undergoing IVF treatment typically produce an increased number of oocytes, which are often of poor quality, leading to a lower fertilization rate and a higher miscarriage rate [3]. They also face a higher risk of moderate/severe ovarian hyperstimulation syndrome (OHSS) [4, 5].

Thanks to the progress of vitrification, oral progestin has been successfully used to prevent premature LH surges in women undergoing ovarian stimulation [6–8]. This progestin-primed ovarian stimulation (PPOS) yields a comparable pregnancy outcome, although it consumes a slightly higher gonadotropin dosage than conventional short protocols [6]. PPOS is approved its efficacy and safety in the population of low-ovarian-reserve, normal-ovarian-reserve and PCOS women [8–10], so PPOS in combination with a freeze-only policy shows good potential to compete with conventional protocols. The existing data from clinical trials often use the equal initiating doses of gonadotropin for women with or without PCOS, but relevant data are lacking about how to individualize the gonadotropin dose and regimen for PCOS women undergoing ovarian stimulation.

Clomiphene citrate (CC) has been a first-line drug for ovulation induction for anovulatory infertility. Its advantages include its oral route, low costs and easy access compared to gonadotropins [11, 12]. CC is also used in GnRH antagonist protocols, and the combination of CC and GnRH antagonist is likely to reduce the risk of OHSS, medication costs and gonadotropin duration compared to those without CC, but it accompanies with an increased risk of premature LH surges [13–15]. Limited data are available about the role of CC in PPOS for PCOS women [16]. In this trial, we attempted to test the hypothesis that in women with PCOS, the milder stimulation of PPOS in combination with CC would provide an acceptable clinical outcome compared with standard PPOS protocol using conventional initiating dose of gonadotropin. Our ultimate aim was to optimize the PPOS protocol and make it more patient-friendly.

Methods

Study setting and subjects

A retrospective cohort trial was conducted at the department of assisted reproduction of the Ninth People's Hospital of Shanghai Jiaotong University School of Medicine. This study was approval by the Ethics Committee (Institutional Review Board) of Shanghai Ninth People's Hospital. The PCOS diagnosis criteria followed the Rotterdam consensus. PCOS was diagnosed by the presence of menstrual disturbance combined with either hyperandrogenism (hirsutism or hyperandrogenaemia) or polycystic ovary on ultrasonography (defined as an ovary that contained ≥12 antral follicles) and excluded other causes of hyperandrogenism (congenital adrenal hyperplasia, Cushing's syndrome, androgen-producing tumours) and ovulation dysfunction (hyperprolactinaemia and thyroid dysfunction). In addition, this study only included women no more than 40 years of age and with baseline serum FSH no more than 10 mIU/ml. Women with functional cysts on the ovaries or medical conditions that contraindicated assisted reproductive technology and/or pregnancy were excluded. A total of 220 infertile women with PCOS from April 2014 to November 2015 were included and classified into the study group (HMG + MPA + CC) and the control group (HMG + MPA). A flowchart of the study is shown in Fig. 1.

Ovarian stimulation protocol

In the study group, a low dose of HMG (150 IU daily), CC 50 mg and MPA 10 mg daily were started from cycle day 3 or after an episode of withdrawal bleeding. MPA was used to prevent premature ovulation during the ovarian stimulation. Follicle monitoring by transvaginal ultrasound and serum hormone measurements (FSH, LH, E_2 and progesterone) were performed 5 days later. HMG doses were then adjusted according to the ovarian response (range 150–300 IU daily). Oocyte maturation was triggered by triptorelin 0.1 mg (Decapeptyl, Ferring Pharmaceuticals, Germany) and urinary human chorionic gonadotropin (hCG 1000 IU, Lizhu Pharmaceutical Trading Co., China) when at least three follicles reached diameters of 18 mm or more. Cumulus oocyte complexes were collected 36 h later. All follicles larger than 10 mm in diameter were aspirated.

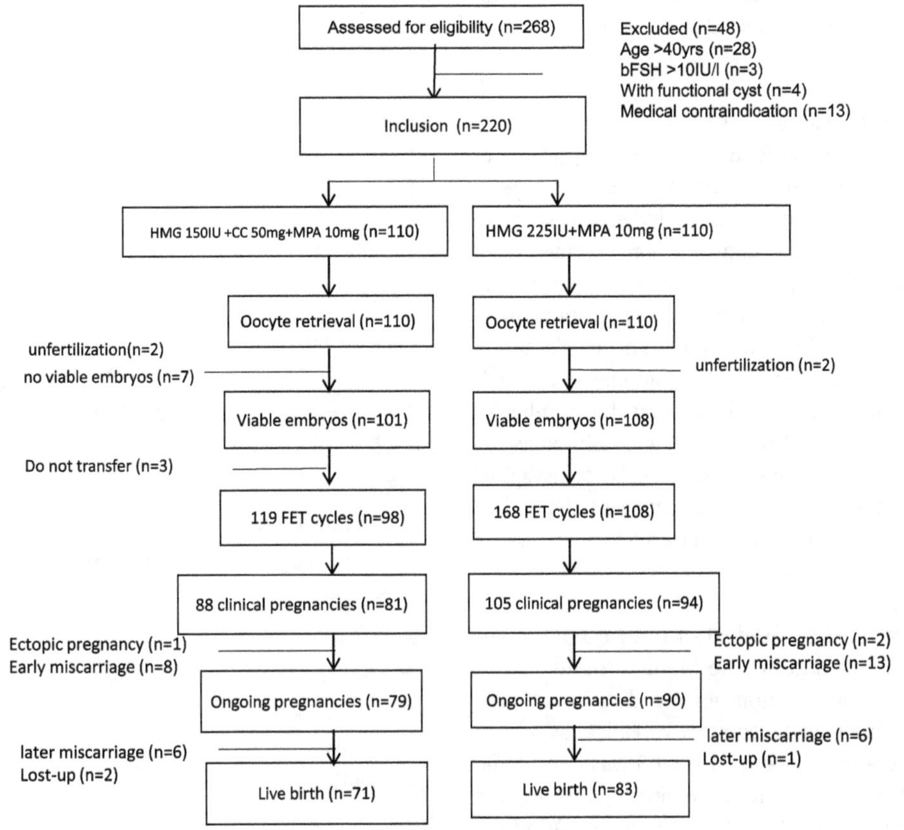

Fig. 1 Study flowchart

In the control group, HMG 225 IU and MPA 10 mg daily were initiated from cycle day 3 or after an episode of withdrawal bleeding. Follicle monitor and hormone assay were performed 5 days later. HMG dose was then adjusted according to the ovarian response, and MPA dose was consistent up to the trigger day. The criteria of mature follicle and the trigger methods were the same as above.

Fertilization was carried out in vitro after oocyte retrieval depending on the semen parameters and previous fertilization situation. Embryos were examined for the number or regularity of blastomeres and the degree of fragmentation. All top-quality cleavage-stage embryos (grade 1 and grade 2, 6-cell embryos and above) were frozen within three days after oocyte retrieval. The non-top-quality embryos were placed in further extended culture, and good-morphology blastocysts were frozen. Cleavage-stage embryos and blastocysts were frozen by vitrification as described previously [17].

Endometrium preparation and FET

Endometrium preparation for FET was arranged on the second cycle after oocyte retrieval. The first choice was using a letrozole-induced- ovulation cycle. Letrozole 5 mg was administered for 5 days, and then, follicle growth was monitored beginning on day 10. At times, a low dose of HMG (75 IU/day) was used to stimulate follicle growth and endometrial lining. The timing of FET was performed 4 or 5 days later, after a spontaneous or hCG-induced LH surge. Hormone replacement treatment was recommended for patients with thin endometrium and patients in whom letrozole failed. Oral ethinyl oestradiol 75 mcg/day was administered from cycle day 3 onwards. Once the endometrial lining was > 8 mm thick, femoston (Solvay Pharmaceuticals B.V.) 8 mg/day was started. The time of thawing and transfer was determined on the third day after femoston administration [17]. Each patient received no more than two embryos at one time. Once pregnancy was achieved, the luteal support was continued until 10 weeks of gestation.

Hormone measurement

Serum FSH, LH, E_2, and progesterone were measured on menstrual cycle day 3, day 8–11 (after 5–7 days of stimulation), the trigger day and the day after trigger. Hormone levels were determined with chemiluminescence (Abbott Biological B.V. Netherlands). The lower limits of sensitivity were as follow: FSH 0.06 mIU/ml, LH 0.09 mIU/ml, E_2 10 pg/ml and progesterone 0.1 ng/ml. The upper limit of E_2 measurement was 5000 pg/ml. If serum E_2 on the trigger day or the day after was higher than the upper limit, it was recorded as 5000 pg/ml.

Outcome variables

The primary measure analysed was the cumulative ongoing pregnancy rate, which was defined as the proportion of patients with ongoing pregnancy after the gestation age of 12 weeks. The secondary measures included the stimulation duration, gonadotropin consumption, incidence of premature LH surge and OHSS, the number of oocytes retrieved, the number of viable embryos, the proportion of mature oocytes and the live birth rate. The implantation rate was calculated as the number of gestational sacs visualized on transvaginal ultrasound divided by the number of transferred embryos. Clinical pregnancy was defined as the presence of foetal cardiac activity confirmed by transvaginal ultrasound. The cumulative live birth rate was defined as the total number of live births divided by all participants.

Statistical analysis

The data were evaluated by Student's t-test for continuous variables of normal distribution, the Mann-Whitney U-test for continuous variables of non-normal distribution, the x^2-test or Fisher's exact for categorical variables, as appropriate. All tests were two-sided, and $P < .05$ was considered statistically significant. All data were analysed using the Statistical Package for the Social Sciences for Windows (SPSS, version 19).

Results

Patient characteristics

The basal demographical and hormonal characteristics are shown in Table 1. A total of 220 patients completed this trial. There were no significant between-group differences in age, body mass index (BMI), previous IVF failures, infertility duration, menstrual cycle, indication for IVF or basal hormonal profile. All women completed one oocyte retrieval cycle, 208 patients had 1–15 viable embryos harvested, and 12 cases were cancelled before transfer due to either non-fertilization or no transferrable embryos. A total of 205 women completed 287 FET cycles in the following two years.

Ovarian stimulation, follicle development, and oocyte performance

Clinical and cycle characteristics of ovarian stimulation in both groups are shown in Table 2. The study group (HMG + MPA + CC protocol) had a similar stimulation duration (9.2 ± 1.3 days vs 9.1 ± 1.2 days, $P > 0.05$) and consumed less HMG (1470.0 ± 360.1 IU vs 1943.8 ± 372.0 IU, $P < 0.05$). The numbers of oocytes retrieved, MII oocytes, and fertilized oocytes in the study group were significantly lower than those in the control group ($P < 0.05$). Consequently, the number of viable embryos in the study group was significantly lower than in the control group (4.8 ± 3.5 vs. 6.2 ± 3.7, $P < 0.05$). No between-group differences were found in the oocyte retrieval rate, but the maturation rate and the proportion of viable embryos per oocyte retrieved were better in the study group (respectively, 87.4% vs 80.3 and 39.5% vs 34.0%, both $P < 0.05$). The cycle cancellation due to zero viable embryos was significantly higher in the study group (9.1% vs 1.8%, $P < 0.05$). One patient experienced moderate or severe OHSS in each group ($P > 0.05$).

Table 1 The basic characteristics of PCOS women in this trial

	Study group (HMG + MPA + CC; *n* = 110)	Control group (HMG + MPA; *n* = 110)
Age (y)	30.5 ± 3.7	30.6 ± 3.4
Duration of infertility (y),	3.5 ± 2.6	3.9 ± 2.3
BMI (kg/m^2) n (%)		
19~ 24.9	80(72.7%)	81(73.6%)
25~ 29.9	25(22.7%)	24(21.8%)
> =30	5(4.5%)	5(4.5%)
Previous IVF failures, n(%)		
0	89(80.9%)	88(80.8%)
1–3	21(19.1%)	22(19.2%)
Indication for IVF n (%)		
PCOS only	27(24.5%)	30(27.3%)
PCOS+ male factor	21(19.1%)	25(22.7%)
PCOS+ tubal factor	52(52.7%)	49(44.5%)
PCOS+ other	4(3.6%)	6(5.5%)
Menstrual cycle n (%)		
Regular	3(2.1%)	3(2.7%)
Oligomenorrhea	82(74.5%)	91(82.7%)
Amenorrhea	25(22.7%)	16(14.5%)
Antral follicle counts	17.9 ± 6.3	18.8 ± 7.1
Baseline hormones		
FSH (mIU/ml)	4.94 ± 1.10	5.0 ± 1.17
LH (mIU/ml)	5.03 ± 3.18	5.61 ± 3.36
E_2(pg/ml)	32.54 ± 10.34	30.32 ± 12.52
P(ng/ml)	0.26 ± 0.19	0.27 ± 0.19
T (ng/ml)	0.35 ± 0.13	0.40 ± 0.19

No significant difference was found between the two groups ($P > 0.05$)

Hormone profile during treatment

The serum concentrations of FSH, LH, E_2 and P in the two groups are presented in Fig. 2. FSH in the study group was slightly lower than in the control group during the mid-follicular phase ($P < 0.05$). LH gradually decreased during ovarian stimulation in the control group; in contrast, LH in the study group showed a slight rise initially, followed by a downward trend, and the mean

Table 2 The cycle characteristics of controlled ovarian stimulation in the two groups

	Study group (HMG + MPA + CC; *n* = 110)	Control group (HMG + MPA; *n* = 110)	*P* value
hMG doses (IU)	1470.0 ± 360.1	1943.8 ± 372.0	< 0.001
hMG duration (days)	9.2 ± 1.3	9.1 ± 1.2	0.594
No. of > 10 mm follicles on trigger day	17.6 ± 8.4	21.2 ± 8.3	0.001
No. of > 14 mm follicles on trigger day	13.8 ± 8.4	17.2 ± 9.3	0.004
No. of oocytes retrieved(n)	12.2 ± 7.4	18.2 ± 9.7	< 0.001
No. of maturation oocytes (n)	10.7 ± 6.3	14.6 ± 8.2	< 0.001
No. of fertilization (n)	8.6 ± 5.6	12.6 ± 7.7	< 0.001
No. of viable embryos(n)	4.8 ± 3.5	6.2 ± 3.7	0.007
Oocyte retrieval rate (%)	58.8% (1343/2285)	60.1% (2006/3335)	0.302
Oocyte maturation rate (%)	87.4% (1174/1343)	80.3% (1610/2006)	< 0.001
The proportion of viable embryo per oocyte retrieved (%)	39.5% (531/1343)	33.8% (678/2006)	0.001
Cancellation for no viable embryos (%)	9.1% (10/110)	1.8% (2/110)	0.018
Incidence of moderate/severe OHSS (%)	0.91% (1/110)	0.91% (1/110)	1.00

LH value on the trigger day was significantly higher than in the control group (4.49 ± 2.49 mIU/ml vs 2.52 ± 2.09 mIU/ml, $P < 0.05$). No endogenous LH surge occurred in either group ($P > 0.05$). The LH value on the post-trigger day showed a dramatic increase in the two groups, with no between-group difference ($P > 0.05$).

E_2 increased gradually, accompanied by with multiple growing follicles during the ovarian stimulation, and no difference was found between the two groups ($P > 0.05$). The measured E_2 values were underestimated in 114 cases due to the upper limit of 5000 pg/ml, so the comparison of E_2 between the two groups was compromised. Serum P showed a gradual increase during ovarian stimulation and increased significantly after trigger in both groups.

Pregnancy outcomes in FET cycles

The pregnancy outcomes from FET are shown in Table 3. A total of 287 FET cycles were completed in the two groups, including 66 women who finished at least two transfers. The control group yielded more embryos, which were able to finish more FET cycles in the following two years. The mean transfer cycles per patient were 1.5 in the control group and 1.1 in the study group in the following two years. A total of 560 embryos were thawed and the survival rate was 99.3% (556/560). The remnant embryos were, respectively, 350 and 303 in the control and study group, which were the suplus embryos in pregnant cases except for three cases in study group without their transfer.

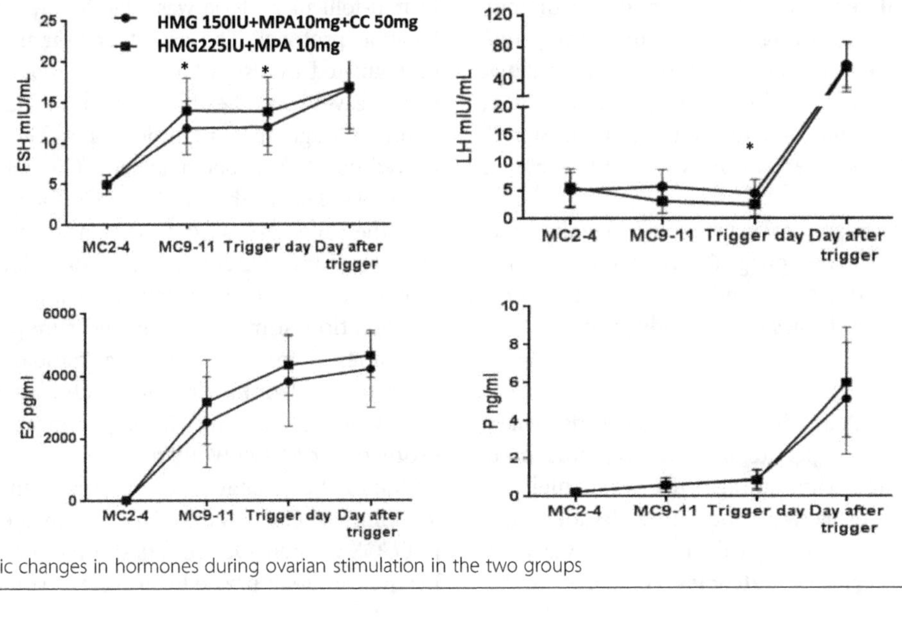

Fig. 2 The dynamic changes in hormones during ovarian stimulation in the two groups

Table 3 Pregnancy and live birth outcomes after FET

	Study group (HMG/MPA/CC)	Control group (HMG/MPA)	Risk Ratio (95% CI)	*P* value
Rates per embryo transfer				
Clinical pregnancy rate	73.9%(88/119)	62.5%(105/168)	1.70 (1.02, 2.85)	0.042
Implantation rate	52.2%(119/228)	42.7%(140/328)	1.47(1.04, 2.06)	0.027
Ectopic pregnancy rate	1.1%(1/88)	1.9%(2/105)	0.59(0.05, 6.64)	0.667
Miscarriage rate				
Early miscarriage	9.1%(8/88)	12.4%(13/105)	0.71(0.28,1.79)	0.465
Later miscarriage	6.8%(6/88)	5.7%(6/105)	1.21(0.38,3.89)	0.752
Ongoing pregnancy rate	66.4%(79/119)	53.6%(90/168)	1.71(1.05,2.78)	0.030
Live-birth rate	59.7%(71/119)[a]	49.4%(83/168)[a]	1.52(0.94,2.44)	0.086
Rates per participant				
Ongoing pregnancy rate	71.8%(79/110)	81.8%(90/110)	0.57(0.30,1.07)	0.079
Live birth rate	64.5%(71/110)[a]	75.5%(83/110)[a]	0.59(0.33,1.06)	0.077
Newborns				
Single birth (n)	50	60		
Single birthweight (g)	3270.4 ± 644.9	3357.0 ± 437.1		0.422
Twin birth (n)	21	23		
Twin birthweight (g)	2371.7 ± 460.7	2460.0 ± 423.5		0.497

[a]3 pregnant women lost to follow up to live birth (2 in study group and 1 in control group)

The synchronization methods of endometrium and embryo were similar between the two groups. The ongoing pregnancy rate per transfer and the implantation rate were significantly higher in the study group (respectively, 66.4% vs 53.6%; 52.2% vs 42.7%, $P < 0.05$) but the live birth rate per transfer was comparable between two groups (59.7% vs 49.4%, $P > 0.05$). Sixty-four women experienced twin pregnancies, including 6 women with vanishing syndrome. One triplet pregnancy occurred in each group, and both resulted in live births after operation of multifetal reduction. The proportions of multiple pregnancies, miscarriage and ectopic pregnancy were similar between groups ($P > 0.05$). The cumulative ongoing pregnancy and live birth rate per patient were lower in the study group but did not reach the significant difference (respectively 71.8% vs 81.8%; 64.5% vs. 75.5%; $P > 0.05$).

All newborns were examined with no congenital malformation except that oesophageal atresia was found in one baby of the control group and ventricular septal defect in one of the twin babies of the study group.

Discussion

Milder stimulation, with its advantages of patient-friendliness, is a good solution for producing an acceptable pregnancy outcome and eliminating OHSS for high responders. This retrospective cohort trial demonstrated that the milder PPOS with CC led to lower oocyte yields and suboptimal pregnancy outcomes compared to the standard PPOS protocol in PCOS women, and the incidence of OHSS was low in both groups (0.91%).

In contrast to the standard protocol of HMG/MPA, the combination protocol of HMG/CC/MPA showed the characteristics of milder stimulation, such as fewer oocytes, fewer embryos, and a higher cancellation rate for non-transferrable embryos, but the harvested embryos showed good developmental potential in terms of implantation rate. This protocol led to fewer oocytes at the cost of low gonadotropin consumption. Serum FSH in mid-follicular phase was slightly lower in the CC combination protocol. The extent of ovarian stimulation may be regulated by using low dose of gonadotropin and CC, which leaves much flexibility for controlled ovarian stimulation. Although the proportion of viable embryos per retrieved oocyte was better in the CC combination protocol (39.5% vs 33.8%), the number of viable embryos was less than the 1.5 embryos from the standard protocol. The total number of transferrable embryos originating from the CC group was significantly lower, meaning the milder CC combination stimulation yielded suboptimal pregnancy outcomes compared with the standard protocol. But these results from a CC combination regimen may provide a new insight for develop a more patient-friendly protocol for PCOS women.

One of the strengths of this trial is that it verified the feasibility of CC co-administration in the PPOS protocol in PCOS women. Our results showed that the endogenous LH was well-suppressed during ovarian stimulation, and no spontaneous LH surge occurred in either group. CC increased endogenous gonadotropin secretion by blocking oestrogen's negative feedback mechanism [11], as evidenced by a relatively higher LH level during the stimulation with CC in this trial. More important, no spontaneous LH surge occurred even with the relatively higher LH, which indicated that P's suppression of pituitary function was still dominant. This phenomenon has also occurred in normo-ovulatory women using a CC combination protocol of PPOS [18]. These data indicate that, although CC and progesterone have separate action sites and pathways, the changed LH trend was the result of their collaborative action, so the two drugs may act independently and have the possibility to act collaboratively.

In PCOS women, multiple follicle growth in controlled ovarian stimulation leads to a higher risk of OHSS due to the higher sensibility and exaggerated response to gonadotropins. The incidence of moderate or severe OHSS in PCOS women is approximately 3.0 to 8.0% [5, 19]. Therefore, it is important to decide the initiating gonadotropin dosage to avoid OHSS. The goal of the CC combination protocol using a low dose of initiating gonadotropin is to maximize the advantages of CC administration. Although CC milder stimulation has the theoretical advantages of a low risk of OHSS, less gonadotropin consumption, and avoiding the resource wastage of cryopreserving more embryos, but in this trial, only 0.91% of patients had OHSS, with no difference between the two groups. This is due to multiple preventive treatments used in this trial: 150–225 IU HMG initiation, a co-trigger using GnRHa and low-dose hCG and a freeze-only strategy. The current data indicate that CC made it possible to reduce the gonadotropin initiating dose in the PPOS protocol in PCOS women, which is helpful to establish a new, milder stimulation regimen with CC and yields an acceptable pregnancy outcome with the benefit of lower gonadotropin dosage.

It is worth noting that most PCOS women in China have a relatively low BMI. The proportion of higher-BMI (> 25 kg/m^2) women among PCOS patients is approximately one third. Previous studies reported an association between obesity and an increased gonadotropin requirement [20, 21], so we must be cautious about generalizing our conclusions, especially on the choice of the HMG initiating dose for obese PCOS women. This trial had a relative small sample size, with insufficient power to compare the live birth rate and incidence of OHSS, so a large-sample, prospective randomized controlled trial using milder PPOS with CC is needed to further confirm our conclusions.

Conclusions

This retrospective cohort trial showed that the milder PPOS protocol with CC in PCOS women led to lower oocyte yields and suboptimal pregnancy outcomes compared to the standard PPOS protocol. The two regimens both achieved a low incidence of OHSS. Milder PPOS with the CC combination regimen showed a higher cancellation rate in exchange for low gonadotropin consumption, but the proportion of viable embryos per oocyte and the implantation rate were higher. Our findings from this CC combination regimen provide a new insight for developing a more patient-friendly protocol for PCOS women.

Abbreviations

AFC: Antral follicle count; CC: Clomiphene citrate; FET: Frozen embryo transfer; FSH: Follicle-stimulating hormone; ICSI: Intracytoplasmic sperm injection; IVF: In vitro fertilization; LH: Luteinizing hormone; MPA: Medroxyprogesterone acetate; OHSS: Ovarian hyperstimulation; P: Progestin; PCOS: Polycystic ovarian syndrome; PPOS: Progestin-primed ovarian stimulation

Acknowledgements

We thank the entire staff of the Department of Assisted Reproduction, Shanghai Ninth People's Hospital, for their support in this trial.

Funding

This study was funded by the National Natural Science Foundation of China (grant numbers: 81671520 and 81571397) and the Natural Science Foundation of Shanghai (grant numbers: 16411963800).

Authors' contributions

Dr. Sun, Dr. Ye and Dr. Chen were the chief investigators who completed the entire study, including procedures, conception, design and completion. Dr. Tian, Dr. Lyu and Dr. He were responsible for the collection of data. Dr. Ye and Dr. Chen analysed the data and drafted the manuscript together. Professor Kuang supervised the study. All authors participated in the ultimate interpretation of the study data and manuscript revisions. All authors read and approved the final manuscript.

Competing interests

The authors declare that they have no competing interests.

References

1. March WA, Moore VM, Willson KJ, Phillips DI, Norman RJ, Davies MJ. The prevalence of polycystic ovary syndrome in a community sample assessed under contrasting diagnostic criteria. Hum Reprod. 2010;25:544–51.
2. Li R, Zhang Q, Yang D, Li S, Lu S, Wu X, Wei Z, Song X, Wang X, Fu S, Lin J, Zhu Y, Jiang Y, Feng HL, Qiao J. Prevalence of polycystic ovary syndrome in women in China: a large community-based study. Hum Reprod. 2013;28:2562–9.
3. Fulvia M, Rosa T, Francisca M, Coroleu B, Rodríguez I, Barri PN. Gonadotrophin-releasing hormone-antagonists vs long agonist in in-vitro fertilization patients with polycystic ovary syndrome: a meta-analysis. Gynecol Endocrinol. 2011;27:150–5.
4. Heijnen EM, Eijkemans MJ, Hughes EG, Laven JS, Macklon NS, Fauser BC. A meta-analysis of outcomes of conventional IVF in women with polycystic ovary syndrome. Hum Reprod Update. 2006;12:13–21.
5. Chen ZJ, Shi Y, Sun Y, Zhang B, Liang X, Cao Y, Yang J, Liu J, Wei D, Weng N, Tian L, Hao C, Yang D, Zhou F, Shi J, Xu Y, Li J, Yan J, Qin Y, Zhao H, Zhang H, Legro RS. Fresh versus frozen embryos for infertility in the polycystic ovary syndrome. N Engl J Med. 2016;375:523–33.
6. Kuang Y, Chen Q, Fu Y, Wang Y, Hong Q, Lyu Q, Ai A, Shoham Z. Medroxyprogesterone acetate is an effective oral alternative for preventing

premature luteinizing hormone surges in women undergoing controlled ovarian hyperstimulation for in vitro fertilization. Fertil Steril, 2015. 104:62–70.
7. Dong J, Wang Y, Chai WR, Hong QQ, Wang NL, Sun LH, Long H, Wang L, Tian H, Lyu QF, Lu XF, Chen QJ, Kuang YP. The pregnancy outcome of progesterone-primed ovarian stimulation using medroxyprogesterone acetate 4 mg versus 10mg daily in infertile women undergoing in vitro fertilization: a randomized controlled trial. B J Obstet Gynaecol. 2017;124: 1048–55.
8. Massin N. New stimulation regimens: endogenous and exogenous progesterone use to block the LH surge during ovarian stimulation for IVF. Hum Reprod Update. 2017;23:211–20.
9. Chen Q, Wang Y, Sun L, Zhang S, Chai W, Hong Q, Long H, Wang L, Lyu Q, Kuang Y. Controlled ovulation of the dominant follicle using progestin in minimal stimulation in poor responders. Reprod Biol Endocrinol. 2017;15:71.
10. Zhu XX, Ye HJ, Fu YL. The Utrogestan and hMG protocol in patients with polycystic ovarian syndrome undergoing controlled ovarian hyperstimulation during IVF/ICSI treatments. Medicine. 2016;95:e4193.
11. Kerin JF, Liu JH, Phillipou G, Yen SS. Evidence for a hypothalamic site of action of clomiphene citrate in women. J Clin Endocrinol Metab. 1985;61:265–8.
12. Casper RF. Letrozole versus clomiphene citrate: which is better for ovulation induction? Fertil Steril. 2009;92:858–9.
13. Tavaniotou A, Albano C, Smitz J, Devroey P. Effect of clomiphene citrate on follicular and luteal phase luteinizing hormone concentrations in in vitro fertilization cycles stimulated with gonadotropins and gonadotropin-releasing hormone antagonist. Fertil Steril. 2002;77:73.
14. Engel JB, Ludwig M, Felberbaum R, Albano C, Devroey P, Diedrich K. Use of cetrorelix in combination with clomiphene citrate and gonadotrophins: a suitable approach to 'friendly IVF'? Hum Reprod. 2002;17:2022–6.
15. Figueiredo JB, Nastri CO, Vieira AD, Martins WP. Clomiphene combined with gonadotropins and GnRH antagonist versus conventional controlled ovarian hyperstimulation without clomiphene in women undergoing assisted reproductive techniques: systematic review and meta-analysis. Arch Gynecol Obstet. 2013;287:779–90.
16. Jiang S, Kuang Y. Clomiphene citrate is associated with favorable cycle characteristics but impaired outcomes of obese women with polycystic ovarian syndrome undergoing ovarian stimulation for in vitro fertilization. Medicine (Baltimore). 2017;96:e7540.
17. Kuang Y, Hong Q, Chen Q, Fu Y, Ai A, Shoham Z. Luteal-phase ovarian stimulation is feasible for producing competent oocytes in women undergoing invitro fertilization/intracytoplasmic sperm injection treatment, with optimal pregnancy outcomes in frozen-thawed embryo transfer cycles. Fertil Steril. 2014;101:105–11.
18. Liu Y, Chen Q, Yu S, Wang Y, He W, Chang HY-N, Wang B, Gao H, Long H, Wang L, Lyu Q, Ai A, Kuang Y. Progestin-primed ovarian stimulation with or without clomiphene citrate supplementation in normal ovulatory women undergoing IVF/ICSI: a prospective randomized controlled trial. Clinical Endocrinology. 2018;88:442–52.
19. Mourad S, Brown J, Farquhar C. Interventions for the prevention of OHSS in ART cycles: an overview of Cochrane reviews. Cochrane Database Syst Rev. 2017;1:CD012103.
20. Fedorcsák P, Dale PO, Storeng R, Ertzeid G, Bjercke S, Oldereid N, Omland AK, Abyholm T, Tanbo T. Impact of overweight and underweight on assisted reproduction treatment. Hum Reprod. 2004;19:2523–8.
21. Orvieto R, Meltcer SR, Rabinson J, Rabinson J, Anteby EY, Ashkenazi J. The influence of body mass index on in vitro fertilization outcome. Int J Gynecol Obstet. 2009;104:53–5.

8

In vitro maturation of oocytes from excised ovarian tissue in a patient with autoimmune ovarian insufficiency possibly associated with Epstein-Barr virus infection

Irma Virant-Klun* and Andrej Vogler

Abstract

Background: Some reports show that it is possible to isolate immature oocytes from human ovarian tissue retrieved by a cortex biopsy or ovariectomy of non-stimulated ovaries and mature them in vitro. The mature oocytes can be vitrified and stored for in vitro fertilization, which, along with ovarian tissue cryopreservation, is mostly practiced in young cancer patients to preserve their fertility. There is much less data on this new approach in women with a natural ovarian insufficiency, which can be caused by different factors, including viral infection. In this case report this advanced methodology was used in a young patient suffering from ovarian insufficiency which was possibly associated with Epstein-Barr virus and infectious mononucleosis (glandular fever).

Methods: This case report included a 27-year-old patient who attended our infertility clinic because of ovarian failure as a part of autoimmune polyendocrinopathy that occurred after Epstein-Barr virus infection, which has rarely been reported until now. Although antral follicles were observed in her ovaries by ultrasound monitoring, she was amenorrhoeic with menopausal concentrations of follicle-stimulating hormone (FSH) and without mature follicles. Therefore, a small biopsy of ovarian cortex tissue was performed using laparoscopy to retrieve immature oocytes. The retrieved oocytes were matured in vitro, cryopreserved, and stored for in vitro fertilization and potential pregnancy.

Results: Four immature, germinal vesicle (GV) oocytes were found and removed from tissue, denuded mechanically by a pipette, and matured in vitro in a maturation medium with added FSH and hCG as well as in co-culture with cumulus cells, which were retrieved by their denudation. Three oocytes matured in vitro to the metaphase II (MII) stage and were vitrified for in vitro fertilization along with ovarian tissue cryopreservation.

Conclusion: Our results show that Epstein-Barr infection is possibly associated with autoimmune ovarian failure. The devastating impact on fertility in such disorder can be successfully avoided by in vitro maturation of oocytes from excised ovarian tissue.

Keywords: Case report, Epstein-Barr virus, In vitro maturation, Laparoscopic biopsy, Oocyte, Ovarian failure, Vitrification

* Correspondence: irma.virant@kclj.si
Reproductive Unit, Department of Obstetrics and Gynecology, University Medical Centre Ljubljana, Zaloska cesta 002, 1000 Ljubljana, SI, Slovenia

Background

Recent reports have demonstrated that it is possible to isolate antral follicles and immature oocytes from human ovarian tissue retrieved by a cortex biopsy or ovariectomy of non-stimulated ovaries and mature them in vitro [1–15]. The retrieved oocytes, which mature in vitro, can be vitrified and stored for in vitro fertilization. This is mostly practiced in young cancer patients, including those with borderline ovarian cancer [4], progressed ovarian cancer [12], and endometrial carcinoma [11], who cryostore their ovarian tissue before chemo- and radiotherapy to preserve their fertility. This cancer treatment is quite advanced and enhances the long-term survival of patients.

In vitro maturation and vitrification of oocytes retrieved from non-stimulated ovaries is usually performed along with ovarian tissue cryopreservation, which is performed to restore fertility by autotransplantation of

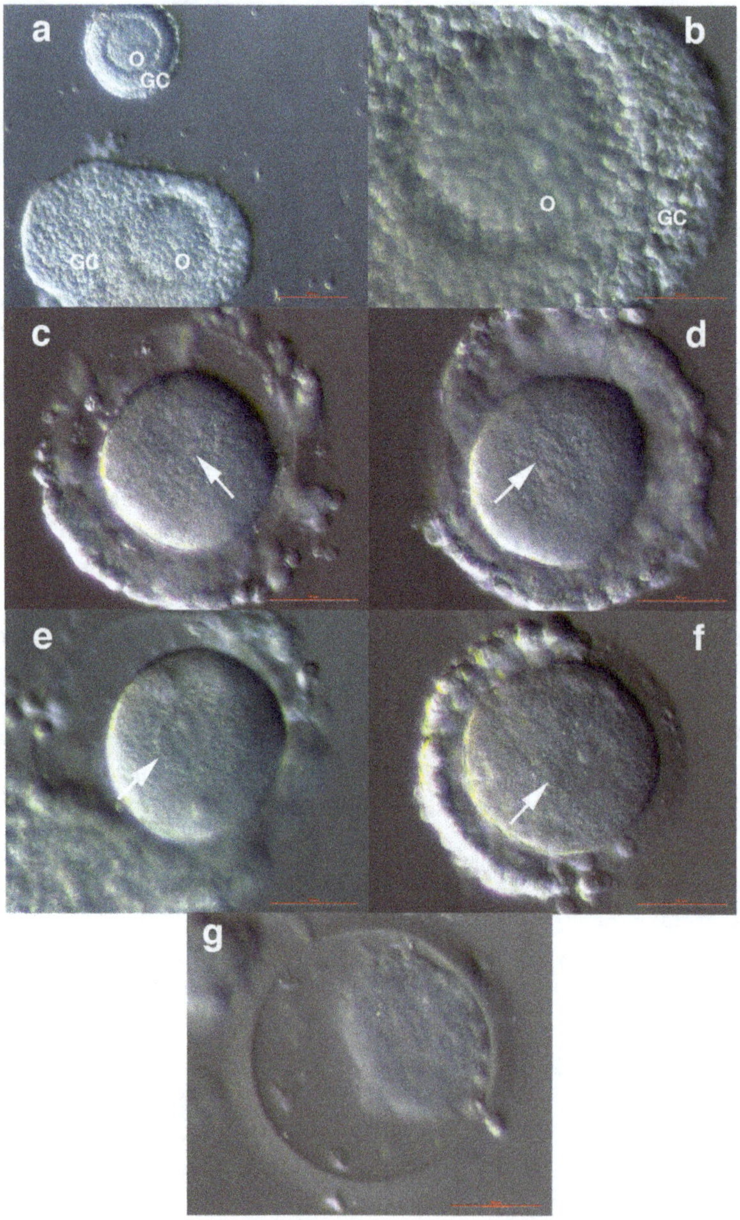

Fig. 1 Immature oocytes expressing a germinal vesicle (arrows) and an immature follicle from the excised ovarian cortex tissue of a patient with ovarian insufficiency. Along with the immature follicle, (**a**) one oocyte appeared to have a follicle-like structure (**a, b**) and was denuded (**c**) to remove granulosa cells. Three oocytes were surrounded by a relatively thin layer of granulosa cells (**d-f**). One oocyte was degenerated (**g**). (Inverted microscope, magnification 40× for **a** and 100× for **b-g**). *Legend*: O-immature oocyte and GC-granulosa cells. *Red Bar*: 100 μm for **a** and 50 μm for **b-g**

tissue after cancer therapy [16]. It is less complicated and safer to preserve fertility in this way than autotransplantation of ovarian tissue, which cannot completely exclude the reintroduction of malignant cells into the body; future transplantation of ovarian tissue is not recommended for several cancer types, such as leukemia, due to high risks of reintroducing malignant cells [17–19]. There are also some reports on the in vitro maturation and cryopreservation of oocytes retrieved from intra-operative aspiration during cancer surgery (e.g., second enucleation of ovarian tumors) [20].

It has been shown that a significant number of immature oocytes can be collected from excised ovarian tissue regardless of the menstrual cycle phases and age of the patient, even for prepubertal girls [8]. Recent findings show that it is possible to isolate immature oocytes even from surplus ovarian medulla tissue and to mature them in vitro [21, 22]. Moreover, first pregnancies and the birth of a healthy baby achieved in this way have been reported recently, which make this new technology beneficial and promising for oncological patients and infertile women [12–14]. This new methodology can also be supported by advanced preimplantation and prenatal genetic testing.

There is not much data on this new approach in women who are infertile because of a natural ovarian insufficiency except for mosaic Turner syndrome [5] and an insufficiency following therapeutic embolization of the left uterine and right ovarian artery because of an arteriovenous malformation [13]. This case report included a 27-year-old patient who attended our infertility clinic because of premature ovarian failure (POF) which was possibly associated with Epstein-Barr virus and infectious mononucleosis (glandular fever). Epstein-Barr virus is rarely related to female infertility in the literature [23]; it may be related to altered immunophenotypic parameters and peripheral immunostimulation in women with a history of infertility [24].

Methods

The 27-year-old patient was referred to our institution by her endocrinologist due to typical signs and symptoms of POF as a part of an autoimmune polyendocrinopathy that occurred after Epstein-Barr virus infection 3 years ago. At that time, she did not desire to become pregnant, but planned to conceive in the next couple of years. In addition to POF, she had Addison's disease and thrombocytopenia, but normal thyroid function. For the last 2 years, she has not received hormonal replacement therapy (HRT); she was amenorrhoeic with menopausal concentrations of FSH (82.5 IU/L and 99.7 IU/L, respectively). Vaginal ultrasound examination 3 months after HRT (combination of estradiol valerate 2 mg and norgestrel 0.5 mg) withdrawal revealed a normal ovarian appearance with more than 10 antral follicles in each ovary without a dominant follicle. Genetic testing showed normal female karyotype and no fragile X-associated ovarian insufficiency (FXOI).

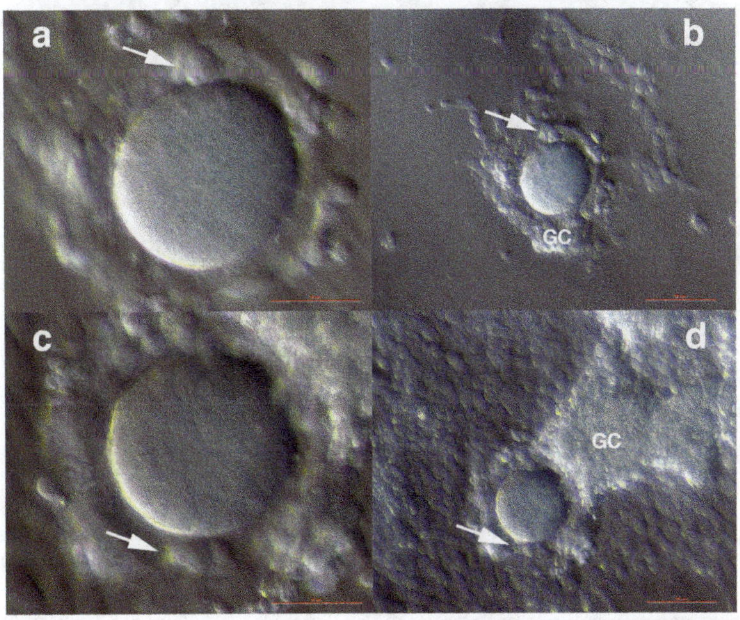

Fig. 2 In vitro maturation of oocytes in a maturation medium with added FSH and hCG and in a co-culture with follicular (granulosa) cells retrieved by mechanical denudation of the same oocytes before in vitro maturation. Oocytes were covered by granulosa cells, forming a primitive follicle-like structure. Two oocytes matured in vitro to the metaphase II (MII) stage and extruded a polar body (arrow) (**a**-**d**). (Inverted microscope, magnification 100× for **a**, **c** and 40× for **b**, **d**). *Legend*: GC-granulosa cells. *Red Bar*: 50 μm for **a**, **c** and 100 μm for **b**, **d**

To retrieve ovarian tissue with possible immature oocytes, mature them in vitro, and vitrify them to perform a later in vitro fertilization along with ovarian tissue cryopreservation, laparoscopy was performed. During laparoscopy, the ovaries were normal in size with small follicles throughout the surface. With cold endoscopic scissors, a 10 × 5 mm section of the ovarian cortex was excided from each ovary opposite to the ovarian hilum. After washing the ovaries, hemostasis was achieved by placing a suture on the defect without using any thermal energy. The ovarian cortex tissue was stored in a sterile physiological saline (B. Braun, Melsungen AG, Germany) at room temperature and immediately brought into the laboratory to find possible immature oocytes, mature them in vitro, and vitrify them to perform a later in vitro fertilization along with ovarian tissue cryopreservation. At the same time a small specimen of each ovarian tissue was taken for histopathological examination. Pathology report showed active parenchyma of the right ovary with some primordial follicles and ovarian parenchyma of the left ovary with numerous primordial and some primary follicles.

This was approved by the Slovenian National Medical Ethical Committee (approval 0120–222/2016–2, KME 115/04/16), and the patient provided informed consent for voluntary participation.

Oocyte retrieval

A section of ovarian tissue was transferred to the IVF Laboratory, placed into Universal IVF Medium (Origio, Denmark), minced by a surgical blade (Tro-Microcision, Troge, Germany) and searched for follicles and oocytes. All oocytes were removed from tissue and denuded mechanically by a denudation pipette with a diameter of

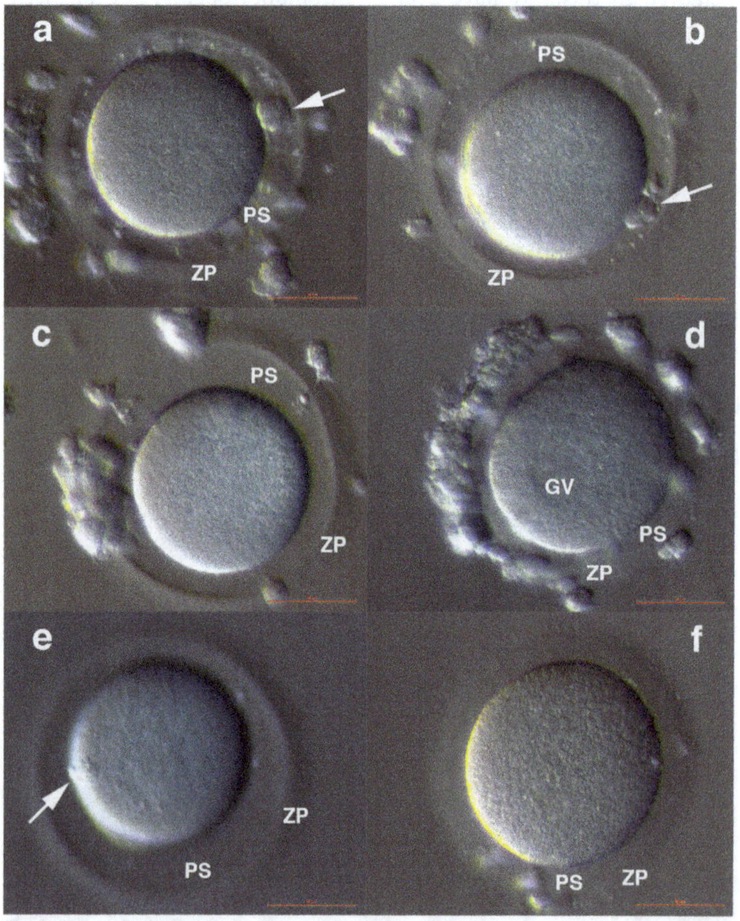

Fig. 3 Oocytes after in vitro maturation were removed from co-cultured granulosa cells and denuded mechanically to remove the granulosa cells. Two oocytes matured to the MII stage after 38–42 h of maturation and extruded a polar body of normal morphology (arrow) (**a**, **b**), while two other oocytes did not mature in vitro over this time frame (**c**, **d**); one oocyte was at the metaphase I (MI) stage (**c**), and another oocyte continued to express a germinal vesicle (GV) (**d**). After another 6-h maturation in vitro, the MI stage oocyte matured to the MII stage and extruded a polar body (arrow) (**e**). The in vitro matured oocytes were of normal dimensions and morphology except for a slightly higher perivitelline space (PS) and thinner zona pellucida (ZP) in comparison to oocytes from the conventional in vitro fertilization procedure after the hormonal stimulation of ovaries (**f**). (Inverted microscope, magnification 100×). *Legend*: GV-germinal vesicle, PS-perivitelline space, and ZP-zona pellucida. *Red Bar*: 50 μm

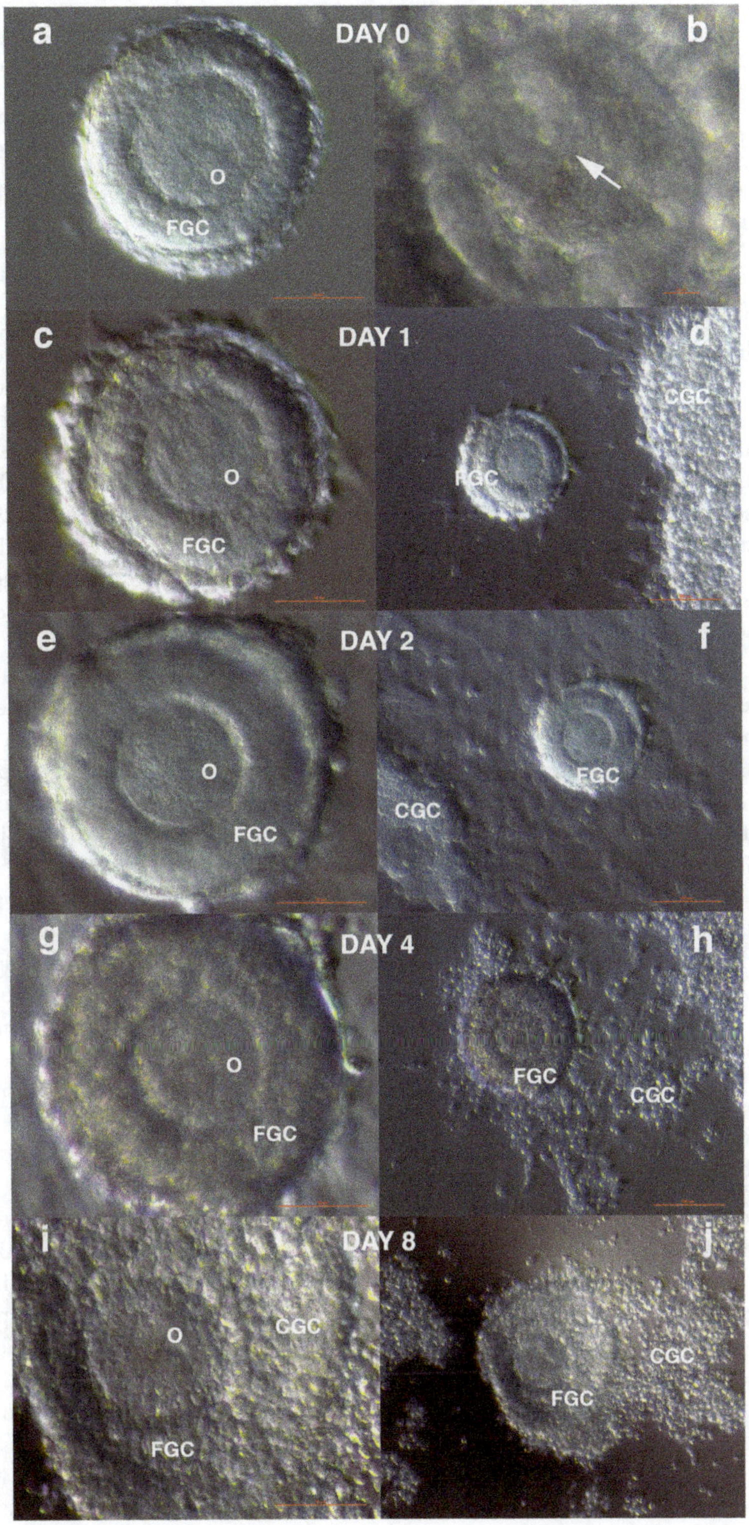

Fig. 4 (See legend on next page.)

(See figure on previous page.)

Fig. 4 In vitro maturation of the immature follicle: the day of retrieval (**a**) of an oocyte that expressed a germinal vesicle (arrow) (**b**); on day 1, a slightly thicker layer of granulosa cells around the oocyte (**c**) in the co-culture with granulosa cells that approached the follicle (**d**); on day 2, a significantly thicker zona pellucida (**e**) in the co-culture with granulosa cells that spread over the follicle (**f**); on day 4, a thicker layer of granulosa cells around the oocyte (**g**) in the co-culture with granulosa cells, which started to incorporate into the layer of the granulosa cells around the oocyte (**h**); and on day 8, a massive layer of granulosa cells around the oocyte (**i**) in the co-culture with granulosa cells, which was massively incorporated into the layer of granulosa cells around the oocyte (**j**). (Inverted microscope, magnification 200× for **b**, 100× for **a**, **c**, **e**, **g**, **i**, and 40× for **d**, **f**, **h**, **j**). *Legend*: O-oocyte, FGC-granulosa cells around the oocyte in the follicle and CGC-co-cultured granulosa cells retrieved by denudation of oocytes in the patient. *Red Bar*: 10 μm for **b**, 50 μm for **a**, **c**, **e**, **g**, **i**, and 100 μm for **d**, **f**, **h**, **j**

134–145 μm and length 75–85 mm (ref. 14,301, Vitrolife, Sweden). Surrounding follicular cells with predominating granulosa cells were removed easily and stored for co-culture during the in vitro maturation procedure to provide an ovarian niche to some extent. The remaining ovarian cortex tissue was cut into smaller pieces and cryopreserved using a propanediol as a cryoprotectant and finally stored in liquid nitrogen (− 196 °C) to perform in vitro activation of follicles and autotransplantation of ovarian tissue beneath the serosa of both fallopian tubes in the future [25].

Oocyte in vitro maturation

For the maturation of oocytes, the certified MediCult IVM System (Origio, Målov, Denmark) was used, which consisted of two solutions: 1.) LAG medium (conditioning) and 2.) in vitro maturation (IVM) medium, which consisted of 100 μl of recFSH solution (75 mIU/ml; Puregon, Merck Sharp & Dohme Gmbh, Haar, Germany), 10 μl of hCG solution (100 mIU/ml; Pregnyl, Organon, Oss, Netherland) and 10 ml of basic IVM medium. Each oocyte was separately matured in a 60 μm drop of maturation medium covered by mineral oil in a UGPS-500 dish (Universal GPS® dish, LifeGlobal Group, Guilford, CT 06437, USA) at 37 °C in an atmosphere of air with 6% CO_2 and 95% humidity. First, they were incubated for 2–3 h in the LAG medium and then for up to 48 h in the maturation medium with added FSH and hCG. Oocytes were co-cultured with granulosa cells retrieved by the previous denudation of oocytes to provide an ovarian niche to some extent; in usual practice, denuded human oocytes are matured in vitro without a granulosa cell co-culture.

Results

Five immature germinal vesicle (GV) oocytes were found in the tissue: one oocyte was embedded in the follicle-like structure (Fig. 1a-c), similarly to a publication by Huang [5]. Three oocytes appeared with a thinner layer of follicular cells around them (Fig. 1d-f), and one oocyte was degenerated (Fig. 1g). In addition to oocytes, one immature follicle was found and isolated from the tissue (Fig. 1a).

Oocytes were matured in vitro. During the maturation process, cumulus/granulosa cells spread over the oocytes, forming primitive follicle-like structures (Fig. 2). Two out of four oocytes matured in vitro to the metaphase II (MII) stage and extruded the first polar body between 38 to 42 h of incubation in the maturation medium (Fig. 3a, b). These two oocytes were vitrified (Kitazato Cryotop®Oocyte Vitrification System, Japan) and stored in liquid nitrogen (− 196 °C) to be used for in vitro fertilization in the future. The remaining two oocytes did not mature in vitro (Fig. 3c, d) and were further matured in vitro for up to 48 h. One of the oocytes matured and extruded the polar body (Fig. 3e); it was also vitrified and stored in liquid nitrogen for a later in vitro fertilization. Another oocyte did not mature at all and was discarded. All of the in vitro matured oocytes that were vitrified had normal polar bodies as well as normal dimensions (diameters of ≈ 100 μm), normal shape and cytoplasm granularity in comparison with oocytes retrieved after controlled ovarian stimulation in the usual in vitro fertilization program (Fig. 3f). The immature follicle was matured in the same maturation medium, but did not mature (Fig. 4). The vitrified oocytes will be stored in liquid nitrogen for 10 years. If not used by a patient during this time period, the oocytes will be further stored or discarded after her written consent. After laparoscopy the hormonal status of patient did not change.

Discussion

Our data show that infection with Epstein-Barr virus, also known as human herpesvirus 4, possibly triggered the polyendocrinopathy (most likely autoimmune) including POF. The devastating impact on fertility in such disorder can be successfully avoided by in vitro maturation of oocytes from excised ovarian tissue.

Ovarian insufficiency or premature ovarian failure (POF) is characterized by loss of function of the ovaries before age 40 characterized with amenorrhoea, hypergonadotropism and hypoestrogenism being one of the most serious causes of infertility [26]. It affects approximately one out of 100 women. Only 5–10% of women diagnosed with POF can achieve a spontaneous pregnancy, while most of them require medical intervention [27]. There is no generally accepted treatment to increase fertility in women with ovarian insufficiency, and the use of donor eggs with in vitro fertilization (IVF) and adoption remain the only options for achieving parenthood for women with POF. The etiology of ovarian insufficiency is still poorly understood, and most cases remain unexplained. According to our data the infection with Epstein-Barr virus with infectious mononucleosis (glandular fever) and autoimmune polyendocrinopathy is considered to be a potential trigger of ovarian failure.

The majority of the human adult population is infected with Epstein-Barr virus, and the majority of infected individuals tolerate the infection well, without any further symptoms after primary infection [28]. Normally, the virus stays in the body and remains dormant throughout life. However, this is not always the case, and a serious Epstein-Barr virus-related illness may develop later in life, especially different autoimmune diseases, such as systemic lupus erythematosus, multiple sclerosis, rheumatoid arthritis, Sjögren's syndrome, autoimmune hepatitis, and autoimmune thyroid disorders [29]. Although this virus is not the only agent responsible for the development of autoimmune diseases, it can be considered to be the main contributory factor.

According to our knowledge, there is not much data on the association between Epstein-Barr virus infection and autoimmune ovarian insufficiency in the literature, but POF is quite frequently associated with Addison's disease which can be in rare cases caused by the virus [30–32].

The patient included in this study had primordial and primary follicles in her ovaries, which did not mature and produce mature oocytes. By performing in vitro maturation of oocytes from excised ovarian tissue, we avoided an autoimmune disorder and cryopreserved the mature oocytes for a later in vitro fertilization along with ovarian tissue cryopreservation. This approach can be beneficial also for other patients with autoimmune POF and non-maturing follicles/oocytes in the ovaries to preserve their fertility, while it cannot help patients with POF and without follicles in the ovaries. The most limiting factor is conventional oocyte in vitro maturation procedure in the presence of reproductive hormones only, which is suboptimal and results in a relatively low number of matured oocytes. Therefore the maturating oocytes in this patient were co-cultured with cumulus cells to provide an ovarian niche as well as with substances released by cumulus cells, which are important for human oocyte maturation [33] and are usually lacking when oocytes are matured in vitro in a conventional way without a co-culture.

Conclusion

Infection with Epstein-Barr virus with severe infectious mononucleosis (glandular fever) and autoimmune polyendocrinopathy need to be considered to be possibly associated with ovarian failure. Further histological, animal and molecular studies will be required for a final conclusion.

As in the patient included in this study, the ovaries of women with autoimmune POF need to be carefully examined for the presence of follicles because it is possible to isolate immature oocytes from excised ovarian tissue, mature them in vitro and vitrify and store them for a later in vitro fertilization along with ovarian tissue cryopreservation. The patient suffering with POF can safeguard her fertility by cryopreserving these excised oocytes. Co-culturing maturing oocytes with cumulus cells may be beneficial to provide an ovarian niche during the maturation process and improve the quality of matured oocytes.

Abbreviations

FSH: Follicle-stimulating hormone; GV: Germinal vesicle (immature oocyte); hCG: Human chorionic gonadotropin; IVM : In vitro maturation; MII: Metaphase II stage (mature oocyte); POF: Premature ovarian failure

Acknowledgements

We acknowledge the colleagues of Reproductive Unit, Department of Obstetrics and Gynecology, University Medical Centre Ljubljana for their collaboration.

Funding

This work was financially supported by the University Medical Centre Ljubljana as grant offered to Prof. Irma Virant-Klun (Tertiary Research Project No. 20150005).

Authors' contributions

IVK performed the retrieval of oocytes from the excised ovarian tissue, maturation of oocytes in vitro, and cryopreservation of ovarian tissue; identified the results; and wrote this case report. AV performed the laparoscopical retrieval of ovarian cortex tissue, provided extended medical information to the patient, and edited this case report. Both authors read and approved the final manuscript.

Competing interests

The authors declare that they have no competing interests.

References

1. Revel A, Koler M, Simon A, Lewin A, Laufer N, Safran A. Oocyte collection during cryopreservation of the ovarian cortex. Fertil Steril. 2003;79:1237–9.
2. Revel A, Revel-Vilk S, Aizenman E, Porat-Katz A, Safran A, Ben-Meir A, et al. At what age can human oocytes be obtained? Fertil Steril. 2009;92:458–63.
3. Isachenko E, Rahimi G, Isachenko V, Nawroth F. In-vitro maturation of germinal-vesicle oocytes and cryopreservation in metaphase I/II: a possible additional option to preserve fertility during ovarian tissue cryopreservation. Reprod BioMed Online. 2004;8:553–7.
4. Huang JY, Buckett WM, Gilbert L, Tan SL, Chian RC. Retrieval of immature oocytes followed by in vitro maturation and vitrification: a case report on a new strategy of fertility preservation in women with borderline ovarian malignancy. Gynecol Oncol. 2007;105:542–4.
5. Huang JY, Tulandi T, Holzer H, Lau NM, Macdonald S, Tan SL, et al. Cryopreservation of ovarian tissue and in vitro matured oocytes in a female with mosaic Turner syndrome: case report. Hum Reprod. 2008;23:336–9.

6. Huang JY, Tulandi T, Holzer H, Tan SL, Chian RC. Combining ovarian tissue cryobanking with retrieval of immature oocytes followed by in vitro maturation and vitrification: an additional strategy of fertility preservation. Fertil Steril. 2008;89:567–72.
7. Gonzalez C, Devesa M, Boada M, Coroleu B, Veiga A, Barri PN. Combined strategy for fertility preservation in an oncologic patient: vitrification of in vitro matured oocytes and ovarian tissue freezing. J Assist Reprod Genet. 2011;28:1147–9.
8. Fasano G, Moffa F, Dechène J, Englert Y, Demeestere I. Vitrification of in vitro matured oocytes collected from antral follicles at the time of ovarian tissue cryopreservation. Reprod Biol Endocrin. 2011;9:150.
9. Escriba MJ, Grau N, Escrich L, Novella-Maestre E, Sanchez-Serrano M. Spontaneous in vitro maturation of oocytes prior to ovarian tissue cryopreservation in natural cycles of oncologic patients. J Assist Reprod Genet. 2012;29:1261–5.
10. Imesch P, Scheiner D, Xie M, Fink D, Macas E, Dubey R, et al. Developmental potential of human oocytes matured in vitro followed by vitrification and activation. J Ovarian Res. 2013;6:30.
11. Shirasawa H, Kumagai J, Sato W, Kumazawa Y, Sato N, Terada Y. Retrieval and in vitro maturation of human oocytes from ovaries removed during surgery for endometrial carcinoma: a novel strategy for human oocyte research. J Assist Reprod Genet. 2013;30:1227–30.
12. Prasath EB, Chan ML, Wong WH, Lim CJ, Tharmalingam MD, Hendricks M, et al. First pregnancy and live birth resulting from cryopreserved embryos obtained from in vitro matured oocytes after oophorectomy in an ovarian cancer patient. Hum Reprod. 2014;29:276–8.
13. Segers I, Mateizel I, Van Moer E, Smitz J, Tournaye H, Verheyem G, et al. In vitro maturation (IVM) of oocytes recovered from ovariectomy specimens in the laboratory: a promising "ex vivo" method of oocyte cryopreservation resulting in the first report of an ongoing pregnancy in Europe. J Assist Reprod Genet. 2015;32:1221–31.
14. Uzelac PS, Delaney AA, Christensen GL, Bohler HC, Nakajima ST. Live birth following in vitro maturation of oocytes retrieved from extracorporeal ovarian tissue aspiration and embryo cryopreservation for 5 years. Fertil Steril. 2015;104:1258–60.
15. Hourvitz A, Yerushalmi GM, Maman E, Raanani H, Elizur S, Brengauz M, et al. Combination of ovarian tissue harvesting and immature oocyte collection for fertility preservation increases preservation yield. Reprod BioMed Online. 2015; 31:497–505.
16. Donnez J, Dolmans MM. Ovarian cortex transplantation: 60 reported live births brings the success and worldwide expansion of the technique towards routine clinical practice. J Assist Reprod Genet. 2015;32(8):1167–70.
17. Dolmans MM, Marinescu C, Saussoy P, Van Langendonckt A, Amorim C, Donnez J. Reimplantation of cryopreserved ovarian tissue from patients with acute lymphoblastic leukemia is potentially unsafe. Blood. 2010;116:2908–14.
18. Rosendahl M, Greve T, Andersen CY. The safety of transplanting cryopreserved ovarian tissue in cancer patients: a review of the literature. J Assist Reprod Genet. 2013;30:11–24.
19. Bastings L, Beerendonk CC, Westphal JR, Massuger LF, Kaal SE, van Leeuwen FE, et al. Autotransplantation of cryopreserved ovarian tissue in cancer survivors and the risk of reintroducing malignancy: a systematic review. Hum Reprod Update. 2013;19:483–506.
20. Shirasawa H, Kumazawa Y, Sato W, Ono N, Terada Y. In vitro maturation and cryopreservation of oocytes retrieved from intra-operative aspiration during second enucleation for ovarian tumor: a case report. Gynecol Oncol Rep. 2016; 19:1–4.
21. Wilken-Jensen HN, Kristensen SG, Jeppesen JV, Yding AC. Developmental competence of oocytes isolated from surplus medulla tissue in connection with cryopreservation of ovarian tissue for fertility preservation. Acta Obstet Gynecol Scand. 2014;93:32–7.
22. Yin H, Jiang H, Kristensen SG, Andersen CY. Vitrification of in vitro matured oocytes collected from surplus ovarian medulla tissue resulting from fertility preservation of ovarian cortex tissue. J Assist Reprod Genet. 2016;33:741–6.
23. Kundsin RB, Falk L, Hertig AT, Horne HW Jr. Mycoplasma, chlamydia, Epstein-Barr, herpes I and II, and AIDS infections among 100 consecutive infertile female patients and husbands: diagnosis, treatment, and results. Int J Fertil. 1986;31:356–9.
24. Thomas D, Michou V, Moustakarias T, Aleporou V, Matzavinos T, Mitsakos-Barbagiannis K, et al. Altered immunophenotypic parameters in infertile women. Possible role of herpes viremia. Am J Reprod Immunol. 2005;54: 101–11.

with cryopreservation of ovarian tissue for fertility preservation. Acta Obstet Gynecol Scand. 2014;93:32–7.
22. Yin H, Jiang H, Kristensen SG, Andersen CY. Vitrification of in vitro matured oocytes collected from surplus ovarian medulla tissue resulting from fertility preservation of ovarian cortex tissue. J Assist Reprod Genet. 2016;33:741–6.
23. Kundsin RB, Falk L, Hertig AT, Horne HW Jr. Mycoplasma, chlamydia, Epstein-Barr, herpes I and II, and AIDS infections among 100 consecutive infertile female patients and husbands: diagnosis, treatment, and results. Int J Fertil. 1986;31:356–9.
24. Thomas D, Michou V, Moustakarias T, Aleporou V, Matzavinos T, Mitsakos-Barbagiannis K, et al. Altered immunophenotypic parameters in infertile women. Possible role of herpes viremia. Am J Reprod Immunol. 2005;54: 101–11.

25. Zhai J, Yao G, Dong F, Bu Z, Cheng Y, Sato Y, et al. In vitro activation of follicles and fresh tissue auto-transplantation in primary ovarian insufficiency patients. J Clin Endocrinol Metab. 2016;101:4405–12.
26. Woad KJ, Watkins WJ, Prendergast D, Shelling AN. The genetic basis of premature ovarian failure. Aust N Z J Obstet Gynaecol. 2006;46:242–4.
27. Van Kasteren Y, Schoemaker J. Premature ovarian failure: a systematic review on therapeutic interventions to restore ovarian function and achieve pregnancy. Hum Reprod Update. 1999;5:483–92.
28. Niller HH, Bauer G. Epstein-Barr virus: clinical diagnostics. Methods Mol Biol. 2017;1532:33–55.
29. Dittfeld A, Gwizdek K, Michalski M, Wojnicz R. A possible link between the Epstein-Barr virus infection and autoimmune thyroid disorders. Cent Eur J Immunol. 2016;41:297–301.
30. Reato G, Morlin L, Chen S, Furmaniak J, Rees Smith B, Masiero S, et al. Premature ovarian failure in patients with autoimmune Addison's disease: clinical, genetic, and immunological evaluation. J Clin Endocrinol Metab. 2011;96:E1255–61.
31. Saeger W. Adrenalitis. Pathologe. 2016;37:238–44.
32. Paolo WF Jr, Nosanchuk JD. Adrenal infections. Int J Infect Dis. 2006;10:343–53.
33. Hassan HA. 2001. Cumulus cell contribution to cytoplasmic maturation and oocyte developmental competence in vitro. J Assist Reprod Genet. 2001;18: 539–43.

9

Comparison of the enzymatic efficiency of Liberase TM and tumor dissociation enzyme: effect on the viability of cells digested from fresh and cryopreserved human ovarian cortex

Viola Maria Schmidt[1], Vladimir Isachenko[1], Gunter Rappl[2], Gohar Rahimi[1], Bettina Hanstein[1], Bernd Morgenstern[1], Peter Mallmann[1] and Evgenia Isachenko[1*]

Abstract

Background: The aim of this study was to examine the effectiveness of Tumor Dissociation Enzyme (TDE) on the viability of follicles after digestion of fresh and cryopreserved ovarian cortex fragments (OCFs).

Methods: Fresh and thawed OCF from 14 patients (29 ± 6 years), sized 20 to 210 mm^3 were randomly distributed into four treatment groups and digested with 16% TDE or 0.05 mg/ml Liberase TM: Group 1, frozen OCF digested with TDE; Group 2, frozen OCF digested with LiberaseTM; Group 3, fresh OCF digested with TDE; and Group 4, fresh OCF digested with Liberase TM. Evaluation of follicle viability was performed under light microscope after staining with Neutral red. For visualization of viable and dead cells under a confocal laser scanning microscope, the follicles were stained with Calcein AM and ethidium homodimer-1.

Results: The results showed that the number of retrieved follicles was significantly higher (990 vs 487; $P < 0.01$) in the TDE-treatment group compared to the Liberase TM-group. The presence of intense neutral red stained follicles was significantly higher in Group 1 and Group 3 compared to Group 2 and Group 4 (70.3% ± +/− 6.22 vs 53,1% ± 2.03 and 94.2% ± 6.6 vs 79.1% ± 2.1; $P < 0.01$). The percentage of Calcein AM stained follicles of class V1 was significantly higher in Group 1 and Group 3 compared to Group 2 and Group 4 (95.97% ± 7.8 vs 87.87% ± 2.4; 97.1% ± 6.8 vs 91.3% ± 2.3; $P < 0.01$).

Conclusion: The enzymatic digestion of ovarian cortex with TDE provides recovery of a higher number of healthy preantral follicles in contrast to earlier described Liberase TM procedure.

Keywords: Artificial ovary, Follicle, Ovarian tissue, Enzymatic isolation, Cryopreservation, Liberase TM, Tumor dissociation enzyme

* Correspondence: e.isachenko@yahoo.de
[1]Research Group for Reproductive Medicine and IVF-Laboratory, Department of Obstetrics and Gynaecology, University Maternal Hospital, Cologne University, Kerpener Str. 34, 50931 Cologne, Germany
Full list of author information is available at the end of the article

Background

Over the last decades, research in medicine has made a great progress in cancer therapy. Long-time survival of cancer patients has increased significantly [1, 2] and after convalescence many patients can lead normal lives. However, highly aggressive and gonadotoxic chemotherapy and radiotherapy have strong side effects such as premature ovarian failure and infertility [3, 4]. At present, the only possibility to maintain fertility as well as hormonal cyclicity and endocrinological function is the cryopreservation and autologous re-transplantation of ovarian cortical fragments taken before chemotherapy or radiotherapy. This method has resulted in large number of live births worldwide [5, 6].

However, this procedure runs the risk of re-transplanting of malignant cells, which makes it unsuitable for patients suffering from neoplastic diseases whose malignant cells are likely to metastasize into the ovary. Cancers that are considered to have a high risk for ovarian metastases are leukaemia, lymphoma, carcinoma coli and cervical as well as uterine cancers [7–10]. In the same time, the re-transplantation of isolated primordial follicles could be an alternative to safe fertility restoration in women with premature ovarian failure [11–13]. It is possible because the basal lamina surrounding the follicles separates them from the surrounding ovarian stroma, blood vessels and nerves, which prevents the invasion of metastatic cells [14]. Therefore, primordial follicles can be isolated and used for the generation of a transplantable artificial human ovary [15, 16]. Construction of an artificial ovary could be the optimal way of preserving fertility as well as protecting female cancer patients, against the re-transplantation of malignant cells, independent from type of neoplastic diseases [9].

This possibility was shown by Laronda et al. [17]. It was demonstrated the real possibility for successful re-transplantation of follicles seeded with scaffolds to SCID-mice with subsequent pups born through natural mating. Successful isolation of preantral follicles from cryopreserved tissue is especially important in global practice: a large amount of ovarian tissues have been already conserved from patients with different types of cancers. According to data, preantral follicles can be successfully cryopreserved before or after their isolation without impairing their ability to survive and grow in vitro [18, 19].

The important step of the artificial ovary creation from preantral follicles is the isolation of these follicles from fresh or cryopreserved (frozen and thawed) ovarian tissues.

In fact, ovarian stromal cells play an important role in the process of development of preantral follicles. According to Young and McNeilly [20], the thecal cells around the secondary preantral follicles appear to be recruited from the surrounding stromal tissue layer by factors that are secreted by activated primary follicles. The growth and development of secondary follicles is affected by steroid hormones that are produced by interactions between granulosa and thecal cells [21, 22]. Ovarian medulla is composed by dense fibrotic stroma consisted from spindle-shaped cells (fibroblasts) and follicles of different stages of maturity [23]. Development of follicles, their ovulation and luteinisation are finely controlled by physiologic hormonal milieu. Therefore, stromal cells of adult ovary actively contribute to the synthesis and phase remodelling both extracellular matrix and blood vessels [23]. Ovarian stromal and endothelial cells are essential to ensure graft survival and quality [24].

In fact, two arteries (*arteria ovarica* and the branch of the *arteria uterina*) penetrate the ovarian *hilus* and form network of blood vessels [23]. They are an opening port for malignant cells [24] which could preferentially generate special kind of stroma cells for aberrant proliferation and invasion [24]. In this case the including of stromal cells by creating of an artificial ovary plays important role only for healthy patients, because of the risk of transfer of malignant cells included in ovarian stroma [7, 8]. The fibroblasts and some other cell types (for example, pre-vascular cells and mesenchymal stem cells) potentially include cancer-associated fibroblasts [25].

At present, for isolation of preantral follicles from human and animal ovarian cortex, a number of mechanical, enzymatic and a combination of both methods have been described [26–40].

The human ovarian tissue has a relatively high density and the current mechanical isolation of follicles demonstrates unsatisfactory performance. However, the combination of mechanical isolation technique with enzymatic digestion significantly improved the viability of isolated follicles [36, 41, 42].

Our own experience supports the effectiveness of the use of a commercial enzyme -cocktail "Tumor Dissociation Enzyme Reagent" (TDE, Innovative Diagnostic Systems Dr. Christian Sartori, Hamburg, Germany) for enzymatic digestion of gynaecological solid tumors with good viability and developmental rate of cancer -and non -cancer cells (non-published data).

This especially designed commercial enzyme - cocktail was developed for gentle enzymatic digestion of solid tumors [43–45] and allows to isolate tumor cells without appearance of apoptosis or necrosis. Despite the highly secured composition of TDE due to patent [46], it was discerned that the contents of this drug are various types of highly purified collagenase (personal communication with Dr. Christian Sartori Labor, Hamburg, Germany) that allowed the digested tissue suspensions to be not sticky and not viscous, and easy to handle and thus, can obtain a good number of viable cells.

The aim of our experiments was to study the Tumor Dissociation Enzyme effects on the integrity and viability of cell -complexes (follicles) after digesting of these cells from cryopreserved ovarian cortex.

Methods

Except where otherwise stated, all chemicals were obtained from Sigma (Sigma-Aldrich Chemie, GmbH, Schnelldorf, Germany).

Tissue collection, dissection, and distribution into groups

This study was approved by the Ethics Boards of Cologne University (applications 99,184 and 13–147).

Written informed consents were obtained from all study participants aged 18 and over.

Tissues were obtained from 14 patients aged between 22 and 39 (29.1± 5.9) years. According to our approved protocol, 10% of ovarian tissues (ovarian tissue biopsies, OTBs) collected from patients were used for 'patient-oriented' research. This refers to research done in order to assess the viability of the tissues for re-transplantation.

The patients with following diseases were indicated: breast cancer (3 patients), Hodgkin lymphoma (2 patients), non-Hodgkin lymphoma (2 patients), acute lymphoblastic leukemia (3 patient), uterine cancer (1 patient), nasopharyngeal cancer (1 patient) and soft tissue sarcoma (2 patient). For our research, the OTBs from three patients were used after surgery without cryopreservation, and OTBs for patient-oriented research from eight patients were cryopreserved long before these experiments.

The medium used for OTBs transport and dissection (the basal medium) was composed by Leibovitz L-15 with 5% Dextran Serum Substitute (Irvine Scientific, Santa Ana, USA). After collection, fresh ovarian tissue fragments were transported at 32 °C to 34 °C to the laboratory within 20 min of surgery.

Using sterile surgical tweezers and no. 22 scalpels, the medullary part of the fragment was removed to achieve ~ 1 mm thickness of the cortical part. A small piece of fragment (~ 1 mm^3) was fixed in Bouin solution for histological evaluation and served as a fresh control. Depending on the size of ovarian fragment intended for this research, the size of OCFs for patient-oriented research was ranged from 20 to 210 mm^3 (Table 1). Each OCF from each patient was cut into two equal parts and cooled to 5 °C for 24 h. After this, the cooled OCF was enzymatically digested or frozen (one OCF per cryo-vial) with subsequent storage in liquid nitrogen until thawing and use. Before each enzymatic treatment, the OCF was weighted using analytical balance.

Histological examination of ovarian tissue cortex

For histological investigation, the OCFs were fixed in Bouin' solution, imbedded in paraffin wax, serially sectioned at 5 mm, stained with haematoxylin/eosin, and analyzed under a light inverted stereomicroscope Nikon SMZ1270 (Nikon, Düsseldorf, Germany) under 400× magnification. The following types of preantral follicles were evaluated: (1) primordial follicles composed of an oocyte surrounded by a layer of flattened follicular cells, (2) primary and secondary follicles that are similar to primordial follicles, but in which the oocyte is surrounded by one to two layers of cuboidal granulosa cells. Morphology of the follicles was evaluated on the basis of parameters previously described [47]. The number of viable and damaged follicles was counted. To avoid overcounting of the same follicles, only the section with a visible oocyte nucleus was counted. Normality of follicles was evaluated based on the parameters previously described by Paynter et al. [47]. Three types of follicles were distinguished: Type I follicle is spherical with randomly distributed granulosa cells around the oocytes. The cytoplasm is homogenous with slightly granulated nucleus, in the center of which condensed chromatin is detected in the form of dense spherical structure. Type II follicle is spherical; however, granulosa cells do not cover the oocytes regularly. The oocytes can be flat, and condensed chromatin is not detected in the cytoplasm. Type III follicle has partly or fully disrupted cytoplasm and pyknotic nucleus. The cytoplasm of granulosa cells has damages similar to oocytes. Follicles of Type I and Type II were denoted as normal, and those of Type III were denoted as degenerated.

Tissue cryopreservation (freezing and thawing)

This procedure was performed as published previously [48–58]. In our protocol, we used DMSO and ethylene glycol as cryoprotective cocktail to support a multi-cellular structure of ovarian tissues to protect all types of cells [59]. On the day of freezing, OCFs were placed for 30 min at room temperature in a 20-ml freezing medium composed of basal medium supplemented with 6% dimethyl sulfoxide, 6% ethylene glycol and 0.15-M sucrose. Then pieces were put into a standard 5-ml cryo-vials (Thermo Fisher Scientific, Rochester, NY, USA) previously filled by 4.5 ml freezing medium and frozen in an IceCube 14S freezer (Sy-Lab, Neupurkersdorf, Austria). The slow cooling profile started at – 6 °C, and the samples were then cooled from – 6 °C to – 34 °C at a rate of 0.3 °C/min. At – 34 °C, the cryo-vials were finally plunged into liquid nitrogen and stored until thawing. The freezing protocol for cryopreservation of this ovarian tissue included an auto-seeding step at – 6 °C.

To thaw the samples, cryo-vials were removed from liquid nitrogen and held for 30 s at room temperature; they were then immersed in a 100 °C (boiling) water bath for 60 s. The exposure time in the boiling water was visually controlled by the presence of ice in the

Table 1 Total number of follicles isolated from frozen/thawed ovarian tissues after enzymatic digestion with different kinds of enzymes in 14 experiments

Number of patient	Patient age (years)	Treatment of ovarian cortex	Enzymatic digestion (follicles number)		Volume of piece (mm^3)	Byopsy weight (g)			Follicle density/ (mm^3)
			TDE**	Liberase TM***		Whole byopsy weight	Byopsy for TDE digestion	Byopsy for Liberase TM digestion	
1	26	frozen	10	5	20	0.0192	0.0090	0.0102	8
2	29	frozen	15	7	30	0.0738	0.0378	0.0360	7
3	33	frozen	23	6	45	0.0941	0.0460	0.0482	7
4	22	frozen	43	20	40	0.0973	0.0479	0.0494	12
5	31	frozen	12	9	22	0.0257	0.0125	0.0132	7
6	39	frozen	14	7	36	0.0854	0.0440	0.0414	5
7	23	frozen	55	13	180	0.2805	0.1396	0.1409	5
8	29	frozen	34	6	55	0.1342	0.0665	0.0677	8
9	34	frozen	125	84	165	0.2348	0.116	0.1188	10
10	20	frozen	321	168	144	0.2220	0.116	0.106	24
11	34	frozen	216	115	157	0.2253	0.1114	0.1139	17
12	32	fresh	44	16	200	0.4592	0.2310	0.2286	4
13	34	fresh	30	12	210	0.5775	0.2905	0.2870	2
14	28	fresh	48	19	55	0.1401	0.0691	0.0710	11
Total	–	–	990	487	–	–			
Mean ± SD			70.7 ± 87.7*	34.8 ± 48.7	81.2 ± 71.8	0.18 ± 0.17	0.096 ± 0.1	0.095 ± 0.1	9.1 ± 5.5

*asterisk corresponding the statistical ($P < 0.01$)
**TDE (Dr. Christian Sartori, Labour, Hamburg, Germany) is a commercial Enzyme-cocktail (Patent Nr. WO 2006031867 A2, 2004)
***Liberase TM Research grade belongs to the group of Liberase Research Grade Purified Enzyme Blends with reduced endotoxine levels and are mixtures of highly purified Collagenase I and Collagenase II, and with a medium concentration of Thermolysin

medium; as soon as the ice was 2 to 1 mm apex, the cryo-vial was removed from the boiling water, at which point the final temperature of the medium was between 4 °C and 10 °C. Within 5–10 s after thawing, the pieces from the cryo-vials were transferred to a 10 ml thawing solution (basal medium containing 0.5-M sucrose) in a 100 ml specimen container (Sarstedt, Nümbrecht, Germany). For stepwise dilution of cryoprotectants, the container was placed on a shaker and continuously agitated with 200 osc/min for 15 min at room temperature.

Rehydration of the tissue by stepwise rehydration followed. This was also performed using the same, previously published [5, 48–58] 'dropping' methodology: slow addition of basal medium to the solution of sucrose with ovarian pieces. For 'dropping', we used 50-ml of basal medium in a 50-ml tube (Greiner Bio-One GmbH, Frickenhausen, Germany). The final sucrose concentration was 0.083-M, resulting in almost isotonic conditions [5, 48–58]. The last step involved three washes in a basal medium for 10 min immediately prior to preparation.

Preparation of fresh and thawed ovarian tissue and isolation of follicles

We compared the influence of the enzyme Liberase TM Research Grade (Thermolysin Medium Concentration, Roche Diagnostics GmbH, Roche Applied Science, Mannheim, Germany) with the Tumor Dissociation Enzyme (TDE) from the DCS ATP-Chemo-sensitivity Assay Kit (DCS Innovative Diagnostik-Systeme, Dr. Christian Sartori Labor, Hamburg, Germany) on the survival of different stages of isolated follicles after enzymatic digestion of fresh and cryopreserved human ovarian cortex.

The TDE (commercially purchased from the Firma Dr. Christian Sartori Labor, Hamburg, Germany) is a commercial enzyme -cocktail for enzymatic digestion of any solid tumors [43–45].

All enzyme solutions were prepared on Leibovitz L-15 medium of appropriate concentrations in combination with 50 μg/ml neutral red dye, a vitality dye that shows a deep red colour in acid cell structures for the express-visualization of viable follicles (Fig. 1a, b).

Twenty-two frozen/thawed and six fresh OCFs obtained from 11 patients were divided into four treatment groups: Group 1: 11 frozen OCFs for enzymatic digestion with TDE; Group 2: 11 frozen OCFs for enzymatic digestion with Liberase TM: and two fresh control groups: Group 3: 3 fresh OCFs for enzymatic digestion with TDE; Group 4: 3 fresh OCFs for enzymatic digestion with Liberase TM (Fig. 2).

The treatment procedure was performed as previously described [60] with some modification. OCFs were mechanically cut into ~ 0.5 × 1 to 1 × 1 mm^3 pieces onto

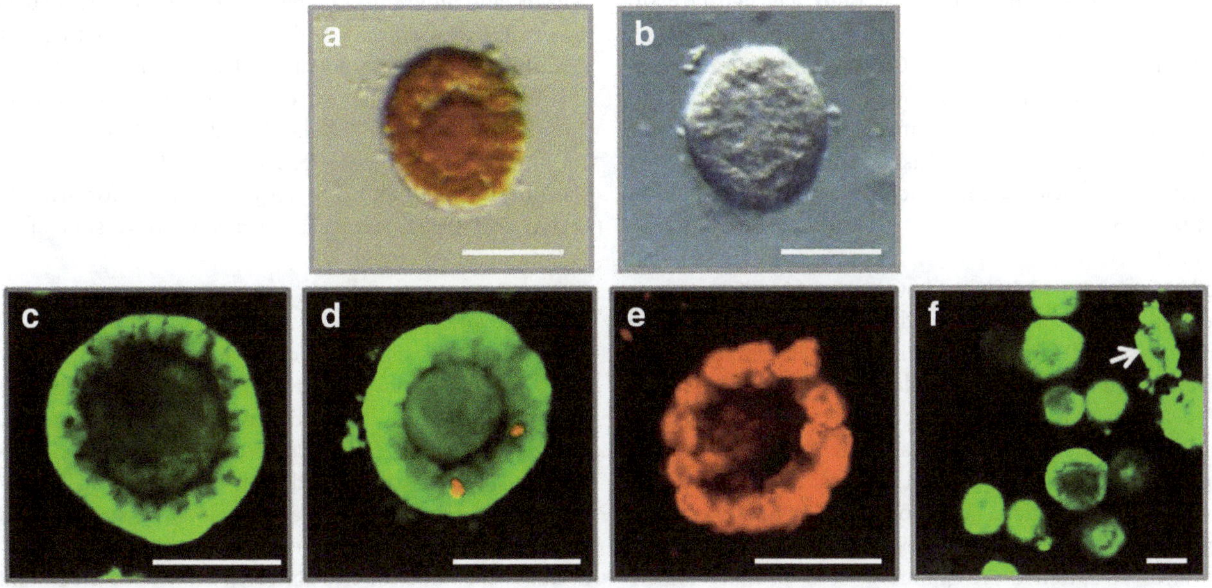

Fig. 1 Example of follicles treated with neutral red dye and live/dead fluorochrome assay. **a** neutral red positive follicle; **b** B neutral red negative follicle. Neutral red dye is a viability stain which shows a deep red colour in acid cell structures like lysosomes. **c** V1, fully viable isolated follicle (granulosa cells as well as oocyte show bright green fluorescence) positive to Calcein AM, negative to ethidium homodimer-1; **d** V2, minimally damaged follicle with two cells positive (bright red colour) to ethidium homodimer-1; **e** negative control: dead follicle showing bright red fluorescence (positive to ethidium homodimer-1, negative to Calcein AM); **f** group of follicles, mostly V1, arrow indicates a follicle that was mechanically disrupted during the manipulation process. Bar = 50 μm

a sterile 100 mm Falcon Petri dish (Falcon, Corning Incorporated-Life Science, Corning, USA) pre-cooled on ice to + 4 °C and put onto a cold plate to stabilize the temperature. The cutting of OCFs was performed with quick simultaneous movements of two scalpels no. 22. The ovarian tissue pieces were then suspended in basal medium containing 16% TDE (Group 1 and Group 3) or in basal medium containing 0.05 mg/ml Liberase TM (Group 2 and Group 4). The optimal concentration for digestion with TDE was titrated in previous experiments (unpublished data). Incubation with enzymes was performed in CO_2 -incubator at 37 °C on KS 260 basic shaker (IKA, Staufen, Germany) with 100 rotations/min for 75 min. Enzymatic digestion was inhibited by the addition of an equal volume of 4 °C cold Leibovitz L-15 medium containing 20% fetal calf serum (FCS). The cell

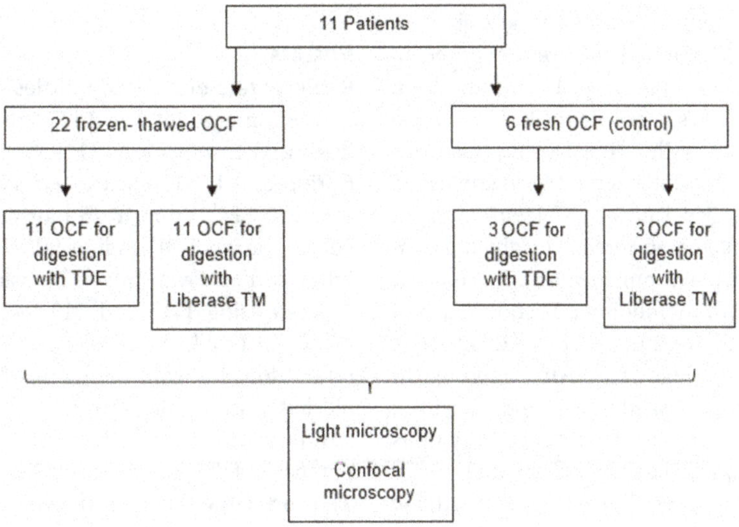

Fig. 2 Experimental design

suspension was immediately put onto ice, gently aspirated up and down with a 1-ml pipette, filtered through 100-μm cell strainers (Falcon, Corning Incorporated-Life Science, NY, USA) and examined by two experienced co-workers under a light inverted stereomicroscope Nikon SMZ1270 (Nikon, Düsseldorf, Germany) in the presence of follicles stained and non-stained with neutral red follicles.

Collection and morphological evaluation of follicles

Isolated follicles were collected with 135 μm V-denuded capillaries (Vitromed GmbH, Jena, Germany) and washed four times in pre-cooled to 4 °C basal medium to discard stromal cells. The number of stained and unstained follicles was calculated for both groups. To identify the isolated primordial follicles, the classification described by Gougeon and Fortune [61, 62] was used: primordial follicle (< 60 μm), oocytes surrounded by a single layer of flattened pre-granulosa cells; primary follicle (> 60 μm - ≤75 μm), oocytes with single layer of cuboidal granulosa cells; secondary follicle (> 75 μm - < 200 μm).

Immediately after isolation of follicles, they were observed under Nikon microscope SMZ25. The follicle diameter was measured by Program Zen (Nikon, Düsseldorf, Germany).

Confocal laser scanning microscopy

The neutral red staining method provides a fairly rough estimation of viability. However, dead granulose cells are difficult to identify [39] and we have chosen a live/dead fluorochrome assay for exact analysis of viability using confocal laser scanning microscopy. To check the viability of cellular structures of isolated ovarian follicles (oocytes surrounded by flat or cubical follicular cells) collected follicles were stained with Calcein AM for visualization of viable cells and ethidium homodimer-1 for visualization of dead cells as previously described by Cortvrindt and Smitz [63]. The follicles were exposed to 2 μM of Calcein AM and 5 μM of ethidium homodimer-1 in Dulbecco's phosphate buffer saline (DPBS) for 15 min at 37 °C in the dark. During this time, living cells for intracellular esterase activity converted the non -fluorescent cell-permeable Calcein AM in fluorescent Calcein producing an intense bright uniform green fluorescence (ex/em, 495 nm/515 nm). In contrast to Calcein AM, ethidium homodimer-1 shows a red fluorescence when bound to the DNA of dead cells (ex/em, 528 nm/617 nm) (Fig. 1c-f). After exposure to these dyes, the follicles were washed in PBS and visualized using a confocal laser scanning microscope Olympus Fluoview FV 1000 (Olympus, Hamburg, Germany) with a multi-line argon laser (458, 488, 515 nm) to record the fluorescent images. Follicle viability was done as described by Paulini [64], as follows. Viable follicles of class V1: oocytes and all granulose cells are viable; minimally damaged follicles of class V2: the presence of less than 10% dead follicular cells; moderately damaged follicles of class V3: 10–50% dead follicular cells; and follicles of class V4: both the oocytes and all follicular cells are dead.

Confocal images were processed and analyzed using the program Fiji, an open-source platform for scientific image processing, which is an advanced version of the commonly used Image J.

Statistical analysis

The enzymatic digestion of ovarian cortex with two types of enzymes was repeated at least three times on different days. Results were expressed as mean ± standard deviation (SD). Statistical evaluation of flow cytometrical results was performed with the GraphPad Prism 5 software package (GraphPad, La Jolla, USA), applying D'Agostino's K2 test to assess Gaussian distribution. To evaluate the effect of two different enzymatic treatments on the cellular viability of ovarian cortex (stromal cells and follicles) immediately after digestion, a T-test for equal variances was performed. P-values less than 0.05 were considered statistically significant.

The correlation test (EXCEL – 2010) was performed for multi-variables (recovered follicle number, patient's age, size and volume of biopsies) to investigate the relationship between these parameters. The value of correlation coefficient (r) was always between + 1 and – 1 inclusive, where 1 is total positive linear correlation, 0 is no linear correlation, and – 1 is total negative linear correlation. A commonly used scale for the interpretation of correlation coefficient is the following: no correlation: r from 0 to 0.1 or from 0 to – 0.1; weak correlation exists: r from 0.1 to 0.3 or from – 0.1 to – 0.3; moderate correlation exists: r from 0.3 to 0.5 or from – 0.3 to – 0.5; and strong correlation exists: r from 0.5 to 1 or from – 0.5 to – 1.

Results

Retrieval rate of isolated follicles

In experiments total of 1477 follicles were isolated from fresh and frozen OCFs (169 follicles were isolated from 6 fresh and 1308 follicles were isolated from 22 cryopreserved OCFs). From fresh biopsies, 122 follicles were recovered using TDE and 46 follicles were recovered using Liberase TM. From frozen biopsies, 868 follicles were recovered using TDE and 440 follicles using Liberase TM ($P < 0.05$) (Table 1). It was established that the retrieval rate of follicles from the biopsies of patients 22–39 years old has a strong negative ($r = -0.6$) correlation with age. However, the relationship between the patient age and number of follicles per 1 mm^3 had no correlation ($r = 0.06$). The correlation between the volume of biopsies and number of retrieved follicles is a moderate positive ($r = 0.3$). The same moderate correlation ($r = 0.4$) was found between the volume of biopsies and number of follicles per 1 mm^3. The correlation between the weight of biopsies and number of retrieved follicles was very weak ($r = 0.1$). However, between the weight of biopsies and number of follicles per 1 mm^3, medium correlation ($r = 0.$) was found. Between the age of patient and volume of biopsies or weight of biopsies, the same very weak correlation ($r = 0.1$ and $r = 0.2$, respectively) was observed. However, the relationship between the weight of biopsies and its volume has a strong positive correlation ($r = 1$) (Table 1).

Quantity and morphology of isolated follicles

As shown in Fig. 3a the most of follicles in Group 1 are fully isolated ($P < 0.01$).

Compared to digestion with TDE, the digestion with Liberase TM (Fig. 3b) has resulted in incomplete tissue digestion (black arrows). Extruded oocytes were found in both treatment groups, but it was extremely rare (< 3%). Note that apart from the good three-dimensional structure, the general morphology of isolated follicles was well maintained independently from the type of enzymatic treatment. After evaluation of isolated follicles under an inverted microscope, it was noted their normal spherical form with mostly one layer of granulosa cells around the oocyte. The data for the quantity of retrieved follicles of different maturity inside each treatment are shown (Fig. 4a). It was also demonstrated that the number of retrieved follicles independently from their maturity was significantly ($P < 0.01$) higher in the TDE -treatment group in comparison with Liberase TM groups (Group 1[$n = 122$] vs Group 2 [$n = 46$], Group 3 [$n = 868$] vs Group 4 [$n = 440$]. However, these differences in all treatment groups were no significant ($P > 0.1$) in the distribution of follicles according to their maturity (Fig. 4b).

Viability of follicles

The viability assessment of follicles was performed using two techniques: (1) express technique for visualization of live follicles with the application of neutral red dye and subsequent evaluation of follicles under a light inverted stereomicroscope and (2) by fluorescence-staining technique with Calcein AM and ethidium homodimer-1 for visualization of viable and dead cells under a confocal laser microscope.

Express technique for visualization of follicle vitality

Immediately after enzymatic treatment and simultaneous staining with Neutral red dye, the suspension of ovarian stromal cells and follicles were examined under an inverted microscope. Follicles were collected and neutral red -uptake was investigated based on the optical presence of their red staining.

The data on Fig. 5a show that the presence of intense red -stained follicles in the suspension from fresh ovarian tissues digested with TDE was significantly higher than in the suspension of tissues digested with Liberase TM (94.2 ± 6.6% in Group 1 vs 79.1 ± 2.1% in Group 2, respectively).

The percent of light red- stained follicles was significantly higher ($P < 0.05$) in the suspension of tissues digested with Liberase TM than after digestion with TDE (Group 2 vs Group 1: 16.6 ± 0.6% vs 4.3 ± 0.4%, respectively), while the presence of non -stained follicles was not significantly different in these groups (Group 2 vs Group 1: 4.2 ± 0.3% vs 1.4 ± 0.3%, respectively). The presence of intense red -stained follicles in the suspension of cryopreserved ovarian tissues digested with TDE was significantly higher ($P < 0.05$) in frozen ovarian tissues (70.3 ± 6.2% in Group 3 vs 53.1 ± 2.0% in Group 4, respectively) than in the suspension of tissues digested with Liberase TM

The amount of light red -stained follicles was not significantly different ($P > 0.1$) between Group 3 and Group 4 (17.7 ± 1.5% vs 20.2 ± 1.0%, respectively), while the presence of non-stained follicles was significantly higher ($P < 0.05$) (12.0 ± 1.3% in Group 3 vs 26.8 ± 0.9% in Group 4, respectively) in the suspension of tissues digested with Liberase TM. The data on Fig. 5b (digested

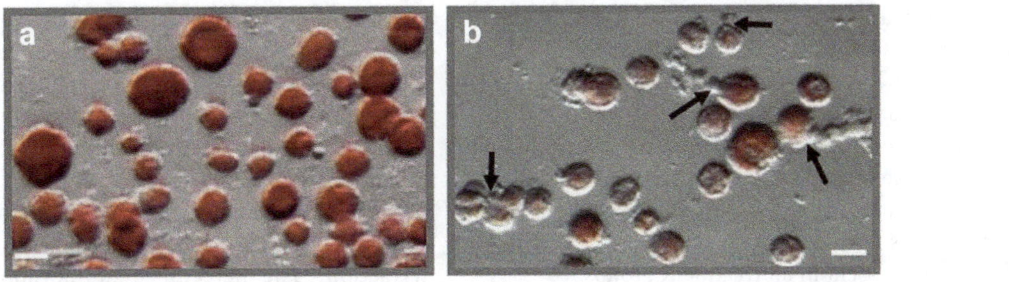

Fig. 3 Typical view of follicle suspension after enzymatic digestion. **a** follicles isolated from frozen ovarian cortex with TDE-enzyme cocktail; **b** follicles isolated from frozen ovarian cortex with Liberase TM. The black arrows show the clustered and partially isolated from incompletely digested stroma follicles. Bar = 50 μm

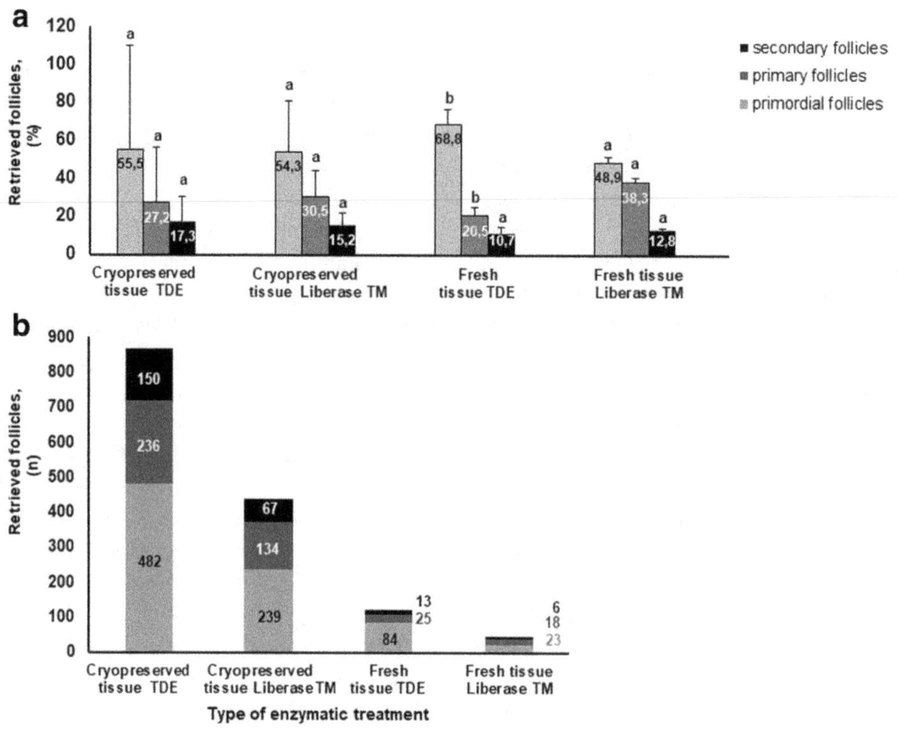

Fig. 4 Distribution of follicles according to their maturity in each treatment group. **a** Percent of retrieved follicles of different maturity inside of each treatment group. **b** Number of retrieved follicles of different maturity inside of each treatment group. Bars (mean ± SD) with different superscripts in respective treatment group represent significant differences ($P < 0.05$)

fresh tissue) and Fig. 5c (digested frozen tissue) characterize the vitality of follicles according to their maturity. No significant difference ($P > 0.1$) according to the vitality of different maturity stages of follicles between treatment groups was found.

Vitality visualisation with confocal laser scanning microscopy

All isolated follicles after assessment of vitality using the Neutral red dye were stained with fluorescent dye to identify the presence of living and dead cells in each follicle. The data on Fig. 6a show that the percent of recovered class V1 follicles in the suspension from fresh ovarian tissues are not significantly different between Group 1 and Group 2 (97.1 ± 6.8% vs 91.3 ± 2.1%, respectively) ($P > 0.1$). However, a significantly higher rate (96.0 ± 7.8% vs 87.9 ± 2.4%, respectively) ($P < 0.05$) of recovered follicles of class V1 in Group 3 (cortical tissue suspension digested with TDE) compared to Group 4 was found. The amount of class V2 and V3 follicles in all treatment groups was not significantly different ($P > 0.1$). Class V4 follicles were absent in all treatment groups.

The data on Fig. 6b (digested fresh tissue) and Fig. 6c (digested frozen tissue) characterize the vitality of follicles according to their maturity stage.

No significant difference ($P > 0.1$) between class V1 primordial follicles was found in ovarian tissues of Group 1 (fresh, TDE-digested ovarian tissues) (58.5 ± 4.2%), Group 2 (fresh, Liberase TM-digested ovarian tissues) (55.8 ± 1.3%), Group 3 (frozen, TDE-digested ovarian tissues) (53.9 ± 4.2%), and Group 4 (frozen, Liberase TM-digested ovarian tissues) (52.1 ± 1.3%).

The presence of class V2 and V3 follicles was not significantly different between all treatment groups, independent of the stage of preantral follicles, ($P > 0.1$). Class V4 preantral follicles in all treatment groups were absent.

Histological evaluation of fresh and frozen ovarian tissue

Histological evaluation of non-treated pieces of ovarian cortex (fresh control) shows that the most of exanimated follicles (96.8 ± 2.5%) were morphologically normal.

Histologic analysis of haematoxylin-eosin stained ovarian cortical tissues showed morphologically normal preantral follicles. The follicles were surrounded by non-disrupted intact basement membrane. The oocytes were slightly stained, without signs of degeneration or retraction. The percentage of morphologically normal follicles was not significantly different ($P > 0.1$) between the fresh and frozen ovarian tissues samples (96.8 ± 2.5% vs 97.1 ± 5.1%, respectively).

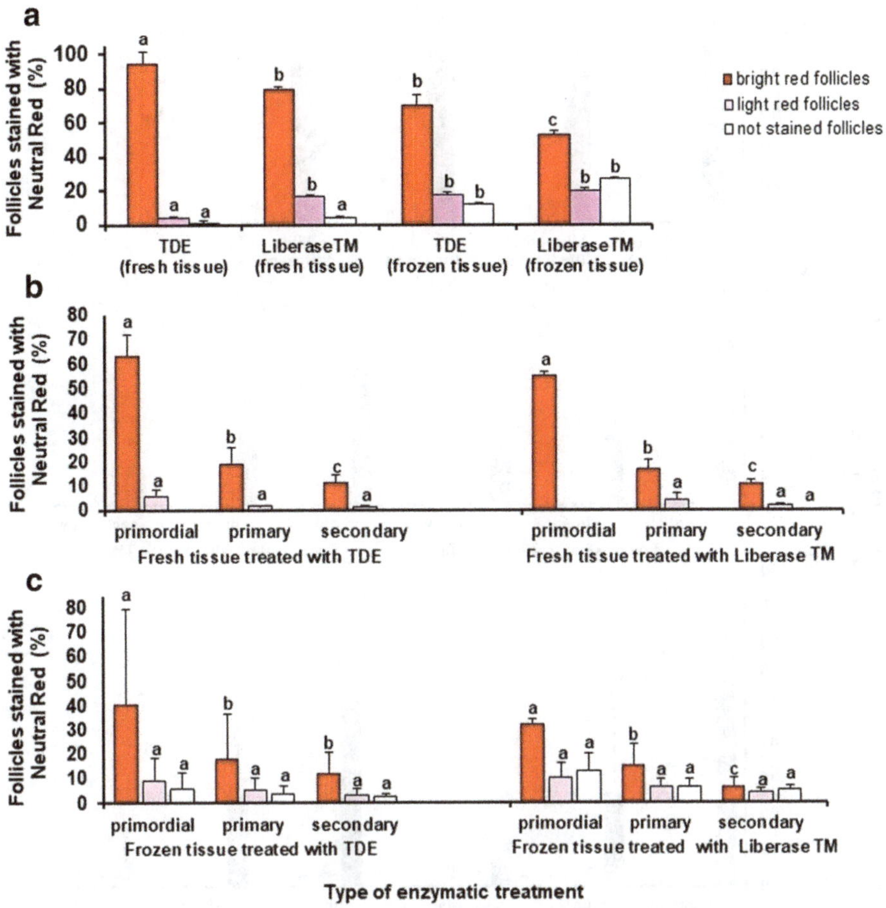

Fig. 5 Influence of the type of enzymatic treatment of ovarian cortex on the vitality of isolated follicles of different maturity tested applying of Neutral Red dye. **a** Vitality of follicles in different treatment groups independent of their maturity stage; **b** Comparison of follicle vitality in Group 1 (fresh ovarian tissues digested with TDE) compared to Group 2 (fresh ovarian tissues digested with Liberase TM) depending on their maturity stage, **c** Comparison of follicle vitality in Group 3 (frozen ovarian tissues digested with TDE) compared to Group 4 (frozen ovarian tissues digested with Liberase TM) depending on their maturity stage. Bars (mean ± SD) with different superscripts in respective treatment group represent significant differences ($P < 0.05$)

Discussion

The latest work in the field of follicle isolation from human and animal ovarian cortical tissue indicates their excellent survival after thawing and the ability to further development both in culture and after xenotransplantation [18, 19, 64, 65]. An important task is isolation of the follicles from ovarian cortex to recover a maximal number of high quality viable follicles.

In this work, we applied our original routine cryopreservation protocol for human ovarian tissue, which presupposes the long-time tissue pre-cooling step before freezing. The reason is our previous establishment that the 24 h cooling to 5 °C before cryopreservation is beneficial for the cryopreservation of human ovarian tissues, especially of follicles [5, 48–58].

Enzymatic digestion is commonly used for tissue dissociation and cell harvesting and offers the advantages of unattended quick sample preparation, potential automation, and is low cost with the possibility to obtain more cells of interest [66–68]. The feasibility of enzymatic digestion is a good alternative tissue sample preparation method to the technique of mechanical tissue dissection.

It is well known that the human ovarian cortex possesses a highly dense and fibrous structure. Therefore, using of special enzymatic digestion technique is necessary for effective isolation of the follicles from the surrounding tissue.

The widely used enzyme collagenase is known to degrade connective tissues to allow tissue dissolution and to get the single-celled suspensions. However, enzymatic digestion with the use of collagenase also has serious disadvantages. These disadvantages are well described [69] on the example of hepatocytes.

Thus, it is known that most isolation protocols result in damage of cell junctions, cell membranes, to cell surface receptors and antigens, and cytosolic contents [70, 71].

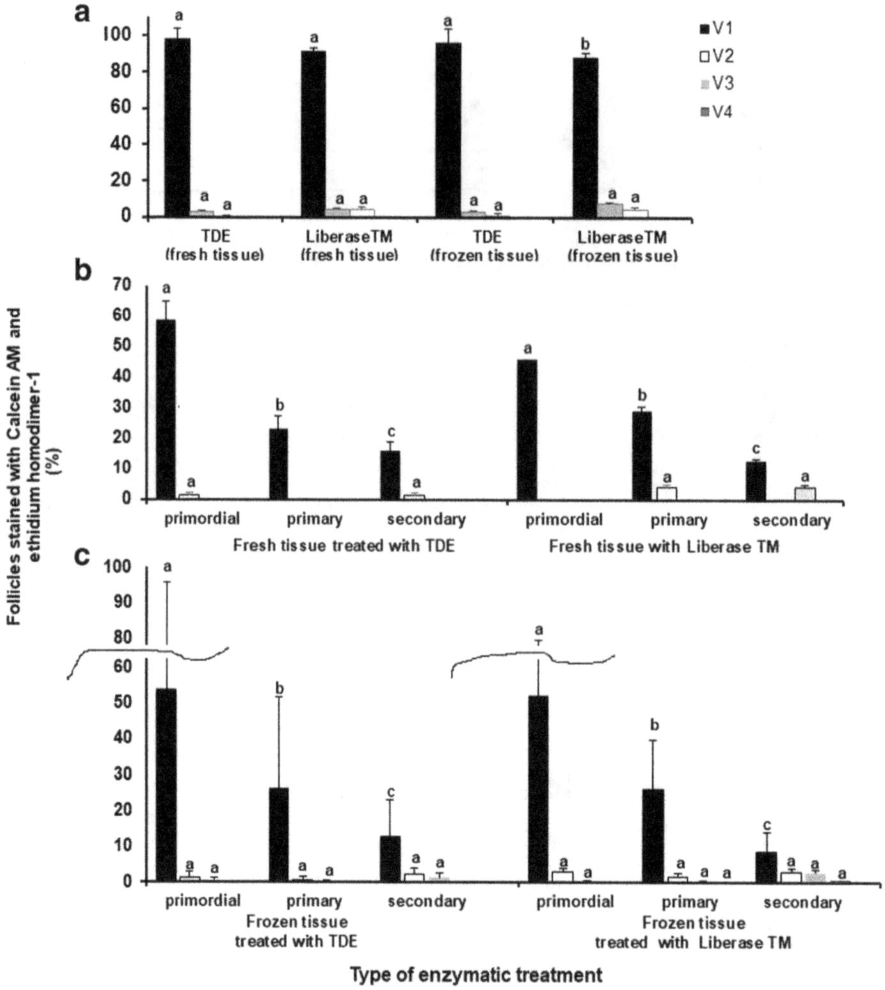

Fig. 6 Influence of the type of enzymatic treatment of ovarian cortex on the vitality of isolated follicles of different maturity tested using of Calcein AM for visualization of viable cells and ethidium homodimer-1 for visualization of dead cells. **a** Viability of follicles in different treatment groups. **b** Comparison of follicle vitality in Group 1 (fresh ovarian tissues digested with TDE) compared to Group 2 (fresh ovarian tissues digested with Liberase TM) depending on their maturity stage, **c** Comparison of follicle vitality in Group 3 (frozen ovarian tissues digested with TDE) compared to Group 4 (frozen ovarian tissues digested with Liberase TM) depending on their maturity stage. Bars (mean ± SD) with different superscripts in respective treatment group represent significant differences ($P < 0.05$)

By enzymatic follicle isolation, the basal membrane disruption occurs often [72]. Collagenase digestion also induces oxidative stress observed 4-8 h after isolation of hepatocytes, leading to a loss of cytochrome enzyme activity [73].

This could be why many isolated preantral follicles degenerate within the first 24 h of in vitro culture and only a few of them could reach the early antral stage [34, 35, 38, 41].

In attempts to standardize the protocol of enzymatic digestion and to improve the quality of isolated follicles, the various types of collagenase (Ia, II, IX, XI) alone [36, 37, 39, 74–76] or in combinations with DNA-se [35, 38, 41, 76–78] were used. However, it was reported about increased amount of lipid droplets in granulosa cells of isolated follicles (collagenase IX and deoxyribonuclease IV, [35]) and about high amounts of premature oocyte extrusions from the enzymatically isolated follicles (collagenase Type II) [37] that shows that the enzyme collagenase has a batch-to-batch variation in effectiveness [79].

According to the latest data [36, 40, 42, 80], the viability of enzymatically isolated follicles depends on the level of purity, the type of collagenase and on combination with other enzymes, which could reduce its toxicity. Such products are Liberase Research Grade Purified Enzyme Blends and are mixtures of highly purified collagenase and neutral protease enzymes, formulated for efficient, gentle, and reproducible dissociation of tissues from a wide variety of sources (Roche Diagnostics GmbH, Mannheim, Germany).

The works of Dolmans et al. [36], Vanacker [40] and Kristensen [39] have shown the beneficial role of different types of Liberase for follicle isolation during enzymatic digestion. In the work of Lierman [60] both Liberase TM combined with collagenase IV and Liberase DH were shown to be better for isolating high-quality primordial follicles, compared with mono-enzyme collagenase IV. The Liberase TM (Thermolysin Medium, 0.04 mg/ml, Roche Diagnostics GmbH, Mannheim, Germany), we used in our experiments belongs to the group of Liberase Research Grade Purified Enzyme Blends with reduced endotoxin levels and is a mixture of highly purified Collagenase I and Collagenase II with a medium concentration of Thermolysin (a non-clostridial neutral extremely stable Zn-metalloendopeptidase (www.Sigma-Aldrich.de) formulated for efficient, gentle, and reproducible dissociation of tissues from a wide variety of sources (http://www.roche-applied-science.com; Worthington Enzyme Manual, V Worthington Biochemical Corporation). Their activity is directed to break the peptide bonds in collagen (Collagenase), fibronectin, collagen IV, and to a lower extent collagen I, however, it does not cleave collagen V or laminin of neutral protease (V Worthington Biochemical Corporation).

Compared to Liberase TM, TDE is a commercial enzyme -cocktail [46] for enzymatic digestion of any solid tumors [43–45]. Due to highly secured patenting [46], we could not obtain the full composition of this enzyme cocktail and we can only assume, according to the quality of the digested material (not sticky, not viscous, and easy to handle), that this cocktail, together with highly purified types of collagenase, may also include enzymes such as protease, dispase or DNA-se.

The comparison of two digestion protocols according to the quality of digestion of stromal tissues showed that TDE allows complete digestion of the stromal tissue with good preservation of follicle integrity. The digested tissue suspension is easy to handle, not sticky and able to obtain a good number of viable follicles. In contrast, the tissue digested with Liberase TM remained poorly dissolved, was sticky and stretchy, and many follicles were still tightly embedded in the tissue and was very difficult to isolate, and this support the finding described [39]. The comparison of the two treatment groups also showed that the number of fully isolated follicles in the TDE groups was significantly higher than in the Liberase TM groups both for fresh and frozen tissues, considering that the size of digested ovarian cortex was similar in both groups.

For evaluation of the quality of recovered follicles from cryopreserved ovarian cortex, we used two techniques: (1) vital staining with neutral red dye for visualization of live follicles and (2) fluorescence -staining of follicles with Calcein AM and ethidium homodimer-1 for visualization of viable and dead cells under a confocal laser microscope.

We have decided to apply the neutral red dye in our experiments, because this vital dye has no deleterious effects on enzymatic activity within cellular organelles [81] and proves to be nontoxic with no long-term negative effects on the follicles [39, 82]. Neutral red (toluylene red, Basic Red 5, or C.I. 50,040) is a eurhodin dye used for many staining methods in histology. Neutral red is used also as a vital stain because the live cells incorporate neutral red into their lysosomes [83]. As cells begin to die, their ability to incorporate neutral red diminishes [84, 85]. This vital dye allows also easy visualization of the follicles in cell suspension. This technique was first applied by Kristensen [39] for follicle visualization and their vitality assessment, and it allows accelerating the process of follicle collection. Our results show that the presence of intense red stained follicles in the ovarian cortical tissue suspension digested with TDE for both fresh and frozen ovarian tissues was significantly higher than in the suspension of tissues digested with Liberase TM.

Visualization of viable and dead cells under a confocal laser scanning microscopy with Calcein AM and ethidium homodimer-1 showed that digestion ovarian tissue with TDE for both fresh and frozen samples provides a significantly higher integrity rate of recovered follicles (class V1) compared to the Liberase TM -groups. The effectiveness of the TDE technique is similar to the data for the Liberase follicles isolated from fresh cortical tissues [36] and with the data for follicles isolated from frozen tissues [18, 86–88].

According to the latest research data, the best survival of the cells of an oocyte-granulosa-cells complex immediately after enzymatic isolation of preantral follicles from fresh ovarian tissue with subsequent one-week in vitro culture provides the Liberase DH enzymatic cocktail [40]. Our data presented here with use of TDE commercial enzyme-cocktail for isolation of preantral follicles are not principally different from the results achieved with use of Liberase DH for digestion of fresh ovarian tissue (95% TDE vs 95% Liberase DH, $P > 0.5$) [40]. The use of highly purified commercial enzyme-cocktails allows eliminating the possibility of obtaining undesirable results through the fault of the drug manufacturer [35, 37, 41, 79]. In fact, there are not principal differences between these two enzymatic cocktails: they content seemingly different types of collagenase.

In the future work we suppose to perform a comparative evaluation of effectiveness of these two commercial enzymatic cocktails (TDE and Liberase DH) with detailed investigation of all apoptotic degenerations (early apoptotic, late apoptotic and necrotic cells) which could take place in enzymatically isolated follicles using specific surface markers for follicular cells by applying flow cytometry and confocal microscopy.

Conclusion

New method for isolation of preantral follicles with tumor dissociation enzyme (TDE) that can be used for the construction of artificial ovary, provides a higher number of healthy preantral follicles from cryopreserved ovarian cortex in contrast with the earlier described Liberase Thermolysin Medium method.

Abbreviations

DNA: Deoxyribonucleic acid; Liberase TM: Liberase Thermolysin Medium; OCF: Ovarian tissue cortical fragment; OTB: 24 ovarian tissue biopsies; PBS: Phosphate buffer saline Dulbecco; SD: Standard deviation; TDE: Tumor dissociation enzyme

Acknowledgements

Supported by Alexander von Humboldt Foundation.

Funding

The authors did not receive any specific funding for this study.

Authors' contributions

Conceived and designed the experiments: EI, VS, GR, VI, PM; performed the experiments: VS, EI, GR; analyzed the data: GR, GR, BH, BM; contributed materials/analysis tools: GR, VS, PM, wrote the manuscript: EI, VI, VS; manuscript drafting and critical discussion: EI, VI, VS, GR; finally approved of the version to be published: EI, VI. All authors read and approved the final manuscript.

Competing interests

The authors declare that they have no competing interests.

Author details

[1]Research Group for Reproductive Medicine and IVF-Laboratory, Department of Obstetrics and Gynaecology, University Maternal Hospital, Cologne University, Kerpener Str. 34, 50931 Cologne, Germany. [2]Cell Sort Service Department, Center for Molecular Medicine Cologne University (CMMC), Robert Koch Str. 21, 50931 Cologne, Germany.

References

1. Abir R, Nitke S, Ben-Haroush A, Fisch B. In vitro maturation of human primordial ovarian follicles: clinical significance, progress in mammals, and methods for growth evaluation. Histol Histopathol. 2006;21:887–98.
2. Feigin E, Freud E, Fisch B, Orvieto R, Kravarusic D, Avrahami G. Fertility preservation in female adolescents with malignancies. In: Cancer in Female Adolescents. Hauppauge: USA Science Publishers Inc; 2008. p. 38–101.
3. Donnez J, Jadoul P, Squifflet J, van Langendonckt A, Donnez O, Van Eyck AS, et al. Ovarian tissue cryopreservation and transplantation in cancer patients. Best Pract Res Clin Obstet Gynaecol. 2010;24:87–100.
4. Wallace WH, Thomson AB, Saran F, Kelsey TW. Predicting age of ovarian failure after radiation to a field that includes the ovaries. Int J Radiat Oncol Biol Phys. 2005;62:738–44.
5. Isachenko V, Todorov P, Isachenko E, Rahimi G, Tchorbanov A, Mihaylova N, et al. Long-time cooling before cryopreservation decreased translocation of phosphatidylserine (Ptd-L-Ser) in human ovarian tissue. PLoS One. 2015;10:e0129108.
6. Donnez J, Dolmans MM. Fertility preservation in women. N Engl J Med. 2017;377:1657–65.
7. Meirow D, Hardan I, Dor J, Fridman E, Elizur S, Ra'anani H, et al. Searching for evidence of disease and malignant cell contamination in ovarian tissue store from hematologic cancer patients. Hum Reprod Oxf Engl. 2008;23:1007–13.
8. Dolmans MM, Marinescu C, Saussoy P, Van Langendonckt A, Amorim C, Donnez J. Reimplantation of cryopreserved ovarian tissue from patients with acute lymphoblastic leukemia is potentially unsafe. Blood. 2010;116:2908–14.
9. Dolmans MM, Jadoul P, Gilliaux S, Amorim CA, Luyckx V, Squifflet J, et al. A review of 15 years of ovarian tissue bank activities. J Assist Reprod Genet. 2013;30:305–14.
10. Rosendahl M, Andersen MT, Ralfkiaer E, Kjeldsen L, Andersen MK, Andersen CY. Evidence of residual disease in cryopreserved ovarian cortex from female patients with leukemia. Fertil Steril. 2010;94:2186–90.
11. Amorim CA, Van Langendonckt A, David A, Dolmans MM, Donnez J. Survival of human pre-antral follicles after cryopreservation of ovarian tissue, follicular isolation and in vitro culture in a calcium alginate matrix. Hum Reprod. 2009;24:92–9.
12. Soares M, Saussoy P, Maskens M, Reul H, Amorim CA, Donnez J, et al. Eliminating malignant cells from cryopreserved ovarian tissue is possible in leukaemia patients. Br J Haematol. 2017;178:231–9.
13. Amorim CA, Shikanov A. The artificial ovary: current status and future perspectives. Future Oncol. 2016;12:2323–32.
14. Rodgers RJ, Irving-Rodgers HF, Russell DL. Extracellular matrix of the developing ovarian follicle. Reproduction. 2003;126:415–24.
15. Luyckx V, Dolmans MM, Vanacker J, Scalercio SR, Donnez J, Amorim CA. First step in developing a 3D biodegradable fibrin scaffold for an artificial ovary. J Ovar Res. 2013;6:83–92.
16. Camboni A, Van Langendonckt A, Donnez J, Vanacker J, Dolmans MM, Amorim CA. Alginate beads as a tool to handle, cryopreserve and culture isolated human primordial/ primary follicles. Cryobiology. 2013;67:64–9.
17. Laronda MM, Rutz AL, Xiao S, Whelan KA, Duncan FE, Roth EW, et al. A bioprosthetic ovary created using 3D printed microporous scaffolds restores ovarian function in sterilized mice. Nat Commun. 2017;8:15261.
18. Vanacker J, Luyckx V, Amorim C, Dolmans MM, Van Langendonckt A, Donnez J, et al. Should we isolate human preantral follicles before or after cryopreservation of ovarian tissue? Fertil Steril. 2013;99:1363–8.
19. Lunardi FO, de Aguiar FL, Duarte AB, Araújo VR, de Lima LF, Ribeiro de Sá NA, et al. Ovine secondary follicles vitrified out the ovarian tissue grow and develop in vitro better than those vitrified into the ovarian fragments. Theriogenology. 2016;85:1203–10.
20. Young JM, McNeilly AS. Theca: the forgotten cell of the ovarian follicle. Reproduction. 2010;140:489–504.
21. Kent J, Ryle M. Histochemical studies on three gonadotrophin-responsive enzymes in the infantile mouse ovary. J Reprod Fertil. 1975;42:519–36.
22. Blanco LZ Jr, Kuhn E, Morrison JC, Bahadirli-Talbott A, Smith-Sehdev A, Kurman RJ. Steroid hormone synthesis by the ovarian stroma surrounding epithelial ovarian tumors: a potential mechanism in ovarian tumorigenesis. Mod Pathol. 2017;30:563–76.
23. Female reproductive system. In. Sorenson RL, Brelje TC, editors. Atlas of human histology. A guide to microscopic structure of cells, tissues and organs. 2014. Minneapolis: University of Minnesota Bookstore; p. 305–28.
24. Furuya M. Ovarian cancer stroma: pathophysiology and the roles in cancer development. Cancers. 2012;4:701–24.
25. Xouri G, Christian S. Origin and function of tumor stroma fibroblasts. Semin Cell Dev Biol. 2010;21:40–6.
26. Figueiredo JR, Hulshof SC, Van den Hurk R, Ectors FJ, Fontes RS, Nusgens B, et al. Development of a combined new mechanical and enzymatic method for the isolation of intact preantral follicles from fetal, calf and adult bovine ovaries. Theriogenology. 1993;40:789–99.
27. Carambula SF, Goncalves PB, Costa LF, Figueiredo JR, Wheeler MB, Neves JP, et al. Effect of fetal age and method of recovery on isolation of preantral follicles from bovine ovaries. Theriogenology. 1999;52:563–71.
28. Amorim CA, Lucci CM, Rodrigues AP, Carvalho FC, Figueiredo JR, Rondina D, et al. Quantitative and qualitative analysis of the effectiveness of a mechanical method for the isolation of preantral follicles from ovine ovaries. Theriogenology. 2000;53:1251–62.
29. Yin H, Kristensen SG, Jiang H, Rasmussen A, Andersen CY. Survival and growth of isolated pre-antral follicles from human ovarian medulla tissue during long-term 3D culture. Hum Reprod. 2016;31:1531–9.
30. Demeestere I, Delbaere A, Gervy C, Van Den Bergh M, Devreker F, Englert Y. Effect of preantral follicle isolation technique on in-vitro follicular growth, oocyte maturation and embryo development in mice. Hum Reprod. 2002;17:2152–9.

31. Santos SS, Biondi FC, Cordeiro MS, Miranda MS, Dantas JK, Figueiredo JR, et al. Isolation, follicular density, and culture of preantral follicles of buffalo fetuses of different ages. Anim Reprod Sci. 2006;95:1–15.
32. Nagano M, Atabay EP, Atabay EC, Hishinuma M, Katagiri S, Takahashi Y. Effects of isolation method and pre-treatment with ethylene glycol or raffinose before vitrification on in vitro viability of mouse preantral follicles. Biomed Res. 2007;28:153–60.
33. Aerts JM, Martinez-Madrid B, Flothmann K, De Clercq JB, Van Aelst S, Bols PE. Quantification and viability assessment of isolated bovine primordial and primary ovarian follicles retrieved through a standardized biopsy pick-up procedure. Reprod Domest Anim. 2008;43:360–6.
34. Abir R, Franks S, Mobberley MA, Moore PA, Margara RA, Winston RM. Mechanical isolation and in vitro growth of preantral and small antral human follicles. Fertil Steril. 1997;68:682–8.
35. Abir R, Fisch B, Nitke S, Okon E, Raz A, Ben Rafael Z. Morphological study of fully and partially isolated early human follicles. Fertil Steril. 2001;75:141–6.
36. Dolmans MM, Michaux N, Camboni A, Martinez-Madrid B, Van Langendonckt A, Nottola SA, et al. Evaluation of Liberase, a purified enzyme blend, for the isolation of human primordial and primary ovarian follicles. Hum Reprod. 2006;21:413–20.
37. Hovatta O, Wright C, Krausz T, Hardy K, Winston RM. Human primordial, primary and secondary ovarian follicles in long-term culture: effect of partial isolation. Hum Reprod. 1999;14:2519–24.
38. Roy SK, Treacy BJ. Isolation and long-term culture of human preantral follicles. Fertil Steril. 1993;59:783–90.
39. Kristensen SG, Rasmussen A, Byskov AG, Andersen CY. Isolation of pre-antral follicles from human ovarian medulla tissue. Hum Reprod. 2011;26:157–66.
40. Vanacker J, Camboni A, Dath C, Van Langendonckt A, Dolmans MM, Donnez J, et al. Enzymatic isolation of human primordial and primary ovarian follicles with Liberase DH: protocol for application in a clinical setting. Fertil Steril. 2011;96:379–83.
41. Abir R, Roizman P, Fisch B, Nitke S, Okon E, Orvieto R, et al. Pilot study of isolated early human follicles cultured in collagen gels for 24 hours. Hum Reprod. 1999;14:1299–301.
42. Rice S, Ojha K, Mason H. Human ovarian biopsies as a viable source of pre-antral follicles. Hum Reprod. 2008;23:600–5.
43. Andreotti PK, Cree IA, Kurbacher CM, Hartmann DM, Linder D, Harel G, et al. Chemosensitivity testing of human tumors using a microplate adenosine triphosphate luminescence assay: clinical correlation for cisplatin resistance of ovarian carcinoma. Cancer Res. 1995;55:52w76–5282.
44. Kurbacher CM, Cree IA, Bruckner HW, Brenne U, Kurbacher JA, Müller K, et al. Use of an ex vivo ATP luminescence assay to direct chemotherapy for recurrent ovarian cancer. Anticancer Drug Des. 1998;9:51–7.
45. Nicolantonio FD. Multidrug resistance in solid tumours. A thesis submitted to the University of London for the degree of Doctor of Philosophy in the Faculty of Medicine Department of Pathology Institute of Ophthalmology, University of London, 2004. p. 372.
46. Bruckner HW. Methods and systems for guiding selection of chemotherapeutic agents. Patent US20060058966A1, 2006.
47. Paynter SJ, Cooper A, Fuller BJ, Shaw RW. Cryopreservation of bovine ovarian tissue: structural normality of follicles after thawing and culture in vitro. Cryobiology. 1999;38:301–9.
48. Isachenko V, Isachenko E, Reinsberg J, Montag M, van der Ven K, Dorn C, et al. Cryopreservation of human ovarian tissue: comparison of rapid and conventional freezing. Cryobiology. 2007;55:261–8.
49. Isachenko V, Isachenko E, Mallmann P, Rahimi G. Long-time cooling of human ovarian tissue before cryopreservation as obvious procedure: stimulation of follicular development and neo-vascularisation. Clin Lab. 2012;58:1293–300.
50. Isachenko V, Isachenko E, Mallmann P, Rahimi G. Increasing follicular and stromal cell proliferation in cryopreserved human ovarian tissue after long-term precooling prior to freezing: in vitro versus chorioallantoic membrane (CAM) xenotransplantation. Cell Transplant. 2013;22:2053–61.
51. Isachenko V, Isachenko E, Reinsberg J, Montag M, Braun F, van der Ven H. Cryopreservation of human ovarian tissue: effect of spontaneous and initiated ice formation. Reprod BioMed Online. 2008;16:336–45.
52. Isachenko V, Isachenko E, Reinsberg J, Montag M, Weiss J, Braun F, van der Ven H. Simplified technique of human ovarian tissue freezing: quick cooling from −36-degree C. CryoLetters. 2008;29:261–8.
53. Isachenko V, Lapidus I, Isachenko E, Krivokharchenko A, Kreienberg R, Woriedh M, et al. Human ovarian tissue vitrification versus conventional freezing: morphological, endocrinological, and molecular biological evaluation. Reproduction. 2009;138:319–27.
54. Isachenko V, Isachenko E, Weiss JM, Todorov P, Kreienberg R. Cryobanking of human ovarian tissue for anti-cancer treatment: comparison of vitrification and conventional freezing. CryoLetters. 2009;30:449–54.
55. Isachenko V, Mallmann P, Petrunkina AM, Rahimi G, Nawroth F, Hancke K, Felberbaum R, Genze F, Damjanoski I, Isachenko E. Comparison of in vitro- and chorioallantoic membrane (CAM)-culture systems for cryopreserved medulla-contained human ovarian tissue. PLoS One. 2012;7:e32549.
56. Isachenko V, Dittrich R, Keck G, Isachenko E, Rahimi G, van der Ven H, et al. Cryopreservation of ovarian tissue: detailed description of methods for transport, freezing and thawing. Geburtsh Frauenheilk. 2012;72:927–32.
57. Isachenko V, Isachenko E, Keck G, Dittrich R, Montag M, van der Ven H, et al. First live birth in Germany after re-transplantation of cryopreserved ovarian tissue: original device for initiation of ice formation. Clin Lab. 2012;58:933–8.
58. Isachenko V, Todorov P, Isachenko E, Rahimi G, Hanstein B, Salama M, et al. Cryopreservation and xenografting of human ovarian fragments: medulla decreases the phosphatidylserine translocation rate. Reprod Biol Endocrin. 2016;14:79.
59. Gook DA, Edgar DH. Ovarian tissue cryopreservation. In: Donnez J, Kim S, editors. Principles and practice of fertility preservation. New York: Cambridge University Press; 2011. p. 342–56.
60. Lierman S, Tilleman K, Cornelissen M, De Vos WH, Weyers S, T'Sjoen G, et al. Follicles of various maturation stages react differently to enzymatic isolation: a comparison of different isolation protocols. Reprod BioMed Online. 2015;30:181–90.
61. Gougeon A. Regulation of ovarian follicular development in primates: facts and hypotheses. Endocr Rev. 1996;17:121–55.
62. Fortune JE. The early stages of follicular development: activation of primordial follicles and growth of preantral follicles. Anim Reprod Sci. 2003;78:135–63. 43
63. Cortvrindt RG, Smitz JE. Fluorescent probes allow rapid and precise recording of follicle density and staging in human ovarian cortical biopsy samples. Fertil Steril. 2001;75:588–93.
64. Paulini F, Vilela JM, Chiti MC, Donnez J, Jadoul P, Dolmans MM, et al. Survival and growth of human preantral follicles after cryopreservation of ovarian tissue, follicle isolation and short-term xenografting. Reprod BioMed Online. 2016;33:425–32.
65. Sampaio da Silva AM, Bruno JB, de Lima LF, Ribeiro de Sá NA, Lunardi FO, Ferreira AC, et al. Connexin 37 and 43 gene and protein expression and developmental competence of isolated ovine secondary follicles cultured in vitro after vitrification of ovarian tissue. Theriogenology. 2016;85:1457–67.
66. Yu C, Penn LD, Hollembaek J, Li W, Cohen LH. Enzymatic tissue digestion as an alternative sample preparation approach for quantitative analysis using liquid chromatography-tandem mass spectrometry. Anal Chem. 2004;76:1761–7.
67. Telfer EE, Zelinski MB. Ovarian follicle culture: advances and challenges for human and non-human Primates. Fertil Steril. 2013;99:1523–33.
68. Hornick JE, Duncan FE, Shea LD, Woodruff TK. Multiple follicle culture supports primary follicle growth through paracrine-acting signals. Reproduction. 2013;145:19–32.
69. Soldatow VY, LeCluyse EL, Griffith LG, Rusyn I. In vitro models for liver toxicity testing. Toxicol Res (Camb). 2013;2:23–39.
70. Jauregui HO, McMillan PN, Hevey K, Naik S. A quantitative analysis of lectin binding to adult rat hepatocyte cell surfaces. In vitro Cell Dev Biol. 1988;24:401–12.
71. Lerche-Langrand C, Toutain HJ. Precision-cut liver slices: characteristics and use for in vitro pharmaco-toxicology. Toxicology. 2000;153:221–53.
72. Demeestere I, Delbaere A, Gervy C, Englert Y. Effect of pre-antral follicle isolation technique on follicular growth, oocyte maturation and fertilization in vitro in the mouse. Hum Reprod. 2000;15(Abst. book 1):89–90.
73. Tirmenstein MA, Nicholls-Grzemski FA, Schmittgen TD, Zakrajsek BA, Fariss MW. Characterization of nitric oxide production following isolation of rat hepatocytes. Toxicol Sci. 2000;53:56–62.
74. Merdassi G, Mazoyer C, Guerin JF, Saad A, Salle B, Lornage J. Examination of viability and quality of ovarian tissue after cryopreservation using simple laboratory methods in ewe. Reprod Biol Endocrinol. 2011;9:78. https://doi.org/10.1186/1477-7827-9-78.
75. Courbiere B, Odagescu V, Baudot A, Massardier J, Mazoyer C, Salle B, et al. Cryopreservation of the ovary by vitrification as an alternative to slow-cooling protocols. Fertil Steril. 2006;86(4 Suppl):1243–51.

76. Milenkovic M, Wallin A, Ghahremani M, Brännström M. Whole sheep ovary cryopreservation: evaluation of a slow freezing protocol with dimethylsulphoxide. J Assist Reprod Genet. 2011;28:7–14.
77. Abir R, Garor R, Felz C, Nitke S, Krissi H, Fisch B. Growth hormone and its receptor in human ovaries from fetuses and adults. Fertil Steril. 2008;90(Suppl):1333–9.
78. Oktay K, Nugent D, Newton H, Salha O, Chatterjee P, Gosden RG. Isolation and characterization of primordial follicles from fresh and cryopreserved human ovarian tissue. Fertil Steril. 1997;67:481–6.
79. McShane P, Sutton R, Gray DW, Morris PJ. Protease activity in pancreatic islet isolation by enzymatic digestion. Diabetes. 1989;38(Suppl 1):126–8.
80. Hornick JE, Duncan FE, Shea LD, Woodruff TK. Isolated primate primordial follicles require a rigid physical environment to survive and grow in vitro. Hum Reprod. 2012;27:1801–10.
81. Nemes Z, Dietz R, Luth JB, Gomba S, Hackenthal E, Gross F. The pharmacological relevance of vital staining with neutral red. Experientia. 1979;35:1475–6.
82. Chambers EL, Gosden RG, YapC PHM. In situ identification of follicles in ovarian cortex as a tool for quantifying follicle, viability and developmental potential in strategies to preserve female fertility. Hum Reprod. 2010;25:2559–68.
83. Winckler J. Vital staining of lysosomes and other cell organelles of the rat with neutral red. Prog Histochem Cytochem. 1974;6:1–89.
84. Park DH, Zeikus JG. Utilization of electrically reduced neutral red by Actinobacillus succinogenes: physiological function of neutral red in membrane-driven fumarate reduction and energy conservation. J Bacteriol. 1999;181:2403–10.
85. Repetto G, del Peso A, Zurita JL. Neutral red uptake assay for the estimation of cellviability/cytotoxicity. Nat Protoc. 2008;3:1125–31.
86. Soares M, Sahrari K, Amorim CA, Saussoy P, Donnez J, Dolmans MM. Evaluation of a human ovarian follicle isolation technique to obtain disease-free follicle suspensions before safely grafting to cancer patients. Fertil Steril. 2015;104:672–80.
87. Amorim CA. Artificial ovary. In: Donnez J, Kim S, editors. Principles and practice of fertility preservation. New York: Cambridge University Press; 2011. p. 448–58.
88. Amorim CA, David A, Dolmans MM, Camboni A, Donnez J, van Langendonckt A. Impact of freezing and thawing of human ovarian tissue on follicular growth after long term xenotransplantation. J Assist Reprod Genet. 2011;28:1157–65.

ART manipulation after controlled ovarian stimulation may not increase the risk of abnormal expression and DNA methylation at some CpG sites of H19, IGF2 and SNRPN in foetuses

Menglu Ji[†], Xingling Wang[*†], Wenbin Wu, Yichun Guan, Jing Liu, Jingyan Wang, Wenxia Liu and Chunyan Shen

Abstract

Background: To examine the effects of IVF, ICSI and FET, as well as in vitro culture, on the safety of offspring, this study was conducted from the perspective of genetic imprinting to investigate whether assisted reproductive technology would influence the parental and maternal imprinting genes.

Methods: Eighteen foetuses were collected from multifoetal reduction and divided into 6 groups: multifoetal reduction after IVF fresh transferred D3 embryos ($n = 3$), multifoetal reduction after IVF frozen transferred D3 embryos ($n = 3$), multifoetal reduction after IVF frozen transferred D5 embryos ($n = 3$), multifoetal reduction after ICSI fresh transferred D3 embryos ($n = 3$), multifoetal reduction after ICSI frozen transferred D3 embryos ($n = 3$), and multifoetal reduction after controlled ovarian hyperstimulation (COH) ($n = 3$). The imprinted genes H19, IGF2 and SNRPN were selected for analysis. The expression and DNA methylation at some CpG sites of H19, IGF2, and SNRPN were examined using real-time quantitative polymerase chain reaction (PCR) and pyrosequencing.

Results: There were no significant differences in the mRNA expression levels among the groups. The mean percentage of H19 methylation (eight CpG sites), IGF2 methylation (five CpG sites) and SNRPN methylation (nine CpG sites) did not differ significantly.

Conclusions: The results suggest that ARTs after controlled ovarian stimulation (IVF, ICSI, cryopreservation and duration of in vitro culture) may not increase the risk of abnormal expression and DNA methylation at some CpG sites of H19, IGF2 and SNRPN in foetuses. Further study with strict design, expanded sample size and CpG sites is essential.

Keywords: Assisted reproductive technology (ART), Imprinted gene, DNA methylation, Multifoetal reduction, Human foetuses

* Correspondence: wangxl1818@126.com
[†]Menglu Ji and Xingling Wang contributed equally to this work.
Department of Reproductive Medical Center, Third Affiliated Hospital of Zhengzhou University, 7 Kangfuqian Road, Zhengzhou 450052, Henan, People's Republic of China

Background

Since the birth of the first IVF infant in the world in 1978 and the first intracytoplasmic sperm injection (ICSI) infant in 1992, assisted reproductive technology (ART) has grown rapidly, and increasing numbers of babies are born using it. ART has been shown to be associated with preterm birth, low birth weight, congenital malformations and rare imprinting disorders [1]. Therefore, increasing numbers of scholars have begun to pay attention to the safety of ART and have conducted relevant research.

Epigenetic modification is a ubiquitous method of gene regulation in life, and it is crucial to maintaining the normal life activities of mammals. Abnormal epigenetic modification of the embryonic stage may induce a variety of diseases in the embryo or even later in adulthood. DNA methylation is one of the main methods of epigenetic modification. The main modification sites occur on the CpG islands of DNA, which are also susceptible to many environmental factors. In mammals, there are special types of genes called imprinted genes. They are located in differentially methylated regions (DMRs), a particular region of DNA where the maternal and paternal alleles are methylated differentially for the purpose of controlling gene expression [2]. Aberrant expression of imprinted genes triggers a variety of human diseases, affects the growth and development of embryos and foetuses, and induces cancer [3]. During mammalian development, there are two large-scale recoding stages of genomic information, which are primarily changes in epigenetic modifications. The first period is in the primordial germ cell development, when DNA demethylation abrogates epigenetic modifications that are then remethylated during gametogenesis with the addition of the mark. The second period occurs in the preimplantation stage; although the DNA undergoes large-scale demethylation changes during this period, the level of methylation of the imprinted genes does not change. However, ART occurs at the time of the removal and at the establishment and maintenance of the imprinted genes. Therefore, any ART may interfere with the expression of the imprinted genes and may have an impact on the offspring.

Chen et al. [4] found that the in vitro environment may affect the maintenance of gene imprinting, and the H19 gene in human day 3 embryos with poor quality (unsuitable for transplantation or cryopreservation) showed demethylation or hypomethylation patterns after in vitro culture. Wang et al. [5] have reported that mouse embryo vitrification tests exacerbate the H19 gene loss and increase expression. A recent meta-analysis found that any imprinting disorder such as Angelman syndrome, Prader-Willi syndrome and Beckwith-Wiedemann syndrome in children conceived through ART had almost fourfold higher incidence than that in children conceived naturally [6]. While overcoming reproductive disorders, ART has the potential to affect the methylation process and affect the health of offspring [7].

Due to the scarcity of embryos used for research and the related ethical restrictions, few reports have been reported on the gene expression of early human foetuses. Most studies use animal models to assess early embryonic development. To the best of the authors' knowledge, no study so far has addressed the impact of various stages of ART on imprinted genes. Therefore, 18 foetuses from multifoetal reduction were collected and divided into 6 groups. H19, IGF2 and SNRPN, which are well-studied imprinted genes, were selected for analysis. In humans, H19 is paternally imprinted, whereas IGF2 and SNRPN are maternally imprinted. The expression and DNA methylation of genes were analysed using real-time quantitative polymerase chain reaction (PCR) and pyrosequencing. The aim of the present study was to discuss the impact of ART on the safety of offspring from the perspective of genetic imprinting.

Methods

Sample collection

The study protocol was approved by the Third Affiliated Hospital of Zhengzhou University Institutional Ethics Committee, and informed consent was obtained from all patients. Between January 2014 and December 2016, 18 multifoetal reduction foetuses were obtained from 18 patients respectively for this study. The inclusion criteria for this study were single gestational sacs and 6–9 weeks of pregnancy. The preoperative B ultrasounds showed intrauterine live births. Preoperative examinations of all the patients were carried out with routine blood examinations, routine urine analysis, routine leukorrheal analysis, hepatic and renal functions tests, infectious diseases examinations, TORCH screens, coagulation analyses and other tests. All the results were normal. During the reduction, the principle of aseptic technique was strictly observed, and the foetal fraction was aspirated first if possible. Then, further confirmation was obtained using the OLYMPUS SZX16 microscope to remove other parts such as the chorionic tissue. Finally, the foetuses (the foetal fraction) were rinsed under iced saline to wash off the blood and then packed for cryopreservation in liquid nitrogen. The foetuses were transferred to a – 80 degree C refrigerator for later use (AllProtect™ Nucleic Acid and Protein Stabilization Reagent for Animal Tissue was added).

All the samples were divided into six groups according to the source as follows: 1) multifoetal reduction after IVF fresh transferred D3 embryos ($n = 3$); 2) multifoetal reduction after IVF frozen transferred D3 embryos ($n = 3$); 3) multifoetal reduction after IVF frozen transferred D5 embryos ($n = 3$); 4) multifoetal reduction after ICSI fresh transferred D3 embryos ($n = 3$); 5) multifoetal reduction after ICSI frozen transferred D3 embryos ($n = 3$); and 6) multifoetal reduction after controlled ovarian stimulation (COS) ($n = 3$). Patients in groups 1–5 were those who received assisted reproductive therapy in the study centre; patients in group 6 were those who had ovulatory disorders and were treated with controlled ovarian stimulation in primary hospitals followed by spontaneous pregnancy, and all patients performed multifoetal pregnancy reduction in the study centre. The patient characteristics are shown in Table 1.

Comparisons between groups 1–5 and group 6 were mainly used to investigate the effects of ART on foetuses after controlled ovarian stimulation; comparisons between group 1 and group 2 and between group 4 and group 5 were used to research the effect of cryopreservation on foetuses; comparisons between group 1 and group 4 and between group 2 and group 5 were used to study the effect of IVF and ICSI on the foetuses; and the comparison between group 2 and group 3 was used to examine the effect of the duration of in vitro culture.

RNA expression analysis

Using the mirVana miRNA Isolation Kit (Ambion), total RNA was isolated from the foetus according to the manufacturer's instructions and checked with an Agilent 2100 Bioanalyzer. Then, the ReverTra Ace qPCR Kit (TOYOBO) was used for reverse transcription as described by the manufacturer (ref). The reverse transcription reaction started with 15-min at 37 °C, ended after a 5-min at 98 °C and was held at 4 °C. PCR was performed with one denature cycle at 50 °C for 2 min and 95 °C for 10 min, 40 amplification cycles at 95 °C for 15 s and 60 °C for 1 min, using ABI Power SYBR Green PCR Master Mix (ABI, USA) on the 7900 HT Sequence Detection System (ABI, USA) according to the manufacturer's protocol. The housekeeping gene Gapdh was used as the reference gene. Finally, the dissolution curve was added, and the result of the dissolution curve analysis showed a single peak, indicating that the PCR amplification specificity was excellent. The repeatability of the data of three replicates was good. Data were analysed using the ΔΔCt method. Primer sequences for these genes are shown in Table 2.

Table 1 Characteristics of multifoetal reduction patients

Sample no.	Source	Maternal age(y)	Gestational age(d)
1	IVF-ET-D3	35	52
2	IVF-ET-D3	32	51
3	IVF-ET-D3	28	53
4	IVF-FET-D3	28	49
5	IVF-FET-D3	36	48
6	IVF-FET-D3	28	50
7	IVF-FET-D5	30	50
8	IVF-FET-D5	30	50
9	IVF-FET-D5	29	52
10	ICSI-ET-D3	32	56
11	ICSI-ET-D3	27	54
12	ICSI-ET-D3	25	55
13	ICSI-FET-D3	26	52
14	ICSI-FET-D3	33	59
15	ICSI-FET-D3	35	51
16	COS	31	50
17	COS	28	55
18	COS	29	59

DNA methylation analysis

The promoter region sequences of targeted imprinted genes H19, IGF2 and SNRPN were searched from UCSC and NCBI and imported into PyroMark Assay Design 2.0 software for primer design. According to the primer design scores, Tm and %GC, the corresponding primer sequences were designed for the three imprinted genes. Primer sequences used for pyrosequencing and the analysed sequences are shown in Additional file 1.

Genomic DNA was extracted using the OMEGA TISSUE DNA Kit (200) according to the manufacturer's instructions and quantified using agarose gel electrophoresis before the follow-up reaction. Each 0.5–1 μg DNA sample was transformed with the EZ DNA Methylation-Gold ™ Kit. Using the transformed DNA sample as a template, PCR amplification was performed as described by manufacturer (ref). Thermocycling conditions consisted of 35 cycles of 98 °C for 10 s, 55 °C for 30 s, and 72 °C for 30 s; then a one-minute extension at 72 °C, and finally samples were held at 4 °C. Pyrosequencing was performed on the PyroMark Q96 Real-Time Quantitative Pyrosequencing Analyser (Qiagen) by taking 15–20 μL of PCR products for each sample.

Statistical analysis

All statistics were performed with IBM SPSS Statistics 23.0. Quantitative data were calculated as the mean ± SD. The Kruskal-Wallis H test was used to evaluate the results among the six groups. A difference was considered significant when $P \leq 0.05$.

Results

Patient characteristics

A total of 18 foetuses from multifoetal reduction of 18 patients respectively were included in this study. The specific grouping was as described above. There was no significant difference in the maternal age between all groups ($P = 0.791$); and there was also no significant difference in gestational age between groups ($P = 0.068$).

Table 2 Primers for real-time quantitative polymerase chain reaction (PCR)

Gene		Primer sequence(5'to3')		Product size(bp)
H19	ID:283120	Forward	TCAAAGCCTCCACGACTCTGT	88
		Reverse	GCCGTCTCCACAACTCCAA	
IGF2	ID:3481	Forward	TGAGATCCAAAACGCTTCGA	87
		Reverse	CGGCGAGGCAGAATATAACAC	
SNRPN	ID:6638	Forward	CGTCCACCAAGACCTTAGCATAC	100
		Reverse	AACAAAAAGCTCACAAACACTCTACAC	
Gapdh	ID:2597	Forward	TGACTTCAACAGCGACACCCA	100
		Reverse	CACCCTGTTGCTGTAGCCAAA	

Changes in the expression levels of genes

The result showed that no significant differences in expression were detected for H19, IGF2 and SNRPN genes (H19: $P = 0.688$; IGF2: $P = 0.527$; SNRPN: $P = 0.295$). The results for gene expression are shown in Table 3.

DNA methylation status of H19, IGF2 and SNRPN

The mean percentage of H19 methylation (eight CpG sites), IGF2 methylation (five CpG sites) and SNRPN methylation (nine CpG sites) showed no significant differences in all groups (H19: $P = 0.169$; IGF2: $P = 0.058$; SNRPN: $P = 0.748$). The specific mean percentages of gene methylation is shown in Table 4.

Discussion

Although ART is an important method in the treatment of many infertile couples, the safety of these procedures has raised many concerns. Hormone stimulation, in vitro fertilization, intracytoplasmic sperm injection, cryopreservation, the timing of embryo transfer and many other techniques in ART must occur in a specific window of time to establish and maintain the correct genomic imprints. Whether these large numbers of non-physiological operations lead to the abnormal epigenetic modification of the embryo and whether it will increase the risk of foetal defects are the important issues that need to be thoroughly investigated.

Some studies indicated an increased risk of birth defects in ART [8, 9], while others showed the opposite [10–12]. It remains a controversial question. The mechanisms that cause imprinted abnormalities in ART offspring are unclear. Possible factors include infertility itself, ovulation induction, mechanical damage of IVF/ICSI, cryopreservation and in vitro culture. It has been shown that superovulation affects the expression of imprinted genes. Loss of SNRPN and gain of H19 imprinted methylation were observed in superovulation [13]. Animal experiments [14] showed that imprinted genes H19 and SNRPN were unaffected in either the placentae or the embryos from the superovulated females. However, the paternally expressed imprinted gene IGF2 had significantly more variable mRNA levels. Due to the application of hormones, superovulation will interfere with the status of imprinted genes on account of the non-physiological endocrine environment. However, the impact of various stages of ART after superovulation on the imprinted genes remains to be investigated, so this study was conducted.

At present, there are not enough reports on human embryo methylation, especially on the methylation status of imprinted genes after embryo implantation of ART. This pilot study collected multifoetal reduction foetuses for examination, thus offsetting the deficiencies in this area. Due to the different time of establishment and different sensitivity to external factors in imprinted genes, the parental imprinting gene H19 and maternal imprinting genes IGF2 and SNRPN were selected to conduct a more comprehensive analysis on the impact of different steps of ART on the foetus.

In this study, there were no significant differences in the maternal age and gestational age, indicating that the collected samples were well balanced. None of the 3 studied imprinted genes (H19, IGF2 and SNRPN) differed significantly in the mRNA expression levels and the mean percentage of methylation at some CpG sites.

Table 3 The $2^{-\Delta Ct}$ value of genes among groups

Value of $2^{-\Delta Ct}$	Group 1 ($n = 3$)	Group 2 ($n = 3$)	Group 3 ($n = 3$)	Group 4 ($n = 3$)	Group 5 ($n = 3$)	Group 6 ($n = 3$)
H19	1.06 ± 0.15	1.31 ± 0.20	1.62 ± 0.94	1.22 ± 0.58	1.29 ± 0.61	1.36 ± 0.07
IGF2	0.59 ± 0.01	0.46 ± 0.14	0.81 ± 0.56	0.58 ± 0.18	0.47 ± 0.23	0.65 ± 0.14
SNRPN	0.13 ± 0.01	0.11 ± 0.03	0.16 ± 0.03	0.14 ± 0.01	0.14 ± 0.04	0.12 ± 0.02

Group 1: multifoetal reduction after IVF fresh transferred D3 embryos ($n = 3$); Group 2: multifoetal reduction after IVF frozen transferred D3 embryos ($n = 3$); Group 3: multifoetal reduction after IVF frozen transferred D5 embryos ($n = 3$); Group 4: multifoetal reduction after ICSI fresh transferred D3 embryos ($n = 3$); Group 5: multifoetal reduction after ICSI frozen transferred D3 embryos ($n = 3$); Group 6: multifoetal reduction after controlled ovarian stimulation (COS) ($n = 3$)

Table 4 The mean percentage of gene methylation among groups

Mean value of methylation (%)	Group 1 ($n = 3$)	Group 2 ($n = 3$)	Group 3 ($n = 3$)	Group 4 ($n = 3$)	Group 5 ($n = 3$)	Group 6 ($n = 3$)
H19	38.21 ± 7.10	36.58 ± 6.66	37.79 ± 8.84	38.96 ± 7.37	32.67 ± 11.91	39.21 ± 7.10
IGF2	1.87 ± 1.25	3.73 ± 2.22	3.73 ± 2.96	2.33 ± 1.29	3.07 ± 3.63	1.93 ± 0.59
SNRPN	45.96 ± 5.47	47.67 ± 2.77	47.19 ± 3.01	46.93 ± 3.52	46.63 ± 3.83	47.44 ± 3.50

Group 1: multifoetal reduction after IVF fresh transferred D3 embryos ($n = 3$); Group 2: multifoetal reduction after IVF frozen transferred D3 embryos ($n = 3$); Group 3: multifoetal reduction after IVF frozen transferred D5 embryos ($n = 3$); Group 4: multifoetal reduction after ICSI fresh transferred D3 embryos ($n = 3$); Group 5: multifoetal reduction after ICSI frozen transferred D3 embryos ($n = 3$); Group 6: multifoetal reduction after controlled ovarian stimulation (COS) ($n = 3$)

It illustrated that cryopreservation may have no negative effect on the foetus (group 1 vs. group 2; group 4 vs. group 5). Similar to the current findings, Derakhshan-Horeh et al. reported that the H19/IGF2 DMR methylation status of day 3 embryos appeared not to be affected by vitrification [15]. As for the duration of in vitro culture, one study that considered extended culture did not show that it posed a greater risk for imprinting errors than short culture [16]. The same conclusion was reached when comparing group 2 with group 3. Mechanical manipulations of IVF and ICSI also did not result in changes in imprinted genes (group 1 vs. group 4; group 2 vs. group 5). In addition, the comparisons between groups 1–5 and group 6 further demonstrate that post-superovulation manipulations have no effect on DNA methylation of the imprinted gene and do not cause a change in the corresponding mRNA levels. The IGF2 gene (five CpG sites) exhibited a slight difference in the mean percentage of methylation among groups ($P = 0.058$), but it was not statistically significant. Owing to the fact that imprinted genes can show considerable methylation variation among normal individuals [17], it is difficult to judge whether this phenomenon is caused by individual differences or caused by ART technology. The sample size must be further expanded to conduct more effective research.

Previous studies have demonstrated that children conceived by ART do not show a higher degree of imprint variability and do not have a higher risk of DNA-methylation defects [11, 18, 19], which were consistent with the results of the current study. A study conducted by Li et al. found no significant increase in imprint variability at H19/IGF2 DMR [20]. Another study from Wong et al. showed that ART might not affect proper imprinting of H19 and IGF2 in the placenta [21]. However, Sakian et al. reported that H19 expression was significantly increased in both IVF and ICSI placentas and IGF2 was significantly decreased when compared to controls [22]. However, these studies did not discuss the role of superovulation and the mechanical manipulation of IVF and ICSI separately, so it is not possible to differentiate whether hormone-induced or ART technology itself made changes in gene expression. This research takes this point into full consideration.

In the past, a large number of studies used the BSP sequencing method. Although this method can clearly show the methylation status of each CpG site in the promoter region, it requires large amounts cloning, complicated operations, it is expensive and it is difficult to carry out en masse. In addition, the degree of methylation quantified depends on the number of clones selected, so this method can only be regarded as a semi-quantitative technology. Pyrosequencing, however, is characterized by its high throughput, low cost, rapidity and visualization. Pyrosequencing is a sequencing-by-synthesis method that allows the accurate evaluation of DNA methylation at CpG sites with high quantitative resolution [23]. However, the length of the sequenced fragment is relatively short. The current study used this new method to study the methylation status of imprinted genes. Although fewer CpG sites were selected, their methylation status could be reflected in a more realistic and accurate way. Further research is needed to expand the studied scope of CpG sites in imprinted gene promoter regions.

This research shows that ARTs after controlled ovarian stimulation (IVF, ICSI, cryopreservation and duration of in vitro culture) may not increase the risk of imprinting defects in the offspring. The increase in imprinted diseases does not seem to be directly affected by ART but the increased fertility problems of the parents [24] or the use of superovulation hormone. This hypothesis should be confirmed by further study. Another possible reason for these research results is that the use of good-quality embryos for transplantation was not excluded. Poor-quality embryos with a high methylation error rate [25] have been eliminated artificially by the time of initial transplantation.

Although the current study suffers from a small sample size (3 foetuses in each group), it is the first research to discuss the post-superovulation procedures in ART separately. Further studies are needed to extend the analysis to more foetuses and subjoin the quality of the transplanted embryos.

Conclusions

To date, ART has been born and has been used clinically for 39 years. The impact of ART on offspring has not yet been clearly revealed. For infertile couples, the most important thing is to nurture a healthy baby. This article only discusses the effect of ART on DNA methylation, and no significant abnormality was found at some CpG sites. Although the results are reassuring, the limitations of this study suggest that additional large studies are needed. Furthermore, other epigenetic mechanisms such as histone post-translational modifications and chromatin remodelling have been implicated in the regulation of these imprinted genes [26, 27]. These also remain to be elucidated. Thus, the safety of ART should be investigated in further studies, and a stricter study design is essential.

Abbreviations

ART: Assisted reproductive technology; FET: Frozen embryo transfer; ICSI: Intracytoplasmic sperm injection; IVF: In vitro fertilization; PCR: Polymerase chain reaction

Acknowledgements

The authors thank all the patients for participating in the study and thank American Journal Experts (AJE) for English language editing. This manuscript was edited for English language by American Journal Experts (AJE).

Funding

The study was supported by Horizontal Research Projects of Zhengzhou University (20170188A).

Authors' contributions

JML, WXL and WWB conducted the literature searches, participated in the design of the study and collection of samples. JML, WXL, WWB, GYC, LJ, WJY, LWX and SCY performed the laboratory work. JML, WXL, WWB and GYC examined the data, made forms and performed analyses. JML was involved in drafting the manuscript. All authors read and approved the final manuscript.

Competing interests

The authors declare that they have no competing interests.

References

1. Skora D, Frankfurter D. Adverse perinatal events associated with ART. Semin Reprod Med. 2012;30:84–91.
2. Williamson CM, Turner MD, Ball ST, Nottingham WT, Glenister P, Fray M, et al. Identification of an imprinting control region affecting the expression of all transcripts in the Gnas cluster. Nat Genet. 2006;38:350–5.
3. Jaenisch R, Bird A. Epigenetic regulation of gene expression: how the genome integrates intrinsic and environmental signals. Nat Genet. 2003;33:245–54.
4. Chen SL, Shi XY, Zheng HY, Wu FR, Luo C. Aberrant DNA methylation of imprinted H19 gene in human preimplantation embryos. Fertil Steril. 2010;94:2356–8.
5. Wang Z, Xu L, He F. Embryo vitrification affects the methylation of the H19/Igf2 differentially methylated domain and the expression of H19 and Igf2. Fertil Steril. 2010;93:2729–33.
6. Lazaraviciute G, Kauser M, Bhattacharya S, Haggarty P, Bhattacharya S. A systematic review and meta-analysis of DNA methylation levels and imprinting disorders in children conceived by IVF/ICSI compared with children conceived spontaneously. Hum Reprod Update. 2014;20:840–52.
7. van Montfoort AP, Hanssen LL, de Sutter P, Viville S, Geraedts JP, de Boer P. Assisted reproduction treatment and epigenetic inheritance. Hum Reprod Update. 2012;18:171–97.
8. Hansen M, Bower C, Milne E, de Klerk N, Kurinczuk JJ. Assisted reproductive technologies and the risk of birth defects–a systematic review. Hum Reprod. 2005;20:328–38.
9. Källén B, Finnström O, Lindam A, Nilsson E, Nygren KG, Otterblad PO. Congenital malformations in infants born after in vitro fertilization in Sweden. Birth Defects Res A Clin Mol Teratol. 2010;88:137–43.
10. Shi X, Ni Y, Zheng H, Chen S, Zhong M, Wu F, et al. Abnormal methylation patterns at the IGF2/H19 imprinting control region in phenotypicallynormal babies conceived by assisted reproductive technologies. Eur J Obstet Gynecol Reprod Biol. 2011;158:52–5.
11. Tierling S, Souren NY, Gries J, Loporto C, Groth M, Lutsik P, et al. Assisted reproductive technologies do not enhance the variability of DNA methylation imprints in human. J Med Genet. 2010;47(6):371.
12. Oliver VF, Miles HL, Cutfield WS, Hofman PL, Ludgate JL, Morison IM. Defects in imprinting and genome-wide DNA methylation are not common in the in vitro fertilization population. Fertil Steril. 2012;97:147–53. e7
13. Market-Velker BA, Zhang L, Magri LS, Bonvissuto AC, Mann MR. Dual effects of superovulation: loss of maternal and paternal imprinted methylation in a dose-dependent manner. Hum Mol Genet. 2010;19:36–51.
14. Fortier AL, McGraw S, Lopes FL, Niles KM, Landry M, Trasler JM. Modulation of imprinted gene expression following superovulation. Mol Cell Endocrinol. 2014;388:51–7.
15. Derakhshan-Horeh M, Abolhassani F, Jafarpour F, Moini A, Karbalaie K, Hosseini SM, et al. Vitrification at Day3 stage appears not to affect the methylation status of H19/IGF2 differentiallymethylated region of in vitro produced human blastocysts. Cryobiology. 2016;73:168–74.
16. White CR, Denomme MM, Tekpetey FR, Feyles V, Power SG, Mann MR. High frequency of imprinted methylation errors in human Preimplantation embryos. Sci Rep. 2015;5:17311.
17. Schneider E, Pliushch G, El Hajj N, Galetzka D, Puhl A, Schorsch M, et al. Spatial, temporal and interindividual epigenetic variation of functionally important DNAmethylation patterns. Nucleic Acids Res. 2010;38:3880–90.
18. Manning M, Lissens W, Bonduelle M, Camus M, De Rijcke M, Liebaers I, et al. Study of DNA-methylation patterns at chromosome 15q11-q13 in children born after ICSI reveals no imprinting defects. Mol Hum Reprod. 2000;6:1049–53.
19. Zheng HY, Shi XY, Wang LL, Wu YQ, Chen SL, Zhang L. Study of DNA methylation patterns of imprinted genes in children born after assisted reproductive technologies reveals no imprinting errors: a pilot study. Exp Ther Med. 2011;2:751–5.
20. Li L, Wang L, Le F, Liu X, Yu P, Sheng J,et al. Evaluation of DNA methylation status at differentially methylated regions in IVF-conceived newborn twins. Fertil Steril .2011;95:1975–1979.
21. Wong EC, Hatakeyama C, Robinson WP, Ma S. DNA methylation at H19/IGF2 ICR1 in the placenta of pregnancies conceived by in vitrofertilization and intracytoplasmic sperm injection. Fertil Steril. 2011;95:2524–6. e1–3
22. Sakian S, Louie K, Wong EC, Havelock J, Kashyap S, Rowe T, et al. Altered gene expression of H19 and IGF2 in placentas from ART pregnancies. Placenta. 2015;36:1100–5.
23. Tost J, Gut IG. DNA methylation analysis by pyrosequencing. Nat Protoc. 2007;2:2265–75.
24. Doornbos ME, Maas SM, McDonnell J, Vermeiden JP, Hennekam RC. Infertility, assisted reproduction technologies and imprinting disturbances: a Dutch study. Hum Reprod. 2007;22:2476–80.
25. Shi X, Chen S, Zheng H, Wang L, Wu Y. Abnormal DNA methylation of imprinted loci in human Preimplantation embryos. Reprod Sci. 2014;21:978–83.
26. Pedone PV, Pikaart MJ, Cerrato F, Vernucci M, Ungaro P, Bruni CB, et al. Role of histone acetylation and DNA methylation in the maintenance of the imprinted expression of the H19 and Igf2 genes. FEBS Lett. 1999;458:45–50.
27. Ito Y, Nativio R, Murrell A. Induced DNA demethylation can reshape chromatin topology at the IGF2-H19 locus. Nucleic Acids Res. 2013;41:5290–302.

11

An extremely patient-friendly and efficient stimulation protocol for assisted reproductive technology in normal and high responders

Chen-Yu Huang[1,3†], Guan-Yeu Chen[1†], Miawh-Lirng Shieh[1] and Hsin-Yang Li[1,2*]

Abstract

Background: The use of oral progestin has been shown to effectively prevent luteining hormone (LH) surge during ovarian stimulation with daily human menopausal gonadotropin injections. This study was aimed to investigate the efficacy of long-acting follicle stimulating hormone (long-acting FSH; corifollitropin alfa, Elonva®) use in progestin-primed ovarian stimulation for normal and high responders undergoing IVF/ICSI.

Methods: This is a retrospective and proof-of-concept study. We developed an extremely patient-friendly protocol to be applied to forty-five normal or high responders, in which a single injection of corifollitropin alfa (Elonva®) was administered and medroxyprogesterone acetate (MPA) was taken orally every day from the day after Elonva injection to the day of trigger. Seven days after Elonva injection, folliculometry and hormone tests were performed, followed by short-acting daily FSH/LH injections, if needed, until the day before trigger. Duration of stimulation, number of injections and visits before trigger, incidence of premature LH surge, the number of oocytes retrieved, fertilization rate, cleavage rate, the rate of day 2 good embryos available, and cumulative ongoing pregnancy rate per retrieval were assessed.

Results: The average age of the population was 34.7 years. Duration of stimulation was 9.4 days in average. Before trigger, only 3.6 injection shots and 1.4 visits were needed on average. There was no case of premature LH surge. Number of oocytes retrieved was 13.7, fertilization rate was 79.04%, cleavage rate was 91.11%, and day 2 good embryo rate was 64.34%, in average respectively. There was no case of ovarian hyperstimulation syndrome. The cumulative ongoing pregnancy rate per oocyte retrieval achieved a satisfactory level as 53.1%.

Conclusions: Our protocol consisting of long-acting FSH injection and oral MPA preventing LH surge reduces the number of injections and visits to an extreme and achieves a satisfactory reproductive outcome, and, therefore, is a really patient-friendly and effective approach to ovarian stimulation.

Keywords: Patient-friendly, Long-acting FSH, PPOS

* Correspondence: lihy@vghtpe.gov.tw
†Equal contributors
[1]Division of Reproductive Endocrinology and Infertility, Department of Obstetrics and Gynecology, Taipei Veterans General Hospital, 201, Shih-Pai Road Section 2, Taipei 112, Taiwan, Republic of China
[2]Division of Obstetrics and Gynecology, Faculty of Medicine, School of Medicine, National Yang-Ming University, Taipei, Taiwan, Republic of China
Full list of author information is available at the end of the article

Background

Prevention of premature luteinizing hormone (LH) surge is the vital component of controlled ovarian stimulation for IVF/ICSI cycles, which is caused by increasing plasma estradiol produced by multiple growing follicles. In the early days, the GnRH agonist down-regulation protocol, which comprises plenty of injections and is therefore named long protocol, was the mainstream to prevent LH elevation [1]. Over the past decade, it was gradually replaced by GnRH antagonist protocol, which is characterized by rapid suppression of LH with fewer injections and reduced risk of ovarian hyperstimulation syndrome (OHSS) [2]. More recently, with improvements in techniques of cryopreservation and thawing, i.e., vitrification of embryos and oocytes, luteal phase stimulation has been adopted [3–5] and achieved satisfactory pregnancy outcomes [6–8]. Stemming from the experiences of luteal phase stimulation, moreover, progestin-primed ovarian stimulation (PPOS) was developed, in which oral progestogen was taken since the first day of ovarian stimulation in the early follicular phase to prevent LH surge; therefore, injections of GnRH analogues can be omitted [9, 10].

Daily injection of FSH/LH was needed in conventional ovarian stimulation. Utilizing recombinant DNA technologies, one single injection of long-acting follicular stimulation hormone (FSH), wherein the FSH β-subunit is extended by a carboxy-terminal peptide (CTP) of the human chorionic gonadotropin (hCG) β-subunit [11], is able to substitute as the first seven daily FSH injections with comparable outcomes in assisted reproduction [12]. Inspired by aforementioned evolutions, we designed an extremely patient-friendly protocol by the combination of long-acting FSH for ovarian stimulation and oral progestin for LH rise prevention. Previous studies on ovarian stimulation protocols using either endogenous or exogenous progestogen to suppress LH surge all utilized daily gonadotropin injection such as human menopausal gonadotropin (HMG) or recombinant FSH (rFSH) [13]. Whether long-acting FSH can be applied in PPOS has not been reported. In this paper, we reported a very patient-friendly and efficient protocol in which an average of 3.6 shots and 1.4 visits were needed before trigger, and this newly developed protocol achieved a cumulative pregnancy rate per retrieval above 50%.

Methods

Study setting and patients

A retrospective study was conducted at the Center for Reproductive Medicine in Taipei Veterans General Hospital, and processed by chart review. All patients were counseled and informed consents for the stimulation protocol and related procedures were provided by infertility specialists. Patients with one of the following conditions were not eligible for this protocol: (i) age above forty years, (ii) hypogonadotropic hypogonadism, (iii) basal FSH above 10 IU/L, (iv) antral follicle count (AFC) below 7, (v) body mass index (BMI) above 30, and (vi) uterine abnormalities.

Treatment protocol of ovarian stimulation and oocyte retrieval

A simplified schematic description of the treatment protocol is shown in Fig. 1. On the menstrual cycle day 2, 3 or 4, transvaginal sonography and serum hormone levels (FSH, LH, estradiol [E2], progesterone [P]) were checked. If the patients met the aforementioned criteria, ovarian stimulation was started on the same day with a single injection of corifollitropin alfa (Elonva®; MSD), of which the dosage was determined by the patient's body

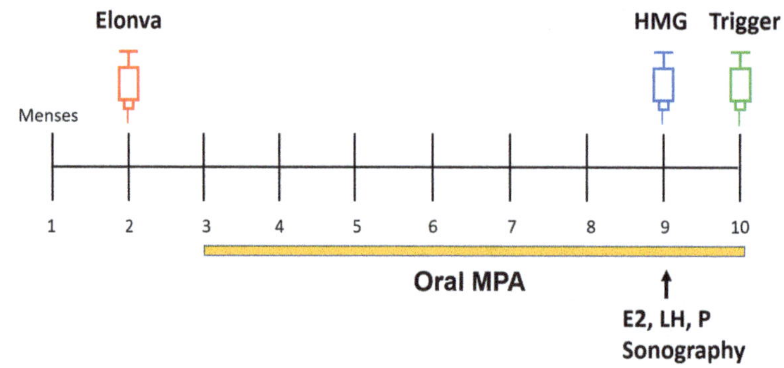

Fig. 1 Treatment protocol of ovarian stimulation. On the menstrual cycle day 2, 3 or 4, ovarian stimulation was started with a single injection of corifollitropin alfa (Elonva®; MSD), of which the dosage was determined by the patient's body weight (150 μg for > 60 kg and 100 μg for ≦ 60 kg). Medroxyprogesterone acetate (MPA) (Provera® 5 mg/tablet; Pfizer) 5 mg twice a day was initiated orally from the day after Elonva injection. Seven days after Elonva injection, follicle development was monitored by transvaginal sonography as well as serum hormone levels of E2, LH and P. The patients received trigger at night if at least three leading follicles reached above 17 mm in diameter, and the final tablet of MPA was taken in the morning of the trigger day. If the folliculogenesis was insufficient for trigger, additional HMG (Menopur®, Ferring) 150 ~ 225 IU/day would be administered for days until the requirement for trigger was met

weight (150 μg for > 60 kg and 100 μg for ≦ 60 kg; [14]). Medroxyprogesterone acetate (MPA) (Provera® 5 mg/tablet; Pfizer) 5 mg twice a day was initiated orally from the day after corifollitropin alfa injection. Seven days after corifollitropin alfa injection, follicle development was monitored by transvaginal sonography as well as serum hormone levels of E2, LH and P. The patients received trigger at night if at least three leading follicles reached above 17 mm in diameter, and the final tablet of MPA was taken in the morning of the trigger day. If the folliculogenesis was insufficient for trigger, additional HMG (Menopur®, Ferring) 150 ~ 225 IU/day would be administered for days depending on the prediction according to the measurement on stimulation day 8. If necessary, follicle monitoring would be performed again every 2–3 days to assess whether the requirement for trigger was met. Triggering was performed by subcutaneous injection of Triptorelin (Decapeptyl® 0.1 mg/ml; Ferring) 0.2 mg with or without hCG 1500~ 6500 IU (Pregnyl®; MSD or Ovidrel®; Merck Sereno), depending on the risk evaluation for early onset OHSS.

Oocytes were retrieved 34–38 h after triggering, followed by in vitro fertilization (IVF) and/or intracytoplasmic sperm injection (ICSI) according to the conditions of the sperm. All embryos were vitrified at pronuclear stage, or on day 2, or on day 3, or on day 5 after retrieval depending on the number of fertilized oocytes available.

Endometrial preparation for frozen-thawed embryo transfer

In frozen-thawed embryo transfer (FET) cycles, oral estradiol valerate (Estrade® 2 mg/tablet; Synmosa) 6 mg twice per day was prescribed from menstrual cycle day 2~ 4 onwards. After oral Estrade supplement had been taken for 10 ~ 14 days, endometrial thickness was measured via transvaginal ultrasound. In addition, hormone measurement (E2, LH, P) was done to confirm that no spontaneous follicle growth and ovulation occurred. Once the endometrial thickness was greater than 7 mm, oral Estrade supplement was continued and the patient began to receive vaginal micronized progesterone gel 90 mg twice a day (Crinone® 8% 90 mg/applicator; Merck Serono) and vaginal micronized progesterone soft capsules 400 mg per night (Utrogestan®100 mg/capsule; Besins) until either ten weeks of gestation or confirmed failure of pregnancy. The timing of thawing and transfer of cryopreserved embryos was determined according to the stage they were vitrified, synchronized with the duration of progesterone exposure to the endometrium. Embryos frozen at the pronuclear stage were warmed after one day of vaginal progesterone administration, followed by transfer one or two days later based on the number of viable embryos. Embryos vitrified on day 2 or day 3 or day 5 post oocyte retrieval were thawed after 2 days or 3 days or 5 days of luteal support, respectively, and were transferred on the same day. Serum β-hCG level was tested after 14 days of luteal support. If the serum β-hCG titer was above 10 IU/L, transvaginal ultrasound was performed three weeks later to detect the site of gestational sacs along with the fetal heart beat.

Outcome measures

Demographic variables recorded for each patient included the following items: age, BMI, serum levels of basal E2, P, FSH and LH, AFC, and the indication for IVF/ICSI treatments. Parameters in terms of ovarian stimulation, oocytes, embryos, and pregnancy outcomes from FET were listed below: duration of stimulation, the number of shots and visits before trigger, incidence of premature LH surge, the number of oocytes retrieved, fertilization rate, cleavage rate, the rate of good embryos available, incidence of OHSS, and cumulative ongoing pregnancy rate per retrieval. In the study, peak E_2 levels and LH levels on the trigger day were not necessarily measured due to freeze-all strategy.

A serum LH concentration exceeding 10 IU/L or rising above twice the basal level before trigger day was considered as premature LH surge. Embryos developing to 2–4 cells on one day after pronuclear stage with a grade of I or II morphology [15], were considered as good embryos. Cumulative ongoing pregnancy rate was counted as pregnancies ≧10 weeks with intrauterine fetal heart beat detected divided by the number of retrieval cycles whose embryos were all transferred or confirmation of intrauterine pregnancies with active fetal heartbeat.

Results

From February to June in 2017, we have applied long-acting FSH in PPOS with MPA followed by embryo vitrification in 45 normal or high responders. The average age was 34.7 years (range, 28–39 years). The average BMI was 21.4 kg/m^2 (range, 17.51–27.31 kg/m^2). The basal AFC was 19.5 in average (range, 8–64). The basal FSH was 6.43 IU/L (range, 4.1–9.2 IU/L) and the basal LH was 4.296 IU/L (range, 0.57–11.22 IU/L), in average. The average basal E2 was 33.19 pg/ml (range, 16.8–61.7 pg/ml). All the demographic data were presented in Table 1. Indications for IVF/ICSI were also shown in Table 1.

Duration of stimulation was 9.4 days on average (range, 8–15). The average number of injections before trigger was 3.6 shots (range, 2–9). The average number of visits between Elonva shot and trigger was 1.4 (range, 1–2). There were no premature LH surge for all cases. The mean number of retrieved oocytes was 13.7, and the mean fertilization rate was 79.04% (Table 2). The mean cleavage rate and good embryo rate were 91.11% and 64.34%, respectively. There was no case of OHSS.

Table 1 Demographic data of patients ($n = 45$)

	Mean ± standard deviation
Age (years)	34.7 ± 2.4
BMI (kg/m^2)	21.4 ± 2.51
AFC	19.5 ± 11.7
Basal E2 (pg/ml)	33.19 ± 10.71
Basal FSH (IU/L)	6.43 ± 1.23
Basal LH (IU/L)	4.296 ± 2.090
Indications for IVF/ICSI	
Endometriosis	6
Male factor	18
PCOS	8
Tubal factor	5
Unexplained	5
Combined factors	3

Till submission of this work, 32 patients have either transferred all their cryopreserved embryos without pregnancy or achieved intrauterine pregnancy with good fetal heartbeat. Seventeen of these 32 patients conceived through FET and continued to be pregnant at 10 weeks of gestation with good fetal heartbeat. Therefore, the cumulative pregnancy rate per ovum pickup was 53.1%.

Discussion

Previous studies confirmed that progestogen administration during follicular phase slowed LH pulse frequency, augmented pulse amplitude, and reduced mean plasma LH levels as compared with those in untreated women studied at the same cycle phase [16]. In animal models, the suppression effect of progestogen on pre-ovulatory GnRH/LH surge is mediated by progesterone receptors in the hypothalamus, and the inhibition is reversible after progestogen discontinuation [17, 18]. Progestogen-induced suppression of LH surge has been applied to develop oral contraceptives, but has not been utilized in ovarian stimulation for IVF until significant improvement of cryopreservation/thawing results brought about by vitrification. "Freeze all strategy" is the prerequisite of PPOS. More and more benefits were discovered about FET under superior techniques of vitrification, including reduced risk of OHSS without compromising implantation rate [19].

Table 2 Stimulation and oocyte/embryo outcomes

	Mean ± standard deviation
Duration of stimulation (days)	9.4 ± 1.4
No. of injections before trigger (shots)	3.6 ± 1.3
No. of visits between Elonva shot and trigger	1.4 ± 0.5
Premature LH surge	0
No. of oocytes retrieved	13.7 ± 7.8
Fertilization rate (%)	79.04 ± 17.61
Cleavage rate (%)	91.11 ± 10.54
Day 2 good embryo rate (%)	64.34 ± 21.43
OHSS	0

MPA has been validated as an effective oral substitute for GnRH analogue injections to prevent LH peak. The use of GnRH antagonist may not completely block the positive feedback of E2 during ovarian stimulation for normal responders [20], and the incidence of untimely LH surge in GnRH antagonist protocols was reported between 0.34% [21] and 35% [22] in different practices. As for the first study presenting MPA use to block LH elevation, a low premature LH surge rate (1/150) was observed in the MPA group. The only case of premature luteinization indicated that in the presence of high basal E2 levels (85 pg/ml), MPA could not prevent imminent LH surge on day 5 of stimulation; however, subsequent folliculogenesis was not affected and no further LH surge occurred (4 oocytes were retrieved from 5 follicles and four embryos were vitrified) [9]. In our study, the basal E2 ranged from 16.8 to 61.7 pg/mL, and we arbitrarily started MPA from one day after corifollitropin alfa injection. As a result, no premature LH surge occurred. In further investigations by the aforementioned group in China, there was zero case of premature LH surge in PCOS patients receiving daily MPA 10 mg for PPOS [23], as well as in normal responders co-administered with either 4 mg or 10 mg MPA per day during ovarian stimulation [24]. Poor ovarian reserve has been noted as a predominant risk factor for a breakthrough LH surge in antagonist protocol [21]. As regards patients with diminished ovarian reserve in PPOS, the incidence of spontaneous LH surge under MPA 10 mg per day was 1.0% in the study including 204 poor responders [25].

Corifollitropin alfa is an rFSH analogue composed of the human FSH α-subunit and a hybrid subunit consisting of the carboxyl-terminal peptide of the β-subunit of hCG coupled with the FSH β-subunit, which is able to sustain follicle-stimulating activity equal to the circulating FSH level above the threshold necessary for multiple follicle growth throughout an entire week [26]. Seven daily FSH injections can thus be replaced by one single shot of corifollitropin alfa. Corifollitropin alfa has no LH activity, so the major difference between our protocol and current regimens using progestogen as a blockade of premature luteinization is whether the remaining LH activity under progestin suppression is adequate for ovarian stimulation in the first 7 days. Still widely debated is the necessity of LH supplementation for patients undergoing IVF/ICSI cycles. The uncertainty about the role of LH in ovarian stimulation continued due to conflicting results from different trials [27, 28].

The updated Cochrane meta-analysis showed no clear evidence of a difference between rLH combined with rFSH and rFSH alone in live birth rates despite more ongoing pregnancies under LH supplementation, in which the benefits appeared to be stronger for low responders [29]. Therefore, we applied the Elonva plus MPA regimen only in normal and high responders.

Earlier studies upon luteal phase stimulation using pure FSH components [3, 30, 31] usually started daily GnRH antagonist from the first day of follicle stimulation due to insufficient knowledge about the effect of endogenous progesterone on the prevention of LH surge. The combined suppressive effect of GnRH antagonists and endogenous progesterone in these regimens led to much more profound pituitary suppression and therefore might need higher dosage of FSH or longer stimulation duration, which is a totally different scenario from our protocol. Under PPOS without GnRH antagonist, the level of pituitary suppression is still to be elucidated. Hormone measurement in the PPOS study by Kuang et al. [9] demonstrated that the LH values gradually declined during ovarian stimulation, and the LH levels were suppressed after 5 days of MPA administration, which was compatible with prior contraception studies [32]. In our study, following 7 days of ovarian stimulation with a single shot of corifollitropin alfa and subsequent 6 days of MPA suppression, the LH levels were measured to be 2.70 ± 1.84 IU/L (data not shown), which was considered to be enough for folliculogenesis. After that, HMG was added until trigger criteria were met. Consequently, LH deficit may not be a critical issue in our protocol. Of course, further randomized controlled trials are needed to compare the pregnancy outcomes for our protocol and other published protocols.

To decrease the physical and mental stress from injection, various regimens were developed in the past. A single depot dose of long-acting GnRH agonist was expected to be superior to short-acting ones. Although no significant difference was concluded in the meta-analysis [33], the long-acting group was associated with not only higher OHSS risk but also inferior outcomes regarding superior-quality embryo rate and implantation rate in a retrospective study enrolling 478 patients [34]. Moreover, daily injection of gonadotropins are needed in the aforementioned down-regulation protocols. Wang et al. [35] proposed a patient-friendly corifollitropin alfa protocol using GnRH antagonist occasionally only when serum LH was ≧ 6 IU/L to reduce injections as much as possible. However, this method needs frequent blood withdrawals to monitor hormone levels for timely initiation of antagonist injection once LH rose above 6 IU/L, which is inconvenient and stressful on the other hand. Even under close follow-up, moreover, some LH peaks might have been missed. After all, according to the previous literature, there was a 20–25% of LH premature surge rate during ovarian stimulation without any preventative treatment [36]. In our regimen, the first visit was arranged at 7 days after corifollitropin alfa injection, and only an average of 1.4 visits were needed before trigger, which is convenient and friendly for the patients.

The unique advantage of our protocol is that seven daily injections are replaced by one shot of corifollitropin alfa as well as many injections of GnRH analogue can be omitted under oral MPA cotreatment, which is friendly for patients in many aspects including not only reduced mental/physical stress and time-consuming visits but also less cost (MPA vs. GnRH antagonist) and more convenience. We have also applied our corifollitropin alfa plus progestogen protocol in a random start fashion, which is needed on several occasions, e.g., emergent oocyte/embryo cryopreservation before chemotherapy and personal scheduling of patients themselves. Caution should be taken about the possibility of spontaneous pregnancy when ovarian stimulation is commenced in the late follicular and luteal phase. For most patients, we would recommend to initiate stimulation in early follicular phase.

Our study is limited by its study design that it is only an observational and proof-of-concept study. Further comparison studies, preferably randomized controlled trials, are required to clarify whether pregnancy outcomes of our friendly method are not inferior to those of conventional protocols.

Conclusions

We have established a patient-friendly stimulation protocol for normal and high responders based on long-acting FSH and progestin, with an average of 3.6 shots and 1.4 visits before trigger and satisfactory reproductive outcomes.

Abbreviations

AFC: antral follicle count; BMI: body mass index; CTP: carboxy-terminal peptide; DNA: Deoxyribonucleic acid; E2: estradiol; FET: frozen-thawed embryo transfer; FSH: follicular stimulation hormone; GnRH: Gonadotropin-releasing hormone; hCG: human chorionic gonadotropin; HMG: human menopausal gonadotropin; ICSI: intracytoplasmic sperm injection; IU: international unit; IVF: in vitro fertilization; Kg: kilogram; L: liter; LH: luteinizing hormone; MPA: Medroxyprogesterone acetate; OHSS: ovarian hyperstimulation syndrome; P: progesterone; PCOS: polycystic ovarian syndrome; PPOS: progestin-primed ovarian stimulation; rFSH: recombinant FSH

Acknowledgements

The authors thank Dr. Shang-Liang Wu at Biostatistics Task Force and Dr. Chi-Mou Juang at Department of Obstetrics and Gynecology, Taipei Veterans General Hospital for their statistical advice.

Funding

This work has been supported, in part, by the Ministry of Science and Technology (MOST 105-2314-B-010-045) and Taipei Veterans General Hospital (V105C-150).

Authors' contributions

CY Huang wrote the original draft. GY Chen collected and analyzed the data. Conceptualization and draft revision: HY Li Investigation: ML Shieh. All authors read and approved the final manuscript.

Competing interests
The authors report no financial or commercial conflicts of interest.

Author details
[1]Division of Reproductive Endocrinology and Infertility, Department of Obstetrics and Gynecology, Taipei Veterans General Hospital, 201, Shih-Pai Road Section 2, Taipei 112, Taiwan, Republic of China. [2]Division of Obstetrics and Gynecology, Faculty of Medicine, School of Medicine, National Yang-Ming University, Taipei, Taiwan, Republic of China. [3]Institute of Clinical Medicine, National Yang-Ming University, Taipei, Taiwan, Republic of China.

References
1. Maheshwari A, Gibreel A, Siristatidis CS, Bhattacharya S. Gonadotrophin-releasing hormone agonist protocols for pituitary suppression in assisted reproduction. Cochrane Database Syst Rev. 2011; https://doi.org/10.1002/14651858.CD006919.pub3.
2. Al-Inany HG, Youssef MA, Ayeleke RO, Brown J, Lam WS, Broekmans FJ. Gonadotrophin-releasing hormone antagonists for assisted reproductive technology. Cochrane Database Syst Rev. 2016; https://doi.org/10.1002/14651858.CD001750.pub4.
3. von Wolff M, Thaler CJ, Frambach T, Zeeb C, Lawrenz B, Popovici RM, Strowitzki T. Ovarian stimulation to cryopreserve fertilized oocytes in cancer patients can be started in the luteal phase. Fertil Steril. 2009;92(4):1360–5. https://doi.org/10.1016/j.fertnstert.2008.08.011.
4. Wang N, Wang Y, Chen Q, Dong J, Tian H, Fu Y, Ai A, Lyu Q, Kuang Y. Luteal-phase ovarian stimulation vs conventional ovarian stimulation in patients with normal ovarian reserve treated for IVF: a large retrospective cohort study. Clin Endocrinol. 2016;84(5):720–8. https://doi.org/10.1111/cen.12983.
5. Boots CE, Meister M, Cooper AR, Hardi A, Jungheim ES. Ovarian stimulation in the luteal phase: systematic review and meta-analysis. J Assist Reprod Genet. 2016;33(8):971–80. https://doi.org/10.1007/s10815-016-0721-5.
6. Kuang Y, Chen Q, Hong Q, Lyu Q, Fu Y, Ai A, Shoham Z. Luteal-phase ovarian stimulation case report: three-year follow-up of a twin birth. J IVF Reprod Med Genet. 2013;1:106. https://doi.org/10.4172/2375-4508.1000106.
7. Kuang Y, Hong Q, Chen Q, Lyu Q, Ai A, Fu Y, Shoham Z. Luteal-phase ovarian stimulation is feasible for producing competent oocytes in women undergoing in vitro fertilization/intracytoplasmic sperm injection treatment, with optimal pregnancy outcomes in frozen-thawed embryo transfer cycles. Fertil Steril. 2014;101(1):105–11. https://doi.org/10.1016/j.fertnstert.2013.09.007.
8. Chen H, Wang Y, Lyu Q, Ai A, Fu Y, Tian H, Cai R, Hong Q, Chen Q, Shoham Z, Kuang Y. Comparison of live-birth defects after luteal-phase ovarian stimulation vs. conventional ovarian stimulation for in vitro fertilization and vitrified embryo transfer cycles. Fertil Steril. 2015;103(5):1194–1201.e2. https://doi.org/10.1016/j.fertnstert.2015.02.020.
9. Kuang Y, Chen Q, Fu Y, Wang Y, Hong Q, Lyu Q, Ai A, Shoham Z. Medroxyprogesterone acetate is an effective oral alternative for preventing premature luteinizing hormone surges in women undergoing controlled ovarian hyperstimulation for in vitro fertilization. Fertil Steril. 2015;104(1):62–70.e3. https://doi.org/10.1016/j.fertnstert.2015.03.022.
10. Zhu X, Zhang X, Fu Y. Utrogestan as an effective oral alternative for preventing premature luteinizing hormone surges in women undergoing controlled ovarian hyperstimulation for in vitro fertilization. Medicine (Baltimore). 2015;94(21):e909. https://doi.org/10.1097/MD.0000000000000909.
11. Fares FA, Suganuma N, Nishimori K, LaPolt PS, Hsueh AJ, Boime I. Design of a long-acting follitropin agonist by fusing the C-terminal sequence of the chorionic gonadotropin beta subunit to the follitropin beta subunit. Proc Natl Acad Sci U S A. 1992;89(10):4304–8.
12. Pouwer AW, Farquhar C, Kremer JA. Long-acting FSH versus daily FSH for women undergoing assisted reproduction. Cochrane Database Syst Rev. 2015; https://doi.org/10.1002/14651858.CD009577.pub3.
13. Massin N. New stimulation regimens: endogenous and exogenous progesterone use to block the LH surge during ovarian stimulation for IVF. Hum Reprod Update. 2017;23(2):211–20. https://doi.org/10.1093/humupd/dmw047.
14. de Greef R, Zandvliet A, de Haan AF, Ijzerman-Boon PC, Marintcheva-Petrova M, Mannaerts BM. Dose selection of corifollitropin alfa by modeling and simulation in controlled ovarian stimulation. Clin Pharmacol Ther. 2010;88(1):79–87. https://doi.org/10.1038/clpt.2010.54.
15. Veeck LL. An atlas of human gametes and conceptuses. New York: Parthenon; 1998. p. 40–5.
16. Soules MR, Steiner RA, Clifton DK, Cohen NL, Aksel S, Bremner WJ. Progestin modulation of pulsatile luteinizing hormone secretion in normal women. J Clin Endocrinol Metab. 1984;58(2):378–83. https://doi.org/10.1210/jcem-58-2-378.
17. Wildt L, Hutchison JS, Marshall G, Pohl CR, Knobil E. On the site of action of progesterone in the blockade of the estradiol-induced gonadotropin discharge in the rhesus monkey. Endocrinology. 1981;109(4):1293–4. https://doi.org/10.1210/endo-109-4-1293.
18. Richter TA, Robinson JE, Lozano JM, Evans NP. Progesterone can block the preovulatory gonadotropin-releasing hormone/luteinising hormone surge in the ewe by a direct inhibitory action on oestradiol-responsive cells within the hypothalamus. J Neuroendocrinol. 2005;17(3):161–9. https://doi.org/10.1111/j.1365-2826.2005.01287.x.
19. Blockeel C, Drakopoulos P, Santos-Ribeiro S, Polyzos NP, Tournaye H. A fresh look at the freeze-all protocol: a SWOT analysis. Hum Reprod. 2016;31(3):491–7. https://doi.org/10.1093/humrep/dev339.
20. Messinis IE, Vanakara P, Zavos A, Verikouki C, Georgoulias P, Dafopoulos K. Failure of the GnRH antagonist ganirelix to block the positive feedback effect of exogenous estrogen in normal women. Fertil Steril. 2010;94(4):1554–6. https://doi.org/10.1016/j.fertnstert.2009.12.055.
21. Reichman DE, Zakarin L, Chao K, Meyer L, Davis OK, Rosenwarks Z. Diminished ovarian reserve is the predominant risk factor for gonadotropin-releasing hormone antagonist failure resulting in breakthrough luteinizing hormone surges in in vitro fertilization cycles. Fertil Steril. 2014;102(1):99–102. https://doi.org/10.1016/j.fertnstert.2014.04.010.
22. Messinis IE, Loutradis D, Domali E, Kotsovassilis CP, Papastergiopoulou L, Kallitsaris A, Drakakis P, Dafopoulos K, Milingos S. Alternate day and daily administration of GnRH antagonist may prevent premature luteinization to a similar extent during FSH treatment. Hum Reprod. 2005;20(11):3192–7. https://doi.org/10.1093/humrep/dei210.
23. Wang Y, Chen Q, Wang N, Chen H, Lyu Q, Kuang Y. Controlled ovarian stimulation using Medroxyprogesterone acetate and hMG in patients with polycystic ovary syndrome treated for IVF: a double-blind randomized crossover clinical trial. Medicine (Baltimore). 2016;95(9):e2939. https://doi.org/10.1097/MD.0000000000002939.
24. Dong J, Wang Y, Chai WR, Hong QQ, Wang NL, Sun LH, Long H, Wang L, Tian H, Lyu QF, Lu XF, Chen QJ, Kuang YP. The pregnancy outcome of progestin-primed ovarian stimulation using 4 versus 10 mg of medroxyprogesterone acetate per day in infertile women undergoing in vitro fertilisation: a randomised controlled trial. BJOG. 2017;124(7):1048–55. https://doi.org/10.1111/1471-0528.14622.
25. Chen Q, Wang Y, Sun L, Zhang S, Chai W, Hong Q, Long H, Wang L, Lyu Q, Kuang Y. Controlled ovulation of the dominant follicle using progestin in minimal stimulation in poor responders. Reprod Biol Endocrinol. 2017;15(1):71. https://doi.org/10.1186/s12958-017-0291-0.
26. Fauser BC, Mannaerts BM, Devroey P, Leader A, Boime I, Baird DT. Advances in recombinant DNA technology: corifollitropin alfa, a hybrid molecule with sustained follicle-stimulating activity and reduced injection frequency. Hum Reprod Update. 2009;15(3):309–21. https://doi.org/10.1093/humupd/dmn065.
27. Hill MJ, Levens ED, Levy G, Ryan ME, Csokmay JM, DeCherney AH, Whitcomb BW. The use of recombinant luteinizing hormone in patients undergoing assisted reproductive techniques with advanced reproductive age: a systematic review and meta-analysis. Fertil Steril. 2012;97(5):1108–14.e1. https://doi.org/10.1016/j.fertnstert.2012.01.130.
28. Xiong Y, Bu Z, Dai W, Zhang M, Bao X, Sun Y. Recombinant luteinizing hormone supplementation in women undergoing in vitro fertilization/intracytoplasmic sperm injection with gonadotropin releasing hormone antagonist protocol: a systematic review and meta-analysis. Reprod Biol Endocrinol. 2014;12:109. https://doi.org/10.1186/1477-7827-12-109.
29. Mochtar MH, Danhof NA, Ayeleke RO, Van der Veen F, van Wely M. Recombinant luteinizing hormone (rLH) and recombinant follicle stimulating hormone (rFSH) for ovarian stimulation in IVF/ICSI cycles. Cochrane Database Syst Rev. 2017; https://doi.org/10.1002/14651858.CD005070.pub3.
30. Buendgen NK, Schultze-Mosgau A, Cordes T, Diedrich K, Griesinger G. Initiation of ovarian stimulation independent of the menstrual cycle: a case-control study. Arch Gynecol Obstet. 2013;288(4):901–4. https://doi.org/10.1007/s00404-013-2794-z.

12

Is there a correlation between follicle size and gene expression in cumulus cells and is gene expression an indicator of embryo development?

Semra Kahraman[1*], Caroline Pirkevi Çetinkaya[1], Murat Çetinkaya[1], Mehmet Ali Tüfekçi[1], Cumhur Gökhan Ekmekçi[1] and Markus Montag[2]

Abstract

Background: In an article published in 2017, we discussed the results of the first part of our study into the morphokinetic development of embryos in relation to follicle diameter and homogeneity of follicular development. Our findings showed that embryos coming from small follicles in heterogeneous cycles had significantly higher rates of arrest or failure to reach blastocyst than embryos coming from large follicles in homogenous cycles. The aim of this further study was to investigate the relationship between follicular size and gene expression of cumulus cells (CCs) and evaluate whether gene expression could be an indicator of embryo development.

Methods: This study was based on 2495 COCs from 184 patients. CC expressions of five genes (*TNFAIP6*, *PTGS2*, *HAS2*, *PTX3* and *GDF9*) were studied by generalized linear mixed models (GLMMs) regarding follicular size. CC expressions were then separately analysed regarding patient-specific variables (age, BMI, AMH and follicular size) in relation to embryos reaching blastocyst (eRB) or top or good quality blastocysts (TQ + GQ) using GLMMs with logit link.

Results: Follicular size significantly correlated with the potential of an oocyte to develop into a blastocyst: oocytes developing from large follicles were more than twice as likely to develop into an eRB than oocytes from small follicles ($p < 0.001$). Gene expression of *HAS2* and *GDF9* correlated with blastocyst quality when separately evaluated with follicular size and the patient specific variables of age, BMI and AMH. However, no such correlation was found in other gene expressions studied.

Conclusions: Our findings suggest that differences in the expression of genes studied could be related to follicular size rather than to embryo quality. Although gene expression of *HAS2* and *GDF9* correlated with blastocyst quality, the only variable correlating with eRB and TQ and GQ blastocysts for each of these five models was follicular size.

Keywords: Gene expression, Cumulus cells, Follicular size, Blastocyst

* Correspondence: semkahraman@gmail.com
[1]Istanbul Memorial Hospital, Assisted Reproductive Technologies and Reproductive Genetics Centre, Piyale Pasa Bulvari 34385 Okmeydani Sisli, Istanbul, Turkey
Full list of author information is available at the end of the article

Background

We conducted a project between July 2014 and September 2015 investigating the relationship between the follicular size and oocyte competence using the morphokinetic and gene expression analyses of the same patient group.

In an article published in 2017, we discussed the results of the first part of our study into the morphokinetic development of embryos in relation to follicle diameter and homogeneity of follicular development [1]. Our findings showed that embryos coming from small follicles in heterogeneous cycles had significantly higher rates of arrest or failure to reach blastocyst than embryos coming from large follicles in homogenous cycles. Subsequently, we conducted this further study to compare gene expression between cumulus cells (CCs) obtained from follicles of different sizes, evaluating RNA concentrations of five well described genes involved in cumulus expansion/ ovulation (*HAS2, PTGS2, PTX3, TNFAIP6* and *GDF9*) [2–13].

There is increasing evidence that CCs play a crucial role in folliculogenesis and oocyte developmental competence acquisition [14–18]. Therefore, many studies correlating cumulus gene expression with different outcome measures such as oocyte maturity, fertilization, embryo development, implantation and pregnancy have been performed [2, 3, 16–24]. However, few investigate the relationship between gene expression and follicular size and embryo development to the blastocyst stage [25–27]. Recently, Nivet and colleagues [24], hypothesized that the combination of a follicle's size and transcriptomic signature provide a reliable method to predict embryonic development. They concluded that follicular size had an impact on oocyte quality as measured by embryonic development and demonstrated that medium follicles yielded a better percentage of transferable embryos than large or small follicles.

The CC-derived candidate genes selected for the study were those which have been identified in previous studies as regulated by oocyte signals and as having important functions in cumulus expansion and metabolism [28–30].

These were: hyaluronan synthase 2 (*HAS2*), prostaglandin-endoperoxide synthase 2 (*PTGS2*), pentraxin-related protein 3 (*PTX3*), tumour necrosis factor alpha induced protein 6 (*TNFAIP6*) and growth differentiation factor 9 (*GDF9*).

HAS2 is critical for the formation and expansion of the CC mass and expression levels correlate with early embryological development [2, 4]. Furthermore, *HAS2* is one of the four genes contained in the ranking method evaluated by Ekart and colleagues [19] for identifying good quality metaphase II (MII) oocytes that will ultimately provide a significantly better outcome regarding good blastocyst development and live birth compared with random selection. The measurement of *HAS2* and *GREM1* levels in CCs would reliably complement the morphological evaluation providing a useful tool for selecting oocytes with greater chances to be fertilized and develop in vitro. Furthermore, *HAS2* is considered to be a human pregnancy or live birth candidate biomarker with conflicting differential mRNA expression by qRT-PCR [2, 19, 31, 32].

In bovine and mice, *PTGS2* has a role in promoting cumulus expansion and oocyte competence [5–8]. In a landmark study comprising eight patients, *PTGS2*, like *HAS2*, was found to correlate with the morphology of human day-3 embryos [2]. The median expression for *PTGS2* was found to be threefold higher in CCs of oocytes that resulted in pregnancy [31]. Moreover, *PTGS2* expression was found to be significantly higher in CCs from oocytes that achieved term birth compared with those that failed to result in a successful pregnancy [31]. Previous studies have suggested that *PTGS2* expression in bovine and primate COCs may participate in the timing of maturation [7, 33] and oocyte quality [6]. Other studies have found an association between *PTGS2* and embryo morphological grade [2]. In mice, *Ptgs2* and the resultant prostaglandin E2 facilitate cumulus expansion through induction of cumulus matrix genes [5] and are important in the survival of mouse cumulus cells [8].

The *PTX3* gene product is another extracellular matrix protein that interacts with hyaluronan in the expanded cumulus matrix [34–36]. *PTX3* gene expression in CCs has been associated with oocyte/embryo competence and was determined as a potentially reliable predictor of embryo developmental competence [3]. Elevated *PTX3* expression has been found in CCs from oocytes that developed into normal appearing embryos on day 3 compared with those from oocytes that failed to fertilize in 16 patients [3]. However, another study failed to establish a correlation between *PTX3* expression and embryos with good or poor morphology [21]. Nonetheless, in other studies, expression of *PTX3* tended toward an association with pregnancy outcome [31, 37].

TNFAIP6 is synthesized by cumulus and granulosa cells in the preovulatory follicle [9, 10]. It was selected because it is a *GDF9*-induced gene in periovulatory granulosa cells although its expression does not differ as a function of embryo quality and oocyte competence [2, 38, 39].

GDF9 is an oocyte-secreted factor playing a key role in the process of follicular development from the recruitment of the primordial follicle to ovulation and even in corpus luteum formation [11–13]. It has been confirmed by many studies that *GDF9* is expressed both in oocytes and cumulus granulosa cells [40–42]. Increased levels of *GDF9* and *BMP15* expression have both been associated with positive pregnancy as well as with mature oocytes, fertilization rate and embryo quality [43].

The aim of our study was to investigate the relationship between follicular size and gene expression of CCs assessing these five candidate genes and to evaluate whether gene expression is an indicator of embryo development.

Methods

Patients

This prospective cohort study was registered at clinicaltrials.gov (NCT02230449) and received funding from the Grant for Fertility Innovation (GFI) in July 2014. It was conducted in a private IVF clinic between July 2014 and September 2015 and the analysis was based on 2495 COCs belonging to 184 patients, with culture until day 5. Our previous study on follicular size and morphokinetics analysed 2526 oocytes [1]. However, in this study three patients and their 31 oocytes were excluded from the expression analysis because their CC samples did not give interpretable results due to technical issues. The patients presented various infertility causes, all protocols were approved by the institutional review board and all patients gave their informed consent prior to their inclusion in the study. Patients were selected with inclusion criteria as similar as possible to the first part of the study [1]. Furthermore, the inclusion criteria specified good prognosis patients with at least 8 COCs in order to provide us with a sufficient number of blastocysts for statistical analyses.

Patients were selected based on inclusion criteria (age ≤ 39 years, body mass index (BMI) < 30 kg/m^2, ≥ 8 COCs retrieved, < 2 previous treatment cycles, hCG trigger) and exclusion criteria (recurrent pregnancy loss, severe endometriosis, PGD or PGS, COC > 24, embryo transfer before day 5, PCOS, uterine anomaly, very severe sperm morphological abnormality such as dominantly macrocephal or globozoospermic sample or cryptozoospermia, ≤ 1million motile sperm cells in total ejaculate). In order to minimize bias, PCOS patients with an abnormally high number of COCs were excluded [44]. Patient characteristics are shown in Additional file 1: Table S1.

Female ages ranged between 18 and 38, with an average of 30.81 ± 4.26 years. AMH measurements ranged from 0.17 to 8.6 with a mean of 3.15 ± 1.80. BMI measurements ranged from 16.3 to 29.7 kg/m^2 with a mean of 23.68 ± 3.00 kg/m^2. This cycle was the first for 66.3% of the patients (n = 122) and the second for 33.7% of the patients (n = 62). Biochemical pregnancy was observed in 66.3% of the patients (n = 122), 53.3% (n = 98) had an ongoing pregnancy and finally, the live birth rate was 51.1% (n = 94).

Ovarian stimulation

Ovarian stimulation was performed as described previously [1]. Briefly, recombinant FSH (rFSH; Gonal-F®; Merck Serono, Switzerland) was used at a dosage of 150 to 225 IU, depending on clinical and hormonal evaluations. A daily administration of 0.25 mg GnRH antagonist (Cetrotide®; Merck Serono, Switzerland) was started when at least one follicle reached 12–13 mm in size. Then, 250 μg recombinant hCG (Ovitrelle®; Merck Serono, Switzerland) was administered to achieve final oocyte maturation when at least three follicles reached a minimum mean diameter of 17 mm. Transvaginal ultrasound-guided oocyte retrieval was scheduled for 36 h later.

Follicular size

Follicular size was defined as large, ≥17 mm and small, < 17 mm at the time of oocyte pick-up (OPU), as a pilot study of more than 2300 oocytes previously performed in our ART centre in 2012 suggested that 17 mm was the size where statistically significant differences were observed. This preliminary study showed a relative increase of 80% for the good and top-quality blastocyst rate (TQ + GQ) of oocytes deriving from large follicles when compared to small follicles if the cut-off was set as 17 mm. This difference disappeared when the cut-off was taken as 20 mm. Each follicular aspiration was performed by the same doctor to reduce any possible inaccuracy of measurement to a minimum.

Cumulus oocyte complex (COC) collection and embryology

Oocyte retrieval, denudation, ICSI and embryo culture were performed as described previously [1]. In summary, on the day of OPU, follicles were aspirated individually. The gynaecologist who performed the pick-up notified the embryologist regarding the size of the follicle for each punctate. A second embryologist assisted the procedure to document the process of isolation, identification and positioning of COCs in the culture dish. Denudation was carried out by mechanical pipetting in ICSI cumulase® (Origio, Måløv, Denmark). Each COC was denuded separately and the maturation status was determined after denudation. Oocytes coming from large and small follicles were incubated separately in different dishes in the same incubator [1]. ICSI was performed at 400× magnification using Olympus IX70 and Olympus IX71 inverted microscopes. Embryo culture was carried out in a single step culture medium (Life Global®, Brussels, Belgium), supplemented with 10% plasmanate (Life Global®, Brussels, Belgium) in a time-lapse incubator (EmbryoScope™). Blastocysts were scored according to Gardner's classification (114–120 h post-ICSI) and selected for transfer based on the final morphology and the score obtained from the morphokinetic ratios published by Çetinkaya and colleagues [45].

Embryo transfer and outcomes of treatment cycles

After embryo transfer, for luteal phase support, patients received a twice daily dose of progesterone gel to be administered intravaginally (Crinone® 8%; Merck Serono, Switzerland). When pregnancy occurred, a daily dose was continued until the 10th week of gestation. Fourteen days after pick-up, serum β-hCG was measured. At 7 weeks, a transvaginal ultrasound was performed to monitor early pregnancy. The implantation rate was calculated by dividing the number of implanted embryos by the total number of transferred embryos. However, for analyses purposes, patients with two transferred embryos but resulting with only one sac were excluded from the analysis as we could not know which embryo had implanted and therefore would not have been able to analyse any possible correlation between follicular size, gene expression and embryo development. Implantation analysis was performed on transferred embryos where the number of gestational sacs matched the number of transferred embryos and on embryos where no biochemical pregnancy was achieved.

Total RNA isolation from cumulus cells and reverse transcription

The CCs of each oocytes were separately numbered, frozen, and cryostored at − 20 °C in Cryo.S ™ Freezing Tubes (Greiner Bio-One, Germany) containing 150 μL of RNA *later* Stabilization Reagent (Qiagen, Germany). CCs were first incubated overnight in the reagent at 2–8 °C, then transferred to − 20 °C for storage until RNA extraction. Total RNA extraction of individual CCs was carried out using the Total RNA Purification kit (NORGEN, BIOTEK CORP., Canada) as recommended by the manufacturer and final elution of the total RNA was performed using 32 μl of RNase free water. Total RNA was quantified using a NanoDrop 2000c UV-Vis spectrophotometer (Thermo-Scientific, USA). The mean quantity of RNA per CC sample was 102.5 ± 44.3 ng. RNA from each sample was used to generate cDNA using the Transcriptor High Fidelity cDNA Synthesis Kit (Roche Diagnostics GmbH, Mannheim, Germany) with random hexamers, following the manufacturer's instructions. Total RNA and/ or cDNA samples were stored at − 80 °C until use.

Real-time PCR

Real-time PCR amplification reactions were carried out using a LightCycler 480 (Roche Diagnostics GmbH, Mannheim, Germany) with the LightCycler FastStart DNA Master SYBR Green I Kits (Roche Diagnostics GmbH, Mannheim, Germany). Real-time PCR was used to quantify the mRNA transcripts levels of *HAS2*, *PTGS2*, *PTX3*, *TNFAIP6* and *GDF9*. Oligonucleotide primer sequences are listed in Additional file 1: Table S2. Primers were designed to cross an exon-exon junction to avoid amplification of genomic DNA.

Primers were synthesized by Metabion International AG (Martinsried, Germany). Real-time RT-qPCR assays were performed in duplicate in 96-well plates. The thermal cycling conditions were 95 °C for 5 min for polymerase activation and the initial denaturation step, followed by 45 cycles with denaturation at 95 °C for 10s, annealing at 60 °C for 10s and extension at 72 °C for 10s. A melting curve analysis was recorded at the end of the amplification to evaluate the absence of contaminants or primer dimers. For each CC sample, gene expression levels of *HAS2*, *PTGS2*, *PTX3*, *TNFAIP6* and *GDF9* were calculated as fold-changes relative to *B2M* level calculated by $2^{-\Delta\Delta CT}$ method [46]. Depending on the transcript targeted, cumulus samples that did not reveal any expression data, either because of an amplification failure or because they did not show any expression of the five genes studied, were excluded from the analysis.

Statistical analysis

NCSS (Number Cruncher Statistical System) 2007 (Kaysville, Utah, USA) program was used for statistical analysis. Data was reported as mean, standard deviation, standard error, frequency, percentage, minimum, maximum. Due to the paired nature of the data, generalized linear mixed models (GLMMs) were conducted.

First, to analyse if there was any correlation between follicular size, the potential of embryos to reach the blastocyst stage, blastocyst quality and gene expression levels, separate GLMMs were conducted. In these models, expression levels of genes were introduced as target variables, follicular size, the potential of embryos to reach blastocyst stage and blastocyst quality as fixed factors and subject id as a random factor.

Second, separate GLMMs with logit link were conducted to analyse the factors affecting embryos development into eRBs or into TQ or GQ blastocysts. In these models, eRB and blastocyst quality were introduced as target variables; age, BMI, AMH, follicular size and expression levels of genes as fixed factors and subject id as a random factor.

Third, separate GLMMs with logit link were conducted to analyse any correlation between gene expression levels and implantation. In these models, implantation was introduced as a target variable; age, BMI, AMH, follicular size and expression levels of genes as fixed factors and subject id as a random factor.

A p value of $p < 0.05$ was accepted as statistically significant.

Results

Follicular size and CC gene expression

When expression levels of genes were evaluated according to follicular size only, *PTGS2* was found to be significantly up-regulated in CCs deriving from large follicles when compared to small follicles ($p < 0.001$) (Table 1).

CC gene expression, embryos reaching blastocyst stage and follicular size

Expression levels of the five genes were analysed in embryos that reached blastocyst stage (eRB) regarding follicular size. For embryos developing to blastocyst and originating from large follicles, *HAS2* and *PTGS2* expressions were significantly up-regulated in the associated CCs when compared to those originating from small follicles ($p < 0.001$; $p = 0.036$, respectively) (Table 1).

CC gene expression, blastocyst quality and follicular size

For embryos becoming TQ or GQ blastocysts and originating from large follicles, *PTGS2* expression was up-regulated in the associated CCs when compared to small follicles ($p = 0.002$) (Table 1). However, a significant up-regulation for *PTGS2* was also observed in CCs of oocytes originating from large follicles and that developed to BQ blastocysts or arrested embryos, when compared to small follicles ($p = 0.003$) (Table 1). Again, a significant up-regulation for *PTGS2* was also observed for CCs of eFRB embryos originating from large follicles when compared to small follicles ($p = 0.010$) (Table 1).

CC gene expressions evaluated with patient-specific variables regarding eRB or TQ + GQ blastocysts

Generalized Linear Mixed Models (GLMMs) with logit link were conducted to analyse the factors correlating with the development to an eRB and to TQ + GQ blastocysts. In these models, which were separately done for the five selected genes, age, BMI, AMH and follicular size were

Table 1 CC gene expression levels regarding follicular size and embryo development on day5

Concentrations		*TNFAIP6*	*PTGS2*	*HAS2*	*PTX3*	*GDF9*
		Mean (se)	Mean (se)	Mean (se)	Mean (se)	Mean (se)
Follicular size	n	1195	1205	1212	1110	742
	Small	0.629 (0.564)	0.281 (0.027)	0.631 (0.287)	0.011 (0.004)	1.075 (0.297)
	n	1061	1066	1072	975	648
	Large	0.956 (0.784)	0.434 (0.047)	0.922 (0.350)	0.014 (0.003)	0.997 (0.255)
p[a]		0.204	< 0.001**	0.193	0.371	0.847
eRB	n	472	478	482	439	295
	Small	1.163 (1.065)	0.284 (0.027)	0.710 (0.339)	0.010 (0.003)	1.217 (0.533)
	n	605	609	612	559	370
	Large	0.790 (0.637)	0.399 (0.038)	0.811 (0.356)	0.013 (0.003)	0.966 (0.347)
p[a]		0.451	< 0.001**	0.036*	0.344	0.701
eFRB	n	723	727	730	671	447
	Small	0.235 (0.245)	0.270 (0.031)	0.538 (0.254)	0.013 (0.006)	0.987 (0.356)
	n	456	457	460	416	278
	Large	1.376 (1.193)	0.480 (0.082)	1.172 (0.562)	0.016 (0.005)	1.047 (0.383)
p[a]		0.274	0.010*	0.249	0.266	0.911
TQ or GQ Blastocysts	n	253	258	260	237	151
	Small	0.726 (0.506)	0.275 (0.031)	0.514 (0.127)	0.011 (0.003)	0.415 (0.323)
	n	349	353	354	325	212
	Large	0.727 (0.506)	0.388 (0.040)	0.562 (0.126)	0.013 (0.005)	0.410 (0.211)
p[a]		0.562	0.002**	0.060	0.714	0.956
Arrested embryos or BQ Blastocysts	n	942	947	952	873	591
	Small	0.684 (0.631)	0.274 (0.030)	0.649 (0.345)	0.011 (0.004)	1.243 (0.361)
	n	712	713	718	650	436
	Large	0.978 (0.841)	0.445 (0.059)	1.001 (0.414)	0.013 (0.003)	1.282 (0.369)
p[a]		0.217	0.003**	0.323	0.466	0.942

Studied genes are: tumour necrosis factor alpha induced protein 6 (*TNFAIP6*), prostaglandin-endoperoxide synthase 2 (*PTGS2*), hyaluronan synthase 2 (*HAS2*), pentraxin-related protein 3 (*PTX3*) and growth differentiation factor 9 (*GDF9*)

eRB embryos reaching blastocyst, *eFRB* embryos failed to reach blastocyst, *TQ* top quality blastocyst, *GQ* good quality blastocyst, *BQ* bad quality blastocyst

**$p < 0.01$; *$p<0.05$

[a]GLMM (Generalized linear mixed model) se: standard error

introduced as patient-specific variables and were simultaneously analysed with each CC gene expression.

For the model analyzing the factors affecting the development to an eRB, CC expression levels of *TNFAIP6, PTGS2, PTX3, HAS2* and *GDF9* were not found to be significant (Table 2). The only variable correlating with eRB for each of these five models was the follicular size ($p < 0.001$) (Table 2).

Generalized Linear Mixed Models (GLMMs) with logit link were also conducted to analyse the factors correlating with blastocyst quality (TQ + GQ). Follicular size was found to be significantly correlated with TQ + GQ in all of these five models ($p < 0.001$), whereas AMH was found to be a variable correlated with the potential of embryos becoming TQ + GQ blastocysts in only three models out of five (*TNFAIP6* ($p = 0.043$); *PTX3* ($p = 0.026$) and *HAS2* ($p = 0.037$)) (Table 2). Blastocyst quality was significantly associated with CC gene expression of *HAS2* and *GDF9* (p = 0.043; $p = 0.049$, respectively) but not with that of *TNFAIP6, PTGS2* and *PTX3* (Table 2).

Follicle size, CC gene expression and implantation

Before starting our two-part study, we conducted a pilot study in order to calculate the minimum number of fertilized oocytes which would be sufficient to detect a significant difference between follicle size and blastulation rates. The results revealed that top and good quality blastocyst rates for large and small follicles were 45 and 32%, respectively. A power analysis indicated that, for an alpha level of 0.05 and a beta level of 0.20 (power = 0.80), 438 fertilized oocytes were sufficient to detect a significant difference between follicle size groups in terms of blastulation rate [1]. But, in spite of the large cohort, the number of resultant blastocysts with known

Table 2 CC expression of the studied genes regarding clinical variables and development into eRBs and TQ + GQs

		eRB		TQ + GQ	
		p	OR (95% CI)	*p*	OR (95% CI)
TNFAIP6	Age	0.790	0.996 (0.965, 1.028)	0.178	0.979 (0.948, 1.010)
	BMI	0.837	1.005 (0.957, 1.055)	0.324	1.025 (0.976, 1.075)
	AMH	0.195	1.045 (0.977, 1.118)	0.043*	1.083 (1.003, 1.169)
	[a]Follicle size (large)	< 0.001**	2.146 (1.760, 2.617)	< 0.001**	1.877 (1.512, 2.329)
	TNFAIP6	0.438	1.001 (0.997, 1.005)	0.081	0.988 (0.974, 1.002)
PTGS2	Age	0.817	0.996 (0.966, 1.027)	0.179	0.979 (0.950, 1.010)
	BMI	0.976	1.001 (0.953, 1.051)	0.435	1.019 (0.971, 1.070)
	AMH	0.214	1.043 (0.975, 1.116)	0.060	1.076 (0.997, 1.160)
	[a]Follicle size (large)	< 0.001**	2.147 (1.760, 2.618)	< 0.001**	1.863 (1.503, 2.308)
	PTGS2	0.439	0.966 (0.887, 1.054)	0.670	0.978 (0.881, 1.085)
PTX3	Age	0.873	0.997 (0.966, 1.029)	0.084	0.973 (0.943, 1.004)
	BMI	0.831	0.995 (0.948, 1.044)	0.492	1.017 (0.969, 1.068)
	AMH	0.149	1.051 (0.982, 1.126)	0.026*	1.089 (1.010, 1.174)
	[a]Follicle size (large)	< 0.001**	2.162 (1.751, 2.671)	< 0.001**	1.880 (1.506, 2.346)
	PTX3	0.720	0.698 (0.097, 4.998)	0.847	0.831 (0.126, 5.446)
HAS2	Age	0.831	0.997 (0.967, 1.028)	0.147	0.978 (0.949, 1.008)
	BMI	0.982	1.001 (0.954, 1.050)	0.401	1.021 (0.973, 1.070)
	AMH	0.163	1.048 (0.981, 1.120)	0.037*	1.081 (1.005, 1.163)
	[a]Follicle size (large)	< 0.001**	2.120 (1.741, 2.582)	< 0.001**	1.859 (1.504, 2.297)
	HAS2	0.511	0.995 (0.982, 1.009)	0.043*	0.955 (0.913, 0.998)
GDF9	Age	0.785	0.995 (0.960, 1.031)	0.208	0.976 (0.939, 1.014)
	BMI	0.715	0.990 (0.937, 1.045)	0.348	1.027 (0.971, 1.085)
	AMH	0.103	1.078 (0.985, 1.180)	0.067	1.088 (0.994, 1.190)
	[a]Follicle size (large)	< 0.001**	2.145 (1.683, 2.734)	< 0.001**	1.913 (1.461, 2.505)
	GDF9	0.912	1.001 (0.987, 1.015)	0.049*	0.975 (0.952, 0.999)

(Studied genes are: tumour necrosis factor alpha induced protein 6 (*TNFAIP6*), prostaglandin-endoperoxide synthase 2 (*PTGS2*), hyaluronan synthase 2 (*HAS2*), pentraxin-related protein 3 (*PTX3*) and growth differentiation factor 9 (*GDF9*)). Embryos reaching blastocyst stage (eRB); top (TQ) or good quality (GQ) blastocysts
$^{*}p < 0.05$; $^{**}p < 0.01$
[a]Small follicular size was selected as a reference category

implantation data would probably not be sufficient to detect a significant correlation between follicular size, gene expression and implantation. However, recognizing that implantation rates are of interest, further separate GLMMs with logit link were conducted to analyse any correlation between gene expression levels, patient-specific variables (age, BMI, AMH and follicular size) and implantation. Results from these models indicated that neither patient-specific variables nor the five studied CC gene expressions had a statistically significant correlation with implantation ($p > 0.05$). This supports our previous findings, published in an article of 2017 [1], where we discussed the results of the first part of this study into the morphokinetic development of embryos in relation to follicle diameter and homogeneity of follicular development. Although oocytes developing from large follicles were more than twice as likely to develop into an eRB than oocytes from small follicles, once the blastocyst stage was achieved, implantation rates were not significantly different between embryos coming from large or small follicles (Additional file 1: Table S3).

Discussion

Morphological criteria which are currently used to describe intra- and extra-cytoplasmic features of human oocytes are not sufficient to accurately and non-invasively predict developmentally competent oocytes [47]. Defined gene expression signatures of oocyte competence acquired during maturation by the surrounding somatic cells would be valuable in predicting the developmental potential of oocytes. The developmental competence of oocytes is indeed acquired progressively during folliculogenesis and is well-known to rely on the bidirectional communication between oocyte and CCs, which deliver nutrients and regulatory molecular signals to promote both oocyte nuclear and cytoplasmic maturation. Our study investigates if there is any association between putative oocyte competence markers in CCs and the developmental competence of oocytes as evaluated by the quality of blastocysts.

Cumulus expansion in vivo is induced by the preovulatory LH surge and requires expression of transcripts encoding hyaluronan synthase 2 (*HAS2*), prostaglandin-endoperoxide synthase 2 (*PTGS2*), pentraxin-related protein 3 (*PTX3*) and tumour necrosis factor alpha induced protein 6 (*TNFAIP6*) [48]. During maturation, oocyte secretory factors (*GDF9* and *BMP15*) act upon CCs and up-regulate mRNA expressions of the above-mentioned cumulus expansion enabling factors [49].

Nivet and colleagues [24], evaluated the relationship between the embryonic outcome of oocytes, follicle volume and transcriptomic signature and concluded that transcriptional characteristics of follicles varied according to their size and that size should be considered to better discriminate between follicles containing oocytes with high developmental competence. In the present study reporting a series of 2495 COCs punctured from 184 young and good prognosis patients, follicular size significantly correlated with the potential of an oocyte to develop into blastocyst: oocytes developing from large follicles were more than twice as likely to develop into an eRB than oocytes from small follicles ($p < 0.001$).

When expression levels of genes were evaluated according to follicular size only, *PTGS2* was significantly up-regulated in large follicles whereas no such significant difference in gene expression was observed in *TNFAIP6, HAS2, PTX3* and *GDF9* (Table 1, Follicular size). Again, when evaluating gene expression levels while taking follicular size into account, significant differences were found only in *PTGS2* and *HAS2* in embryos originating from large follicles and reaching to blastocyst stage (Table 1, eRB). Only *PTGS2* was significantly up-regulated in top or good quality blastocysts originating from oocytes coming from large follicles (Table 1, TQ or GQ Blastocysts). However, *PTGS2* was also upregulated in embryos failing to reach blastocyst, bad quality blastocysts and arrested embryos (Table 1).

Thus, *PTGS2* expression in CCs correlated significantly with follicular size being up regulated in large follicles regardless of whether embryos arrested or were slow growing or whether blastocyst stage was reached or not and whether blastocysts were poor, good or top quality. These findings seem to indicate that differences of gene expression of *PTGS2* were related to follicular size rather than to embryo quality. This demonstrates that up-regulation of *PTGS2* in large follicles does not necessarily indicate oocyte competence.

In a study by Ekart and colleagues [19], in which a group of 25 women below the age of 38 underwent an rFSH-stimulated ICSI treatment, a total of 270 COCs were analysed. The authors found that 99.7% of COC retrieved within each woman involved in their study were significantly different from each other regarding CC mRNA levels of eight candidate genes (*HAS2, FSHR, SLC2A4, ALCAM, SFRP2, VCAN, NRP1* and *PR*) and cell composition [19]. The authors associate this heterogeneity either with an artefact during the mechanical isolation and enzymatic dissection process or to variations in granulosa cell numbers in developing follicles. Our study may indicate that this heterogeneity could also be related to size discrepancies within a follicular cohort stimulated exogenously by gonadotropins.

Two genes, *HAS2* and *GDF9*, showed significantly higher expression in CCs from oocytes that progressed to TQ or GQ blastocysts. Our results support a relationship between *HAS2* and *GDF9* expression in CCs and the developmental competence of oocytes. According to the GLMMs with logit link, one unit increase in *HAS2* decreased the probability of obtaining a TQ + GQ

blastocyst by 8.7%. Similarly, one unit increase in *GDF9* decreased the probability of obtaining a TQ + GQ blastocyst by 2.5%. No such correlation was found in other gene expressions studied. However, once again this correlation was seen only when the genes were evaluated together with follicular size and the patient specific variables of age, BMI and AMH. Although gene expression of *HAS2* and *GDF9* correlated with blastocyst quality, the only variable correlating with eRB and TQ and GQ blastocysts for each of the five GLMM models was follicular size. Furthermore, the correlation was stronger. These findings support the clinical implications of the first part of our study [1] that follicle size is a strong in-
blastocyst.
dicator of the likelihood of an embryo proceeding to

As the nuclear and cytoplasmic competence are acquired during follicular growth, which requires the bidirectional cross-talk between the oocyte itself and CCs, CC gene expression of essential genes can be expected to be altered. Thus, it can be speculated that follicular size is fundamental when analysing CC expression data and that markers of oocyte competence based on CC
accurate.
studies have to include follicular size to be rigorously

The complexity related to modifiers of gene expression is illustrated in the recent literature [32]. In a randomized study, Cruz and colleagues (2017) showed that the type of gonadotropin used during controlled ovarian stimulation (follicle-stimulating hormone (FSH), urinary FSH, or human menopausal gonadotropin (hMG)) induce differential gene expression in human CCs [50]. Moreover, *PTGS2* was shown to be down-regulated in CCs of infertile women with endometriosis [51]. Patient age affects differential mRNA gene expression in CCs [52–54]. Patient BMI is also a modifier of CC gene expression in both polycystic ovarian syndrome (PCOS) [44] and non-PCOS women [54]. CC gene expression from different patients were studied, and it is known that factors such as different stimulation protocols, patient characteristics and transfer techniques may impact either CC gene expression or implantation [44, 50–56].

Therefore, in our study, patients were selected with inclusion criteria as similar as was possible in a clinical context. Although some minor variations (e.g. BMI) were unavoidable, bias in the participants selection was minimized by including only antagonist cycles in the study, by administering GnRH antagonist when the size of the follicle was at least 12 mm, but never exceeding 13 mm. Although there was some variation in the FSH dose (150–225 IU) depending on BMI, cases with more extreme dosages were not included. Furthermore, PCOS patients with an abnormally high number of COCs were excluded [44], because abnormal gene expression profiles in human ovaries from polycystic ovary syndrome patients have been described in the literature [57]. Finally, severe male infertility cases, where sperm might have played a critical role, were excluded.

Thus, this study was conducted using a homogeneous group of young and good prognosis patients and generalized linear mixed models (GLMMs) were applied in order to correct the expression data of each oocyte regarding the clinical characteristics of each patient included in the study. Hence, unlike a more basic statistical evaluation in which each oocyte is considered to be independent, this paired analysis corrected for the follicular cohort effect, giving more reliable results.

A correlation was found in this study between blastocyst quality and CC gene expressions of *HAS2* and *GDF9* by GLMM analyses. Increased levels of *GDF9* and *BMP15* expression have both been associated with positive pregnancy as well as with mature oocytes, fertilization rate and embryo quality [43]. Analyzing *GDF9* and *BMP15* expression by qRT-PCR, Li and colleagues [32] utilized one of the largest samples sizes to date, using 2426 CC masses from 196 patients. Furthermore, *HAS2* is considered to be a human pregnancy or live birth candidate biomarker with conflicting differential mRNA expression by qRT-PCR [2, 19, 31, 32].

Finally, to answer the questions asked when beginning the study; although gene expression of *HAS2* and *GDF9* correlated with blastocyst quality when separately evaluated with follicular size and the patient specific variables of age, BMI and AMH, the only variable correlating with eRB and TQ and GQ blastocysts for each of these five models was follicular size. Furthermore, the correlation was stronger.

Conclusions

In conclusion, follicular size correlated significantly with blastocyst quality and viability. Embryos coming from large follicles were almost twice as likely as those coming from small follicles to develop into TQ + GQ blastocysts suitable for transfer or freezing. There was also a correlation between blastocyst quality and CC gene expressions of *HAS2* and *GDF9*, but only when evaluated together with follicular size, age, BMI and AMH, no such correlation was found in the case of other gene expressions studied. The only variable correlating with eRB and TQ and GQ blastocysts for each of the five models including the expression levels of the five genes studied was follicular size. Our findings suggest that differences in gene expression could be related to follicular size rather than to embryo quality.

Abbreviations
BMI: Body Mass Index; BQ: Bad Quality blastocyst; CCs: Cumulus Cells; COC: Cumulus Oocyte Complex; eFRB: embryos Failed to Reach Blastocyst; eRB: embryos Reaching Blastocyst; *GDF9*: Growth Differentiation Factor 9; GLMMs: Generalized linear mixed models; GQ: Good quality blastocyst; *HAS2*: Hyaluronan Synthase 2; MII: Metaphase II oocyte; OPU: Oocyte Pick-Up; *PTGS2*: Prostaglandin-Endoperoxide Synthase 2; *PTX3*: Pentraxin-related protein 3; *TNFAIP6*: Tumour Necrosis Factor Alpha Induced Protein 6; TQ: Top quality blastocyst

Funding
The study was supported by the Grant for Fertility Innovation (GFI 2014) provided by Merck KGaA, Darmstadt, Germany. The funding body had no role either in the design of the study and collection, analysis, and interpretation of data or in writing the manuscript.

Authors' contributions
CPC and MC made substantial contributions to conception and design, analysis and interpretation of data and have been involved in drafting the manuscript and revising it critically for important intellectual content; MA and CGE made substantial contributions to conception and design, analysis and acquisition of data; SK and MM made substantial contributions to conception and design and have been involved in drafting the manuscript and revising it critically for important intellectual content; SK has given final approval of the version to be published. All authors read and approved the final manuscript.

Competing interests
SK has received a research grant from the Grant for Fertility Innovation (GFI 2014) provided by Merck KGaA, Darmstadt, Germany. MM has received consultancy fees from Vitrolife AB Sweden. CPC, MC, MA and CGE declare that they have no conflict of interest.

Author details
[1]Istanbul Memorial Hospital, Assisted Reproductive Technologies and Reproductive Genetics Centre, Piyale Pasa Bulvari 34385 Okmeydani Sisli, Istanbul, Turkey. [2]ilabcomm GmbH, Eisenachstr. 34, 53757 Sankt Augustin, Germany.

References
1. Kahraman S, Cetinkaya CP, Cetinkaya M, Yelke H, Colakoglu YK, Aygun M, et al. The effect of follicle size and homogeneity of follicular development on the morphokinetics of human embryos. J Assist Reprod Genet. 2017;34(7):895–903.
2. McKenzie LJ, Pangas SA, Carson SA, Kovanci E, Cisneros P, Buster JE, et al. Human cumulus granulosa cell gene expression: a predictor of fertilization and embryo selection in women undergoing IVF. Hum Reprod. 2004;19(12):2869–74.
3. Zhang X, Jafari N, Barnes RB, Confino E, Milad M, Kazer RR. Studies of gene expression in human cumulus cells indicate pentraxin 3 as a possible marker for oocyte quality. Fertil Steril. 2005;83(Suppl 1):1169–79.
4. Cillo F, Brevini TA, Antonini S, Paffoni A, Ragni G, Gandolfi F. Association between human oocyte developmental competence and expression levels of some cumulus genes. Reproduction. 2007;134(5):645–50.
5. Lim H, Paria BC, Das SK, Dinchuk JE, Langenbach R, Trzaskos JM, et al. Multiple female reproductive failures in cyclooxygenase 2-deficient mice. Cell. 1997;91:197–208.
6. Calder MD, Caveney AN, Westhusin ME, Watson AJ. Cyclooxygenase-2 and prostaglandin E(2) (PGE(2)) receptor messenger RNAs are affected by bovine oocyte maturation time and cumulus-oocyte complex quality, and PGE(2) induces moderate expansion of the bovine cumulus in vitro. Biol Reprod. 2001;65:135–40.
7. Sirois J, Sayasith K, Brown KA, Stock AE, Bouchard N, Dore M. Cyclooxygenase-2 and its role in ovulation: a 2004 account. Hum Reprod Update. 2004;10:373–85.
8. Takahashi T, Morrow JD, Wang H, Dey SK. Cyclooxygenase-2-derived prostaglandin E(2) directs oocyte maturation by differentially influencing multiple signaling pathways. J Biol Chem. 2006;281:37117–29.
9. Fulop C, Kamath RV, Li Y, Otto JM, Salustri A, Olsen BR, et al. Coding sequence, exon-intron structure and chromosomal localization of murine TNF-stimulated gene 6 that is specifically expressed by expanding cumulus cell-oocyte complexes. Gene. 1997;202(1–2):95–102.
10. Yoshioka S, Ochsner S, Russell DL, Ujioka T, Fujii S, Richards JS, et al. Expression of tumor necrosis factor-stimulated gene-6 in the rat ovary in response to an ovulatory dose of gonadotropin. Endocrinology. 2000;141(11):4114–9.
11. Trombly DJ, Woodruff TK, Mayo KE. Roles for transforming growth factor beta superfamily proteins in early folliculogenesis. Semin Reprod Med. 2009;27:14–23.
12. Kedem A, Fisch B, Garor R, Ben-Zaken A, Gizunterman T, Felz C, et al. Growth differentiating factor 9 (*GDF9*) and bone morphogenetic protein 15 both activate development of human primordial follicles in vitro, with seemingly more beneficial effects of *GDF9*. J Clin Endocrinol Metab. 2011;96(8):E1246–54.
13. Paulini F, Melo EO. The role of oocyte-secreted factors *GDF9* and BMP15 in follicular development and oogenesis. Reprod Domest Anim. 2011;46:354–61.
14. Albertini DF, Combelles CM, Benecchi E, Carabatsos MJ. Cellular basis for paracrine regulation of ovarian follicle development. Reproduction. 2001;121(5):647–53.
15. Hutt KJ, Albertini DF. An oocentric view of folliculogenesis and embryogenesis. Reprod BioMed Online. 2007;14(6):758–64.
16. Assou S, Haouzi D, Mahmoud K, Aouacheria A, Guillemin Y, Pantesco V, et al. A non-invasive test for assessing embryo potential by gene expression profiles of human cumulus cells: a proof of concept study. Mol Hum Reprod. 2008;14(12):711–9.
17. Assou S, Boumela I, Haouzi D, Anahory T, Dechaud H, De Vos J, et al. Dynamic changes in gene expression during human early embryo development: from fundamental aspects to clinical applications. Hum Reprod Update. 2011;17(2):272–90.
18. Assou S, Haouzi D, Dechaud H, Gala A, Ferrieres A, Hamamah S. Comparative gene expression profiling in human cumulus cells according to ovarian gonadotropin treatments. Biomed Res Int. 2013;2013:354582.
19. Ekart J, McNatty K, Hutton J, Pitman J. Ranking and selection of MII oocytes in human ICSI cycles using gene expression levels from associated cumulus cells. Hum Reprod. 2013;28(11):2930–42.
20. Li Y, Li RQ, Ou SB, Ren L, Zhang NF, Wei LN, et al. Association between the proportion of dominant follicles and oocyte developmental competence. J Assist Reprod Genet. 2014;31(12):1599–604.
21. Li SH, Lin MH, Hwu YM, Lu CH, Yeh LY, Chen YJ, et al. Correlation of cumulus gene expression of GJA1, PRSS35, *PTX3*, and SERPINE2 with oocyte maturation, fertilization, and embryo development. Reprod Biol Endocrinol. 2015;13:93.
22. Assidi M, Montag M, Sirard MA. Use of both cumulus cells' transcriptomic markers and zona pellucida birefringence to select developmentally competent oocytes in human assisted reproductive technologies. BMC Genomics. 2015;16(Suppl 1):S9.
23. Dumesic DA, Meldrum DR, Katz-Jaffe MG, Krisher RL, Schoolcraft WB. Oocyte environment: follicular fluid and cumulus cells are critical for oocyte health. Fertil Steril. 2015;103(2):303–16.
24. Nivet AL, Léveillé MC, Leader A, Sirard MA. Transcriptional characteristics of different sized follicles in relation to embryo transferability: potential role of hepatocyte growth factor signalling. Mol Hum Reprod. 2016;22(7):475–84.
25. Arnot AM, Vandekerckhove P, DeBono MA, Rutherford AJ. Follicular volume and number during in-vitro fertilization: association with oocyte developmental capacity and pregnancy rate. Hum Reprod. 1995;10(2):256–61.
26. Salha O, Nugent D, Dada T, Kaufmann S, Levett S, Jenner L, et al. The relationship between follicular fluid aspirate volume and oocyte maturity in in-vitro fertilization cycles. Hum Reprod. 1998;13(7):1901–6.
27. Farhi J, Orvieto R, Gavish O, Homburg R. The association between follicular size on human chorionic gonadotropin day and pregnancy rate in clomiphene citrate treated polycystic ovary syndrome patients. Gynecol Endocrinol. 2010;26(7):546–8.
28. Matzuk MM, Lamb DJ. The biology of infertility: research advances and clinical challenges. Nat Med. 2008;14(11):1197–213.

29. Chang HM, Qiao J, Leung PC. Oocyte-somatic cell interactions in the human ovary-novel role of bone morphogenetic proteins and growth differentiation factors. Hum Reprod Update. 2016;23(1):1–18.
30. Patino LC, Beau I, Carlosama C, Buitrago JC, Gonzalez R, Suarez CF, et al. New mutations in non-syndromic primary ovarian insufficiency patients identified via whole-exome sequencing. Hum Reprod. 2017;32(7):1512–20.
31. Gebhardt KM, Feil DK, Dunning KR, Lane M, Russell DL. Human cumulus cell gene expression as a biomarker of pregnancy outcome after single embryo transfer. Fertil Steril. 2011;96(1):47–52.e2.
32. Kordus RJ, LaVoie HA. Granulosa cell biomarkers to predict pregnancy in ART: pieces to solve the puzzle. Reproduction. 2017;153(2):R69–83.
33. Duffy DM, Dozier BL, Seachord CL. Prostaglandin dehydrogenase and prostaglandin levels in periovulatory follicles: implications for control of primate ovulation by prostaglandin E2. J Clin Endocrinol Metab. 2005;90:1021–7.
34. Russell DL, Salustri A. Extracellular matrix of the cumulus-oocyte complex. Semin Reprod Med. 2006;24:217–27.
35. Salustri A, Garlanda C, Hirsch E, De Acetis M, Maccagno A, Bottazzi B, et al. PTX3 plays a key role in the organization of the cumulus oophorus extracellular matrix and in in vivo fertilization. Development. 2004;131:1577–86.
36. Varani S, Elvin JA, Yan C, DeMayo J, DeMayo FJ, Horton HF, et al. Knockout of pentraxin 3, a downstream target of growth differentiation factor-9, causes female subfertility. Mol Endocrinol. 2002;16:1154–67.
37. Feuerstein P, Puard V, Chevalier C, Teusan R, Cadoret V, Guerif F, et al. Genomic assessment of human cumulus cell marker genes as predictors of oocyte developmental competence: impact of various experimental factors. PLoS One. 2012;7(7):e40449.
38. Fulop C, Szanto S, Mukhopadhyay D, Bardos T, Kamath RV, Rugg MS, et al. Impaired cumulus mucification and female sterility in tumor necrosis factor-induced protein-6 deficient mice. Development. 2003;130:2253–61.
39. Hamel M, Dufort I, Robert C, Gravel C, Leveille MC, Leader A, et al. Identification of differentially expressed markers in human follicular cells associated with competent oocytes. Hum Reprod. 2008;23(5):1118–27.
40. Silva JR, van den Hurk R, van Tol HT, Roelen BA, Figueiredo JR. Expression of growth differentiation factor 9 (*GDF9*), bone morphogenetic protein 15 (BMP15), and BMP receptors in the ovaries of goats. Mol Reprod Dev. 2005;70:11–9.
41. Zhao SY, Qiao J, Chen YJ, Liu P, Li J, Yan J. Expression of growth differentiation factor-9 and bone morphogenetic protein-15 in oocytes and cumulus granulosa cells of patients with polycystic ovary syndrome. Fertil Steril. 2010;94:261–7.
42. Hosoe M, Kaneyama K, Ushizawa K, Hayashi KG, Takahashi T. Quantitative analysis of bone morphogenetic protein 15 (BMP15) and growth differentiation factor 9 (*GDF9*) gene expression in calf and adult bovine ovaries. Reprod Biol Endocrinol. 2011;9:33.
43. Li Y, Li RQ, Ou SB, Zhang NF, Ren L, Wei LN, et al. Increased GDF9 and BMP15 mRNA levels in cumulus granulosa cells correlate with oocyte maturation, fertilization, and embryo quality in humans. Reprod Biol Endocrinol. 2014;12:81.
44. Kenigsberg S, Bentov Y, Chalifa-Caspi V, Potashnik G, Ofir R, Birk OS. Gene expression microarray profiles of cumulus cells in lean and overweight-obese polycystic ovary syndrome patients. Mol Hum Reprod. 2009;15(2):89–103.
45. Cetinkaya M, Pirkevi C, Yelke H, Colakoglu YK, Atayurt Z, Kahraman S. Relative kinetic expressions defining cleavage synchronicity are better predictors of blastocyst formation and quality than absolute time points. J Assist Reprod Genet. 2015;32(1):27–35.
46. Schmittgen TD, Livak KJ. Analyzing real-time PCR data by the comparative C(T) method. Nat Protoc. 2008;3(6):1101–8.
47. Rienzi L, Vajta G, Ubaldi F. Predictive value of oocyte morphology in human IVF: a systematic review of the literature. Hum Reprod Update. 2011;17(1):34–45.
48. Trounson A, Gosden R, Eichenlaub-Ritter U. Biology and pathology of the oocyte: role in fertility, medicine, and nuclear reprogramming. 2nd ed: Cambridge University Press; 2013.
49. Buccione R, Schroeder AC, Eppig JJ. Interactions between somatic cells and germ cells throughout mammalian oogenesis. Biol Reprod. 1990;43:543–7.
50. Cruz M, Requena A, Agudo D, García-Velasco JA. Type of gonadotropin used during controlled ovarian stimulation induces differential gene expression in human cumulus cells: a randomized study. Eur J Obstet Gynecol Reprod Biol. 2017;215:124–33.
51. da Luz CM, da Broi MG, Donabela FC, Paro de Paz CC, Meola J, Navarro PA. *PTGS2* down-regulation in cumulus cells of infertile women with endometriosis. Reprod BioMed Online. 2017;35(4):379–86.
52. McReynolds S, Dzieciatkowska M, McCallie BR, Mitchell SD, Stevens J, Hansen K, et al. Impact of maternal aging on the molecular signature of human cumulus cells. Fertil Steril. 2012;98(6):1574–80.e5.
53. Al-Edani T, Assou S, Ferrieres A, Bringer Deutsch S, Gala A, Lecellier CH, et al. Female aging alters expression of human cumulus cells genes that are essential for oocyte quality. Biomed Res Int. 2014;2014:964614.
54. Kedem A, Yung Y, Yerushalmi GM, Haas J, Maman E, Hanochi M, et al. Anti Müllerian hormone (AMH) level and expression in mural and cumulus cells in relation to age. J Ovarian Res. 2014;7:113.
55. Robker RL, Akison LK, Bennett BD, Thrupp PN, Chura LR, Russell DL, et al. Obese women exhibit differences in ovarian metabolites, hormones, and gene expression compared with moderate-weight women. J Clin Endocrinol Metab. 2009;94(5):1533–40.
56. Kava-Braverman A, Martínez F, Rodríguez I, Álvarez M, Barri PN, Coroleu B. What is a difficult transfer? Analysis of 7,714 embryo transfers: the impact of maneuvers during embryo transfers on pregnancy rate and a proposal of objective assessment. Fertil Steril. 2017;107(3):657–663.e1.
57. Jansen E, Laven JS, Dommerholt HB, Polman J, van Rijt C, van den Hurk C, et al. Abnormal gene expression profiles in human ovaries from polycystic ovary syndrome patients. Mol Endocrinol. 2004;18(12):3050–63.

13

Efficacy, safety and recurrence of new progestins and selective progesterone receptor modulator for the treatment of endometriosis

Bo Liang[1], Ling Wu[1], Hui Xu[1], Chun Wai Cheung[1], Wen Ying Fung[1], Sze Wai Wong[1] and Chi Chiu Wang[1,2,3*]

Abstract

Background: Current medical treatments for endometriosis are very limited. Progestin and selective progesterone receptor modulators (SPRM) are developed but their efficacy, safety, mechanism and recurrence in endometriosis are not fully studied.

Methods: In order to compare therapeutic, side effects and therapeutic actions of Esmya, Duphaston and Dienogest in endometriosis. Experimental endometriosis was induced by either intraperitoneal or subcutaneous mouse endometrium transplantation. Lesion size, weight and histology at the end of intervention were compared. Expression of related markers in the endometriotic lesions were examined. Body, uterus and ovary weights, endometrial glands and thickness (ETI), and follicle count were measured. For recurrent study, lesion growth before and after intervention was monitored.

Results: After Esmya, Duphaston, Dienogest treatment, lesion size and weight were significantly decreased. Proliferation Pcna expression was significantly decreased in all groups, but proliferation cells were significantly decreased only in Duphaston group. Apoptosis Mapk1 expression and TUNEL-positive cells were significantly increased in Duphaston group. Adhesion Mmp2 and Itgavβ3 expression were significantly increased in Esmya group. Plau, Hif1α and Vegfa expression, peritoneal fluid PGE2 levels, and ERα and ERβ expression were not affected; while PR expression was significantly lower in all groups. Endometrial gland count in uterus was significantly increased in Dienogest group, ETI was significantly decreased in Duphaston group, and AFC were significantly increased in Esmya group. Upon treatment cessation, lesion growth rebound quickly in Dienogest and Duphaston groups, but slowly in Esmya group.

Conclusion: Esmya, Duphaston and Dienogest are effective anti-endometriosis drugs targeting proliferation, apoptosis and adhesion. Esmya, Duphaston and Dienogest are all well tolerable, although endometrial glandular hyperplasia was found in Dienogest, endometrial atrophy in Duphaston, follicle accumulation in Esmya.

Keywords: Progestin, Selective progesterone receptor modulator, Endometrium

* Correspondence: ccwang@cuhk.edu.hk

[1]Department of Obstetrics and Gynaecology, The Chinese University of Hong Kong, c/o 1st Floor, Special Block E, Prince of Wales Hospital, Shatin, Hong Kong

[2]Reproduction and Development Laboratory, Li Ka Shing Institute of Health Sciences, The Chinese University of Hong Kong, Shatin, Hong Kong

Full list of author information is available at the end of the article

Background

Endometriosis is a common and chronic benign gynecological disorder characterized by the presence of endometrial-like tissues outside the uterine cavity. It affects around 10% of reproductive women, and up to 24–50% of infertile women [1, 2]. Although endometriosis is an estrogen-dependent disease, etiological studies showed that pathogenesis of endometriosis is complex and multifactorial [3–6]. The most widely accepted and scientifically supported theory for the occurrence of endometriosis is retrograde menstruation since the anatomical locations and histochemical characteristics of endometriotic lesions [4, 7]. Clinical symptoms of endometriosis include but not limited to pelvic pain, dysmenorrhea, dyspareunia and infertility [8], which have significant impacts on both general and mental health of afflicted individuals [9, 10]. Current available treatment of endometriosis, including removal surgery and hormonal medication [11], are still not ideal for reproductive women who would like to preserve their fecundity without any side-effect and recurrence.

Seeking targeted therapy with minimal side-effect has been going on for several decades, but there is still no better medication. Recently selective progesterone-receptor modulators (SPRM) and new generation progestins have been speculated or indicated as potential treatment for endometriosis [12–14]. For example, Ulipristal acetate (Esmya) is a SPRM, which has been used for uterine fibroids for a while [15]. Esmya can reduce the volume of uterine fibroid by inhibiting proliferation and increasing apoptosis [16, 17]. It may also work on endometriosis, but its therapeutic effects on endometriosis are still not fully evaluated. Duphaston contains dydrogesterone, a progestin derived from 9β,10α-progesterone [18], which can relieve pain in endometriosis and does not interrupt pregnancy during treatment. There is no conclusive evidence to support its therapeutic use in endometriosis [13, 19]. Dienogest is another progestin derived from 19- nortestosterone [18], which have been used to relief symptoms of endometriosis [20]. It can inhibit the endometriotic lesion growth by inducing decidualization [21, 22] and also inhibiting implantation and angiogenesis of endometriotic lesions [23–25]. However, the exact mechanism of Dienogest on endometriotic lesion growth and development is still unclear and the controversial effect on endometrium thickness has been noted [26]. Nevertheless, recurrence of endometriosis after cessation of Esmya, Duphaston and Dienogest had never been studied.

In present study, we aimed to compare anti-endometriotic effects, reproductive side-effects, therapeutic mechanism and recurrence of Esmya, Duphaston and Dienogest in an experimental endometriosis mouse model.

Methods

Chemicals and reagents

17-β-estradiol was purchased from Sigma Chemical Co. (St. Louis, USA). Ketamine, xylazine, and acepromazine were purchased from Alfasan (Netherlands, Holland); Rabbit monoclonal antibody for Ki67 was purchased from Cell signaling technology (D3B5, Danvers, USA). In situ apoptosis detection kit was purchased from Merck Millipore (USA). Reagents for RT-PCR and quantitative PCR were purchased from TaKaRa (TaKaRa Bio, Shiga, Japan). Estradiol and progesterone ELISA kits were obtained from Cayman Chemical, USA. Prostaglandin E2 ELISA kit was purchased from Abcam (Abcam, England).

Animals and endometriosis model

Six to seven weeks female C57BL/6 mice were housed in pathogen-free animal rooms with fixed cycle of 12 h' light and 12 h' dark. Standard laboratory chows and clean water were provided and all mice were allowed to acclimatize at least 1 week prior to experiments. A mixture of ketamine at 100 mg/kg, xylazine at 10 mg/kg and acepromazine at 3 mg/kg was injected intraperitoneally to anesthetize the mice before invasive surgery. Based on different goals of experiments in this study, two different mouse endometriosis models were established as below. Animals' estrous cycle were synchronized by transferring urine-soaked male bedding every 5 days for both IP and SC endometriosis mouse model. [27]. All of the animal experiments were approved from the Animal Experimentation Ethics Committee, The Chinese University of Hong Kong.

Intraperitoneal (IP) endometriosis mouse model for therapeutic safety and mechanistic study

The IP endometriosis model was established with minor modifications as described before [27, 28]. Briefly, mice were randomly divided into two groups, either donors or recipients. In day 0, uterus was dissected out from each donor mouse after sacrificed and washed in PBS for 3 times. Endometrial tissues were prepared from each uterus horn by a 2 mm biopsy punch. After endometrial tissues were prepared, recipient mouse was anesthetized and a 0.5 to 1 cm incision was made on the midline of mouse abdomen wall and peritoneum. Colon was pulled out carefully and kept hydration with sterile PBS. Three pieces of endometrial tissues were sutured on the vessels of mesentery with 6–0 surgical thread in each recipient mouse. Colon were put back to the peritoneal cavity gently; abdomen wall and skin were closed by 5–0 surgical thread individually. Mice were then placed on a warm pad until fully recovered from anesthesia after the surgery.

Subcutaneous (SC) endometriosis mouse model for recurrence study

We established another mouse endometriosis model by SC transplantation to monitor the dynamic change of lesion growth during and after the medical interventions. It has been reported that both of IP and SC model exhibits similar development of endometriosis in respect with the cyst-like growth, and glandular and epithelial structures of the lesions [27, 29]. The same strain C57BL/6 mice were used to establish SC endometriosis mouse model as described before [30, 31]. Briefly, uterus was dissected out from donor mice and endometrial tissues were prepared as IP model mentioned above. Under anesthesia, the abdominal skin was shaved and then a 3 mm skin incision was made on the middle line of abdomen of each recipient mouse and bilateral SC pockets were created carefully without damaging the abdomen wall. One piece of endometrial tissue was placed into each pocket and then the skin incision was closed with 5–0 surgical thread.

Study medications

One week after the surgery, mice were randomly divided into four groups. Either vehicle (the mice were treated with double distill water), Ulipristal acetate (Esmya™, 1 mg/kg, po, PregLem, England), Dydrogesterone (Duphaston™, 5 mg/kg, po, Abbott, USA) or Progestin (Dienogest™, 0.3 mg/kg, po, Bayer, Germany) were administered orally every day. The suggested oral daily dose for human from manufacturer instruction of Esmya, Duphaston and Dienogest were 5 mg, 20-30 mg and 2 mg, respectively. The dosage of each medication for the mice was based on FDA approved clinical dose for human and then converted to animal dose according to the guidelines of FDA calculator based on the surface area of humans and experimental animals [32]. All the medications were dissolved into appropriate volume of double distill water in 100ul.

For IP model, the medication was lasted for 28 days. For SC model, medication lasted for 21 days. The endometriotic lesion growth was determined by measuring longest length and perpendicular width of the lesions every 3 days in SC model and at the end of intervention in IP model using caliper as described before [31]. Then all the mice were sacrificed and lesions were removed and washed in sterilize PBS, then weighted on balance. For all lesions from each mouse, one lesion was fixed with 10% formalin (Sigma) and embedded in paraffin wax for histological analysis; the other lesions were either immersed in RNA later solution (Ambion™) for qPCR analysis or snap-frozen in liquid nitrogen for protein analysis.

Uterus size was estimated by measuring and averaging the longest diameter with caliper in the middle of each uterus horn. Ovaries was considered as ellipsoid and the ovary size was measured and calculated according to formula [33]: $1/6\ \pi \times$ length $\times$ width $\times$ thickness (mm^3). Uterus was dissected and weighed before separated into 3 pieces and stored in the same way as lesions. Ovaries were dissected and then either fixed in 10% formalin for histological analysis or stored in RNA later solution for qPCR analysis.

Hematoxylin and eosin staining

After embedding, 4um serial paraffin sections of lesions, uterus and ovary were prepared on coated slides. Hematoxylin and eosin staining will be carried out in every 10th section to confirm the microscopic structures in the lesions, uterus and ovary [34]. Surface area of the sections under the microscope were measured.

Immunohistochemistry and TUNEL assay

Proliferation of the lesion was evaluated by immunohistochemical staining using rabbit anti mouse Ki-67 antibody (D3B5, Cell signaling technology). After de-paraffin and re-hydration, antigens were retrieved with sodium citrate buffer in microwave for 20 min. The sections were incubated with 1% BSA in PBS at room temperature for 1 h, follow by incubating with Ki-67 antibody in 4 °C for 15 h. After incubation with the primary antibody, sections were incubated with secondary antibody Donkey anti-Rabbit IgG-HRP (sc2313, Santa Cruz) for 1 h at room temperature and then with the colour was developed using DAB kit (k3468, Dako). Finally, the sections were counterstained with hematoxylin and dehydrated in serial concentration ethanol and mounted with coverslips. All the sections were examined under microscope. The cells with strong or moderated brown staining in nuclear were counted.

Apoptotic cells in the lesion were examined using an in situ apoptosis detection kit (ApopTAG®, S7100, Millipore, USA) according to the manufacturer's instruction.

Quantitative PCR analysis

Total RNA in the lesions was extracted by QIAGEN RNeasy Mini Kit (QIAGEN, Germany) according to the manufacturer's protocol. Concentration and quality of RNA were measured by Nanodrop spectrophotometry (Wilmington, USA) and reverse-transcribed with TaKaRa RT-PCR kit (TaKaRa, 6110A, Japan) in ProFlex PCR System (Thermo Fisher Scientific, USA). Quantitative qPCR was carried out with TaKaRa SYBR Green quantitative qPCR kit (SYBR® Premix Ex Taq, TaKaRa) in 7900HT Fast Quantitative PCR system. Forty nanograms of cDNA was added to the reaction system. Primers used in this study are listed in Additional file 1: Table S1. Mouse β-actin gene was used as housekeeping gene. Data were analyzed using relative expression level and comparison was performed between different groups after normalized to the β-actin expression. The markers had been shown to play important role in the pathogenesis of endometriosis were chosen to screen the therapeutic actions [31]. Mmp2 and Plau play key role in breaking down the endometrial stroma and extracellular basement membrane [35, 36]. Integrins αV β3 (Itgav β3) is an adhesion molecule that functions in both cell–cell and cell–substratum adhesion [37]. Vascular endothelial growth factor (Vegf) and hypoxia inducible factor-1α (Hif1α) are key factors in angiogenesis [38]. Both Vegf and Hif1α expression were increased in endometriotic lesions [39]. NF-kB p105 and MAPK1 play a critical role in the regulation of cell proliferation and apoptosis [40, 41]. Pro-caspase 3 (pro-Cas3) is a key factor in caspase related apoptosis. Proliferating cell nuclear antigen (Pcna) is a protein associated with cell proliferation [42].

Uterine gland count and endometrium thickness index

After stained by hematoxylin and eosin and examined under microscope, 6 serial uterine sections were scanned with Leica microscope in 100× magnification. For uterine gland count, all the glands in endometrium layer were counted and averaged for statistical analysis. Endometrium thickness index (ETI) was evaluated as the method described before with some modifications [43]. Briefly, the area of endometrium (A_e) and uterus cavity (A_{uc}) was measured using Image J [44]. ETI was then calculated using the formula $ETI = \sqrt{\frac{A_e}{\pi}} - \sqrt{\frac{A_{uc}}{\pi}}.$

Follicle count

After stained by hematoxylin and eosin and examined under microscope, 3 serial ovarian sections were scanned with Leica microscope in 40× magnification. Follicle classification was based on morphological criteria: primary follicles were defined as follicles which contain oocyte surrounded by single layer of granulosa cells; secondary follicles were defined as follicles which contain oocyte with 2 or more layers of granulosa cells, and antral follicles were defined as follicles contain oocyte which surrounded by several layers of granulosa cells and contain a visible antrum [45, 46]. The follicle count of each classification in each sample was measured and compared.

Enzyme-linked immunosorbent assay

Serum and peritoneal fluid were collected for enzyme-linked immunosorbent assays. Whole blood was collected by 1 ml syringe with 25G needle from mouse heart, and then was centrifuged at 4 °C with 1000×g for 10 min. Serum was collected after centrifuge and stored in -80 °C. Peritoneal fluid was collected as method described before with some modifications [47]. Mice were sacrificed by overdose of anesthetic; skin was opened to expose the abdomen. 3 ml sterilize PBS and 2 ml air were injected into peritoneum using a 5 ml syringe and 21G needle. Then the peritoneal salvage was removed and centrifuged at 4 °C, 1000×g for 10 min, the supernatant was kept in -80 °C prior to analysis. Estradiol (E2) and progesterone (P4) levels in serum and prostaglandin E2 (PGE2) concentration in peritoneal fluid were measured by ELISA kits (Abcam, England) according to manufacturer's instruction.

Statistical analysis

Statistical analysis was carried out with Software Graphpad Prism 5, the differences between the treatment groups and control group were evaluated by One Way ANOVA if data distribution normal or Kruskal–Wallis test if data distribution skewed followed by Dunnett's multiple post-hoc comparisons. Data were expressed as mean ± SEM. $p < 0.05$ was considered as significant.

Results

Ectopic endometriotic lesions growth

After IP transplantation, endometriotic lesions developed in the mesentery (Fig. 1a). Compared to vehicle control (size: 6.744±0.444 mm^2; weight: 12.1±1.383 mg, n = 9), lesion size and weight were significantly decreased after treatment with Esmya (size: 4.171± 0.442 mm^2, p < 0.0001; weight: 6.133±0.907 mg, n = 9, p = 0.0007), Duphaston (size: 4.104±0.262 mm^2, p < 0.0001; weight: 6.747±0.679 mg, n = 9, p = 0.0012) and Dienogest (size: 3.092±0.340 mm^2, p < 0.0001; weight: 5.744±0.621 mg, n = 9, p = 0.001) (Fig. 1b). The cyst-like endometriotic lesion with endometrial glandular and stroma structures were underdeveloped in the treatment groups (Fig. 1c). Cell proliferation in both epithelial and stromal cells of the endometriotic tissues was significantly decreased in Duphaston group when compared with control group (Fig. 1d and e, epithelial: 4.117±0.581 cells/field vs 37.606±2.604 cells/field, n = 9, p < 0.0001; stromal: 14.294±1.305 cells/field vs 23.258±1.783 cells/field, n = 9, p = 0.0095). However, cell proliferation in stromal cells were significantly increased in Dienogest group (37.333±6.179 cells/field vs 23.258±1.783 cells/field, n = 9, p = 0.0202). Apoptotic cells in the endometriotic lesions were significantly increased in Duphaston group. (Fig. 1f and g, 57.333±2.186 cells/field vs 23±8.756 cells/field, n = 9, p = 0.0461).

Therapeutic actions

Only Esmya significantly increased the mRNA expression of adhesion markers Mmp2 (0.174±0.030 vs 0.083±0.006, n = 9, p = 0.0066) and Itgav β3 (0.025 ±0.001 vs 0.015±0.003, n = 9, p = 0.001), but not invasion marker Plau (0.046±0.018 vs 0.058±0.021, n = 9, p = 0.941) (Fig. 2a-c). Only Duphaston significantly increased the mRNA expression of apoptotic

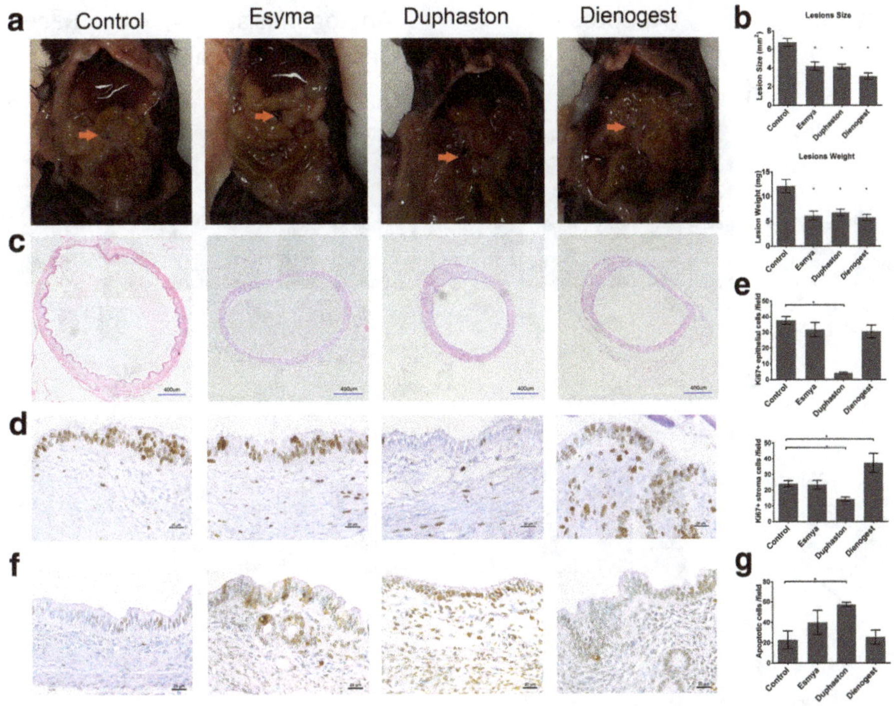

Fig. 1 Esmya, Duphaston and Dienogest suppress the growth and development of endometriotic lesions in mice. **a** Lesion size was measured by caliper at the end of intervention. Representative in situ pictures of the endometriotic lesions in vehicle, Esmya, Duphaston and Dienogest group are shown. Red arrows indicate the locations of the lesions. **b** Endometriotic lesion size and weight. Data are shown as mean ± SEM, $n = 9$ for each group, *: $p < 0.05$ when compared to the control group. **c** Histological change of lesions after medication. This panels show the representative cross-sections of the endometriotic lesion as endometrial cyst-like structure. *Scar bar*: 400um. **d** Proliferation of the endometriotic lesions. Representative pictures of immunohistochemical staining of Ki67 in endometriotic-like lesions in different groups after treatment. *Scar bar*: 200um. **e** Comparison of Ki67 positively stained epithelial and stroma cells in the lesions. **f** Representative pictures of TUNEL staining in endometriotic-like lesions in different groups after treatment. *Scar bar*: 200um. **g** Comparison of TUNEL positively cells in the lesions. Data are shown as mean ± SEM, $n = 3$ for each group, *: $p < 0.05$ when compared to the control group

marker Mapk1 (0.021±0.001 vs 0.013±0.001, $n = 9$, p = 0.0138) but not NF-κB p105 (0.014±0.0002 vs 0.013±0.0012, $n = 9$, p = 0.686) and pro-Casp3 (0.0071±0.0006 vs 0.0068 ±0.0006, n = 9, p = 0.968) (Fig. 2d-f,). All Esmya, Duphaston and Dienogest significantly decreased the mRNA expression of proliferation marker Pcna (0.069±0.007 vs 0.078±0.004 vs 0.066± 0.004 vs 0.108±0.014, p = 0.0079, p = 0.0479, $n = 9$, p = 0.0041; Esmya, Duphaston, Dienogest and control, respectively), but not angiogenesis markers Vegf (0.0745±0.006 vs 0.0942±0.011 vs 0.080±0.009 vs 0.0675 ±0.006, $n = 9$, p = 0.825, p = 0.051, p = 0.777; Esmya, Duphaston, Dienogest and control, respectively) and Hif1α (0.0087±0.0004 vs 0.0097±0.0003 vs 0.0093±0.0005 vs 0.0090±0.0008, $n = 9$, p = 0.967, p = 0.739, p = 0.970; Esmya, Duphaston, Dienogest and control, respectively) (Fig. 2g-i). Esmya, Duphaston and Dienogest also significantly decreased the mRNA expression of progesterone receptor PR (0.0012±0.0001 vs 0.0012±0.00008 vs 0.0014 ±0.00006 vs 0.0023±0.0005, $n = 9$, p = 0.0099, p = 0.0099, p = 0.0168; Esmya, Duphaston, Dienogest and control, respectively) but not estrogen receptor ERα/ERβ ratios (67.151±9.706 vs 60.342±15.704 vs 39.284±11.690 vs 60.861±25.804, n = 9, p = 0.983, p > 0.999, p = 0.668; Esmya, Duphaston, Dienogest and control, respectively) (Fig. 2j-k). Pain mediator PGE2 concentration in peritoneal fluid was not significantly decreased after any treatment (1937.169±250.804 pg/ml vs 1850.524±273.428 pg/ml vs 1476.434±250.292 pg/ml vs 2484.759±466.669 pg/ml, $n = 9$, p = 0.720, p = 0.597 p = 0.152; Esmya, Duphaston, Dienogest and control, respectively) (Fig. 2l).

Safety profiles

All the animals were well-tolerated with the treatment and showed no significant change in body weight (detailed mean±sem and p value was provided in Additional file 1: Table S2) (Fig. 3a). None of the animals exhibited any behavior or signs of stress or toxic reaction throughout the study. Serum estrogen (40.484±3.771 pg/ml vs 43.201±6.825 pg/ml vs 47.674±7.219 pg/ml vs 41.055±6.335 pg/ml, $n = 9$, p = 0.999, p = 0.990, p = 0.792; Esmya, Duphaston, Dienogest and control, respectively) and progesterone (194.489±65.

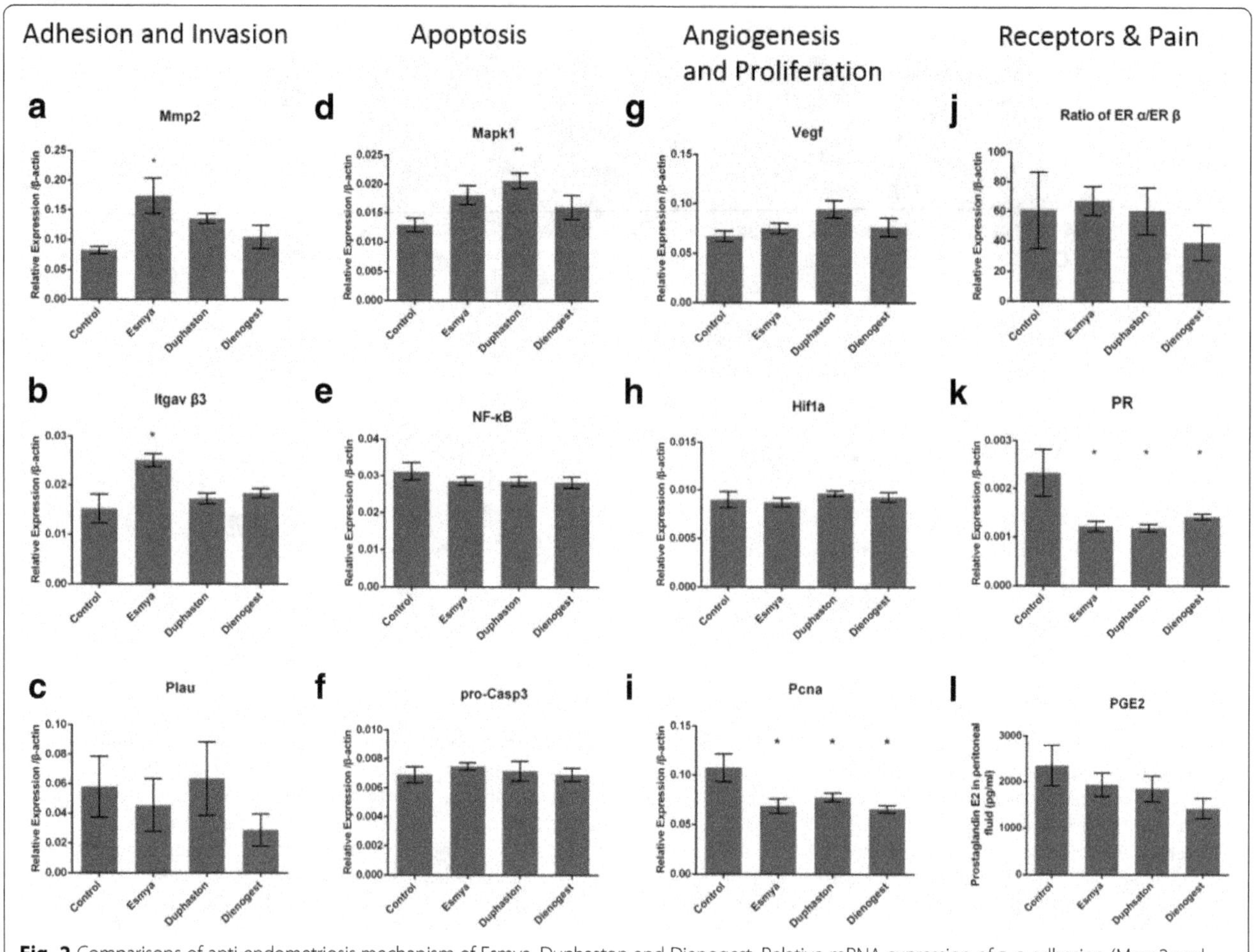

Fig. 2 Comparisons of anti-endometriosis mechanism of Esmya, Duphaston and Dienogest. Relative mRNA expression of **a-c**, adhesion (Mmp2 and Itgav β3) and invasion (Plau) marker genes, **d-f**, apoptosis-related genes (Mapk1, NF-kB p105 and pro-Caspase 3), **g-i**, angiogenesis and proliferation mrakers (Vegf, Hif1α and Pcna) and **j-k**, hormone receptors (ERα/ERβ ratio and PR) in lesions; and ELISA quantitation of **l**, Prostaglandin E2 (PGE2) concentrations in peritoneal fluid. Data are shown as mean ± SEM, n = 9 for each group, *: $p < 0.05$ when compared to the control group

011 pg/ml vs 228.899±33.706 pg/ml vs 209.084±34.224 pg/ml vs 185.480±14.228 pg/ml, $n = 9$, $p = 0.997$, $p = 0.779$, $p = 0.958$; Esmya, Duphaston, Dienogest and control, respectively) levels were not significantly different amongst groups after treatment (Fig. 3b). There is no significant difference in uterus size (2.140±0.102 mm vs 2.143±0.103 mm vs 2.490±0.125 mm vs 2.590±0.254 mm, $n = 9$, $p = 0.344$, $p = 0.350$, $p = 0.978$; Esmya, Duphaston, Dienogest and control, respectively) and weight (3.361±0.341 mg/g vs 2.908±0.159 mg/g vs 3.170±0.260 mg/g vs 3.148±0.193 mg/g, $n = 9$, $p = 0.929$, $p = 0.902$, $p > 0.999$; Esmya, Duphaston, Dienogest and control, respectively), but histological examination showed significant reduced ETI in Duphaston group (0.285±0.024 mm vs 0.376±0.018 mm, $n = 9$, $p = 0.0149$) and significant increased endometrial gland counts in Dienogest group (48.478±2.379 vs 34.637±3.743, $n = 9$, p = 0.0149) (Fig. 3c). Similarly, there was no significant change in ovary size (2.591±0.242 mm^3 vs 2.444±0.153 mm^3 vs 2.463±0.154 mm^3 vs 2.587±0.120 mm^3, n = 9, $p = 0.987$, $p = 0.907$, p = 0.907; Esmya, Duphaston, Dienogest and control, respectively) and weight (0.360±0.015 mg/g vs 0.349±0.018 mg/g vs 0.330±0.023 mg/g vs 0.357±0.015 mg/g, $n = 9$, $p = 0.999$, $p = 0.986$, $p = 669$; Esmya, Duphaston, Dienogest and control, respectively) but the numbers of antral follicle were significantly increased in Esmya group (0.285±0.024 mm vs 0.376±0.017 mm, n = 9, $p = 0.0143$) (Fig. 3d).

Withdrawn recurrence

After SC transplantation, Duphaston significantly decreased the lesion size from day 9 (3.609±0.176 mm^2, $n = 10$, $p = 0.0418$) of treatment, then Dienogest from day 12 (3.397±0.157 mm^2, $n = 10$, $p = 0.0024$) and Esmya from day 15 (3.585±0.160 mm^2, $n = 10$, $p = 0.0223$) when compared with control group (4.689±0.328 mm^2 or 4.843±0.199 mm^2 or 4.844±0.200 mm^2, day 9, day 12, day 15 respectively) (Fig. 4). When treatment was withdrawn in day 21, lesion size of Dienogest group remained significantly smaller only until day 36 (4.686±0.377 mm^2

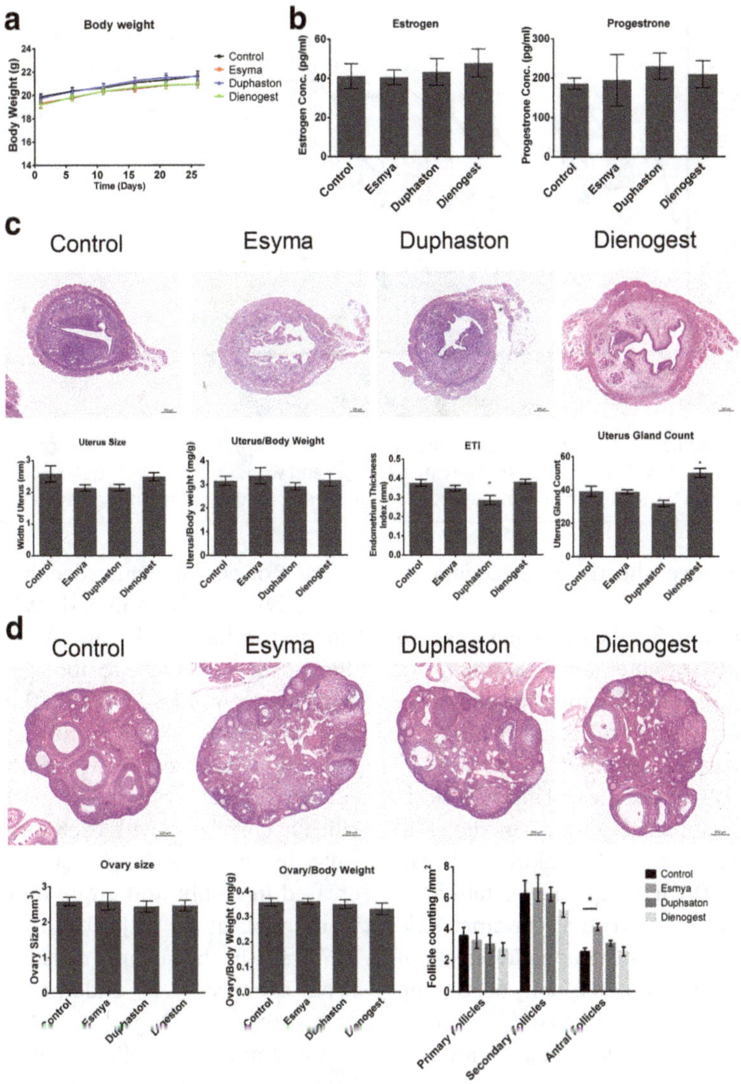

Fig. 3 Safety profiles of Esmya, Duphaston and Dienogest. **a** Body weight changes during the study intervention. Data was recorded every 5 days from day 1 to day 25 after transplantation. **b** Serum estrogen and progesterone concentrations after treatment in the mice. **c** Upper panels show the representative cross section images of uterus, structure of endometrium gland, stroma and lumen cavity. *Scar bar*: 200um. Lower panels compare the uterus size, ratio of uterus and body weight, endometrium thickness index (ETI) and uterus gland count from left to right. **d** Upper panels show the histological change of ovary after treatment. *Scar bar*: 200um. Lower panels compared the ovary size, ratio of ovary and body weight and the follicle count from left to right. Data are shown as mean ± SEM. *: $p < 0.05$ when compared to the control group

vs 6.028±0.394 mm^2, $n = 10$, $p = 0.0168$), 14 days after withdrawal. Lesion size of Duphaston and Esmya groups remained significantly smaller until day 39 (Duphaston vs control: 4.588±0.324 mm^2 vs 6.001±0.233 mm^2, $n = 10$, $p = 0.0255$) and day 48 (Esmya vs control: 4.962±0.556 mm^2 vs 6.577±0.379 mm^2, $n = 10$, $p = 0.0352$), 18 days and 27 days after withdrawal, respectively.

Discussion

This is the first study to compare anti-endometriosis, therapeutic mechanism, safety profile and withdrawn recurrence of Esmya, Duphaston and Dienogest in an experimental endometriosis model in mice. The results showed that Esmya, Duphaston and Dienogest can effectively limit the endometriotic lesion growth and development (Table 1). The therapeutic effects are mainly through inhibition of progesterone receptor and cell proliferation and activation of apoptosis mechanisms. In particularly, Duphaston significantly inhibited the proliferation of both epithelial cells and stroma cells and activated apoptosis in the endometriotic lesions. Although wide safety margin, Duphaston induced endometrial atrophy, Dienogest enhanced endometrial glandular hyperplasia, Esmya increased adhesion of the lesion and antral follicle

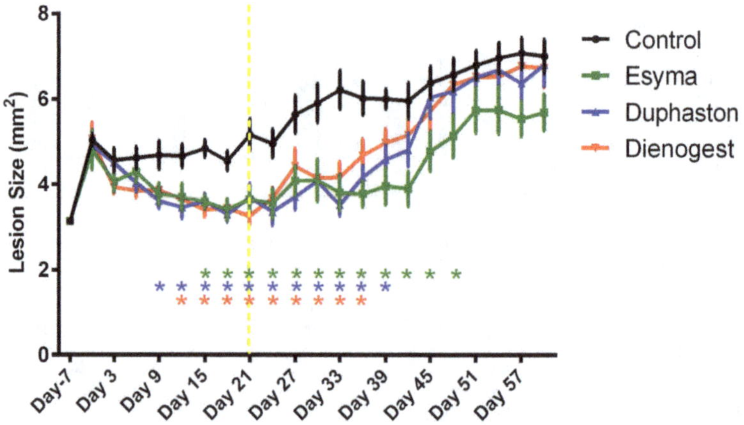

Fig. 4 Dynamic change of endometriotic lesion size during and after treatment of Esmya, Duphaston and Dienogest. The endometriotic lesions were transplanted subcutaneously in day − 7. Intervention was started at day 0 and withdrawn at day 21 (yellow dot line). Data were shown as mean ± SEM, $n = 10$ for each group, *: $p < 0.05$ when compared to the control group in the corresponding days and groups

accumulation, and recurrence shortly after Dienogest and Duphaston withdrawn.

Esmya as a new generation SPRM has been used to treat uterine fibroids and as an emergency contraceptive [48, 49], but it is not yet used for treatment of endometriosis. The major active component of Esmya is ulipristal acetate. The detail mechanism of ulipristal acetate on endometriosis of human is still not clear. Ulipristal acetate had been tested as another brand of medication, ellaOne, on a rat endometriosis model before [50]. According to Huniadi's study, 0.1 mg ulipristal acetate daily for 8 weeks significantly reduced the endometriotic lesion about to 55%. The potential therapeutic effects of ulipristal acetate on increasing apoptosis and decreasing proliferation were also confirmed in this study although its safety was not studied. Compared to our study, the inhibitory effect was similar in terms of the decreased lesion size and proliferation. Although our dose was similar in terms of human equivalent dose, our intervention time was shorter (4 weeks vs 8 weeks). It has been shown that ulipristal acetate increased Bax/Bcl-2 ratio and cytochrome c expression [50] which activated capase-3 and increased apoptosis in the endometriotic lesions [51]. In our study, we did not study cytochrome c and Bax/Bcl-2 but neither apoptotic markers Mapk1, NF-κB p105 or pro-caspase3 expression were significantly increased in the lesions. The limitation of mRNA expression level is that only the pro-caspase-3 rather than activated form caspase-3 can be evaluated. The expression level of pro-caspase-3 on mRNA level can provide one of evidence for the caspase-related apoptosis in endometriotic lesions, however, the definitive regulation of apoptosis of endometriotic lesions should be carried out by protein expression, such as immunohistochemistry or Western blot analysis. Unlike caspase related apoptosis, Mapks involved in the pathophysiological process of endometrium decidualisation [52] and upregulated NF-κB p105 [53, 54]. When compared to Esmya, Duphaston has similar anti-endometriosis efficacy in reducing the lesion size to about 61%. But only Duphaston significantly reduced proliferating cells in both epithelial and stroma cells and significantly increased apoptotic cells and Mapk1 expression in the endometriotic lesions. Although cells proliferation markers Pcna and Ki67 specifically correlated with each other [55, 56], Ki67 positive cells in endometriotic lesions were significantly decreased in Duphaston group only. In contrast to the previous publication [22], Dienogest significantly increased Ki67 cells in the stromal cells but significantly decreased Pcna expression in endometriotic lesions. Compared with Esmya and Duphaston, Dienogest has the strongest anti-endometriosis efficacy in terms of the reduced lesion size up to 61%. Its anti-proliferative and anti-apoptosis effects on the endometriotic lesions were not as good as Esmya and Duphaston, suggesting other more important underlying mechanism may be involved in Dienogest, further study is needed, thus warranting further future studies.

Some common side effects of progestin include, but not limit to hot flushes, irregular uterine bleeding, headache and weight gain [21, 57]. SPRMs have similar side effects, like hot flushes, headache and nausea, but SPRMs significantly reduce abnormal uterine bleeding in uterine fibroid [58]. In our study, no significant change on body weight gain and behavioural changes were observed, indicating wide safety margin amongst Esmya, Duphaston, Dienogest. Increased weight gain after long-term administration of progestin for 6 months or above was demonstrated in other study [59–61], but for short-term treatment as in our study, no significant change in body weight was observed in mice. In uterus, Esmya, Duphaston and Dienogest showed different adverse

Table 1 Summary of significant change after treatment of Esmya, Duphaston and Dienogest

Efficacy	Parameters (methods)		Esyma	Duphaston	Dienogest
Lesions growth	Lesions size, weight,		↓	↓	↓
Lesions growth	Lesions Morphology		The wall of cyst is thin.		
Adhesion	Lesions Mmp2 (q-PCR)		↑		
	Lesions Itgav β3 (q-PCR)		↑		
Proliferation	Lesions Pcna (q-PCR)		↓	↓	↓
	Ki 67 staining	All cells		↓	
		Epithelial cells		↓	
		Stroma cells		↓	↑
Apoptosis	Lesions Mapk1 (q-PCR)			↑	
	Lesions Nf-kb (q-PCR)				
	Lesions pro-Casp3 (q-PCR)				
	Tunel Assay	All cells		↑	
		Epithelial cells		↑	
		Stroma cells			
Angiogenesis	Lesions Hif1α (q-PCR)				
	Lesions Vegf (q-PCR)				
Invasion	Lesions Plau (q-PCR)				
Hormone receptors	ER α (q-PCR)				
	ER β (q-PCR)				
	ER α/ER β ratio (q-PCR)				
	PR (q-PCR)		↓	↓	↓
Pain	PGE2 (ELISA)				
Safety					
Genearl Safety	Body Weight				
Hormone Change	E2 Conc. (ELISA)				
	P4 Conc. (ELISA)				
Side effect in Uterus	Uterus size, Uterus/Body weight ratio				
	Gland Count in uterus				↑
	ETI			↓	
Side effect in Ovary	Ovary size, Ovary/Body weight ratio				
	Antral Follicle		↑		

Red arrows indicate significant increase and blue arrows indicate significant decrease when compared to the vehicle group

effects probably due to different effects of SPRMs and progestin [62]. Ulipristal acetate can control irregular bleeding by inducing amenorrhea [58, 63, 64] while Dienogest may cause irregular uterine bleeding unless cyclic administration or combine estradiol valerate treatment [65, 66]. Due to the progesterone antagonist effect of SPRMs, it is well known that ulipristal acetate can induce the progesterone receptor modulator associated endometrial changes (PEAC) [67], but no significant change in endometrial morphology was observed in Esmya group in our study. It may be due to short-term administration of Esmya in our intervention protocol and the high metabolic and rapid cyclic changes of endometrium in mice [68]. Consistent with previous studies, by inducing withdrawal bleeding Duphaston could suppress endometrial hyperplasia which may lead to lower endometrium thickness [69–71] observed in our study. Similar to Duphaston, Dienogest may also reduce endometrium thickness [72–74], but further study showed that endometrium thickness change under the treatment of Dienogest are mainly dependent on the duration of treatment [26]. In our short-term study, there was no significant endometrium thickness change, but in contrast endometrial glandular hyperplasia was observed in Dienogest group. In ovary, both Duphaston and Dienogest are as effective progestins that can be used as oral contraceptive with different ovulation inhibitory effects [75, 76]. The ovulation inhibitory effect induced by Dienogest could be reverse rapidly by stopping treatment [74]. Interestingly, Duphaston showed different anti-ovulation effect on different species [75]. Whilst Duphaston induces delay effect on ovulation in rats, it only slightly inhibits ovulation in rabbits but has no effect on ovulation in monkeys [75]. No significant change on ovary and follicles development was observed in our Duphaston and Dienogest groups, but antral follicles was significantly increased in Esmya group. The accumulation of antral follicles may be related to delay in follicular rupture induced by ulipristal acetate [49, 77]. On the other hand, recurrence of endometriosis is very common. The reported recurrence rate was high, estimated as 21.5% at 2 years and 40–50% at 5 years [78]. All the pharmacological treatments used are able to control the symptoms but not effectively treating the condition [79]. In our study, the endometriosis growth was still inhibited after withdrawal of Esmya, but not after Duphaston and Dienogest. This may be related to the prolong anti-ovulation effect of Esmya while the anti-endometriosis effects of Duphaston and Dienogest through inhibiting decidualisation and ovulation is rather transient. The detailed mechanism about Duphaston and Dienogest on recurrence of endometriosis is still unknown. Taken together, endometrium side-effects and withdrawn recurrence of Duphaston and Dienogest should be warranted.

Although Dienogest can be used as contraceptive medication, Dienogest showed no significant effect on endometrium in short term treatment in our study and ovulation inhibition could be reversed by stopping intervention in another study [74]. Based on the characteristics of Esmya on delaying ovulation and the suppressive effect of Duphaston on endometrium growth, they maybe not suitable for endometriosis patients who are considering conception. Because of the anti-proliferation effect on endometrium and suppressive effect on endometriotic lesions, Duphaston could be a better option for endometriosis patient during perimenopause, while Esmya is suitable for endometriosis patient who cannot tolerate progesterone effect due to the heavy irregular uterine bleeding. Even though Esmya have been used for contraceptive and it shows suppressive effect on endometriotic lesion growth, the detailed mechanism of anovulation and accumulation of antral follicle after treatment with Esmya is still unknown. Further studies should be carried out to understand the dynamic changes and detailed mechanism of anovulation effect for its further use in endometriosis. For Duphaston, its potential progesterone effect on ovulation is still unknown, so further studies should also be carried out to investigate its detail effect on ovary.

There are three major limitations in our present study. In order to compare the efficacy and safety, all three drugs were tested on an experimental model of endometriosis in mice. The therapeutic effect was tested in an animal which have no menstruation and never develop endometriosis spontaneously. The endometriosis was induced by suturing endometrium tissues on the vessels of mesentery or placing endometrium tissues into SC pocket rather than inducing by IP injection. When compared to the possible pathogenesis process of endometriosis, induced endometriosis by suturing endometrial tissues may cause extra inflammatory reaction on the endometriotic lesions. However, compared to the IP injection model, suturing or placing endometrial tissues to induce endometriosis has a better control on the variation and monitoring of the lesion size and weight. Furthermore, all these medications were tested in only single dosage and only for 4 weeks. The dose was used according to the FDA approved dose for human use and the duration already covered at least 6 estruses cycle of the mice which equivalent to almost half year in human. The purpose of present study was to compare progestins and selective progesterone receptor modulator as new indication for endometriosis, and the results of the study already showed positive therapeutic effects in clinical dose. Hence higher dose and longer treatment duration may not be necessary. The markers were selected to screen the therapeutic actions, not for detailed mechanistic study. Finally, the samples were collected at the end of intervention, therapeutic effect and side effect were compared in only a single time point which is not sufficient to monitor the dynamic change of reproductive organs or the hormone change during intervention.

Conclusion

All Esmya, Duphaston and Dienogest can suppress endometriotic growth on mouse model and Dienogest has the best suppressive effect. Esmya has significant ovulation suppressive effect and Duphaston may suppress endometrium growth while no significant side effect of Dienogest on ovary or endometrium was found. Detail endometriotic lesion suppressive effect and side effect on ovary or endometrium are still not clear and further studies need to be carried out.

Acknowledgments

The authors thank Dr. C.W. Cheung, Dr. W.Y. Fung and Dr. S.W. Wong for the clinical advice and interpretation of the results.

Funding

The Hong Kong Obstetrical and Gynaecological Trust Fund 2018 from The Obstetrical and Gynaecological Society of Hong Kong to CCW and BL.

Authors' contributions

BL and CCW designed the study. BL performed the experiments and the statistical analysis with help from LW, HX. CWC, WYF and SWW provided the provided clinical advice and interpreted the results. BL and CCW wrote the manuscript. All authors reviewed the manuscript. All authors read and approved the final manuscript.

Competing interests

The authors declare that they have no competing interests.

Author details

[1]Department of Obstetrics and Gynaecology, The Chinese University of Hong Kong, c/o 1st Floor, Special Block E, Prince of Wales Hospital, Shatin, Hong Kong. [2]Reproduction and Development Laboratory, Li Ka Shing Institute of Health Sciences, The Chinese University of Hong Kong, Shatin, Hong Kong. [3]School of Biomedical Sciences, The Chinese University of Hong Kong, Shatin, Hong Kong.

References

1. Garcia-Velasco JA, Somigliana E. Management of endometriomas in women requiring IVF: to touch or not to touch. Hum Reprod. 2009;24:496–501.
2. Meuleman C, Vandenabeele B, Fieuws S, Spiessens C, Timmerman D, D'Hooghe T. High prevalence of endometriosis in infertile women with normal ovulation and normospermic partners. Fertil Steril. 2009;92:68–74.
3. Kitawaki J, Kado N, Ishihara H, Koshiba H, Kitaoka Y, Honjo H. Endometriosis: the pathophysiology as an estrogen-dependent disease. J Steroid Biochem Mol Biol. 2002;83:149–55.
4. Sampson JA. Peritoneal endometriosis due to the menstrual dissemination of endometrial tissue into the peritoneal cavity. Am J Obstet Gynecol. 1927, 14:422–69.
5. Zeitoun K, Takayama K, Sasano H, Suzuki T, Moghrabi N, Andersson S, Johns A, Meng L, Putman M, Carr B, Bulun SE. Deficient 17beta-hydroxysteroid dehydrogenase type 2 expression in endometriosis: failure to metabolize 17beta-estradiol. J Clin Endocrinol Metab. 1998;83:4474–80.
6. van der Linden PJ. Theories on the pathogenesis of endometriosis. Human Reprod (Oxford, England). 1996;11(Suppl 3):53–65.
7. Olive DL, Pritts EA. Treatment of endometriosis. N Engl J Med. 2001;345: 266–75.
8. Fuldeore MJ, Soliman AM. Prevalence and symptomatic burden of diagnosed endometriosis in the United States: National Estimates from a cross-sectional survey of 59,411 women. Gynecol Obstet Investig. 2016;
9. De Graaff AA, D'Hooghe TM, GAJ D, Dirksen CD, Hummelshoj L, Simoens S, Bokor A, Brandes I, Brodszky V, Canis M, et al. The significant effect of endometriosis on physical, mental and social wellbeing: results from an international cross-sectional survey. Hum Reprod. 2013;28:2677–85.
10. Fagervold B, Jenssen M, Hummelshoj L, Moen MH. Life after a diagnosis with endometriosis - a 15 years follow-up study. Acta Obstet Gynecol Scand. 2009;88:914–9.
11. Dunselman GaJ, Vermeulen N, Becker C, Calhaz-Jorge C, D'Hooghe T, De Bie B, Heikinheimo O, Horne AW, Kiesel L, Nap A, et al: ESHRE guideline: management of women with endometriosis. Hum Reprod 2014, 29:400–412.
12. Bateman J, Bougie O, Singh S, Islam S. Histomorphological changes in endometriosis in a patient treated with ulipristal: a case report. Pathol Res Pract. 2017;213:79–81.
13. Cornillie FJ, Puttemans P, Brosens IA. Histology and ultrastructure of human endometriotic tissues treated with dydrogesterone (Duphaston). Eur J Obstet Gynecol Reprod Biol. 1987;26:39–55.
14. Schindler AE, Henkel A, Moore C, Oettel M. Effect and safety of high-dose dienogest (20 mg/day) in the treatment of women with endometriosis. Arch Gynecol Obstet. 2009;282:507–14.
15. Donnez J, Tatarchuk TF, Bouchard P, Puscasiu L, Zakharenko NF, Ivanova T, Ugocsai G, Mara M, Jilla MP, Bestel E, et al. Ulipristal acetate versus placebo for fibroid treatment before surgery. N Engl J Med. 2012;366:409–20.
16. Courtoy GE, Donnez J, Marbaix E, Dolmans M-M. In vivo mechanisms of uterine myoma volume reduction with ulipristal acetate treatment. Fertil Steril. 2015;104:426–34. e421
17. Esber N, Le Billan F, Resche-Rigon M, Loosfelt H, Lombès M, Chabbert-Buffet N. Ulipristal acetate inhibits progesterone receptor isoform A-mediated human breast Cancer proliferation and BCl2-L1 expression. PLoS One. 2015; 10:e0140795.
18. Mansour D. Use of the new progestogens in contraception and gynaecology. Obstet Gynaecol. 2006;8:229–34.
19. Overton CE, Lindsay PC, Johal B, Collins SA, Siddle NC, Shaw RW, Barlow DH. A randomized, double-blind, placebo-controlled study of luteal phase dydrogesterone (Duphaston) in women with minimal to mild endometriosis. Fertil Steril. 1994;62:701–7.
20. Casper RF. Progestin-only pills may be a better first-line treatment for endometriosis than combined estrogen-progestin contraceptive pills. Fertil Steril. 2017;107:533–6.
21. Vercellini P, Cortesi I, Crosignani PG. Progestins for symptomatic endometriosis: a critical analysis of the evidence. Fertil Steril. 1997;68:393–401.
22. Okada H, Nakajima T, Yoshimura T, Yasuda K, Kanzaki H. The inhibitory effect of dienogest, a synthetic steroid, on the growth of human endometrial stromal cells in vitro. Mol Hum Reprod. 2001;7:341–7.
23. Laschke MW, Menger MD. Anti-angiogenic treatment strategies for the therapy of endometriosis. Hum Reprod Update. 2012;18:682–702.
24. Makabe T, Koga K, Miyashita M, Takeuchi A, Sue F, Taguchi A, Urata Y, Izumi G, Takamura M, Harada M, et al. Drospirenone reduces inflammatory cytokines, vascular endothelial growth factor (VEGF) and nerve growth factor (NGF) expression in human endometriotic stromal cells. J Reprod Immunol. 2017;119:44–8.
25. Nakamura M, Katsuki Y, Shibutani Y, Oikawa T. Dienogest, a synthetic steroid, suppresses both embryonic and tumor-cell-induced angiogenesis. Eur J Pharmacol. 1999;386:33–40.
26. Tsuchiya T, Katagiri Y, Maemura T, Hayata E, Fukuda Y, Kitamura M, Morita M. Preoperative dienogest to improve the surgical field of view in resectoscopic surgery. Gynecol Minim Invasive Ther. 2016;5:16–9.
27. Pelch KE, Sharpe-Timms KL, Nagel SC. Mouse model of surgically-induced endometriosis by auto-transplantation of uterine tissue. J Vis Exp. 2012:e3396.
28. Bacci M, Capobianco A, Monno A, Cottone L, Di Puppo F, Camisa B, Mariani M, Brignole C, Ponzoni M, Ferrari S, et al. Macrophages are alternatively activated in patients with endometriosis and required for growth and vascularization of lesions in a mouse model of disease. Am J Pathol. 2009;175:547–56.
29. Aoki D, Katsuki Y, Shimizu A, Kakinuma C, Nozawa S. Successful heterotransplantation of human endometrium in SCID mice. Obstet Gynecol. 1994;83:220–8.
30. Wang CC, Xu H, GCW M, Zhang T, Chu KO, Chu CY, JTY C, Li G, He YX, Qin L, et al. Prodrug of green tea epigallocatechin-3-gallate (pro-EGCG) as a potent anti-angiogenesis agent for endometriosis in mice. Angiogenesis. 2013;16:59–69.
31. Xu H, Lui WT, Chu CY, Ng PS, Wang CC, Rogers MS. Anti-angiogenic effects of green tea catechin on an experimental endometriosis mouse model. Hum Reprod. 2009;24:608–18.
32. Rockville. Guidance for industry: estimating the maximum safe starting dose in initial clinical trials for therapeutics in adult healthy volunteers. In: Center for Drug Evaluation and Research (CDER); 2005.
33. Oliveira CR, Salvatori R, Nobrega LM, Carvalho EO, Menezes M, Farias CT, Britto AV, Pereira RM, Aguiar-Oliveira MH. Sizes of abdominal organs in adults with severe short stature due to severe, untreated, congenital GH deficiency caused by a homozygous mutation in the GHRH receptor gene. Clin Endocrinol. 2008;69:153–8.
34. Cardiff RD, Miller CH, Munn RJ: Manual hematoxylin and eosin staining of mouse tissue sections. Cold Spring Harb Protoc 2014, 2014:pdb.prot073411.
35. Kahari VM, Saarialho-Kere U. Matrix metalloproteinases and their inhibitors in tumour growth and invasion. Ann Med. 1999;31:34–45.
36. Rabbani SA. Metalloproteases and urokinase in angiogenesis and tumor progression. In Vivo. 1998;12:135–42.
37. Sheppard D. Integrin-mediated activation of latent transforming growth factor beta. Cancer Metastasis Rev. 2005;24:395–402.

38. Sivridis E, Giatromanolaki A, Gatter KC, Harris AL, Koukourakis MI, for the T, Angiogenesis Research G. Association of hypoxia-inducible factors 1α and 2α with activated angiogenic pathways and prognosis in patients with endometrial carcinoma. Cancer. 2002;95:1055–63.
39. Goteri G, Lucarini G, Montik N, Zizzi A, Stramazzotti D, Fabris G, Tranquilli AL, Ciavattini A. Expression of vascular endothelial growth factor (VEGF), hypoxia inducible factor-1alpha (HIF-1alpha), and microvessel density in endometrial tissue in women with adenomyosis. Int J Gynecol Pathol. 2009; 28:157–63.
40. Joyce D, Albanese C, Steer J, Fu M, Bouzahzah B, Pestell RG. NF-kappaB and cell-cycle regulation: the cyclin connection. Cytokine Growth Factor Rev. 2001;12:73–90.
41. Schwartz SA, Hernandez A, Mark Evers B. The role of NF-kappaB/IkappaB proteins in cancer: implications for novel treatment strategies. Surg Oncol. 1999;8:143–53.
42. Hall PA, Levison DA, Woods AL, Yu CC, Kellock DB, Watkins JA, Barnes DM, Gillett CE, Camplejohn R, Dover R, et al. Proliferating cell nuclear antigen (PCNA) immunolocalization in paraffin sections: an index of cell proliferation with evidence of deregulated expression in some neoplasms. J Pathol. 1990; 162:285–94.
43. Rossi AGZ, Soares Jr JM, Motta ELA, Simões MJ, Oliveira-Filho RM, Haidar MA, Rodrigues de Lima G, Baracat EC. Metoclopramide-induced hyperprolactinemia affects mouse endometrial morphology. Gynecol Obstet Investig. 2003;54:185–90.
44. Schindelin J, Rueden CT, Hiner MC, Eliceiri KW. The ImageJ ecosystem: an open platform for biomedical image analysis. Mol Reprod Dev. 2015;82:518–29.
45. Durlinger ALL, Gruijters MJG, Kramer P, Karels B, Kumar TR, Matzuk MM, Rose UM, de Jong FH, Uilenbroek JTJ, Grootegoed JA, Themmen APN. Anti-Müllerian hormone attenuates the effects of FSH on follicle development in the mouse ovary. Endocrinology. 2001;142:4891–9.
46. Myers M, Britt KL, Wreford NGM, Ebling FJP, Kerr JB. Methods for quantifying follicular numbers within the mouse ovary. Reproduction. 2004;127:569–80.
47. Ray A, Dittel BN. Isolation of mouse peritoneal cavity cells. J Vis Exp. 2010: e1488.
48. Grzechocinska B, Gadomska H, Zygula A, Wielgos M. Application of ulipristal acetate in female patients with uterine fibroids. Neuroendocrinol Lett. 2014; 35:175–8.
49. Brache V, Cochon L, Deniaud M, Croxatto HB. Ulipristal acetate prevents ovulation more effectively than levonorgestrel: analysis of pooled data from three randomized trials of emergency contraception regimens. Contraception. 2013;88:611–8.
50. Huniadi CA, Pop OL, Antal TA, Stamatian F. The effects of ulipristal on Bax/ Bcl-2, cytochrome C, Ki-67 and cyclooxygenase-2 expression in a rat model with surgically induced endometriosis. Eur J Obstet Gynecol Reprod Biol. 2013;169:360–5.
51. Rossé T, Olivier R, Monney L, Rager M, Conus S, Fellay I, Jansen B, Borner C. Bcl-2 prolongs cell survival after Bax-induced release of cytochrome c. Nature. 1998;391:496–9.
52. Yoshino O, Osuga Y, Hirota Y, Koga K, Hirata T, Harada M, Morimoto C, Yano T, Nishii O, Tsutsumi O, Taketani Y. Possible pathophysiological roles of mitogen-activated protein kinases (MAPKs) in endometriosis. Am J Reprod Immunol. 2004;52:306–11.
53. Schulze-Osthoff K, Ferrari D, Riehemann K, Wesselborg S. Regulation of NF-kappa B activation by MAP kinase cascades. Immunobiology. 1997;198:35–49.
54. Wada T, Penninger JM. Mitogen-activated protein kinases in apoptosis regulation. Oncogene. 2004;23:2838–49.
55. Moldovan GL, Pfander B, Jentsch S. PCNA, the maestro of the replication fork. Cell. 2007;129:665–79.
56. Scholzen T, Gerdes J. The Ki-67 protein: from the known and the unknown. J Cell Physiol. 2000;182:311–22.
57. Ylänen K, Laatikainen T, Lähteenmäki P, Moo-Young AJ. Subdermal progestin implant (Nestorone®) in the treatment of endometriosis: clinical response to various doses. Acta Obstet Gynecol Scand. 2003;82:167–72.
58. Donnez J, Hudecek R, Donnez O, Matule D, Arhendt H-J, Zatik J, Kasilovskiene Z, Dumitrascu MC, Fernandez H, Barlow DH, et al. Efficacy and safety of repeated use of ulipristal acetate in uterine fibroids. Fertil Steril. 2015;103:519–27. e513
59. Kim SA, Um MJ, Kim HK, Kim SJ, Moon SJ, Jung H. Study of dienogest for dysmenorrhea and pelvic pain associated with endometriosis. Obstet Gynecol Sci. 2016;59:506–11.
60. Strowitzki T, Marr J, Gerlinger C, Faustmann T, Seitz C. Dienogest is as effective as leuprolide acetate in treating the painful symptoms of endometriosis: a 24-week, randomized, multicentre, open-label trial. Hum Reprod. 2010;25:633–41.
61. Berlanda N, Somigliana E, Frattaruolo MP, Buggio L, Dridi D, Vercellini P. Surgery versus hormonal therapy for deep endometriosis: is it a choice of the physician? Eur J Obstet Gynecol Reprod Biol. 2017;209:67–71.
62. Chwalisz K, Perez MC, Demanno D, Winkel C, Schubert G, Elger W. Selective progesterone receptor modulator development and use in the treatment of leiomyomata and endometriosis. Endocr Rev. 2005;26:423–38.
63. Arendas K, Leyland NA. Use of Ulipristal acetate for the Management of Fibroid-Related Acute Abnormal Uterine Bleeding. J Obstet Gynaecol Can. 2016;38:80–3.
64. Matytsina-Quinlan L, Matytsina L. Abnormal excessive per vagina (PV) bleeding on Esmya-selective progesterone receptor modulator (SPRM) in a symptomatic patient with uterine fibroid. BMJ Case Rep. 2015;2015: bcr2014209015.
65. Nagata C, Yanagida S, Okamoto A, Morikawa A, Sugimoto K, Okamoto S, Ochiai K, Tanaka T. Risk factors of treatment discontinuation due to uterine bleeding in adenomyosis patients treated with dienogest. J Obstet Gynaecol Res. 2012;38:639–44.
66. Micks EA, Jensen JT. Treatment of heavy menstrual bleeding with the estradiol valerate and dienogest oral contraceptive pill. Adv Ther. 2013;30:1–13.
67. Whitaker LHR, Murray AA, Matthews R, Shaw G, Williams ARW, Saunders PTK, Critchley HOD. Selective progesterone receptor modulator (SPRM) ulipristal acetate (UPA) and its effects on the human endometrium. Hum Reprod. 2017;32:531–43.
68. Jesam C, Cochon L, Salvatierra AM, Williams A, Kapp N, Levy-Gompel D, Brache V. A prospective, open-label, multicenter study to assess the pharmacodynamics and safety of repeated use of 30 mg ulipristal acetate. Contraception. 2016;93:310–6.
69. Nakamura S, Douchi T, Oki T, Ijuin H, Yamamoto S, Nagata Y. Relationship between sonographic endometrial thickness and progestin-induced withdrawal bleeding. Obstet Gynecol. 1996;87:722–5.
70. Bergeron C, Fox H. Low incidence of endometrial hyperplasia with acceptable bleeding patterns in women taking sequential hormone replacement therapy with dydrogesterone. Gynecol Endocrinol. 2000;14:275–81.
71. Quereux C, Pornel B, Bergeron C, Ferenczy A. Continuous combined hormone replacement therapy with 1 mg 17β-oestradiol and 5 mg dydrogesterone (Femoston®-conti): endometrial safety and bleeding profile. Maturitas. 2006;53:299–305.
72. Kodama M, Onoue M, Otsuka H, Yada-Hashimoto N, Saeki N, Kodama T, Wakasa T, Funato T. Efficacy of Dienogest in thinning the endometrium before Hysteroscopic surgery. J Minim Invasive Gynecol. 2013;20:790–5.
73. Laganà AS, Vitale SG, Muscia V, Rossetti P, Buscema M, Triolo O, Rapisarda AMC, Giunta L, Palmara V, Granese R, et al. Endometrial preparation with Dienogest before hysteroscopic surgery: a systematic review. Arch Gynecol Obstet. 2017;295:661–7.
74. Klipping C, Duijkers I, Remmers A, Faustmann T, Zurth C, Klein S, Schuett B. Ovulation-inhibiting effects of dienogest in a randomized, dose-controlled pharmacodynamic trial of healthy women. J Clin Pharmacol. 2012;52:1704–13.
75. Claassen V, Morsink L, de Wachter AM. Influence of dydrogesterone (6-dehydroretroprogesterone, Duphaston) on ovulation in the rat, rabbit and monkey. Acta Endocrinol. 1971;67:551–62.
76. Endrikat J, Parke S, Trummer D, Serrani M, Duijkers I, Klipping C. Pituitary, ovarian and additional contraceptive effects of an estradiol-based combined oral contraceptive: results of a randomized, open-label study. Contraception. 2013;87:227–34.
77. Brache V, Cochon L, Jesam C, Maldonado R, Salvatierra AM, Levy DP, Gainer E, Croxatto HB. Immediate pre-ovulatory administration of 30 mg ulipristal acetate significantly delays follicular rupture. Hum Reprod. 2010;25:2256–63.
78. Guo SW. Recurrence of endometriosis and its control. Hum Reprod Update. 2009;15:441–61.
79. Signorile PG, Baldi A. New evidence in endometriosis. Int J Biochem Cell Biol. 2015;60:19–22.

14

Effect of exposure to CeO_2 nanoparticles on ram spermatozoa during storage at 4 °C for 96 hours

Laura Falchi[1*], Grazia Galleri[2], Gian Mario Dore[1], Maria Teresa Zedda[1], Salvatore Pau[1], Luisa Bogliolo[1], Federica Ariu[1], Alessandra Pinna[3], Stefano Nieddu[1], Plinio Innocenzi[4] and Sergio Ledda[1]

Abstract

Background: Cerium oxide nanoparticles (CeO_2 NPs) are able to store and release oxygen, conferring them scavenger activity against oxidative stress. However, their effects in reproductive systems are not yet well understood. The aim of the study was to investigate the effects of exposure of refrigerated ram semen to CeO_2 NPs for 96 h on the main structural and kinematic parameters of spermatozoa.

Methods: The ejaculates of 5 Sarda rams were collected, pooled and diluted in a soybean lecithin extender. Samples were exposed to increasing doses of CeO_2 NPs (0, 44 and 220 μg/mL) and stored at 4 °C for 96 h. Analyses of kinematic parameters (computer assisted sperm analysis, CASA), integrity of membranes (PI/PSA staining), ROS production (H_2DCFDA staining) and DNA damage (sperm chromatin structure assay with acridine orange, SCSA) were performed every 24 h (0, 24, 48, 72 and 96 h of incubation). The experiment was carried out in 6 replicates. Data were analysed by repeated measures ANOVA with Bonferroni's as post hoc test. When the assumption of normality was not met (ROS), non-parametric Kruskal-Wallis rank test was carried out.

Results: Exposure of ram spermatozoa to increasing doses of CeO_2 NPs had a beneficial effect on the main motility parameters from 48 h of incubation onward. Velocity of sperm cells was enhanced in the groups exposed to CeO_2 NPs compared to the control. Incubation with NPs had beneficial effects on the integrity of plasma membranes of spermatozoa, with higher percentage of damaged cells in the control group compared to the exposed ones. Production of ROS was not affected by exposure to NPs and its levels rose at 96 h of incubation. The integrity of DNA remained stable throughout the 96 h of storage regardless of co-incubation with NPs.

Conclusions: We reported beneficial effects of CeO_2 NPs on kinematic and morphologic parameters of ram semen, such as motility and membrane integrity following 96 h of exposure. Furthermore, we also proved no genotoxic effects of CeO_2 NPs. These effects could not be related to an antioxidant activity of CeO_2 NPs, since ROS levels in exposed cells were similar to those of unexposed ones.

Keywords: Acrosome, CASA, DNA, Motility, Nanoparticles, Ovine, Oxidative stress, ROS, Spermatozoa

* Correspondence: lfalchi@uniss.it
[1]Dipartimento di Medicina Veterinaria, Università degli Studi di Sassari, Sassari, Italy
Full list of author information is available at the end of the article

Background

Over the past decades, nanoparticles of Cerium oxide (CeO_2 NPs) have received considerable scientific interest due to their peculiar chemical, physical and biological properties. However, their everyday use in industry, food science and cosmetics is limited by the concerns about potential effects of their distribution and bioaccumulation in the environment [1]. More recently, the use of CeO_2 NPs in biomedicine has been taken into account considering their capacity to store oxygen and consequent scavenger activity against reactive oxygen species (ROS) comparable to that of antioxidant enzymes in biological systems [2–4]. In literature, a large number of articles described a reduction in ROS levels in several tissues or cells following exposure to CeO_2 NPs. Recently, scavenger action has been reported in cortical neurons in rats with spinal injuries [5], human keratinocytes [6], mice endothelial cells and fibroblasts [7], human breast and fibrosarcoma cells [8] and cardiac cells [9]. In contrast, many authors reported pro-oxidant effects especially in pulmonary cells [10, 11] and DNA damage in liver cells and leucocytes [12]. These diverging observations suggest that CeO_2 NPs may show the same paradox activity described for other scavenger substances, perhaps depending on the physical and chemical characteristics of the compound, the concentration, the length of exposure and the biological system involved.

Few studies focussed on the effects of CeO_2 NPs in the reproductive system and the findings are often in contrast. In mice, exposure of oocytes to increasing doses of CeO_2 NPs led to oxidative stress and consequent DNA damage [13]. In the same species, a decrease in fertilization rates and accumulation in granulosa cells and sperm plasma membranes has been described [14]. However, in the ovine, gametes well tolerated co-incubation with CeO_2 NPs. In particular, our research group reported that granulosa cells but not oocytes internalise this compound by endocytosis. Moreover, low concentrations of NPs enhanced in vitro fertilization of oocytes with low developmental competence possibly throughtheir scavenging action and downregulation of genes activated by oxidative stress [15].

Ram spermatozoa exposed to increasing concentrations of CeO_2NPs for 24 h, showed no NPs uptake, occasionally sporadic contacts with plasma membranes and no adverse effects on DNA integrity and motility parameters. Furthermore, the redox balance of the cells was not perturbed by exposure to NPs since both ROS levels and mitochondrial activity remained stable [16]. We hypothesised that, submitting ram spermatozoa to a prolonged stressing condition such as extended storage at 4 °C and exposing them to CeO_2 NPs would have triggered the scavenging action of this compound. Thus, the aim of the study was to investigate the effects of the exposure to increasing doses of CeO_2 NPs on the kinematic parameters, integrity of membranes, DNA fragmentation and oxidative status of ram semen stored at 4 °C for 96 h.

Methods

Experimental design

The experimental design is described in Fig. 1. The ejaculates of 5 rams were collected and selected by mass motility [score ≥ 3 on a scale of 0–5 (0 = no motility, 5 = vigorous swirling waves of movements)], volume (≥ 0.5 mL) and sperm concentration ($3x10^9$spz/mL). After selection, the samples were immediately pooled and diluted 1:5 (final concentration $600x10^6$spz/mL) in soybean lecithin extender OVIXcell (IMV Technologies) at 30 °C. The pool of ejaculates was divided in 3 aliquots that were supplemented with increasing doses of CeO_2 NPs [0 (control), 44 and 220 μg/mL], gradually cooled to 4 °C in 2 h and stored at this temperature for 96 h. At different time points (0, 24, 48, 72 and 96 h), analyses on kinematic parameters, integrity of acrosome and plasma membranes, oxidative stress (ROS production) and DNA integrity were assessed in all 3 groups. The selection of the two doses of NPs was adopted from our previous study [16] and was close to the doses used in studies performed on somatic cells [7, 17] and gametes [15]. The experiment was carried out in 6 replicates.

Animals and semen collection

Five rams of Sarda breed (2–3 years old) housed at the Genetic Centre of AGRIS (Agenzia Regionale per la Ricerca in Agricoltura, Bonassai, Italy) were selected for the present experiment. They were of proven fertility and their sanitary status was checked before starting the trial. Semen was collected by artificial vagina, placed in a 30 °C water bath and processed for initial evaluation (volume, concentration and mass motility) within 5 min.

Cerium dioxide nanoparticles (CeO_2 NPs)

Nanoparticles of CeO_2 were synthesized according to the protocol reported by Falchi et al. [16].

Motility analysis

Motility analysis was performed by computer assisted sperm analysis (CASA, Ivos, Hamilton Thorne, Biosciences). An aliquot of each sample was diluted in warm PBS (Dulbecco's Phosphate Buffered Saline; 37 °C; 10–20 x 10^6spz/mL), a 10 μL drop was placed on a warm slide (Leja slides, 20 μm, IMV Technologies, France) and loaded in the analyser. Six fields were selected and analysed in triplicate for: total motility (TM), progressive motility (PM), average path velocity (VAP), straight line

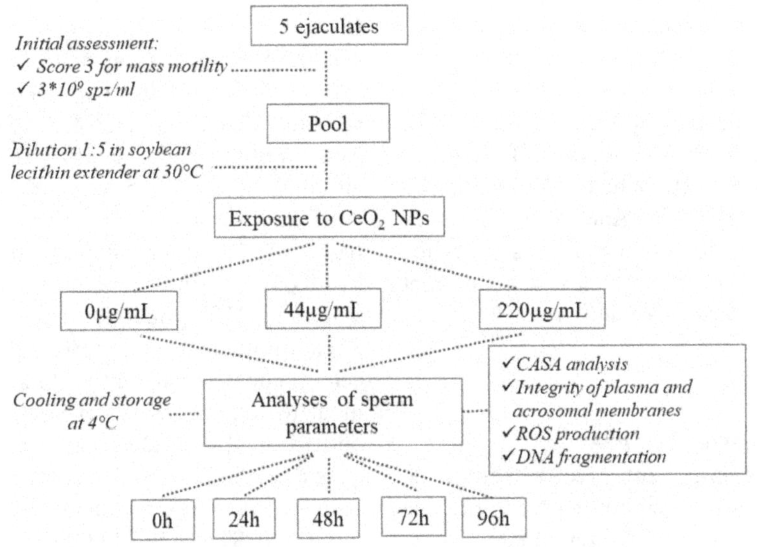

Fig. 1 Experimental plan for the investigation of the effects of CeO_2 NPs on ram semen stored at 4 °C for 96 h

velocity (VSL), curvilinear velocity (VCL), lateral head displacement (ALH), beat cross frequency (BCF), straightness (ratio VSL/VAP, STR), linearity (ratio VSL/VCL, LIN). Elongation (ELONG), area and velocity distribution (rapid, medium, slow and static spermatozoa) were also assessed.

Plasma membrane integrity and acrosome status

Plasma membrane integrity and acrosome status were assessed by differential staining. An aliquot of semen (10 μL) from each group was added to 290 μL PBS (phosphate buffer saline), 4 μL PI (Propidium Iodide, 1 mg/mL; Sigma-Aldrich, USA) and 4 μL FITC-PSA (*Pisum sativum* agglutinin conjugated with fluorescein isothiocyanate; 1 mg/mL; Sigma-Aldrich, USA) and incubated in the dark for 15 min at 37 °C. Each sample was washed twice by centrifugation at 4229 RPM for 3 min. The final pellet was re-suspended in 250 μL PBS. A 10 μL drop was placed on a warm slide with a cover slip and observed under fluorescence microscope (Olympus IX70, Olympus Optical Co. Ltd, Japan). A total of 200 spermatozoa per slide were counted and classified in: viable spermatozoa with intact acrosome, PI-/PSA-; dead spermatozoa with intact acrosome, red, PI+/PSA-; viable spermatozoa with reacted acrosome, green, PI-/PSA+; dead spermatozoa with reacted acrosome, red and green, PI+/PSA+.

Flow cytometer analyses

Flow cytometry was performed using the BD FACS Canto™ platform (BD Biosciences, USA) and the data were analysed by BD FACS DIVA software (BD Biosciences, USA). A total of 20,000 events per sample were acquired.

ROS production

For the assessment of intracellular ROS production, sperm samples were stained with 2′,7′dichlorofluorescein diacetate (H_2DCFDA, Sigma Aldrich, USA). Briefly, an aliquot (25 μL) of each sample was diluted in 1 mL PBS containing 10 μM H_2DCFDA and incubated in the dark for 30 min at 38 °C. Following incubation, samples were centrifuged at 4229 RPM for 3 min, the supernatant was gently discarded, and the pellet was re-suspended in 500 μL of 2% paraformaldehyde and left at 4 °C for 1 h. After fixation, samples were centrifuged again at 4229 RPM for 3 min and supernatant was removed and replaced by 300 μL PBS. Samples were stored in the dark at 4 °C until flow cytometric analysis, which was performed within a month.

Sperm chromatin structure assay

The integrity of DNA was assessed by SCSA. The labelling of fragmented DNA in fresh controls and in samples incubated with CeO_2 NPs was carried out as previously described by Evenson et al. [18]. Briefly, an aliquot of 50 μL of each sample was diluted in 150 μL TNE buffer (0.15 M NaCl, 1 mM EDTA, 10 mM Tris, pH 7.2) at 4 °C, immediately plunged into liquid nitrogen and stored at – 80 °C until analysis. Frozen samples were thawed in crushed ice and 200 μL of sperm/TNE suspension was mixed to 400 μL of Acid Detergent Solution (0.08 M HCl, 0.15 M NaCl, 0.1% Triton X-100, pH 1.4). After 30 s, 1.2 mL of staining solution (0.15 M NaCl, 1 mM EDTA, 10 mM Tris, 0.2 M NA_2HPO_4, 0.1 M citric acid, pH 6) containing 6 μg/mL of Acridine Orange, was added to the mixture. Within 3 min from the staining, the samples were analysed by the flow cytometer. The levels of DNA fragmentation were assessed calculating the DFI (DNA fragmentation index) as the ratio of red fluorescence and total fluorescence (green + red).

Statistical analysis

Statistical analysis was performed using Stata 11.2/IC (StataCorp LP, USA). Normal distribution of data was checked by Shapiro-Wilk test. When the assumption was met, data were analysed by Analysis of Variance with repeated measures with Bonferroni's as post hoc test. When the assumption of normality was not met (ROS), non-parametric Kruskal-Wallis rank test was performed.

Results

Kinematic parameters assessed by CASA

Motility parameters are important predictors of male fertility since they indicate the ability to move into the female genital tract to reach the fertilization site. To assess the potential effects of the exposure of ram spermatozoa to CeO_2 NPs on kinematic parameters, CASA analysis was performed every 24 h for 96 h. The results showed that the exposure to increasing doses of CeO_2 NPs had a significant effect on the main kinematic parameters from 48 to 72 h onward whereas the time of incubation affected all of them ($P < 0.05$).

In detail, most of the main kinematic parameters (PM, VAP, VSL, VCL) showed a sharp decrease in the first 24 h of storage at 4 °C independently of the exposure to CeO_2 NPs. The decline was steeper for PM (around 15% drop) and for VSL (around 30% drop). Total motility had a gradual time-dependent decrease although from 48 h onward sperm cells incubated with 220 μg/mL CeO_2 NPs showed a significantly higher TM and PM compared to the control group ($P < 0.05$). A similar pattern was observed for VAP, VSL and VCL, but the effect was significant from 72 h of incubation onward ($P < 0.05$; Fig. 2). Sperm cells incubated with 44 μg/mL NPs showed an intermediate pattern, with no significant differences from both control and 220 μg/mL groups ($P > 0.05$).

As described in Fig. 3, the incubation with NPs had no influence on most of the secondary kinematic parameters (BCF, STR, LIN, ELONG and AREA) at any time point of the experiment ($P > 0.05$). Lateral head amplitude (ALH) was the only secondary parameter significantly affected by exposure to CeO_2 NPs ($P < 0.05$). However, the effect was visible only at 96 h of incubation, when the control group showed significantly lower ALH compared to exposed groups ($P < 0.05$). The time of exposure significantly affected all secondary

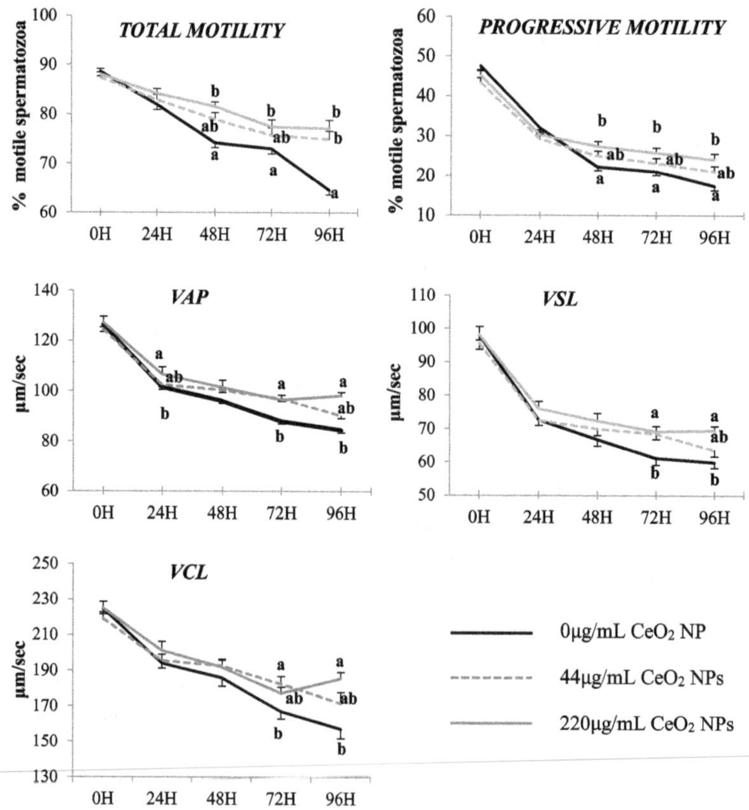

Fig. 2 Main kinematic parameters assessed by CASA of ram spermatozoa exposed to CeO_2 NPs for 96 h at 4 °C. Different letters ([a], [b]) indicate significant differences among treatments within time point ($P < 0.05$). Results are shown as means ± SEM

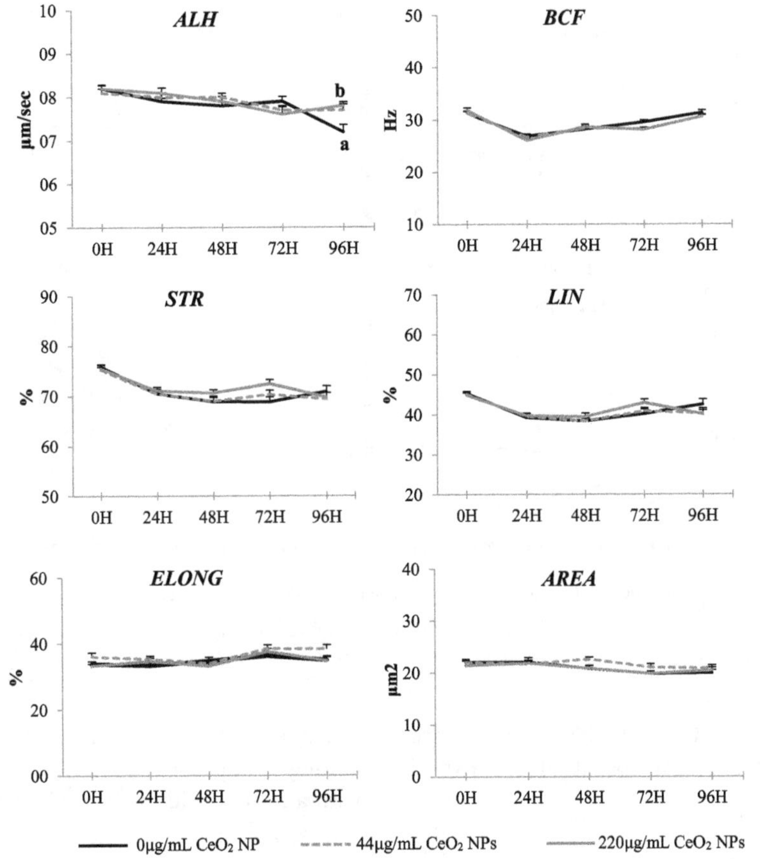

Fig. 3 Secondary kinematic parameters assessed by CASA of ram spermatozoa exposed to CeO_2 NPs for 96 h at 4 °C. Different letters ([a, b]) indicate significant differences among treatments within time points ($P < 0.05$). Time had a significant effect on the analysed parameters ($P < 0.05$). Results are shown as means ± SEM

parameters ($P < 0.05$) except for ELONG and AREA, that remained stable throughout the experiment.

Concerning the analysis of velocity distribution (Fig. 4), the collected data showed a pattern similar to that of TM and PM. In detail, CeO_2 NPs had no influence on velocity distribution during the first 24 h of exposure but, from 48 h onward, sperm cells incubated with 220 µg/mL NPs were consistently more rapid and less static compared to the control group ($P < 0.05$); sperm cells exposed to 44 µg/mL NPs showed an intermediate pattern. No effect of CeO_2 NPs was observed on the percentage of medium cells at any time point of the experiment ($P < 0.05$). The percentage of slow cells gradually increased in all groups in the first 24 h remaining stable in exposed sperm cells from the 48 h onward. Conversely, in control sperm cells, it continued to increase until 96 h showing significantly higher rates compared to exposed groups ($P < 0.05$).

Integrity of plasma membrane and acrosome

In the ram, plasma and acrosomal membranes of sperm cells, that play an important role during sperm capacitation and fertilization, can be easily damaged during storage procedures leading to decrease in semen quality and consequently in fertilizing ability. To test the effects of the exposure to CeO_2 NPs on plasma and acrosomal membranes, the differential staining with PI/PSA was used. As described in Fig. 5, incubation time and CeO_2 NPs exposure had an overall significant effect on the percentage of viable (unstained, PI-/PSA-) sperms and of sperms with damaged plasma membranes (PI+/PSA-; $P < 0.05$). In general, no effect of co-incubation with CeO_2 NPs was observed in the first 48 h of exposure, during which the rates of viable and damaged spermatozoa remained stable. However, at 72 h and 96 h, the 220 µg/mL group had a higher percentage of viable spermatozoa compared to the control ($P < 0.05$); whereas at 96 h a significant difference was also found between the 44 µg/mL and the control group ($P < 0.05$). Conversely, at 72 h and 96 h the percentage of damaged non reacted spermatozoa was significantly higher in the control compared to the 220 µg/mL group ($P < 0.05$). No time and treatment effects were observed in the percentages of reacted

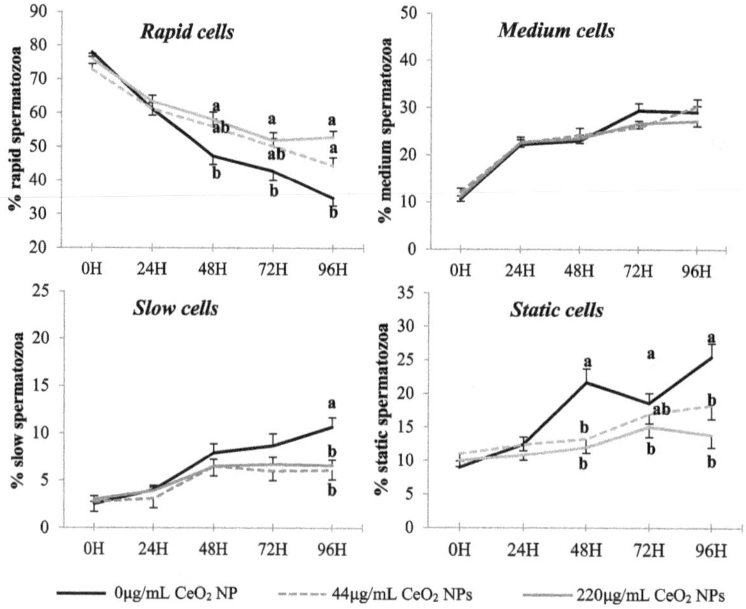

Fig. 4 Velocity distribution of ram spermatozoa exposed to increasing doses of CeO_2 NPs and stored for 96 h at 4 °C. Different letters ([a, b]) indicate significant differences among treatments within time points ($P < 0.05$). Results are shown as means ± SEM

(PI-/PSA+) and dead reacted (PI+/PSA+) spermatozoa among groups at any time point of the experiment ($P > 0.05$; Fig. 5).

Production of ROS

Since ram spermatozoa are susceptible to oxidative stress with overproduction of ROS during storage at low temperatures, we tested the effects of CeO_2 NPs on ROS levels in sperm cells stored for 96 h at 4 °C. The results, represented in Fig. 6, showed that increasing doses of CeO_2 NPs did not affect the production of ROS at any time point of the experiment ($P > 0.05$). Conversely, time of storage had a significant effect on the oxidative status of sperm cells stored for 96 h. In detail, ROS levels remained fairly stable for 72 h with no differences among groups, while the levels rose abruptly at 96 h with a 3- to 4-fold increase ($P < 0.05$; Fig. 6).

DNA fragmentation

Since there is no consensus on the effects of CeO_2 NPs on DNA integrity of somatic cells or gametes, we measured the levels of DNA fragmentation through SCSA in ram sperm cells exposed to NPs for 96 h. The results showed that DNA of sperm cells exposed to NPs well tolerated co-incubation with these compounds. No significant differences in DFI% were found among treated and control groups at any time point of the experimental

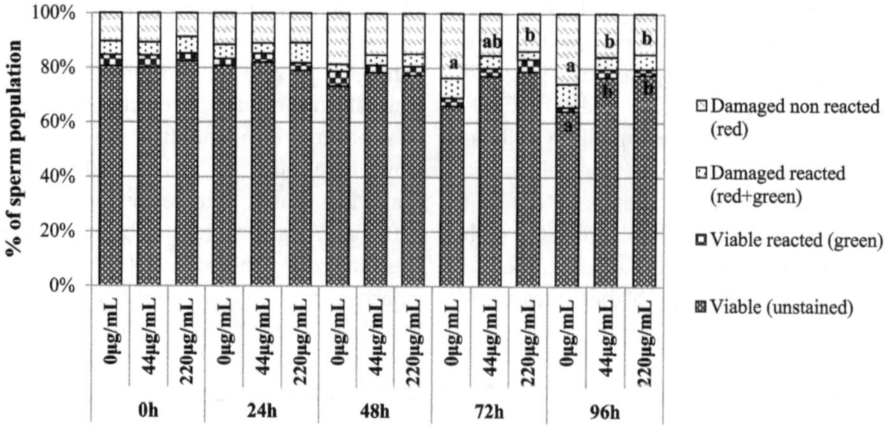

Fig. 5 Integrity of cytoplasmic and acrosomal membranes of spermatozoa incubated with CeO_2 NPs for 96 h at 4 °C. Different superscripts ([a, b]) indicate significant differences for $P < 0.05$ among treatments within time points

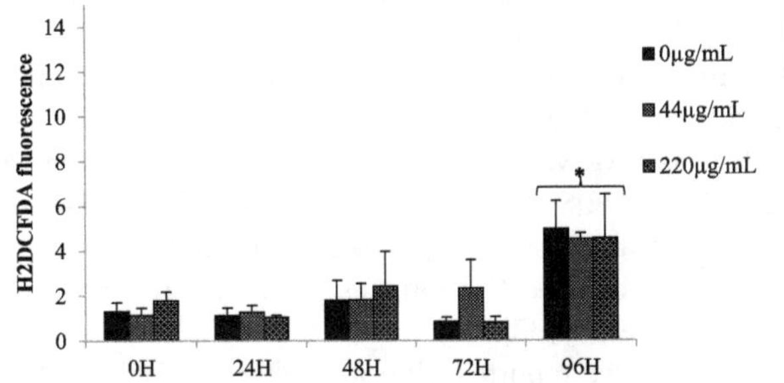

Fig. 6 Reactive oxygen species (ROS) production by ram semen exposed to increasing concentrations of CeO_2 NPs. Results are shown as means ± SEM of fluorescence following H_2DCFDA staining. Asterisk indicates significant difference ($P < 0.05$) between time points

trial ($P > 0.05$). Moreover, time effect was also not significant ($P > 0.05$; Fig. 7).

Discussion

In this study, we reported the effects of exposure to CeO_2 NPs of ram spermatozoa stored for 96 h at 4 °C. The choice of these experimental conditions was based on the hypothesis that CeO_2 NPs, with their catalytic action, might prevent the deleterious effects of storage at low temperatures on ram sperm cells. The decrease in quality of refrigerated semen restricts its application during artificial insemination programs to a short time span, limiting the diffusion of superior genotypes to small geographic areas and to restricted numbers of selected animals. For this reason, the perspective of storing semen for longer times would represent a great benefit in the management of genetic selection and reproduction in sheep breeding systems and a valuable alternative to cryopreserved semen.

Over the past decades many research groups focussed on improving the quality of refrigerated ram semen. The most promising approach is represented by the supplementation of storage extenders with anti-oxidant substances that contrast the deleterious effects of ROS accumulation and oxidative stress on sperm cells. Among others, CeO_2 NPs are gaining increasing interest for their ability to change their oxidation status [19] conferring them promising scavenger properties.

Our research group [16] previously reported that ram spermatozoa stored at 4 °C for 24 h well tolerated concentrations of CeO_2 NPs above those commonly dispersed in the environment (water 0.024 mg/L [20]; soil 1.12 mg/kg [21]) and the results reported in the present study are in agreement with these observation. The potential toxic effects of these compounds have to be carefully assessed and the consequences on the reproductive system are still under investigation. In mice, low concentrations of CeO_2 NPs significantly affected in vitro fertilization and had genotoxic effects on both male and female gametes [13, 14]. In the present study, we can state that none of the sperm parameters analysed was negatively affected by extended exposure of sperm cells to CeO_2 NPs.

Moreover, we described a consistent and significant increase in kinematic parameters of spermatozoa incubated with high concentrations of NPs that has not been reported before. This beneficial effect was mostly evident in spermatozoa exposed to 220 µg/mL NPs from 48 h of incubation onward. In fact, in the first 24 h of the trial, CeO_2 NPs did not exert any effect on any of the analysed parameters. It has been reported that the overall quality of ram semen stored at 4 °C dramatically drops after 3 days [22–24] and we can speculate that the activity of NPs might be stronger in cells with compromised morphologic and structural characteristics under stressing conditions such as storage at low temperatures.

In addition to the enhancement of TM and PM, incubation with NPs promoted the increase in parameters

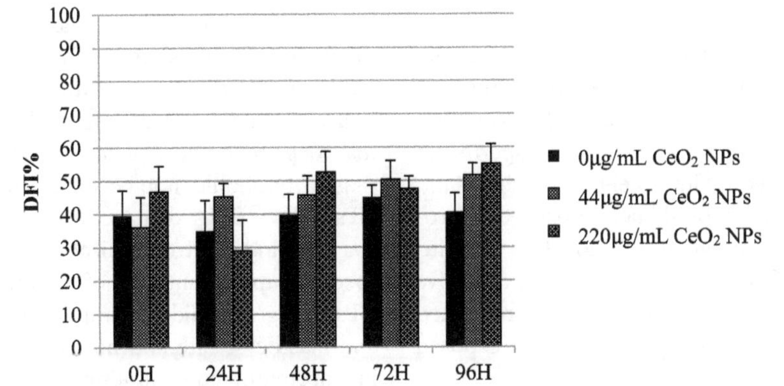

Fig. 7 Sperm chromatin structure assay in ram spermatozoa incubated with increasing concentrations of CeO_2 NPs for 96 h. The DFI% was calculated as the ratio red fluorescent cells (single strand DNA)/total fluorescent cells [red + green (double strand DNA)]. Results are shown as mean percentages ± SEM

related to cells velocity (VAP, VCL and VSL) of around 10 μm/s. It has been reported that these parameters are highly correlated to fertility in several species such as ram [25, 26], bull [27] and boar [28]. Incubation with NPs also changed the rates of rapid spermatozoa in the exposed groups compared to the control with more than 50% of cells having a VAP > 75 μm/s at 72 and 96 h of incubation. These results are in agreement with what previously reported in rats fed with a diet containing citrate-coated CeO_2 NPs (1 mg/kg). After 10 days of diet, the authors reported a significant increase in motility and viability of epididymal spermatozoa in treated animals compared to control group and suggested NPs as a helpful tool in contrasting age-related infertility [29]. A recent study carried out on humans reported an improvement in motility parameters in frozen- thawed semen following supplementation of cryopreservation medium with ZnO NPs [30]. These promising results may pave the way for a use of NPs as preservers of semen quality during storage at low temperatures although further investigations are strictly needed. Preaubert et al. reported no effect of CeO_2 NPs on progressive motility rates in mice spermatozoa [14] and detrimental effects of NPs on sperm motility have been described in bull [31] and human [32], suggesting species-specific effects of these compounds.

Data on motility correlated well with the results obtained by the analysis of the integrity of plasma and acrosomal membranes suggesting a high biocompatibility of CeO_2 NPs. As for kinematic parameters, NPs did not influence the status of the membranes in the first 48 h of exposure, but from 72 h onward, the effects of co-incubation were visible on spermatozoa exposed to NPs, that preserved more efficiently the morphologic structure of plasma membranes compared to unexposed cells. Acrosomes were not affected by exposure to NPs and this suggests a differential sensitivity of sperm membranes to stressing conditions. The absence of membrane alterations during incubation with NPs has been previously observed in the same species [16]. Moreover, no interaction with membranes or up-take but only occasional contacts between NPs and the post-acrosomal region of spermatozoa was described [16], suggesting that the positive effects triggered by NPs on sperm parameters are not mediated by intra-cellular mechanisms.

In this experiment, we exposed spermatozoa to a prolonged stressing factor (storage at 4 °C for 96 h) and investigated the role of CeO_2 NPs in preventing oxidative sperm damage. However, the levels of ROS remained fairly stable until 72 h and then rose at 96 h in exposed and unexposed cells.

During storage procedures at low temperatures, ram spermatozoa are extremely sensitive to oxidative stress due to the high ratio unsaturated/saturated fatty acids in phospholipids of plasma membranes [33]. Disruption of intra-cellular balance of free radicals accumulation leads to impairment of quality parameters such as viability, motility, membranes integrity and consequent fertilizing ability, as reviewed by Bansal and Bilaspuri [34]. On the other side, ROS play a critical role in several essential physiological processes such as sperm binding, capacitation and hyper-activation, as recently reviewed by O'Flaherty et al. [35].

Although we reported a positive effect of CeO_2 NPs in preserving quality traits in semen from 48 h onward, we could not correlate this effect with changes in the levels of ROS. This controversial result suggests that NPs, in the specific experimental conditions of the present trial, acted through pathways that are independent from ROS accumulation in sperm cells.

We could also speculate that CeO_2 NPs might exert their catalytic action in the extra-cellular compound (storage extender) perhaps through their SOD or catalase mimetic behaviour, rather than inside sperm cells. This hypothesis is supported by the previously reported lack of uptake and internalisation of CeO_2 NPs by sperm cells [16]. These external actions possibly depend on chemical and physical characteristics of NPs and interaction with the compounds involved in storing spermatozoa, such as extender and seminal plasma. In physiological conditions, SOD and catalase antioxidant activities have been detected in seminal plasma of several species like bull [36], boar [37] and equine [38], where they are involved in maintaining integrity of membranes and sperm function. We can also suggest that supplementation of storage extender with CeO_2 NPs might have supported the activity of the enzymatic systems formerly present in seminal plasma of rams.

Perrin et al. reported that exposure of human spermatozoa to CeO_2 NPs has genotoxic effects that were limited by the use of an antioxidant (L-Ergothioneine) suggesting a pro-oxidant activity of the NPs [39]. In our experiment, we did not report any genotoxic effect of CeO_2 NPs at any time of the experimental trial. The levels of DNA fragmentation remained stable for up to 96 h and no differences were found with unexposed spermatozoa. This indicates that the biocompatibility of these compounds may depend by several factors; among others, a species sensitivity should not be excluded. In the mouse, CeO_2 NPs induce DNA damage in both oocytes and spermatozoa affecting in vitro fertilization [14] whereas in the ovine species, supplementation of maturation media with CeO_2 NPs (44μg/mL) did not impair but enhanced fertilization and blastocyst rate and no adverse effects were observed in chromatin configuration of oocytes exposed to NPs [15]. On the other side chromatin damage has been reported in mice [40] and bull spermatozoa [41] exposed to silver NPs.

Conclusions

To our knowledge, this is the first report describing beneficial effects of CeO_2 NPs on morphologic and kinematic parameters of ram semen, such as motility and plasma membrane integrity after 96 h of exposure. We also reported no genotoxic effects of these NPs. However, these beneficial effects could not be explained by an intra-cellular antioxidant activity exerted by these compounds, since ROS levels in exposed cells were similar to those of unexposed ones. Eventually, further investigations are needed to support these preliminary results and to pave the way to future applications of these compounds in reproductive biology.

Abbreviations

ALH: Lateral head displacement; BCF: Beat cross frequency; CASA: Computer assisted sperm analysis; DFI: DNA fragmentation index; ELONG: Elongation; H_2DCFDA: Dichlorofluorescein diacetate; LIN: Linearity; NPs: Nanoparticles; PBS: Phosphate buffer saline; PI: Propidium Iodide; PM: Progressive motility; PSA: *Pisum sativum* agglutinin; ROS: Reactive oxygen species; RPM: Revolutions per minute; SCSA: Sperm chromatin structure assay; STR: Straightness; TM: Total motility; TNE: Tris-NaCl-EDTA; VAP: Average path velocity; VCL: Curvilinear velocity; VSL: Straight line velocity

Acknowledgements

The authors would like to thank Dr. G.P. Epifani of Servizio Zootecnico, AGRIS, Agenzia Regionale per la Ricerca in Agricoltura, Bonassai, Italy, for the assistance in providing the animals for the experiment.

Funding

This work was supported by: Fondazione Banco di Sardegna and Centro di Competenza di Biodiversità Animale RAS.

Authors' contributions

LF and SL collaborated in conceiving the experimental design and in writing the manuscript; GG and LF performed flow cytometer analyses; LF, GMD, MTZ, SP, LB, FA, PI and SN contributed in performing the experiments and in collecting and analysing data; AP synthesized CeO_2 NPs; SL supervised the project. All authors contributed in writing the manuscript, read and approved its final version.

Competing interests

The authors report no conflicts of interest that could be perceived as prejudicing the impartiality of the research reported.

Author details

[1]Dipartimento di Medicina Veterinaria, Università degli Studi di Sassari, Sassari, Italy. [2]Dipartimento di Medicina Clinica e Sperimentale, Università degli Studi di Sassari, Sassari, Italy. [3]Department of Materials, Imperial College London, South Kensington Campus, London, UK. [4]Dipartimento di Chimica e Farmacia, Università degli Studi di Sassari, Sassari, Italy.

References

1. Bour A, Mouchet F, Cadarsi S, Silvestre J, Baque D, Gauthier L, et al. CeO_2 nanoparticle fate in environmental conditions and toxicity on a freshwater predator species: a microcosm study. Environ Sci Pollut Res Int. 2017;24:17081–9.
2. Pirmohamed T, Dowding JM, Singh S, Wasserman B, Heckert E, Karakoti AS, et al. Nanoceria exhibit redox state-dependent catalase mimetic activity. Chem Commun (Camb). 2010;46:2736–8.
3. Heckert EG, Karakoti AS, Seal S, Self WT. The role of cerium redox state in the SOD mimetic activity of nanoceria. Biomaterials. 2008;29:2705–9.
4. Korsvik C, Patil S, Seal S, Self WT. Superoxide dismutase mimetic properties exhibited by vacancy engineered ceria nanoparticles. Chem Commun (Camb). 2007:1056–8.
5. Kim JW, Mahapatra C, Hong JY, Kim MS, Leong KW, Kim HW, et al. Functional recovery of contused spinal cord in rat with the injection of optimal-dosed cerium oxide nanoparticles. Adv Sci (Weinh). 2017;4:1700034.
6. Singh R, Karakoti AS, Self W, Seal S, Singh S. Redox-sensitive cerium oxide nanoparticles protect human keratinocytes from oxidative stress induced by glutathione depletion. Langmuir. 2016;32:12202–11.
7. Chigurupati S, Mughal MR, Okun E, Das S, Kumar A, McCaffery M, et al. Effects of cerium oxide nanoparticles on the growth of keratinocytes, fibroblasts and vascular endothelial cells in cutaneous wound healing. Biomaterials. 2013;34:2194–201.
8. Akhtar MJ, Ahamed M, Alhadlaq HA, Khan MAM, Alrokayan SA. Glutathione replenishing potential of CeO(2) nanoparticles in human breast and fibrosarcoma cells. J Colloid Interface Sci. 2015;453:21–7.
9. Pagliari F, Mandoli C, Forte G, Magnani E, Pagliari S, Nardone G, et al. Cerium oxide nanoparticles protect cardiac progenitor cells from oxidative stress. ACS Nano. 2012;6:3767–75.
10. Nemmar A, Al-Salam S, Beegam S, Yuvaraju P, Ali BH. The acute pulmonary and thrombotic effects of cerium oxide nanoparticles after intratracheal instillation in mice. Int J Nanomedicine. 2017;12:2913–22.
11. Ma JY, Mercer RR, Barger M, Schwegler-Berry D, Scabilloni J, Ma JK, et al. Induction of pulmonary fibrosis by cerium oxide nanoparticles. Toxicol Appl Pharmacol. 2012;262:255–64.
12. Kumari M, Kumari SI, Kamal SSK, Grover P. Genotoxicity assessment of cerium oxide nanoparticles in female Wistar rats after acute oral exposure. Mutat Res Gen Toxicol Environ Mutagen. 2014;775–776:7–19.
13. Courbiere B, Auffan M, Rollais R, Tassistro V, Bonnefoy A, Botta A, et al. Ultrastructural interactions and genotoxicity assay of cerium dioxide nanoparticles on mouse oocytes. Int J Mol Sci. 2013;14:21613–28.
14. Preaubert L, Courbiere B, Achard V, Tassistro V, Greco F, Orsiere T, et al. Cerium dioxide nanoparticles affect in vitro fertilization in mice. Nanotoxicology. 2015:1–7.
15. Ariu F, Bogliolo L, Pinna A, Malfatti L, Innocenzi P, Falchi L, et al. Cerium oxide nanoparticles (CeO2 NPs) improve the developmental competence of in vitro-matured prepubertal ovine oocytes. Reprod Fertil Dev. 2017;29:1046–56.
16. Falchi L, Bogliolo L, Galleri G, Ariu F, Zedda MT, Pinna A, et al. Cerium dioxide nanoparticles did not alter the functional and morphologic characteristics of ram sperm during short-term exposure. Theriogenology. 2016;85:1274–81.
17. Zhou X, Wang B, Chen Y, Mao Z, Gao C. Uptake of cerium oxide nanoparticles and their influences on functions of A549 cells. J Nanosci Nanotechnol. 2013;13:204–15.
18. Evenson D. Jost L. sperm chromatin structure assay for fertility assessment. Curr Protoc Cytom. Chapter 7:Unit. 2001;7:13.
19. Migani A, Vayssilov GN, Bromley ST, Illas F, Neyman KM. Greatly facilitated oxygen vacancy formation in ceria nanocrystallites. Chem Commun (Camb). 2010;46:5936–8.
20. O'Brien N, Cummins E. Ranking initial environmental and human health risk resulting from environmentally relevant nanomaterials. J Environ Sci Health A Tox Hazard Subst Environ Eng. 2010;45:992–1007.
21. Park B, Donaldson K, Duffin R, Tran L, Kelly F, Mudway I, et al. Hazard and risk assessment of a nanoparticulate cerium oxide-based diesel fuel additive - a case study. Inhal Toxicol. 2008;20:547–66.
22. O'Hara L, Hanrahan JP, Richardson L, Donovan A, Fair S, Evans AC, et al. Effect of storage duration, storage temperature, and diluent on the viability and fertility of fresh ram sperm. Theriogenology. 2010;73:541–9.
23. Paulenz H, Söderquist L, Pérez-Pé R, Andersen Berg K. Effect of different extenders and storage temperatures on sperm viability of liquid ram semen. Theriogenology. 2002;57:823–36.
24. Gundogan M, Yeni D, Avdatek F, Fidan AF. Influence of sperm concentration on the motility, morphology, membrane and DNA integrity along with oxidative stress parameters of ram sperm during liquid storage. Anim Reprod Sci. 2010;122:200–7.
25. Sanchez-Partida LG, Windsor DP, Eppleston J, Setchell BP, Fertility MWMC. Its relationship to motility characteristics of spermatozoa in ewes after cervical, transcervical, and intrauterine insemination with frozen-thawed ram semen. J Androl. 1999;20:280–8.
26. Robayo I, Montenegro V, Valdés C, Cox JF. CASA assessment of kinematic parameters of ram spermatozoa and their relationship to migration efficiency in ruminant cervical mucus. Reprod Domest Anim. 2008;43:393–9.

27. Farrell PB, Presicce GA, Brockett CC, Foote RH. Quantification of bull sperm characteristics measured by computer-assisted sperm analysis (CASA) and the relationship to fertility. Theriogenology. 1998;49:871–9.
28. Holt C, Holt WV, Moore HD, Reed HC, Curnock RM. Objectively measured boar sperm motility parameters correlate with the outcomes of on-farm inseminations: results of two fertility trials. J Androl. 1997;18:312–23.
29. Kobyliak NM, Falalyeyeva TM, Kuryk OG, Beregova TV, Bodnar PM, Zholobak NM, et al. Antioxidative effects of cerium dioxide nanoparticles ameliorate age-related male infertility: optimistic results in rats and the review of clinical clues for integrative concept of men health and fertility. EPMA J. 2015;6:12.
30. Isaac AV, Kumari S, Nair R, Urs DR, Salian SR, Kalthur G, et al. Supplementing zinc oxide nanoparticles to cryopreservation medium minimizes the freeze-thaw-induced damage to spermatozoa. Biochem Biophys Res Commun. 2017;494:656–62.
31. Taylor U, Barchanski A, Petersen S, Kues WA, Baulain U, Gamrad L, et al. Gold nanoparticles interfere with sperm functionality by membrane adsorption without penetration. Nanotoxicology. 2014;8:118–27.
32. Wiwanitkit V, Sereemaspun A, Rojanathanes R. Effect of gold nanoparticles on spermatozoa: the first world report. Fertil Steril. 2009;91:e7–8.
33. Muiño-Blanco T, Pérez-Pé R, Cebrián-Pérez JA. Seminal plasma proteins and sperm resistance to stress. Reprod Domest Anim. 2008;43:18–31.
34. Bansal AK, Bilaspuri GS. Impacts of oxidative stress and antioxidants on semen functions. Vet Med Int. 2010;doi:https://doi.org/10.4061/2011/686137.
35. O'Flaherty C, Matsushita-Fournier D. Reactive oxygen species and protein modifications in spermatozoa. Biol Reprod. 2017;97:577–85.
36. Gurler H, Calisici O, Bollwein H. Inter- and intra-individual variability of total antioxidant capacity of bovine seminal plasma and relationships with sperm quality before and after cryopreservation. Anim Reprod Sci. 2015;155:99–105.
37. Li J, Barranco I, Tvarijonaviciute A, Molina MF, Martinez EA, Rodriguez-Martinez H, et al. Seminal plasma antioxidants are directly involved in boar sperm cryotolerance. Theriogenology. 2017;107:27–35.
38. Baumber J, Ball BA. Determination of glutathione peroxidase and superoxide dismutase-like activities in equine spermatozoa, seminal plasma, and reproductive tissues. Am J Vet Res. 2005;66:1415–9.
39. Perrin J, Tassistro V, Auffan M, Liu W, Botta A, Sari-Minodier I, et al. Cerium dioxide nanoparticles induce DNA damage in human spermatozoa. Hum Reprod. 2014;29(Suppl 1):8–9.
40. Asare N, Instanes C, Sandberg WJ, Refsnes M, Schwarze P, Kruszewski M, et al. Cytotoxic and genotoxic effects of silver nanoparticles in testicular cells. Toxicology. 2012;291:65–72.
41. Zakhidov ST, Pavlyuchenkova SM, Samoylov AV, Mudzhiri NM, Marshak TL, Rudoy VM, et al. Bovine sperm chromatin is not protected from the effects of ultrasmall gold nanoparticles. Biol Bull. 2013;40:493–9.

15

Prostaglandin E2 involvement in mammalian female fertility: ovulation, fertilization, embryo development and early implantation

Jean Damascene Niringiyumukiza, Hongcai Cai and Wenpei Xiang*

Abstract

Background: Infertility in mammalian females has been a challenge in reproductive medicine. The causes of female infertility include anovulation, ovulated oocyte defects, abnormal fertilization, and insufficient luteal support for embryo development, as well as early implantation. Ovulation induction, in vitro fertilization and luteal support regimens have been performed for decades to increase fertility rates. The identification of proteins and biochemical factors involved in female reproduction is essential to further increase female fertility rates. Evidence has shown that prostaglandins (PGs) might be involved in the female reproductive process, mainly ovulation, fertilization, and implantation. However, only a few studies on individual PGs in female reproduction have been done so far. This review aimed to identify the pivotal role of prostaglandin E2 (PGE2), a predominant PG, in female reproduction to improve fertility, specifically ovulation, fertilization, embryo development and early implantation.

Results: Prostaglandin E2 (PGE2) was shown to play a relevant role in the ovulatory cascade, including meiotic maturation, cumulus expansion and follicle rupture, through inducing ovulatory genes, such as *Areg*, *Ereg*, *Has2* and Tnfaip6, as well as increasing intracellular cAMP levels. PGE2 reduces extracellular matrix viscosity and thereby optimizes the conditions for sperm penetration. PGE2 reduces the phagocytic activity of polymorphonuclear neutrophils (PMNs) against sperm. In the presence of PGE2, sperm function and binding capacity to oocytes are enhanced. PGE2 maintains luteal function for embryo development and early implantation. In addition, it induces chemokine expression for trophoblast apposition and adhesion to the decidua for implantation.

Conclusion: It has been shown that PGE2 positively affects different stages of female fertility. Therefore, PGE2 should be taken into consideration when optimizing reproduction in infertile females. We suggest that in clinical practice, the administration of non-steroidal anti-inflammatory drugs, which are PGE2 synthesis inhibitors, should be reasonable and limited in infertile women. Additionally, assessments of PGE2 protein and receptor expression levels should be taken into consideration.

Keywords: Blastocyst, Cumulus, Chemokine, Extracellular matrix, Fertilization, Implantation, Prostaglandin E2

* Correspondence: wpxiang2010@gmail.com
Family Planning Research Institute/Center of Reproductive Medicine, Tongji Medical College, Huazhong University of Science and Technology, Wuhan 430030, Hubei, China

Background

Many couples suffer from infertility, which is a big challenge not only to them but also to their family, endocrinology and infertility specialists, and embryologists. Different assisted reproductive techniques (ART) are used to enhance fertility rates. However, despite the constant development of sophisticated equipment and procedures, infertility treatment is still complicated and has a low success rate.

Previous studies have provided evidence that prostaglandins (PGs) may play a pivotal role in female reproduction, particularly in ovulation, implantation, and menstruation; however, the mechanisms involved remain elusive [1, 2]. The non-steroidal anti-inflammatory drugs (NSAIDs) aspirin and indomethacin, which inhibit cyclooxygenase (COX), were reported to have adverse effects on gonadotropin-releasing hormone release, ovulation, fertilization and luteolysis [3].

There are five types of PGs (also known as prostanoids): prostaglandin E2 (PGE2), prostaglandin D2 (PGD2), prostaglandin PGF2α (PGF2 Alfa), prostaglandin PGI2 (PGI2) and thromboxane (THA2). These are ubiquitously secreted, mostly from inflamed cells. PGs are synthesized from arachidonic acid by the key enzyme COX, also called prostaglandin synthase protein (PTGS) [4, 5]. Each PG has a specific influence and mechanism in the female reproductive system. However, it is possible that the different PGs also act in a synergistic way to fulfill their biological functions. Although the role of PGs in the female reproductive system has been already described, little is known about the individual PGs as separate functional entities in female reproduction.

PGE2 is the most common and substantial PG found in animal species. A wide range of receptor (EP, also noted as PTGER) subtypes (EP1, EP2, EP3 and EP4) that are bound by PGE2 have a multitude of signal transduction properties [6, 7]. The essential role of PGE2 production in female fertility has been suggested in previous studies [7, 8]. Experiments with PGE2 receptor type2 (EP2)-deficient mice showed disturbances in ovulation, fertilization, embryo development and implantation [9, 10]. Due to the predominance of PGE2 and its broad biological functions mediated by its different types of receptors, this review summarizes the role and mechanisms of PGE2 in ovulation, fertilization, embryo development and successful early implantation (Fig. 1).

Results

PGE2 involvement in the ovulation cascade

The luteinizing hormone (LH) surge was demonstrated to be responsible for oocyte cumulus expansion and meiotic maturation [11, 13]. However, the small amounts of LH receptors expressed in cumulus cells and in the oocyte [12] suggest that LH acts via other mediators. PGE2 is one of the mediators found to promote oocyte cumulus expansion and maturation [14]. Previous studies reported that inhibiting PGE2 production in follicles or genetically knocking out PGE2 and PGE2 receptor expression could prevent ovulation [7, 8]. However, the mechanisms of PGE2 in oocyte cumulus expansion and meiotic maturation remain elusive.

PGE2 enhances cumulus expansion

Ovulation requires adequate cumulus cell expansion to enable cumulus-oocyte complex (COC) detachment from the follicle wall and follicle rupture to release the oocyte into the oviduct. It was found that the LH surge increases PGE2 levels in the dominant follicle to modulate the action of gonadotropin for cumulus cell expansion and the expression of proteases associated with follicle rupture [15–18]. Female mice deficient in EP2, a PGE2 receptor, presented with abnormal cumulus cell expansion and unruptured follicles, which resulted in infertility or subfertility [7, 19].

The essential genes that are induced in COCs and are responsible for expansion include the following: oocyte maturation genes of epidermal growth factor (EGF)-like factors, such as amphiregulin (*Areg*), epiregulin (*Ereg*) and betacellulin (*Btc*) [20, 21]; and matrix-forming and stabilizing elements, such as hyaluronan synthase 2 (*Has2*) and tumor necrosis factor α-induced protein 6 (*Tnfaip6*) [20, 22]. Studies have shown that PGE2 up-regulates the expression of many of these genes, including *Areg*, *Ereg*, *Has2* and *Tnfaip6*, in granulosa and cumulus cells via its receptor EP2 [21, 23]. Moreover, there is evidence that the cAMP pathway induces the expression of the cumulus expansion-related genes *Has2* and *Tnfaip6* in cumulus cells [4] and that PGE2 increases cAMP concentrations in cumulus cells during ovulation [23]; these findings suggest a direct role of PGE2 in cumulus expansion via these growth factors. The role of the protein kinase B and mitogen-activated protein kinases3/1 (PKB-MAPK3/1) pathway in cumulus expansion has also been documented [24, 25], and *PGE2 was found to activate this pathway* for cumulus cell expansion and meiosis resumption [26].

PGE2 has been involved in oocyte meiotic maturation

PGE2 was found to be involved in not only cumulus expansion but also in meiotic maturation [27]. Cyclic adenosine monophosphate (cAMP) is a well-known mediator of meiotic maturation. PGE2 increases cAMP production in follicles, resulting in the maturation and cumulus expansion of oocytes [23, 28]. The PGE2 receptors EP2 and EP4, which are predominant in cumulus and granulosa cells [29], can increase intracellular cAMP levels when they are coupled to adenylate cyclase [30, 31]. In an in vitro study using mouse oocytes, treatment with an agonist selective for EP2 and EP4 increased cAMP production and subsequently increased ovulation rates [32], whereas

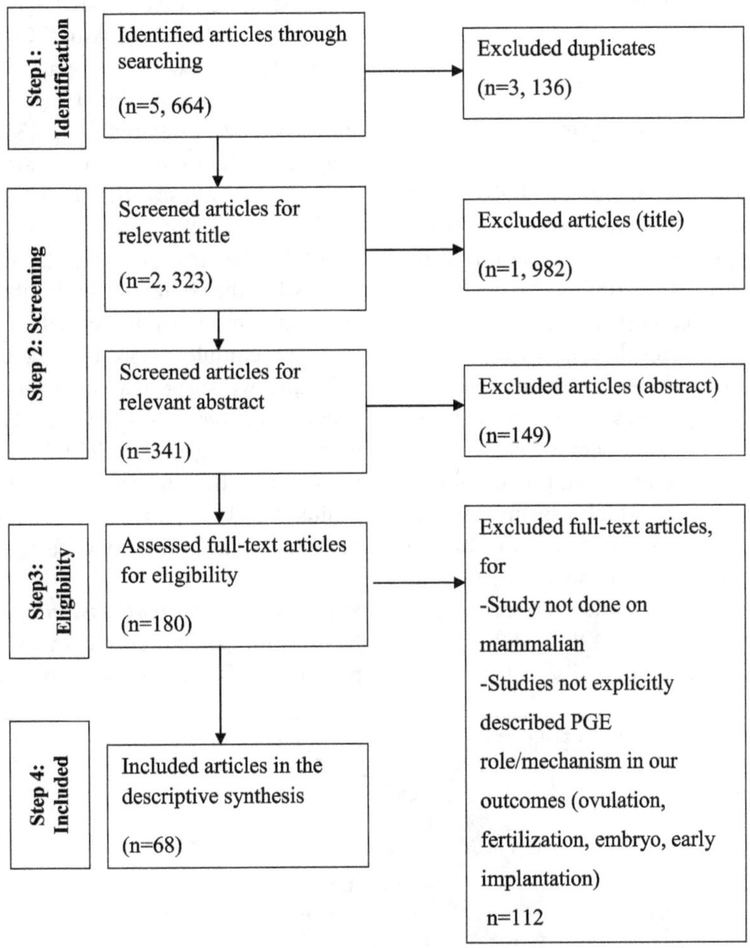

Fig. 1 Selection of articles

the genetic manipulation of genes encoding EP2 and EP4 resulted in the inhibition of meiotic maturation and cumulus expansion [10, 33]. Several factors are responsible for maintaining spindle integrity during meiotic maturation. MAPK regulates spindle integrity during the meiotic maturation of oocytes [34, 35]. MAPK activity depends on phosphorylation. PGE2 was found to be responsible for the phosphorylation of MAPK [36], suggesting that PGE2 activates MAPK and indirectly induces the meiotic maturation of oocytes.

PGE2 was thought to mediate LH signals for meiotic maturation. Angiotensin II stimulation by LH has been reported to promote the meiotic maturation of oocytes by blocking the inhibitory effect of theca cells [37, 38]. It was demonstrated that the effects of angiotensin II in this process are mediated by PGE2 [39–41]. In an in vitro bovine oocyte study, indomethacin supplementation blocked the meiotic maturation of bovine oocytes induced by angiotensin II, whereas PGE2 treatment restored meiotic maturation to levels comparable to those induced by angiotensin II [39]. Human chorionic gonadotropin (hCG), a substitute for LH that stimulates oocyte maturation and ovulation in assisted reproduction, was reported to increase PGE2 and ovulatory gene expression through prostaglandin transport (PGT) in human granulosa cells [42].

Even though LH and PGE2 were shown to trigger cumulus expansion and meiotic maturation separately [11–13], according to the above findings, we suggest similarity and synergetic effects between LH and the PGE2 pathways in regulating cumulus expansion and meiotic maturation. First, LH and PGE2 receptors are members of the G protein-coupled receptor (GPCR) family, and they trigger the ovulation process via activating adenylate cyclases to increase cAMP concentrations [23, 43, 44] for the synthesis of EGF-like factors, including *Areg* and *Ereg*, in granulosa and cumulus cells [23, 44–46]. Because the PGE2/cAMP pathway has been studied in meiotic maturation [23, 28], but not in the stimulation of *Areg* and *Ereg* secretion, we hypothesize that PGE2 induces cAMP pathways to stimulate EGF-like growth factors in cumulus and granulosa cells via its receptors (the same as LH); we propose this since these growth factors are positively involved in both cumulus expansion and oocyte meiotic maturation (Fig. 2).

PGE2 modulates the fertilization process

PGE2 regulates cumulus ECM disassembly for sperm penetration into the oocyte

Cumulus cells synthesize and secrete extracellular matrices (ECMs) composed of mostly hyaluronan deposited in the intercellular space [47, 48]. ECM deposition in the inter-cumulus cell space leads to cumulus expansion, increases ECM viscosity and confers resistance capacity against biochemical and mechanical stress to the cumulus ECM. Chemokines were reported to modulate cumulus ECM consistency [49–51]. It has been demonstrated that upon ovulation, cumulus cells secrete various factors, including chemokine receptors and chemokines, such as CCL7, CCL2, and CCL9, which can increase the ECM viscosity to protect the oocyte from mechanical stress [49, 51]. The increased ECM consistency in cumulus cells by CCL-CCR signals impedes the passage of sperm and prevents fertilization [3, 49]. PGE2-induced activation of the cAMP pathway [50] disassembles and attenuates the ECM consistency [7, 50] by inhibiting the secretion of the chemokines CCL7 and CCL2 [50, 52]; these effects create a free space for sperm penetration.

In addition, interleukin-1β (IL-1β) stimulates the secretion of CCL2 in different cells [53, 54] and granulosa cells [55]. Given that cumulus cells are derived from granulosa cells, we hypothesize that IL-1β also stimulates CCL2 secretion in cumulus cells. It was found that PGE2 inhibits IL-1β in the myometrial cells of pregnant women [56], suggesting that PGE2 also inhibits the expression of CCL2 stimulated by IL-1β. Increased IL-1β expression was identified in cumulus cells lacking the PGE2 receptor EP2 [49], and we suspect a subsequent increase in CCL2 expression in these cells lacking PGE2 receptors. Taken together, we suggest that PGE2 acts via EP2 as a negative regulator of the chemokines CCL7 and CCL2 in the cumulus ECM to enhance ECM disassembly for sperm penetration and subsequent fertilization (Fig. 3a, b).

PGE2 protects sperm against phagocytosis in the oviduct

Neutrophils are mobilized in oviduct in response to the presence of sperm, a process resembling classical

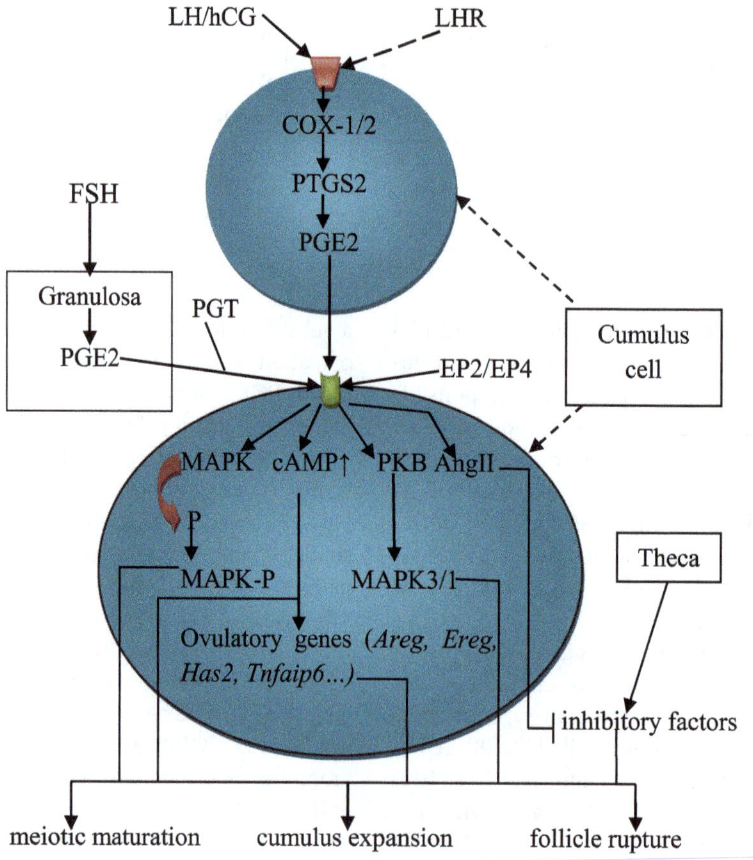

Fig. 2 Ovulatory cascade. LH/hCG induces PGE2 synthesis and secretion in cumulus cells. Additionally, granulosa cells under FSH stimulation release PGE2, which is coupled with PGT and transported to the cumulus cell membrane to bind the PGE2 receptors EP2 and EP4. Via these receptors, PGE2 induces MAPK phosphorylation, increases intracellular cAMP levels and activates the PKB/MAPK3/1 pathway to stimulate ovulatory gene expression. Furthermore, PGE2 stimulates Angiotensin II to inhibit the inhibitory factors against meiotic maturation, released by theca cells

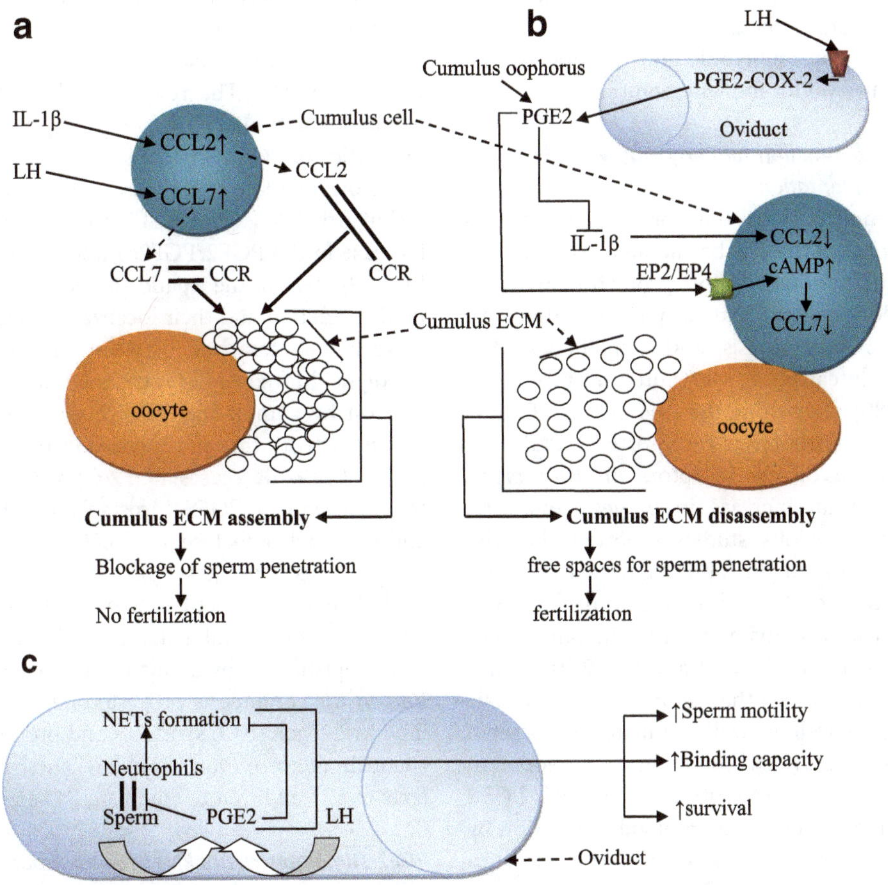

Fig. 3 PGE2 in the fertilization process. PGE2 disassembles the cumulus ECM for sperm penetration and inhibits the phagocytic activity of PMNs against sperm. **a** Cumulus ECM assembly: In cumulus cells, LH and IL-1β respectively induce the expression of the chemokines CCL7 and CCL2. CCL7 and CCL2 bind the chemokine receptor CCR to induce cumulus cell-ECM assembly. **b** Cumulus cell-ECM disassembly: Upon ovulation, there is an increased level of PGE2 secreted by oviduct epithelial cells and the *cumulus oophorus*. PGE2 inhibits IL-1β and increases intracellular cAMP concentrations, respectively, resulting in decreased expression levels of CCL2 and CCL7; these actions subsequently result in the disassembly of the cumulus ECM. The disassembly of the cumulus ECM leaves a free space for sperm penetration into the oocyte for fertilization. **c** In the oviduct, sperm binding to epithelial cells, as well as LH stimulation, induce PGE2 secretion. The released PGE2 inhibits neutrophil binding to the sperm and NET formation. Sperm in the presence of PGE2 have increased mobility, survival and binding capacity to the oocyte

inflammation [57–59]. When protective signals become ineffective, the neutrophils fight against the sperms and reduce their motility and fertilization potential [60–62].

PGE2 exerts immunosuppressive activity [63], which inhibits the phagocytosis of sperm by neutrophils and macrophages [64, 65]. In the oviduct, in addition to the PGE2 secreted after epithelial cell stimulation by LH [66], it was found that sperm binding to the epithelial cells also induces PGE2 release [67], suggesting an auto-defense mechanism exerted by sperm in the oviduct. Via its receptor EP2, PGE2 may protect sperm from the phagocytic activity of polymorphonuclear neutrophils (PMNs) in the oviduct [68–70]. Neutrophils phagocytize spermatozoa either through cell attachment or by entrapping them in neutrophil extracellular traps (NETs) [71, 72]. A previous study demonstrated that PGE2 inhibits NET formation [73]. We suggest that the immunosuppressive potential of PGE2 and its inhibition of NET formation may result in enhanced sperm survival and higher motility and binding capacity of sperm in the oviduct, which subsequently increase the fertilization rate (Fig. 3c).

Essential role of PGE2 in embryo development and early implantation

Various factors mediate the cell proliferation, cleavage and survival of embryonic cells, as well as blastocyst formation and hatching. An embryo in the endometrium stimulates signals that have direct or indirect effects on its development and implantation. In embryos, gradually increasing levels of PGE2 from a 2-cell embryo to blastocyst were identified [74]. PGE2 was demonstrated to promote blastocyst hatching and enhance trophoblast proliferation after embryo transfer [75, 76]. PGE2 is considered to be a mitogenic, anti-apoptotic and angiogenic factor for cell proliferation and survival in other cells [77, 78], which suggests that PGE2 exerts these effects in embryo development, thus enhancing embryonic and trophoblast cell proliferation and survival for implantation (Fig. 4).

PGE2 maintains luteal function for early embryo development and implantation

After ovulation, mechanisms that protect the *corpus luteum* from regression should be initiated to stimulate the continuous production of factors protecting and promoting embryo development and early implantation. An increase in PGE2 biosynthesis and signaling in the uterus during the luteal phase was noted in sheep [79] and pig models [80], suggesting the role of this PG during early pregnancy. Through its receptor EP2, PGE2 induces the expression of LH receptors on the *corpus luteum*, resulting in an increase in progesterone (P4) synthesis [81, 82]. Previous studies reported that decreased blood flow to the luteal-containing ovary and decreased progesterone production result in luteolysis [83]. Blood flow has to be maintained for incoming biochemical factors, including LH, E2 and PGE2, to stimulate the *corpus luteum* to synthesize and secrete various factors, mostly P4, as well as to disseminate the secreted factors in the systemic system for embryo development and early implantation [84]. Via its receptor EP4, PGE2 was shown to enhance utero-ovarian blood circulation by increasing adenylate cyclase (AC) activity, which in turn increases nitric oxide synthase (OS) activity to increase synthesis and nitric oxide (NO) release, a vasodilator [85].

Interferon tau (IFN-t) was reported to reverse the PG secretion profile in endometrial cells during early pregnancy, thus resulting in increased PGE2 secretion and decreased PGF2a secretion [86, 87]. The increased PGE2/PGF2α ratio during early pregnancy is thought to prevent luteolysis and to support the luteal function for embryo development and successful implantation. It was reported that embryos secrete 17-β estradiol (E2) to stimulate continuous P4 production by the *corpus luteum* [88, 89]. The roles of embryo-secreted estradiol would be anti-luteolytic and lyteoprotectant, which are properties of PGE2. Previous studies demonstrated a simultaneous increase in E2 secretion by the embryo [90] and a shift from PGF2α to PGE2 secretion with a subsequent increase in the PGE2/PGF2α ratio during early pregnancy [91, 92]. Given the spatio-temporal pattern of E2 and PGE2 secretion and their localization, we hypothesize that there is an interaction between E2 and PGE2 to inhibit luteolysis. Moreover, E2 was shown to increase PGE2 production by stimulating PTGS2 secretion, which potentiates its activity through increasing the expression of EP2 [93]; E2 also decreases PGF2α production by inhibiting the secretion of PGFS (prostaglandin F2alpha synthase) and carbonyl reductase 1 (CBR1) [93], enzymes involved in PGF2α secretion [94–96].

We hypothesize that PGE2 exerts its anti-luteolytic properties to protect and enhance embryo development and early implantation by inducing LH receptors on the *corpus luteum* for continuous progesterone secretion, by increasing nitric oxide (NO) synthesis and production to maintain adequate utero-ovarian blood flow and by mediating the effects of E2 and IFN-t to stimulate P4 secretion (Fig. 5a).

PGE2 stimulates chemokines for trophoblast apposition and adhesion to the maternal decidua

Different signals, including chemokines and chemokine receptors, produced in the endometrium are essential for embryo development and early implantation. Previous studies found that PGE2 modulates the expression of CXCR4, which is a receptor for the chemokine CXCL12, in hematopoietic stem cells [97] and stromal cells of the endometrium [98]. Embryonic signals were shown to regulate the expression of

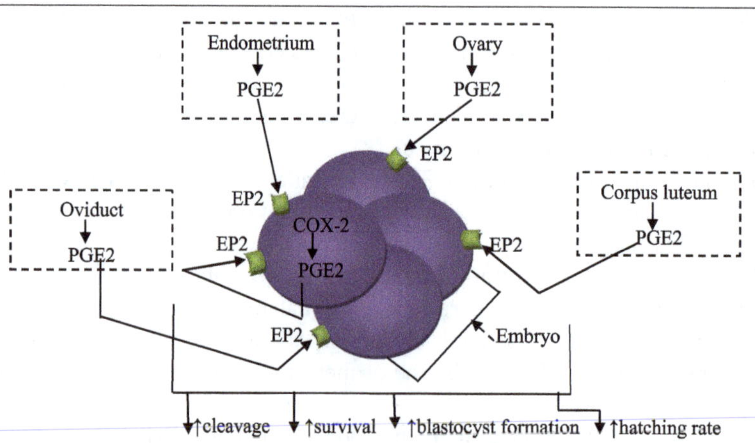

Fig. 4 Role of PGE2 in embryo development. PGE2 is secreted by the embryo, from the 2-cell embryo to the blastocyst stage. The level of PGE2 increases gradually in the embryo pre-implantation. PGE2 secreted by the embryo, ovary, *corpus luteum*, oviduct and endometrium stimulate cleavage, survival, and blastocyst formation and hatching rates in the intrauterine cavity

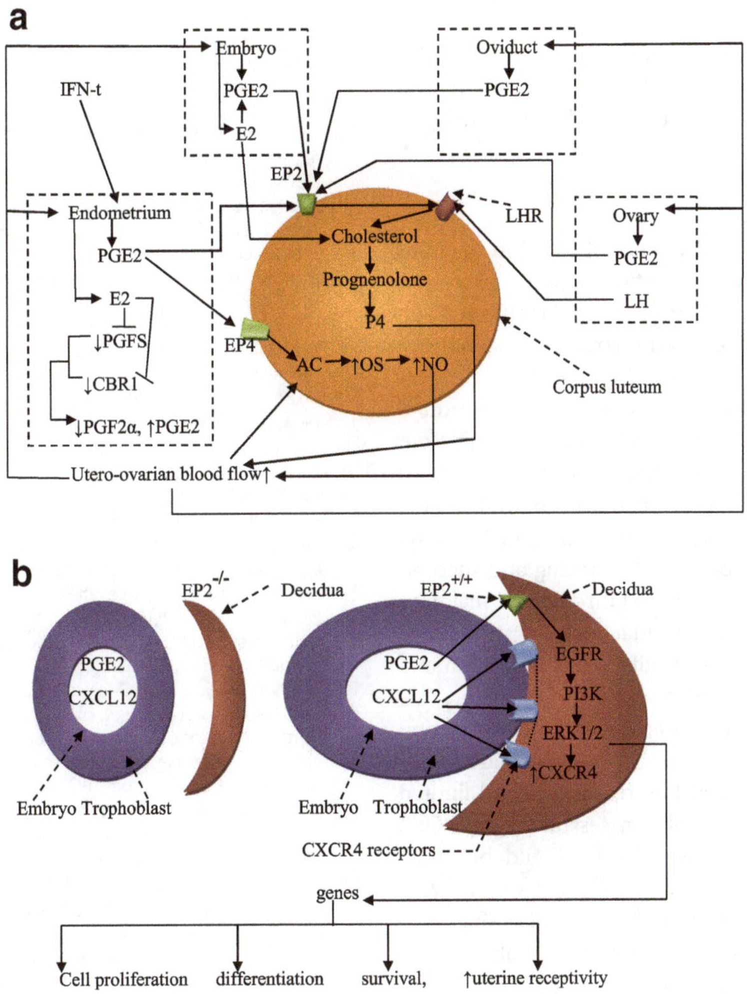

Fig. 5 a PGE2 mediates early implantation. **a** Upon ovulation, PGE2 is secreted by the following reproductive organs: ovaries, endometrium and oviduct, as well as the embryo. EP2 induces LH receptor expression on the *corpus luteum* to secrete P4 and stimulate its continuous release into the in utero-ovarian circulation. P4 exerts positive feedback to the ovaries, endometrium and oviduct to recognize and maintain the ongoing implantation and embryo development. Via EP4, PGE2 increases the activity of adenylate cyclase (AC) and nitric oxide synthase (OS) successivelyto increase synthesis and nitric oxide (NO) release. NO, a vasodilator, increases the utero-ovarian blood flow and the concentration of pro-pregnancy factors. Additionally, E2 secreted by the embryo and endometrium stimulates PGE2/EP2 to increase the secretion of P4 and inhibits PGFS and CRB1, enzymes involved in the synthesis of PGF2α, an antagonist of PGE2. **b** In endometrial cells with EP2 receptors, PGE2 stimulates the expression of CXCR4 via the EGFR-PI3K/ERK1/2 pathway. CXCR4 is bound by the chemokine CXCL12, which is secreted by the embryo. PGE2 also stimulates the EGFR-PI3K/ERK1/2 pathway to induce the expression of genes involved in cell proliferation, differentiation and uterine receptivity

CXCR4 receptors in the endometrium [99], and the chemokine CXCL12 was identified in blastocysts [100].

PGE2 secreted by the embryo [101] binds to EP2 receptors in the endometrium to stimulate CXCR4 via the epidermal growth factor receptor (EGFR)-phosphatidyl inositol-3 kinase (PI3K) and extracellular signal-regulated kinase (ERK1/2) pathways [102]. The EGFR, PI3K and ERK1/2 pathways were shown to mediate early embryo implantation by inducing the expression of genes involved in cell growth, differentiation and uterine receptivity [103–105]. Moreover, high levels of CXCR4 expression were found in endometrium stromal cells at the apposition site of the embryo during the implantation window [106]. Furthermore, the PI3K/ERK1/2 pathways are known as pro-survival pathways that enhance the growth, proliferation, differentiation and survival of embryonic and endometrial cells [107]. We hypothesize that PGE2 secreted by embryos influences the apposition, adhesion and invasion of trophoblastic cells to the decidua by stimulating the expression of the chemokine CXCR4 receptor at the implantation site via the EP2, EGFR, PI3K and ERK1/2 pathways and/or by stimulating the synthesis of the chemokine CXCL12, which in turn will bind to CXCR4 receptors. In addition, we suggest that PGE2 uses the PI3K/ERK1/2 pathways to promote embryonic growth, proliferation, differentiation and survival, as well as endometrial cell growth, proliferation and differentiation in decidual cells.

The above findings indicate that PGE2 is essential for enhancing pre-implantation embryo development and early implantation. However, other mechanisms need to be further investigated (Fig. 5b).

Conclusion

This review explored the involvement of PGE2 in cumulus cell expansion and meiotic maturation; in these processes, PGE2 either mediates LH signaling or directly acts on EGFs, such as Areg and Ereg, and matrix forming and stabilizing factors, such as *Has2* and *Tnfaip6*. PGE2 production in the oviduct reduces cumulus ECM viscosity around the oocyte for sperm penetration, protects the sperm from the phagocytic activity of neutrophils and enhances sperm survival, binding capacity, motility and function to promote successful fertilization. In addition, the effects of PGE2 on embryo development to a blastocyst, hatching and successfully implantation were demonstrated through the maintenance of luteal function and the induction and stimulation of chemokines for trophoblast proliferation, apposition and adhesion to the maternal decidua.

We suggest that in clinical practice, the administration of non-steroidal anti-inflammatory drugs, which are inhibitors of PGE2 synthesis, should be reasonable and limited in infertile women. Additionally, assessments of PGE2 protein and receptor expression levels should be taken into consideration in infertile women. However, we recommend more studies on the mechanisms of PGE2 in female reproduction and randomized clinical trials to draw definite conclusions to support this hypothesis.

Abbreviations

AC: Adenylate cyclase; Areg: Amphiregulin; cAMP: Cyclic adenosine monophospate; CBR1: Carbonyl reductase 1; CCL2: Chemokine ligand 2; CCL7: Chemokine ligand 7; CCR: Chemokine receptor; COX: Cyclo-oxygenase; CXCL12: Chemokine 12; CXCR4: Chemokine receptor type 4; E2: Estradiol; ECM: Cumulus extracellular matrix; EGF: Epidermal growth factor; EGFR: Epidermal growth factor receptor; EP2: Prostaglandin E2 receptor type 2; EP4: Prostaglandin E2 receptor type 4; Ereg: Epiregulin; ERK1/2: Extracellular-regulated kinase 1and 2; FSH: Follicle stimulating hormone; Has2: Hyaluronan synthase 2; hCG: Human chorionic gonadotropin; IFN-t: Interferon-tau; IL-1β: Interleukin-1 beta; LH: Luteinizing hormone; MAPK3/1: Mitogen-activated protein kinases 3 and 1; NETs: Neutrophil extracellular traps; NO: Nitric oxide; OS: Oxide synthase; P4: Progesterone; PG: Prostaglandin; PGE2: Prostaglandin E2; PGF2α: Prostaglandin F2 alfa; PGFS: Prostaglandin F2 alfa synthase; PGT: Prostaglandin transport; PI3K: Phosphatidyl inositol-3 kinase; PKB: Protein kinase B; PTGS: Prostaglandin synthase; Tnaif6: Tumor necrosis factor α-induced protein 6

Authors' contributions

JDN and HC were involved in the conception and design of the study, data acquisition, analysis and manuscript drafting. JDN and WX were involved with data acquisition and analysis. All authors read and approved the final manuscript.

Competing interests

The authors declare that they have no competing interests.

References

1. Jabbour HN, Sales KJ. Prostaglandin receptor signalling and function in human endometrial pathology. Trends Endocrinol Metab. 2004;15(8):398–404.
2. Kang J, et al. Expression of human prostaglandin transporter in the human endometrium across the menstrual cycle. J Clin Endocrinol Metab. 2005; 90(4):2308–13.
3. Sugimoto Y, Inazumi T, Tsuchiya S. Roles of prostaglandin receptors in female reproduction. J Biochem. 2015;157(2):73–80.
4. Helliwell RJ, Adams LF, Mitchell MD. Prostaglandin synthases: recent developments and a novel hypothesis. Prostaglandins Leukot Essent Fatty Acids. 2004;70(2):101–13.
5. Seo MJ, Oh DK. Prostaglandin synthases: molecular characterization and involvement in prostaglandin biosynthesis. Prog Lipid Res. 2017; 66:50–68.
6. Fujino H, Xu W, Regan JW. Prostaglandin E2 induced functional expression of early growth response factor-1 by EP4, but not EP2, prostanoid receptors via the phosphatidylinositol 3-kinase and extracellular signal-regulated kinases. J Biol Chem. 2003;278(14):12151–6.
7. Hizaki H, et al. Abortive expansion of the cumulus and impaired fertility in mice lacking the prostaglandin E receptor subtype EP(2). Proc Natl Acad Sci U S A. 1999;96(18):10501–6.
8. Lim H, et al. Multiple female reproductive failures in cyclooxygenase 2-deficient mice. Cell. 1997;91(2):197–208.
9. Chakraborty I, et al. Developmental expression of the cyclo-oxygenase-1 and cyclo-oxygenase-2 genes in the peri-implantation mouse uterus and their differential regulation by the blastocyst and ovarian steroids. J Mol Endocrinol. 1996;16(2):107–22.
10. Matsumoto H, et al. Diversification of cyclooxygenase-2-derived prostaglandins in ovulation and implantation. Biol Reprod. 2001;64(5):1557–65.
11. Amsterdam A, Rotmensch S. Structure-function relationships during granulosa cell differentiation. Endocr Rev. 1987;8(3):309–37.
12. Peng XR, et al. Localization of luteinizing hormone receptor messenger ribonucleic acid expression in ovarian cell types during follicle development and ovulation. Endocrinology. 1991;129(6):3200–7.
13. Amsterdam A, Rotmensch S, Ben-Ze'ev A. Coordinated regulation of morphological and biochemical differentiation in a steroidogenic cell: the granulosa cell model. Trends Biochem Sci. 1989;14(9):377–82.
14. Sirois J, et al. Cyclooxygenase-2 and its role in ovulation: a 2004 account. Hum Reprod Update. 2004;10(5):373–85.
15. Duffy DM, Stouffer RL. Follicular administration of a cyclooxygenase inhibitor can prevent oocyte release without alteration of normal luteal function in rhesus monkeys. Hum Reprod. 2002;17(11):2825–31.
16. Duffy DM, Stouffer RL. The ovulatory gonadotrophin surge stimulates cyclooxygenase expression and prostaglandin production by the monkey follicle. Mol Hum Reprod. 2001;7(8):731–9.
17. Murdoch WJ, Hansen TR, McPherson LA. A review–role of eicosanoids in vertebrate ovulation. Prostaglandins. 1993;46(2):85–115.
18. Duffy DM, Dozier BL, Seachord CL. Prostaglandin dehydrogenase and prostaglandin levels in periovulatory follicles: implications for control of primate ovulation by prostaglandin E2. J Clin Endocrinol Metab. 2005; 90(2):1021–7.
19. Ochsner SA, et al. Decreased expression of tumor necrosis factor-alpha-stimulated gene 6 in cumulus cells of the cyclooxygenase-2 and EP2 null mice. Endocrinology. 2003;144(3):1008–19.
20. Park JY, et al. EGF-like growth factors as mediators of LH action in the ovulatory follicle. Science. 2004;303(5658):682–4.
21. Liu Z, et al. Targeted disruption of Mapk14 (p38MAPKalpha) in granulosa cells and cumulus cells causes cell-specific changes in gene expression profiles that rescue COC expansion and maintain fertility. Mol Endocrinol. 2010;24(9):1794–804.
22. Fulop C, et al. Impaired cumulus mucification and female sterility in tumor necrosis factor-induced protein-6 deficient mice. Development. 2003; 130(10):2253–61.
23. Ben-Ami I, et al. PGE2 up-regulates EGF-like growth factor biosynthesis in human granulosa cells: new insights into the coordination between PGE2 and LH in ovulation. Mol Hum Reprod. 2006;12(10):593–9.
24. Fan HY, et al. MAPK3/1 (ERK1/2) in ovarian granulosa cells are essential for female fertility. Science. 2009;324(5929):938–41.
25. Prochazka R, Blaha M, Nemcova L. Signaling pathways regulating FSH- and amphiregulin-induced meiotic resumption and cumulus cell expansion in the pig. Reproduction. 2012;144(5):535–46.

26. Blaha M, et al. Prostaglandin E2 stimulates the expression of cumulus expansion-related genes in pigs: the role of protein kinase B. Prostaglandins Other Lipid Mediat. 2017;130:38–46.
27. Yamashita Y, et al. Positive feedback loop between prostaglandin E2 and EGF-like factors is essential for sustainable activation of MAPK3/1 in cumulus cells during in vitro maturation of porcine cumulus oocyte complexes. Biol Reprod. 2011;85(5):1073–82.
28. Downs SM, Hunzicker-Dunn M. Differential regulation of oocyte maturation and cumulus expansion in the mouse oocyte-cumulus cell complex by site-selective analogs of cyclic adenosine monophosphate. Dev Biol. 1995;172(1):72–85.
29. Segi E, et al. Expression of messenger RNA for prostaglandin E receptor subtypes EP4/EP2 and cyclooxygenase isozymes in mouse periovulatory follicles and oviducts during superovulation. Biol Reprod. 2003;68(3):804–11.
30. Sugimoto Y, Narumiya S, Ichikawa A. Distribution and function of prostanoid receptors: studies from knockout mice. Prog Lipid Res. 2000;39(4):289–314.
31. Narumiya S, FitzGerald GA. Genetic and pharmacological analysis of prostanoid receptor function. J Clin Invest. 2001;108(1):25–30.
32. Duffy DM, et al. Mammalian oocytes are targets for prostaglandin E2 (PGE2) action. Reprod Biol Endocrinol. 2010;8:131.
33. Takahashi T, et al. Cyclooxygenase-2-derived prostaglandin E(2) directs oocyte maturation by differentially influencing multiple signaling pathways. J Biol Chem. 2006;281(48):37117–29.
34. Gordo AC, et al. Mitogen activated protein kinase plays a significant role in metaphase II arrest, spindle morphology, and maintenance of maturation promoting factor activity in bovine oocytes. Mol Reprod Dev. 2001;59(1): 106–14.
35. Sun QY, et al. Regulation of mitogen-activated protein kinase phosphorylation, microtubule organization, chromatin behavior, and cell cycle progression by protein phosphatases during pig oocyte maturation and fertilization in vitro. Biol Reprod. 2002;66(3):580–8.
36. Nuttinck F, et al. PTGS2-related PGE2 affects oocyte MAPK phosphorylation and meiosis progression in cattle: late effects on early embryonic development. Biol Reprod. 2011;84(6):1248–57.
37. Li YH, et al. Localization of angiotensin II in pig ovary and its effects on oocyte maturation in vitro. Theriogenology. 2004;61(2):447–59.
38. Giometti IC, et al. Angiotensin II reverses the inhibitory action produced by theca cells on bovine oocyte nuclear maturation. Theriogenology. 2005; 63(4):1014–25.
39. Barreta MH, et al. Evidence that the effect of angiotensin II on bovine oocyte nuclear maturation is mediated by prostaglandins E2 and F2alpha. Reproduction. 2008;136(6):733–40.
40. Siqueira LC, et al. Angiotensin II, progesterone, and prostaglandins are sequential steps in the pathway to bovine oocyte nuclear maturation. Theriogenology. 2012;77(9):1779–87.
41. Ferreira R, et al. The role of angiotensin II in the early stages of bovine ovulation. Reproduction. 2007;134(5):713–9.
42. Yerushalmi GM, et al. The prostaglandin transporter (PGT) as a potential mediator of ovulation. Sci Transl Med. 2016;8(338):338ra68.
43. Furman A, et al. Culture of human granulosa cells from an in vitro fertilization program: effects of extracellular matrix on morphology and cyclic adenosine 3',5' monophosphate production. Fertil Steril. 1986;46(3):514–7.
44. Breyer RM, et al. Prostanoid receptors: subtypes and signaling. Annu Rev Pharmacol Toxicol. 2001;41:661–90.
45. Freimann S, et al. Differential expression of genes coding for EGF-like factors and ADAMTS1 following gonadotropin stimulation in normal and transformed human granulosa cells. Biochem Biophys Res Commun. 2005; 333(3):935–43.
46. Freimann S, et al. EGF-like factor epiregulin and amphiregulin expression is regulated by gonadotropins/cAMP in human ovarian follicular cells. Biochem Biophys Res Commun. 2004;324(2):829–34.
47. Richards JS, et al. Ovulation: new dimensions and new regulators of the inflammatory-like response. Annu Rev Physiol. 2002;64:69–92.
48. Buccione R, et al. FSH-induced expansion of the mouse cumulus oophorus in vitro is dependent upon a specific factor(s) secreted by the oocyte. Dev Biol. 1990;138(1):16–25.
49. Tamba S, et al. Timely interaction between prostaglandin and chemokine signaling is a prerequisite for successful fertilization. Proc Natl Acad Sci U S A. 2008;105(38):14539–44.
50. Yodoi R, et al. RhoA/rho kinase signaling in the cumulus mediates extracellular matrix assembly. Endocrinology. 2009;150(7):3345–52.
51. Isobe T, et al. The effect of RANTES on human sperm chemotaxis. Hum Reprod. 2002;17(6):1441–6.
52. Tamba S, et al. Expression profiling of cumulus cells reveals functional changes during ovulation and central roles of prostaglandin EP2 receptor in cAMP signaling. Biochimie. 2010;92(6):665–75.
53. Sica A, et al. Monocyte chemotactic and activating factor gene expression induced in endothelial cells by IL-1 and tumor necrosis factor. J Immunol. 1990;144(8):3034–8.
54. Reinecker HC, et al. Monocyte-chemoattractant protein 1 gene expression in intestinal epithelial cells and inflammatory bowel disease mucosa. Gastroenterology. 1995;108(1):40–50.
55. Dahm-Kahler P, et al. Monocyte chemotactic protein-1 in the follicle of the menstrual and IVF cycle. Mol Hum Reprod. 2006;12(1):1–6.
56. Mosher AA, et al. Prostaglandin E2 represses interleukin 1 beta-induced inflammatory mediator output from pregnant human myometrial cells through the EP2 and EP4 receptors. Biol Reprod. 2012;87(1):7. 1-10
57. Kaeoket K, Persson E, Dalin AM. Influence of pre-ovulatory insemination and early pregnancy on the infiltration by cells of the immune system in the sow endometrium. Anim Reprod Sci. 2003;75(1–2):55–71.
58. Tremellen KP, Seamark RF, Robertson SA. Seminal transforming growth factor beta1 stimulates granulocyte-macrophage colony-stimulating factor production and inflammatory cell recruitment in the murine uterus. Biol Reprod. 1998;58(5):1217–25.
59. Troedsson MH, Liu IK, Crabo BG. Sperm transport and survival in the mare: a review. Theriogenology. 1998;50(5):807–18.
60. Alghamdi A, et al. Uterine secretion from mares with post-breeding endometritis alters sperm motion characteristics in vitro. Theriogenology. 2001;55(4):1019–28.
61. Alghamdi AS, Foster DN, Troedsson MH. Equine seminal plasma reduces sperm binding to polymorphonuclear neutrophils (PMNs) and improves the fertility of fresh semen inseminated into inflamed uteri. Reproduction. 2004; 127(5):593–600.
62. Wah RM, Anderson DJ, Hill JA. Asymptomatic cervicovaginal leukocytosis in infertile women. Fertil Steril. 1990;54(3):445–50.
63. Kalinski P. Regulation of immune responses by prostaglandin E2. J Immunol. 2012;188(1):21–8.
64. Smith RJ. Modulation of phagocytosis by and lysosomal enzyme secretion from Guinea-pig neutrophils: effect of nonsteroid anti-inflammatory agents and prostaglindins. J Pharmacol Exp Ther. 1977;200(3):647–57.
65. Aronoff DM, Canetti C, Peters-Golden M. Prostaglandin E2 inhibits alveolar macrophage phagocytosis through an E-prostanoid 2 receptor-mediated increase in intracellular cyclic AMP. J Immunol. 2004;173(1):559–65.
66. Wijayagunawardane MP, et al. Local distributions of oviductal estradiol, progesterone, prostaglandins, oxytocin and endothelin-1 in the cyclic cow. Theriogenology. 1998;49(3):607–18.
67. Kodithuwakku SP, Miyamoto A, Wijayagunawardane MP. Spermatozoa stimulate prostaglandin synthesis and secretion in bovine oviductal epithelial cells. Reproduction. 2007;133(6):1087–94.
68. Yousef MS, et al. Sperm binding to oviduct epithelial cells enhances TGFB1 and IL10 expressions in epithelial cells as well as neutrophils in vitro: prostaglandin E2 as a main regulator of anti-inflammatory response in the bovine oviduct. PLoS One. 2016;11(9):e0162309.
69. Talpain E, et al. Characterization of the PGE receptor subtype mediating inhibition of superoxide production in human neutrophils. Br J Pharmacol. 1995;114(7):1459–65.
70. Burelout C, et al. Prostaglandin E2 inhibits the phospholipase D pathway stimulated by formyl-methionyl-leucyl-phenylalanine in human neutrophils. Involvement of EP2 receptors and phosphatidylinositol 3-kinase gamma. Mol Pharmacol. 2004;66(2):293–301.
71. Alghamdi AS, Foster DN. Seminal DNase frees spermatozoa entangled in neutrophil extracellular traps. Biol Reprod. 2005;73(6):1174–81.
72. Brinkmann V, et al. Neutrophil extracellular traps kill bacteria. Science. 2004; 303(5663):1532–5.
73. Marey MA, et al. Bovine oviduct epithelial cells downregulate phagocytosis of sperm by neutrophils: prostaglandin E2 as a major physiological regulator. Reproduction. 2014;147(2):211–9.
74. Tan HN, et al. Cyclooxygenases and prostaglandin E synthases in preimplantation mouse embryos. Zygote. 2005;13(2):103–8.
75. Chan SY. Effects of prostaglandin E2 and F2 alpha on peri-implantation development of mouse embryos in vitro. Prostaglandins. 1991;42(4):321–36.
76. Sayre BL, Lewis GS. Arachidonic acid metabolism during early development of ovine embryos: a possible relationship to shedding of the zona pellucida. Prostaglandins. 1993;45(6):557–69.

77. Jabbour HN, et al. Expression of COX-2 and PGE synthase and synthesis of PGE(2)in endometrial adenocarcinoma: a possible autocrine/paracrine regulation of neoplastic cell function via EP2/EP4 receptors. Br J Cancer. 2001;85(7):1023–31.
78. Sales KJ, et al. Cyclooxygenase-2 expression and prostaglandin E(2) synthesis are up-regulated in carcinomas of the cervix: a possible autocrine/paracrine regulation of neoplastic cell function via EP2/EP4 receptors. J Clin Endocrinol Metab. 2001;86(5):2243–9.
79. Arosh JA, Banu SK, McCracken JA. Novel concepts on the role of prostaglandins on luteal maintenance and maternal recognition and establishment of pregnancy in ruminants. J Dairy Sci. 2016;99(7):5926–40.
80. Wasielak M, Kaminska K, Bogacki M. Effect of the conceptus on uterine prostaglandin-F2alpha and prostaglandin-E2 release and synthesis during the periimplantation period in the pig. Reprod Fertil Dev. 2009;21(5):709–17.
81. Weems YS, et al. Effects of prostaglandin E and F receptor agonists in vivo on luteal function in ewes. Prostaglandins Other Lipid Mediat. 2010; 92(1–4):67–72.
82. Ashley RL, Arreguin-Arevalo JA, Nett TM. Binding characteristics of the ovine membrane progesterone receptor alpha and expression of the receptor during the estrous cycle. Reprod Biol Endocrinol. 2009;7:42.
83. Nett TM, Niswender GD. Luteal blood flow and receptors for LH during PGF2 alpha-induced luteolysis: production of PGE2 and PGF2 alpha during early pregnancy. Acta Vet Scand Suppl. 1981;77:117–30.
84. Ford SP. Control of blood flow to the gravid uterus of domestic livestock species. J Anim Sci. 1995;73(6):1852–60.
85. Hristovska AM, et al. Prostaglandin E2 induces vascular relaxation by E-prostanoid 4 receptor-mediated activation of endothelial nitric oxide synthase. Hypertension. 2007;50(3):525–30.
86. Asselin E, Bazer FW, Fortier MA. Recombinant ovine and bovine interferons tau regulate prostaglandin production and oxytocin response in cultured bovine endometrial cells. Biol Reprod. 1997;56(2):402–8.
87. Guzeloglu A, Michel F, Thatcher WW. Differential effects of interferon-tau on the prostaglandin synthetic pathway in bovine endometrial cells treated with phorbol ester. J Dairy Sci. 2004;87(7):2032–41.
88. Geisert RD, et al. Embryonic steroids and the establishment of pregnancy in pigs. J Reprod Fertil Suppl. 1990;40:293–305.
89. Spencer TE, Bazer FW. Conceptus signals for establishment and maintenance of pregnancy. Reprod Biol Endocrinol. 2004;2:49.
90. Almog B, et al. Promoting implantation by local injury to the endometrium. Fertil Steril. 2010;94(6):2026–9.
91. Waclawik A, et al. Molecular cloning and spatiotemporal expression of prostaglandin F synthase and microsomal prostaglandin E synthase-1 in porcine endometrium. Endocrinology. 2006;147(1):210–21.
92. Waclawik A, Ziecik AJ. Differential expression of prostaglandin (PG) synthesis enzymes in conceptus during peri-implantation period and endometrial expression of carbonyl reductase/PG 9-ketoreductase in the pig. J Endocrinol. 2007;194(3):499–510.
93. Waclawik A, et al. Estradiol-17beta, prostaglandin E2 (PGE2), and the PGE2 receptor are involved in PGE2 positive feedback loop in the porcine endometrium. Endocrinology. 2009;150(8):3823–32.
94. Ghosh D, et al. Porcine carbonyl reductase. Structural basis for a functional monomer in short chain dehydrogenases/reductases. J Biol Chem. 2001; 276(21):18457–63.
95. Ashworth MD, et al. Expression of porcine endometrial prostaglandin synthase during the estrous cycle and early pregnancy, and following endocrine disruption of pregnancy. Biol Reprod. 2006;74(6):1007–15.
96. Blitek A, et al. Expression of cyclooxygenase-1 and -2 in the porcine endometrium during the oestrous cycle and early pregnancy. Reprod Domest Anim. 2006;41(3):251–7.
97. Hoggatt J, et al. Prostaglandin E2 enhances hematopoietic stem cell homing, survival, and proliferation. Blood. 2009;113(22):5444–55.
98. Katoh H, et al. COX-2 and prostaglandin EP3/EP4 signaling regulate the tumor stromal proangiogenic microenvironment via CXCL12-CXCR4 chemokine systems. Am J Pathol. 2010;176(3):1469–83.
99. Sherwin JR, et al. Identification of novel genes regulated by chorionic gonadotropin in baboon endometrium during the window of implantation. Endocrinology. 2007;148(2):618–26.
100. Zhou WH, et al. Chemokine CXCL12 promotes the cross-talk between trophoblasts and decidual stromal cells in human first-trimester pregnancy. Hum Reprod. 2008;23(12):2669–79.
101. Weber JA, et al. Prostaglandin E2 secretion by oviductal transport-stage equine embryos. Biol Reprod. 1991;45(4):540–3.
102. Sales KJ, et al. Chorionic gonadotrophin regulates CXCR4 expression in human endometrium via E-series prostanoid receptor 2 signalling to PI3K-ERK1/2: implications for fetal-maternal crosstalk for embryo implantation. Mol Hum Reprod. 2011;17(1):22–32.
103. Sales KJ, et al. Seminal plasma activates cyclooxygenase-2 and prostaglandin E2 receptor expression and signalling in cervical adenocarcinoma cells. Mol Hum Reprod. 2002;8(12):1065–70.
104. Jabbour HN, Boddy SC. Prostaglandin E2 induces proliferation of glandular epithelial cells of the human endometrium via extracellular regulated kinase 1/2-mediated pathway. J Clin Endocrinol Metab. 2003;88(9):4481–7.
105. Banerjee P, et al. Chorionic gonadotropin regulates prostaglandin E synthase via a phosphatidylinositol 3-kinase-extracellular regulatory kinase pathway in a human endometrial epithelial cell line: implications for endometrial responses for embryo implantation. Endocrinology. 2009;150(9): 4326–37.
106. Dominguez F, et al. Hormonal and embryonic regulation of chemokine receptors CXCR1, CXCR4, CCR5 and CCR2B in the human endometrium and the human blastocyst. Mol Hum Reprod. 2003;9(4):189–98.
107. Gentilini D, et al. PI3K/Akt and ERK1/2 signalling pathways are involved in endometrial cell migration induced by 17beta-estradiol and growth factors. Mol Hum Reprod. 2007;13(5):317–22.

16

Trophoblast differentiation, invasion and hormone secretion in a three-dimensional in vitro implantation model with rhesus monkey embryos

T. Arthur Chang[1,4], Gennadiy I. Bondarenko[1,5], Behzad Gerami-Naini[1,6], Jessica G. Drenzek[1,7], Maureen Durning[1], Mark A. Garthwaite[1], Jenna Kropp Schmidt[1] and Thaddeus G. Golos[1,2,3*]

Abstract

Background: The initiation of primate embryo invasion into the endometrium and the formation of the placenta from trophoblasts, fetal mesenchyme, and vascular components are essential for the establishment of a successful pregnancy. The mechanisms which direct morphogenesis of the chorionic villi, and the interactions between trophectoderm-derived trophoblasts and the fetal mesenchyme to direct these processes during placentation are not well understood due to a dearth of systems to examine and manipulate real-time primate implantation. Here we describe an in vitro three-dimensional (3-D) model to study implantation which utilized IVF-generated rhesus monkey embryos cultured in a Matrigel explant system.

Methods: Blastocyst stage embryos were embedded in a 3-D microenvironment of a Matrigel carrier and co-cultured with a feeder layer of cells generating conditioned medium. Throughout the course of embryo co-culture embryo growth and secretions were monitored. Embedded embryos were then sectioned and stained for markers of trophoblast function and differentiation.

Results: Signs of implantation were observed including enlargement of the embryo mass, and invasion and proliferation of trophoblast outgrowths. Expression of chorionic gonadotropin defined by immunohistochemical staining, and secretion of chorionic gonadotropin and progesterone coincident with the appearance of trophoblast outgrowths, supported the conclusion that a trophoblast cell lineage formed from implanted embryos. Positive staining for selected markers including Ki67, MHC class I, NeuN, CD31, vonWillebrand Factor and Vimentin, suggest growth and differentiation of the embryo following embedding.

Conclusions: This 3-D in vitro system will facilitate further study of primate embryo biology, with potential to provide a platform for study of genes related to implantation defects and trophoblast differentiation.

Keywords: Embryo, Implantation, Trophoblast, Non-human primate

* Correspondence: golos@primate.wisc.edu
[1]Wisconsin National Primate Research Center, University of Wisconsin-Madison, 1223 Capitol Court, Madison, Wisconsin 53715-1299, USA
[2]Department of Comparative Biosciences, School of Veterinary Medicine, University of Wisconsin-Madison, Madison, WI, USA
Full list of author information is available at the end of the article

Background

Implantation is a crucial developmental event for establishing a pregnancy. The central events to implantation are the apposition of the blastocyst to the uterine epithelium, adhesion of the embryo to the uterus, followed by the penetration and invasion of trophoblast cells into the uterine stroma [1]. Abnormal implantation of an embryo is an underlying cause of infertility and has implications in development of placenta-associated pathologies including preclampsia and intrauterine growth restriction. The understanding of the mechanisms driving the key events of human implantation, particularly those that lead to placental pathologies, remains unclear. Given the ethical constraints in assessing human implantation in vivo, animal models and in vitro platforms are needed to study mechanisms underlying the establishment of pregnancy.

Current in vitro models of human implantation mimic interactions between the embryo and endometrium, as reviewed by Hohn and Denker [2] and Weimar et al. [3], however, these models focus on a specific stage of implantation rather than fully recapitulating the entire process. Human in vitro implantation models are comprised of either a human embryo or an embryo surrogate, such as trophoblast spheroids, positioned above either a layer of endometrial stromal and/or epithelial cells, or alternatively, a synthetic basement membrane [3–6]. Although these models garnered valuable knowledge on trophoblast attachment [6–8], migration [9], invasion [4] and molecular interactions at the interface [9, 10], there are also limitations to these models. There are few studies utilizing human embryos due to the ethical constraints surrounding their use. As a substitute, embryo surrogates, such as trophoblast spheroids, derived from immortal cell lines have been utilized to evaluate attachment, invasion and migration [6, 7, 11, 12]. These models are also limited to studying a specific event during implantation and lack a complete representation of all cell types present at the maternal-fetal interface, including immune cells, thus further development of in vitro implantation models that better simulate in vivo implantation are needed.

Animal models are particularly effective for studying implantation both in vivo and in vitro [1, 13], and bypass the challenges posed by human models. However, the degree of penetration and invasion of the embryo into the uterus varies greatly across species [1]. When considering a rodent model, mouse models are useful for assessing genes and gene networks involved in implantation, however, placental organization and the invasion of trophoblasts into the uterine epithelium is relatively shallow in comparison to the human. The placentation and endovascular invasion of the human is more closely paralleled in non-human primates including the great apes, baboons and macaques [13, 14]. Despite the high cost of maintaining primate colonies in comparison to rodents, the use of assisted reproductive technologies can be implemented to increase the number of embryos produced by a single animal. In vitro studies of blastocyst formation in the marmoset [15–17], baboon [18], rhesus monkey [19–21] and human [22] demonstrated the feasibility of embryonic development to the blastocyst stage in vitro following IVF. Such studies also showed that in vitro cultured preimplantation primate embryos could produce chorionic gonadotrophin (CG) [23–25] and syncytiotrophoblast-like cells when cultured beyond the time of normal implantation [18, 24, 26]. This supports the possibility that extended primate embryo culture, under appropriate conditions, could provide a paradigm for development of new approaches to study mechanisms underlying primate peri-implantation development.

A central feature to developing an in vitro model of embryo implantation is creating a microenvironment that supports development similar to that observed in vivo. Three-dimensional culture systems may create a better microenvironment, including an extracellular matrix (ECM) that supports adhesion and regulates cellular proliferation and differentiation [27, 28]. When considering a three-dimensional (3-D) in vivo implantation scenario [29–32], extrapolating results from 2-D models to the physiological situation are likely to be simplistic. In a previous study by Gerami-Naini et al. [33], significant differences between embryoid bodies derived from human embryonic stem cells cultured in 2-D and 3-D systems were observed in the maintenance of a differential trophoblast phenotype, as defined by CG and progesterone secretion. Moreover, that study reported substantial outgrowth of trophoblasts into Matrigel (MG), coincident with elevated CG secretion. Based on this study, we have adopted a 3-D model to study primate embryo development in vitro. The current study presented demonstrates that an in vitro 3-D environment can promote non-human primate embryo development that manifests characteristics of in vivo implantation and pregnancy initiation. Overall, the 3-D implantation model builds on knowledge obtained from traditional 2-D culture environments, and provides a platform to study effects and impact of various growth factors or experimental conditions thought to be critical for the local support of implantation.

Methods

In vitro production of rhesus monkey embryos

Rhesus monkeys (*Macaca mulatta*) were from the colony maintained at the Wisconsin National Primate Research Center. All procedures were performed in accordance with the NIH Guide for the Care and Use of Laboratory Animals and under the approval of the University of Wisconsin Graduate School Animal Care and Use Committee. In vitro production of rhesus macaque embryos was carried out as previously reported by others [34–40] and are described here in brief. Rhesus macaque (*Macaca mulatta*) oocyte donors were hyperstimulated by recombinant human follicle stimulation hormone (FSH; Organon, Oss, Netherlands) 30 IU per injection twice daily for 7 days, followed by a single injection of 1000 IU human chorionic gonadotropin (hCG; Serono S.A., Geneva, Switzerland) on day 8. Cumulus-oocyte complexes were retrieved by laparoscopic follicular aspiration 27–30 h after hCG administration and placed in TL-Hepes medium containing 0.3% bovine serum albumin at 37 °C. Aspirated contents were filtered through an EmCon filter (Veterinary Concepts, Spring Valley, WI) and immediately washed with TL-Hepes media containing hyaluronidase (1 mg/ml). Oocytes were stripped of residual cumulus cells by mechanical pipetting, and placed 10 per 50 μl drop of CMRL-1066 media, supplemented with 20% fetal bovine serum, 0.5 mM sodium pyruvate, 2 mM l-alanyl-l-glutamine, until fertilization. Prior to fertilization, semen was collected from male rhesus monkey donors, washed and capacitated in TL-based capacitation medium (containing 0.1% sodium Pyruvate, 0.01% Polyvinyl alcohol) covered by mineral oil prior to fertilization. Matured oocytes and capacitated sperm were moved to TL-based IVF medium containing 0.5% sodium pyruvate, 1.0% glutamine and 0.01% PVA for fertilization. Fertilized embryos were cultured to the 8-cell stage at 37 °C in 5% CO_2, 5% O_2, and 90% N_2 in chemically defined, protein-free hamster embryo culture medium-9 (HECM-9) media [38, 41, 42] supplemented with amino acids. Embryos at the 8-cell stage were selected and transferred to fresh plates of HECM-9 supplemented with amino acids and 5% fetal bovine serum (FBS; HyClone, Logan, UT) with medium changed every other day. Embryos were cultured for a maximum of 9 days at which point blastocyst stage embryos were embedded into a Matrigel (MG) raft for extended culture.

Preparation of Matrigel rafts and extended embryo culture

As previously described by Gerami-Naini et al. [33], dome-shaped, growth factor-reduced MG (BD-Biosciences, Bedford, MA) carriers were formed by initially pipetting 50–60 μl MG onto sterile glass cover slides, followed by sequential pipetting of additional 30 μl volumes of MG, within 5 min intervals to allow for the previous layer to solidify. Embryos at the morula and blastocyst stages (6 to 8 days post insemination) were transferred by a micropipettor and embedded into the MG raft. A feeder layer of Buffalo Liver Rat (BRL) cells were plated onto the bottom of 35 mm 6-well dishes and cultured for 1 day prior to receiving embryo rafts to establish a conditioned culture environment. Each MG raft containing 1 embryo was placed into one 35 mm well containing BRL-conditioned media and the feeder layer cells (Additional file 1). Morphological assessment of embryo development was performed included the time of hatching, initiation of MG invasion and outgrowth, sizes and shape of outgrowth and changes of outgrowth proliferation, and degradation of outgrowths. Photomicrographic images were captured using a Leica DMIRB microscope and MagnaFire software. Media were collected every 3 days for hormone assays, and the rafts were transferred to fresh feeder dishes at the same time. Collected media were briefly centrifuged and the supernatants were stored at – 20°C until hormone assays were performed. While most embryos were terminated by the end of the third week of culture, some embryos were maintained for up to 45 days in MG.

Hormone assays

Levels of CG in the conditioned embryo media samples were determined by Leydig cell bioassay as previously described [43]. The minimum detectable level was 10 pg of hCG/tube, and the intraassay and interassay coefficients of variation were 5.34% and 9.77% respectively. Progesterone secretion was determined by enzyme immunoassay [44–46]. All hormone determinations were made on duplicate samples.

Immunohistochemistry (IHC)

For histological and IHC analyses, MG-embedded embryos were removed from cover slips at various time points with minimal amount of MG carry over, fixed for 2 h in 2% paraformaldehyde, washed 3 times in PBS, then covered by 1% agarose warmed to 48°C. Agarose containing the MG-embedded embryo was rapidly cooled by placement on ice, dehydrated and embedded in paraffin. Trimmed blocks containing an embryo were sectioned at 5 μm for IHC staining procedures. For CD31 and MHC class I IHC, 5 μm paraffin sections were treated with proteinase K as previously described [33, 47]; for all other IHC experiments, sections were boiled in a microwave oven using sodium citrate buffer (pH 6.0) [33, 47]. Antibodies are listed in Additional file 2. Negative controls were isotype-matched rabbit or mouse IgG (Sigma), at the same concentration as the specific primary antibodies. Endogenous peroxidase activity was quenched using 5% hydrogen peroxide in methanol for 20 min, and sections were blocked by incubation for 30 min with 20% horse serum in 4% TBS/Triton X-100. Positive immunostaining was visualized using an ABC Peroxidase Kit (Vector Labs, Burlingame, CA) and freshly prepared Nova Red substrate (Vector Labs). Sections were counterstained with hematoxylin, mounted in organic mount Cytoseal XYL (both from Richard-Allan Scientific, Kalamazoo, MI), and analyzed by light microscopy.

Results

Morphological observations of embryo development

Embryonic escape from the zona pellucida, or hatching, is a critical step required for implantation and further differentiation and development. In initial experiments, we determined whether embryos transferred and embedded into a "raft", prepared from a 100 μl drop of MG, at the zona-enclosed blastocyst stage were capable of hatching from the zona pellucida. Embryos were morphologically evaluated following embedding in the raft. Embryos that successfully hatched routinely displayed growth of the embryonic mass and outgrowth of cells into the MG, whereas those that did not complete hatching failed to further develop. Representative images of the development of 16 rhesus embryos embedded into MG are shown in Figs. 1, 2 and 4. In pilot experiments, embryos transferred into MG at the zona-enclosed morula or earlier stages did not hatch within the MG; hence no further development was observed. This is not unexpected since embryo implantation does not occur at the morula stage of development. Morula stage embryos that had the zona pellucida removed in vitro and were then embedded into MG likewise did not progress into blastocyst and develop outgrowths (not shown), while blastocysts that underwent assisted hatching continued to develop. Zona-intact blastocysts that received assisted hatching prior to implantation into the MG rafts, developed outgrowth protrusions in the MG, similar to their spontaneously hatched counterparts. Therefore, assisted hatching was applied to all embryos prior to implantation into the MG rafts in subsequent experiments to provide a consistent experimental paradigm.

The initiation of invasion by embryo-derived cells was heralded as a visible spherical enlargement of the embryo mass and a thickened layer of trophectoderm observed after zona escape was completed (Fig. 2b,c). Within the first week post-embedding, the diameter of the embryo mass increased by two to three-fold greater than the hatching stage. This spherical enlargement, accompanied by a thicker layer of cells, putatively derived from the trophectoderm of the blastocyst, was a strong indicator of future development of outgrowths. In addition, the formation of "cystic" structures inside the embryo or appearing at the surface of the embryonic trophectoderm layer was noted (Additional file 3A). Formation of the "cystic" appearing structures began by the end of the first week post-embedding, continued to enlarge during the early stages of protrusion growth, and was retained while further trophoblast outgrowth continued (Fig. 2c; Additional file 3B). The specific identity of cells involved in formation of these cystic structures remains to be defined.

Embryos which successfully expanded typically progressed to show varied levels of development of extraembryonic structures with significant outgrowths of a variety of morphologies, including elongated branches, as well as dense shell-like cellular

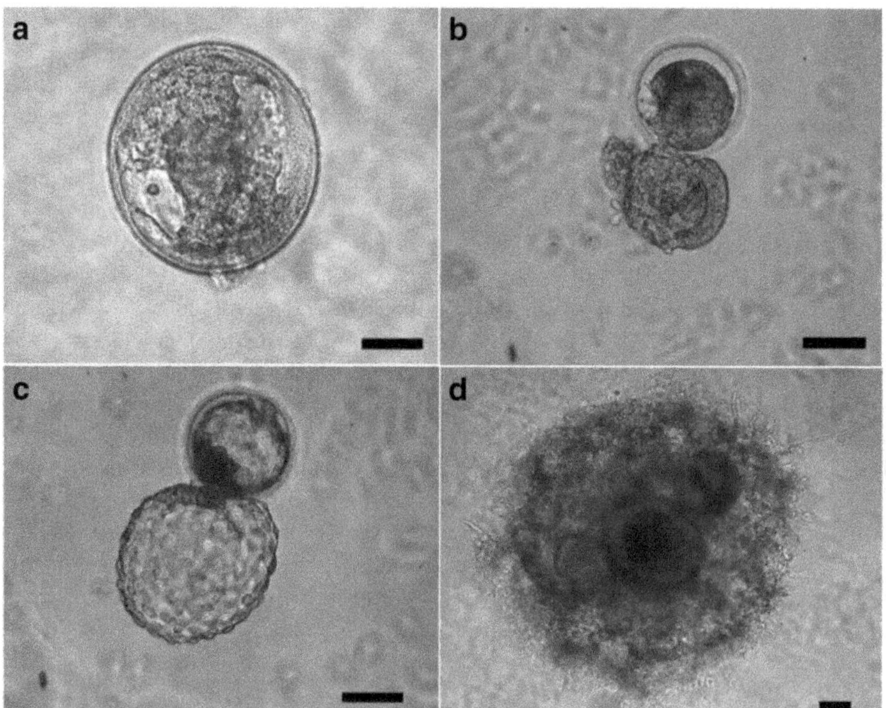

Fig. 1 Growth of Rhesus Embryos in Matrigel Rafts. Embryos that failed to hatch (**a**) or that did not completely hatch (**b**), failed to develop and degenerated. Embryos that completed hatching (**c**) continued to develop (**d**), where within 15 days post embedding trophoblast protrusions and inner cavities formed. Scale bar = 100 μm

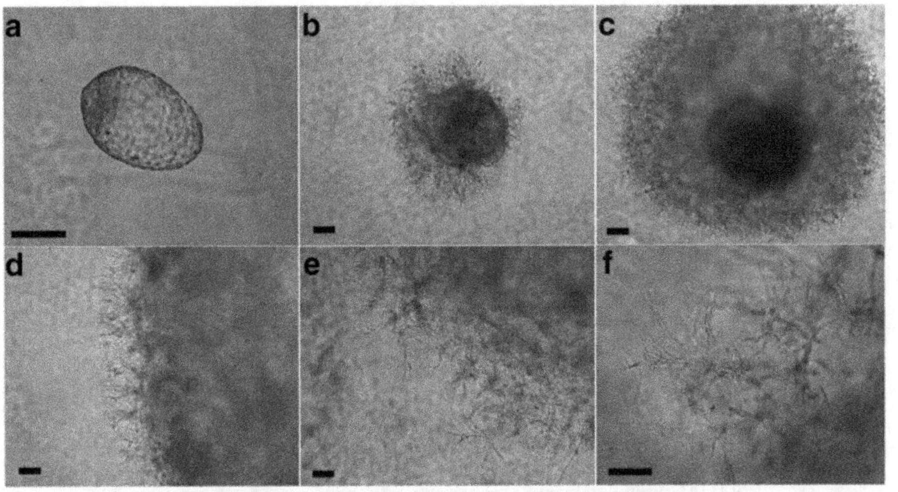

Fig. 2 Development of rhesus blastocysts embedded in Matrigel: (**a**) day 0 post embedding in Matrigel; (**b**) day 6: outgrowths and cystic structure shown; (**c**) day 14: extensive branch-like outgrowths extended from dense extraembryonic mass; (**d**) day 19; (**e**) day 26; (**f**) day 38. Over the course of development post-embedding, trophoblastic protrusions invaded into the Matrigel environment. Scale bar = 100 μm

structures (Fig. 2c, d). Approximately a week after embedding into the MG, 30% of embryos typically began to exhibit these projections (Figs. 1 and 2), which were similar in appearance to trophoblastic outgrowths observed with embryoid bodies derived from human embryonic stem cells [33]. Once initiated, the protrusions typically continue to extend and elongate throughout the culture period, with the length of the embryonic outgrowths extending to 7 mm, although heterogeneity was seen among embryos (Additional file 3). Overall, 15 of 16 embryos with trophoblastic protrusions grew through day 18, 3 were allowed to continue to day 21, and 2 progressed to day 45 at which point embryos were terminated for analysis.

Hormone secretion by cultured embryos into culture media

Culture media were evaluated for secretion by the embryo of both CG and progesterone, which are markers of primate trophoblast differentiation. As illustrated in Fig. 3, secretion of CG and progesterone was detectable in culture media from embryos within the first week post-embedding. Elevated levels of secreted CG were sometimes observed with more developmentally advanced embryos (Fig. 4). We evaluated the secretion of CG in association with embryo growth in Matrigel. Additional file 4 illustrates that there was a trend for peak CG secretion to be correlated with embryo size, however this trend was not statistically significant ($P = 0.09$). Although trophoblastic outgrowths continued to expand throughout culture, levels of CG and progesterone approached basal levels by the end of the third week of culture (Fig. 3).

Histological evaluation of ECM-cultured rhesus embryos

To distinguish cellular structures across various time points of culture, embryos were embedded in paraffin, sectioned and evaluated by hematoxylin and eosin (H&E) and IHC. Embryos terminated around day 45 post-embedding demonstrated extensive outgrowth development of invasive trophoblasts, as indicated by the bright "halo" around the embryo mass, represented in the bright field images of Fig. 5. Sections stained with H&E revealed extensive digestion of the MG environment presumably by the outgrowths expanding and migrating from the surface of the embryo (Fig. 5c). The leading edge of the outgrowths were seen to be individual cells that were migrating away from the embryo proper (Fig. 5b, c), leaving a substantially degraded MG in the vicinity of the embryo, whereas the MG distant from the embryo had a homogeneous, undisturbed, eosinophilic appearance by H&E staining.

Proliferation of embryo-derived cells was evaluated by IHC for Ki67. As the embryo progressed in development, Ki67 was extensively noted primarily in cells at the cytokeratin-positive periphery of the expanded embryonic structure (Fig. 5h), as well as in the migrating cells which had invaded into the MG, and were distant from the embryo proper (Fig. 5f-g).

Characterization of embryonic and extraembryonic differentiation was assessed by IHC of embryos terminated early and late in culture. IHC with an antibody recognizing cytokeratin 7/8 demonstrated multiple areas of epithelial differentiation, including potential trophoblast formation. Consistently, an outer layer of cytokeratin-positive cells was observed at the border of the expanded embryo (Fig. 5i, j). We also observed positive cytokeratin staining of the migrating individual cells

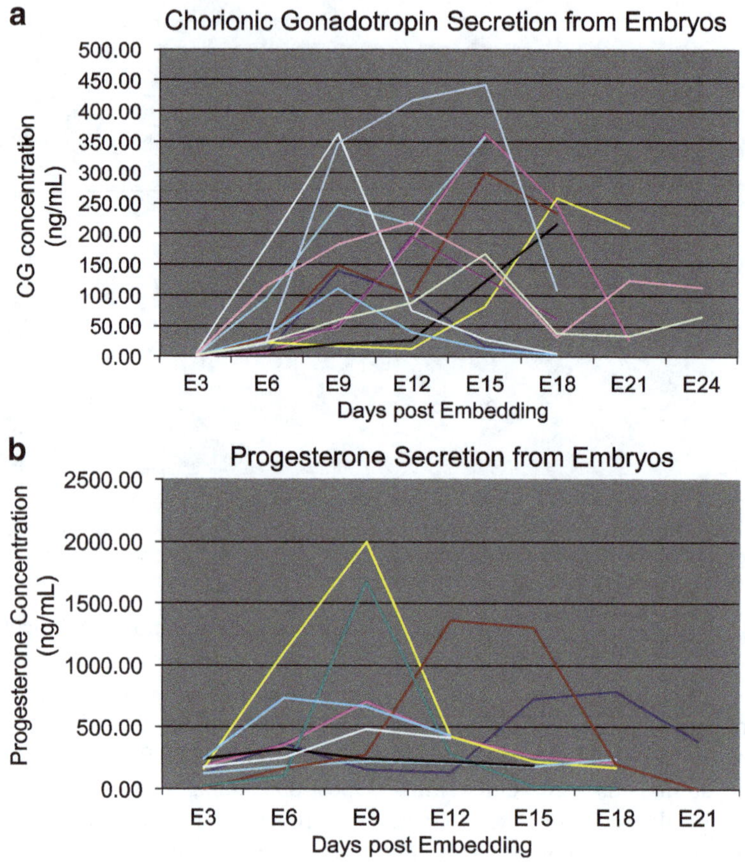

Fig. 3 Hormone secretion from embryos embedded in Matrigel and co-cultured with BRL cells: (**a**) CG, $n = 12$ and (**b**) progesterone secretion, $n = 9$. Each individual colored line represents the secretion profile from an individual embryo, where the same color between (**a**) and (**b**) represent the same embryo

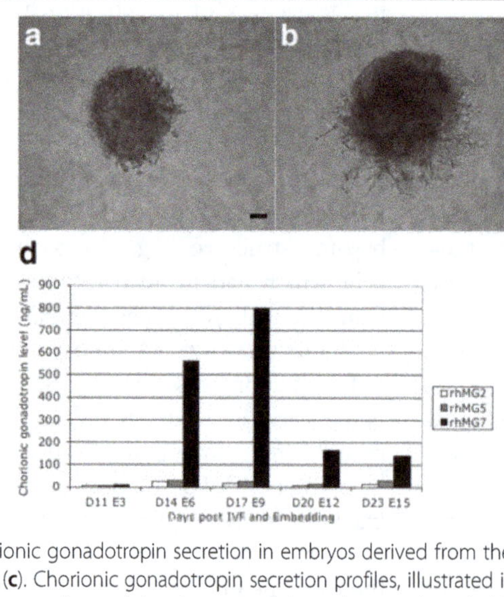

Fig. 4 Comparison of chorionic gonadotropin secretion in embryos derived from the same oocyte donor with less extensive development (**a**, **b**) or advanced development (**c**). Chorionic gonadotropin secretion profiles, illustrated in panel (**d**), from those three embryos showed higher CG secretion coincident with more advanced development of the embryo and trophoblastic shell. Scale bar = 100 μm

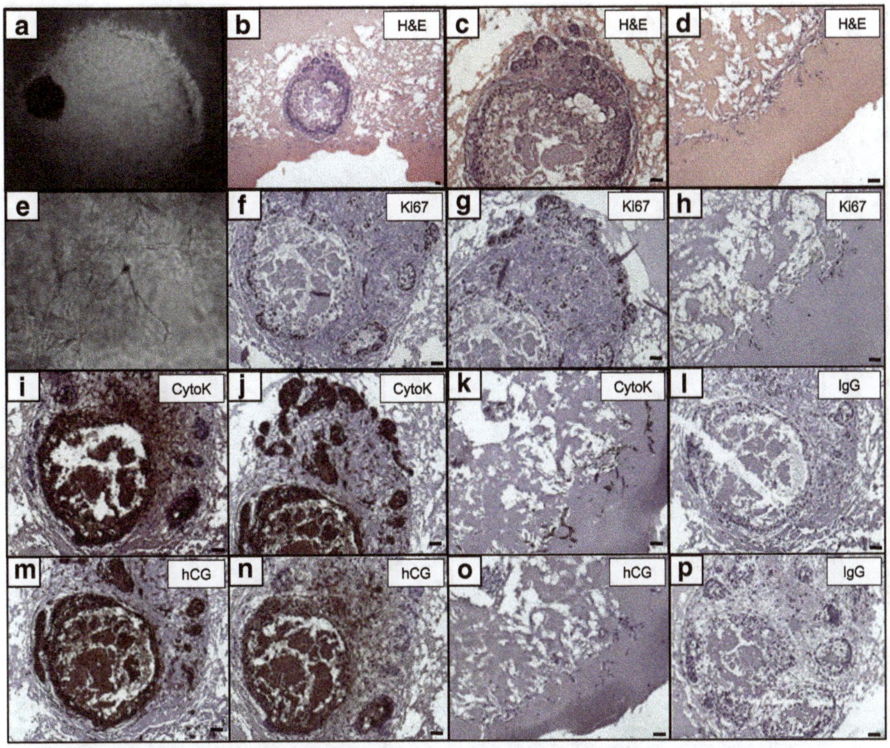

Fig. 5 Histological and immunohistochemical images of paraffin sections of embedded in vitro developed rhesus embryos: (**a**) bright field; (**b-d**) H&E; (**e**) bright field image of trophoblastic outgrowths; (**f-h**) Ki67; (**i-k**) cytokeratin (CytoK); (**l**) IgG negative control for cytokeratin; (**m-o**) CG; and (**p**) IgG negative control for CG. Results representative of 2 embryos. Scale bar = 500 μm

at the outer edge of the overall outgrowth shell (Fig. 5i, j), identifying the protrusions as trophoblast cells mimicking endometrial invasion.

Immunostaining for CG was performed to determine whether CG was expressed within the embryos. Immunostaining with antibodies against CG demonstrated that the primary localization of CG-β subunit expression was in the cytokeratin-positive layer constituting the outer surface of the embryo. As the embryo progressed in development, CG staining was positive in the embryonic structures proper as well as extraembryonic protrusions (Fig. 5m-o), including internal localization of CG within the central cavity of the embryo, which was clearly specific in comparison with staining of nonspecific control IgG (Fig. 5p) or other antibodies (Fig. 5).

To better characterize the cells which comprise the embryo at later stages of development, IHC was performed for several selected markers indicative of differentiation. Evaluation of MHC class I expression by the HC10 antibody identified MHC class I heavy chains widely expressed throughout the embryo (Fig. 6a). Neuroectoderm differentiation was also evaluated by staining with NeuN antibodies, which showed positive staining on embryonic structures (Fig. 6b). CD 31, an endothelial cell marker, and in the rhesus, a marker for differentiated trophoblasts [48], was also used to determine these cell lineages in embryos growing in MG. Staining for CD31 was apparent in the areas surrounding the villous embryonic structure, as well as part of the trophoblast shell (Fig. 6c, d). Positive staining for the endothelial marker, von Willebrand Factor (vWF), was also observed in the outer villous area and cells lining the embryonic structure (Fig. 6e, f), suggesting endothelial cell differentiation. Staining with an anti-vimentin antibody, a marker of mesenchymal cells, showed positive expression in cords of fibroblast-like cells (Fig. 6g, h). Collectively, these results demonstrate that the embryonic cells undergo differentiation, however, a more rigorous characterization is warranted in future studies.

Discussion

Here we describe an experimental platform for long term in vitro rhesus embryo culture using a novel 3-D Matrigel scaffold. Similar to in vivo implantation, extensive trophoblast migration into the extracellular, MG environment was observed. The extensive degradation of the MG at the interface with the embryo, and the migration of these cells suggests the secretion of proteolytic enzymes to facilitate migration, however this remains to be demonstrated formally. Trophoblast differentiation from embryos maintained in MG explants was demonstrated by the secretion of CG and progesterone into the culture medium, and CG

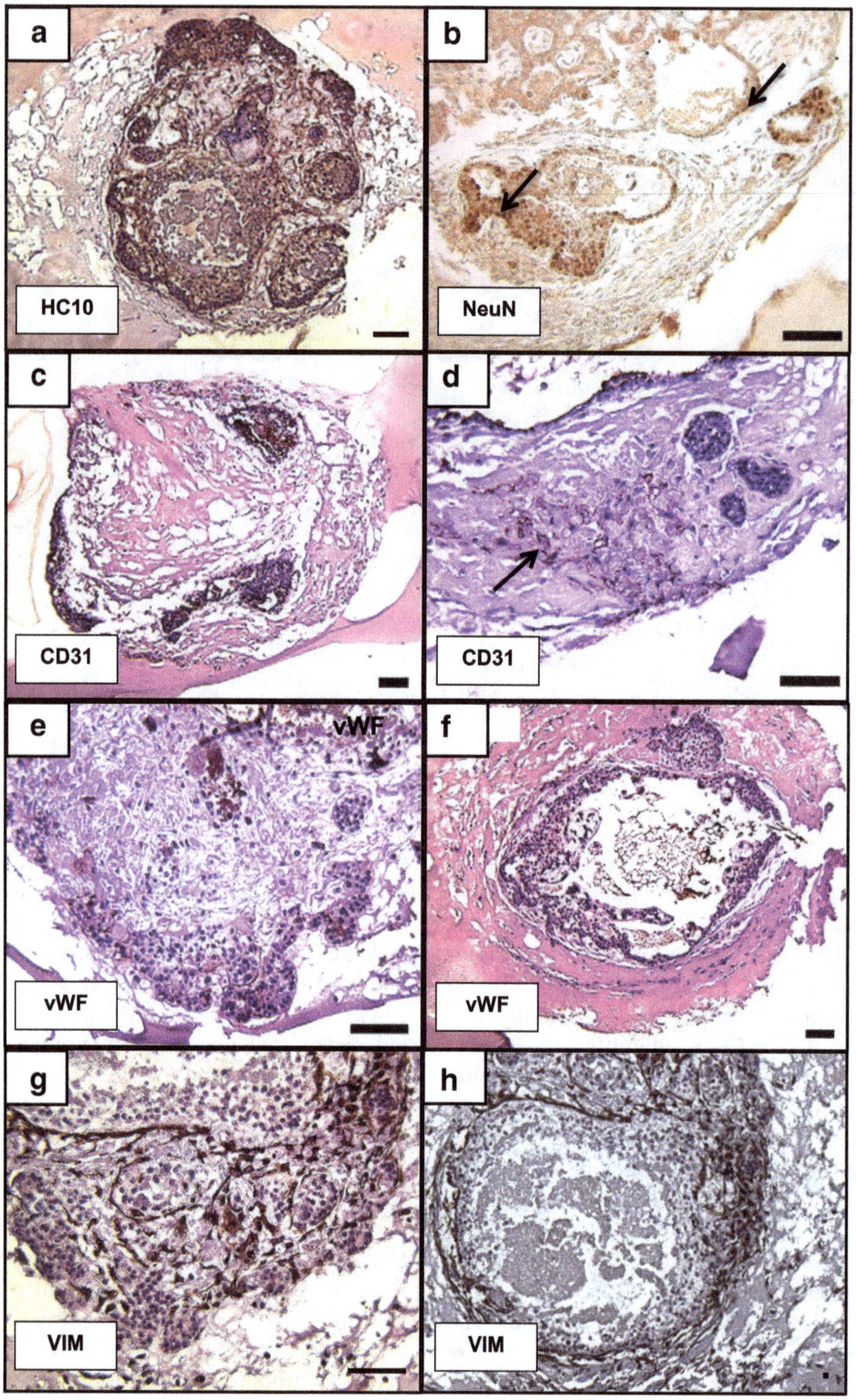

Fig. 6 Immunohistochemical staining for selected markers in Matrigel-embedded embryos: (**a**) HC10, (**b**) neuronal marker NeuN; (**c-d**) CD31, an endothelial and monkey extravillous trophoblast marker; (**e-f**) von Willebrand Factor (vWF), an endothelial marker (arrow); (**g-h**) Vimentin (VIM), a marker of mesenchymal cells. Results representative of 2 embryos. Scale bar = 100 μm

expression was confirmed by IHC analyses. Differentiation within the embryo and the extraembryonic structures, as well as sustained proliferation within these cultured embryos, demonstrates that this 3-D in vitro system provides a unique paradigm to model early events in primate implantation, the initiation of pregnancy, and the determination of trophoblast lineage specification in primate development.

Ethical limitations surrounding the study of human implantation in vivo has driven the need to establish in vitro models of implantation to better understand the molecular mechanisms of implantation. Human in vitro models of implantation include embryos or embryo surrogates, such as a trophoblast spheroid, cultured on a specified ECM, layer(s) of endometrial cells, or placed into a transwell setup or bioreactor [2, 3, 30, 49]. There are limitations to these models, including the ethical concern surrounding the use of human embryos, the use of immortalized trophoblasts and/or endometrial epithelial cell lines compared to primary cells, and the technical challenge of reproducibly isolating populations of primary endometrial epithelial and stromal cells.

To overcome these challenges, our model rather relies on a non-human primate embryo embedded within a synthetic ECM, MG, to define the feasibility of studying embryonic development during primate implantation. Our study illustrated that the embryo itself can interact with its surrounding environment to support embryonic growth, and initiate trophoblast proliferation and differentiation in the absence of endometrial cells. Enders et al. [50] previously reported that 2-dimensional culture of rhesus blastocysts on MG alone resulted in inappropriate development and limited trophectoderm outgrowth. In our 3-D environment, branches and protrusions from the embedded rhesus embryos that rapidly developed in MG as similarly described in human embryoid bodies [33], non-human primate embryos [24], and human embryos [4]. Interaction between the embryo and the MG ECM was observed based on the development of trophoblast columns extending from the embryo proper accompanied by apparent proteolytic degradation of the ECM from the invading trophoblasts. The adhesion of the embryo-derived structures and cells to the MG, and the involvement of specific proteins are beyond the scope of this study, but are important areas for future investigation.

During placenta formation in vivo, the highly proliferative and invasive extravillous trophoblast (EVT) structures migrate and invade the uterus and its vasculature. Previous studies have demonstrated that migration and invasion of human EVTs are regulated by growth factors, their binding proteins, ECM components and adhesion molecules, in autocrine and paracrine manners at the maternal-fetal interface in human pregnancy [51–53]. In the present study, embryonic cell migration was concomitant to degradation of the MG in the area surrounding protrusions was observed. These events were similarly observed for human in vitro first trimester trophoblasts, where upon attachment trophoblasts subsequently migrated through a matrix-substrate [54, 55]. Degradation of the ECM is likely a result of secretion of matrix metalloproteinases (MMPs) from the trophoblast cells as similarly observed in vivo during implantation. A critical process to establishment of pregnancy is trophoblast cell invasion into the uterus and modification of maternal spiral arteries, and one of the major factors contributing to the process is the secretion of MMPs [54, 56].

Extraembryonic cellular differentiation in our model was evident by the secretion of CG, a hallmark of trophoblast differentiation to syncytiotrophoblasts [57]. Consistently elevated CG and progesterone secretion, coincident with the presence of outgrowths confirmed trophoblast differentiation. The presence of trophectodermal growth was absolutely required for the secretion of CG: in occasional embryos which failed to initiate trophectodermal proliferation and expansion, CG was essentially never detectable. Interestingly, CG secretion was sustained for several weeks in embryos, similar to the in vivo hormonal secretion in the rhesus monkey [35]. While the secretion of CG in rhesus monkey embryos has been previously described [40, 58], the present study is the first to report immunohistochemical localization of CG in a 3-D in vitro cultured rhesus embryo model.

Proliferation and differentiation of the embryonic and extraembryonic cells was further confirmed by immunohistochemistry for various selected markers. Cellular proliferation was evidenced by positive staining of Ki67 throughout the interior of the embryonic structures with a greater proportion of positive at the periphery of outgrowth, thus demonstrating continued growth throughout the duration of culture. At the periphery of outgrowth positive Ki67 cells were co-localized with cytokeratin positive cells. Cytokeratin 7 is a well-known marker for the characterization and identification of differentiated trophoblasts in placental cell isolates [59–61]. Conversely, vimentin-positive cells were observed internally in the embryonic structures, complementary to cytokeratin staining. Vimentin is a non-trophoblastic, mesenchymal marker and is expressed in fibroblasts and endothelial cells [62].

Our previous study identified a non-human primate MHC class I gene, Mamu-AG, which has similar characteristics to the human MHC class I gene, HLA-G [63]. The expression of Mamu-AG is restricted to the placenta, although a soluble form is also expressed in the testis of rhesus macaques [64, 65]. Temporal expression pattern of Mamu-AG has been observed at implantation sites of rhesus macaque placentas, where at days 10–14 of pregnancy it is expressed predominantly in cytotrophoblasts and as development progresses there is an accumulation of the glycoprotein at the interface between the decidua and trophoblast by day 36 of pregnancy [47]. Although the paraffin embedding of the embryos precluded specific staining in the present study, the HC10 antibody revealed that MHC Class I molecules are expressed throughout the embryonic structure, including cells at the leading edge, consistent with a differentiated trophoblast phenotype.

Immunohistochemistry confirmed the presence of cellular differentiation by positive staining for other selected markers including CD31, vWF, and NeuN. CD31 and vWF staining on the outer areas of the embryonic structures indicating possible development of endothelial cells as well as differentiated trophoblasts in the post-implantation rhesus macaque embryo. NeuN positive staining on the embryonic structures suggests the formation of neuroectoderm cell lineages in the 3-D model cultured embryo. The presence of cells positive for these markers confirms differentiation, however, further characterization of cellular differentiation representative of the respective germ layers is needed in future studies.

Conclusions

Overall, the results reported here establish a platform for assessing primate implantation in vitro. This non-human primate 3-D model, because of its relative simplicity, isolates the embryonic component during implantation allowing for investigators to assess the impact of additional variables added to the MG, such as growth factors or maternal immune or uterine cells. The 3-D implantation model could be used in an experimental infection paradigm to evaluate the impact of pathogens on trophoblast differentiation and function. Altogether, our 3-D non-human primate model could serve as valuable platform to for study of the mechanisms underpinning human implantation.

Abbreviations

3-D: three-dimensional; BRL cells: Buffalo rat liver cells; CG: Chorionic gonadotropin; ECM: Extracellular matrix; EVT: Extravillous trophoblasts; HECM: Hamster embryo culture medium; IHC: Immunohistochemistry; MG: Matrigel; MMP: Matrix metalloproteases; vWF: von Willebrand Factor

Acknowledgements

We sincerely thank Rick Grendell for assistance with figure preparation and Fritz Wegner and Dan Wittwer of the Wisconsin National Primate Research Center Hormone Assay Laboratory for assistance with chorionic gonadotropin and progesterone assays.

Funding

This work was supported by NIH Grants R24 RR14040, R21HD HD053925 and R01 RR021876 (to T.G.G.), and P51 OD011106 (to the WNPRC). The funding body had no role in the design of the study or collection, analysis and interpretation of the data or writing of the manuscript.

Authors' contributions

TAC, BG-N, JGD and TGG designed the study. TAC and GIB conducted experiments and analyzed samples. TAC, MD, MAG, JKS, and TGG analyzed and interpreted data. TAC, JKS and TGG wrote the manuscript. All authors read and approved the final manuscript.

Competing interests

The authors declare they have no competing interests.

Author details

[1]Wisconsin National Primate Research Center, University of Wisconsin-Madison, 1223 Capitol Court, Madison, Wisconsin 53715-1299, USA. [2]Department of Comparative Biosciences, School of Veterinary Medicine, University of Wisconsin-Madison, Madison, WI, USA. [3]Department of Obstetrics and Gynecology, School of Medicine and Public Health, University of Wisconsin-Madison, Madison, WI, USA. [4]Present address: Department of Obstetrics and Gynecology, University of Texas Health Science Center, San Antonio, TX, USA. [5]Present address: Covance Laboratories, Madison, WI, USA. [6]Present address: School of Dental Medicine, Tufts University, Boston, MA, USA. [7]Present address: Illumina-Madison, Madison, WI, USA.

References

1. Lee KY, DeMayo FJ. Animal models of implantation. Reproduction. 2004;128: 679–95.
2. Hohn HP, Denker HW. Experimental modulation of cell-cell adhesion, invasiveness and differentiation in trophoblast cells. Cells Tissues Organs. 2002;172:218–36.
3. Weimar CH, Post Uiterweer ED, Teklenburg G, Heijnen CJ, Macklon NS. In-vitro model systems for the study of human embryo-endometrium interactions. Reprod BioMed Online. 2013;27:461–76.
4. Carver J, Martin K, Spyropoulou I, Barlow D, Sargent I, Mardon H. An in-vitro model for stromal invasion during implantation of the human blastocyst. Hum Reprod. 2003;18:283–90.
5. Bentin-Ley U, Pedersen B, Lindenberg S, Larsen JF, Hamberger L, Horn T. Isolation and culture of human endometrial cells in a three-dimensional culture system. J Reprod Fertil. 1994;101:327–32.
6. Wang H, Pilla F, Anderson S, Martinez-Escribano S, Herrer I, Moreno-Moya JM, Musti S, Bocca S, Oehninger S, Horcajadas JA. A novel model of human implantation: 3D endometrium-like culture system to study attachment of human trophoblast (jar) cell spheroids. Mol Hum Reprod. 2012;18:33–43.
7. Ho H, Singh H, Aljofan M, Nie G. A high-throughput in vitro model of human embryo attachment. Fertil Steril. 2012;97:974–8.
8. Bentin-Ley U, Horn T, Sjogren A, Sorensen S, Falck Larsen J, Hamberger L. Ultrastructure of human blastocyst-endometrial interactions in vitro. J Reprod Fertil. 2000;120:337–50.
9. Lacey H, Haigh T, Westwood M, Aplin JD. Mesenchymally-derived insulin-like growth factor 1 provides a paracrine stimulus for trophoblast migration. BMC Dev Biol. 2002;2:5.
10. Meseguer M, Aplin JD, Caballero-Campo P, O'Connor JE, Martin JC, Remohi J, Pellicer A, Simon C. Human endometrial mucin MUC1 is up-regulated by progesterone and down-regulated in vitro by the human blastocyst. Biol Reprod. 2001;64:590–601.
11. Holmberg JC, Haddad S, Wunsche V, Yang Y, Aldo PB, Gnainsky Y, Granot I, Dekel N, Mor G. An in vitro model for the study of human implantation. Am J Reprod Immunol. 2012;67:169–78.
12. Hohn HP, Linke M, Denker HW. Adhesion of trophoblast to uterine epithelium as related to the state of trophoblast differentiation: in vitro studies using cell lines. Mol Reprod Dev. 2000;57:135–45.
13. Carter AM. Animal models of human placentation–a review. Placenta. 2007; 28(Suppl A):S41–7.
14. Carter AM, Enders AC, Pijnenborg R. The role of invasive trophoblast in implantation and placentation of primates. Philos Trans R Soc Lond Ser B Biol Sci. 2015;370:20140070.
15. Gilchrist RB, Nayudu PL, Hodges JK. Maturation, fertilization, and development of marmoset monkey oocytes in vitro. Biol Reprod. 1997;56:238–46.
16. Marshall VS, Browne MA, Knowles L, Golos TG, Thomson JA. Ovarian stimulation of marmoset monkeys (Callithrix jacchus) using recombinant human follicle stimulating hormone. J Med Primatol. 2003;32:57–66.
17. Sasaki E, Suemizu H, Shimada A, Hanazawa K, Oiwa R, Kamioka M, Tomioka I, Sotomaru Y, Hirakawa R, Eto T, et al. Generation of transgenic non-human primates with germline transmission. Nature. 2009;459:523–U550.
18. Pope CE, Pope VZ, Beck LR. Development of baboon preimplantation embryos to post-implantation stages in vitro. Biol Reprod. 1982;27:915–23.
19. Wolf DP, Vandevoort CA, Meyer-Haas GR, Zelinski-Wooten MB, Hess DL, Baughman WL, Stouffer RL. In vitro fertilization and embryo transfer in the rhesus monkey. Biol Reprod. 1989;41:335–46.

20. Zhang L, Weston AM, Denniston RS, Goodeaux LL, Godke RA, Wolf DP. Developmental potential of rhesus monkey embryos produced by in vitro fertilization. Biol Reprod. 1994;51:433–40.
21. Bavister BD, Boatman DE, Leibfried L, Loose M, Vernon MW. Fertilization and cleavage of rhesus-monkey oocytes Invitro. Biol Reprod. 1983;28:983–99.
22. Niakan KK, Han J, Pedersen RA, Simon C, Pera RA. Human pre-implantation embryo development. Development. 2012;139:829–41.
23. Fishel SB, Edwards RG, Evans CJ. Human chorionic gonadotropin secreted by preimplantation embryos cultured in vitro. Science. 1984;223:816–8.
24. Lopata A, Kohlman DJ, Bowes LG, Watkins WB. Culture of marmoset blastocysts on matrigel: a model of differentiation during the implantation period. Anat Rec. 1995;241:469–86.
25. Lopata A, Oliva K, Stanton PG, Robertson DM. Analysis of chorionic gonadotrophin secreted by cultured human blastocysts. Mol Hum Reprod. 1997;3:517–21.
26. Enders AC, Boatman D, Morgan P, Bavister BD. Differentiation of blastocysts derived from in vitro-fertilized rhesus monkey ova. Biol Reprod. 1989;41: 715–27.
27. Schindler M, Nur EKA, Ahmed I, Kamal J, Liu HY, Amor N, Ponery AS, Crockett DP, Grafe TH, Chung HY, et al. Living in three dimensions: 3D nanostructured environments for cell culture and regenerative medicine. Cell Biochem Biophys. 2006;45:215–27.
28. Schmeichel KL, Bissell MJ. Modeling tissue-specific signaling and organ function in three dimensions. J Cell Sci. 2003;116:2377–88.
29. Miller RK, Genbacev O, Turner MA, Aplin JD, Caniggia I, Huppertz B. Human placental explants in culture: approaches and assessments. Placenta. 2005; 26:439–48.
30. LaMarca HL, Ott CM, Honer Zu Bentrup K, Leblanc CL, Pierson DL, Nelson AB, Scandurro AB, Whitley GS, Nickerson CA, Morris CA. Three-dimensional growth of extravillous cytotrophoblasts promotes differentiation and invasion. Placenta. 2005;26:709–20.
31. Liu H, Collins SF, Suggs LJ. Three-dimensional culture for expansion and differentiation of mouse embryonic stem cells. Biomaterials. 2006;27: 6004–14.
32. Liu H, Lin J, Roy K. Effect of 3D scaffold and dynamic culture condition on the global gene expression profile of mouse embryonic stem cells. Biomaterials. 2006;27:5978–89.
33. Gerami-Naini B, Dovzhenko OV, Durning M, Wegner FH, Thomson JA, Golos TG. Trophoblast differentiation in embryoid bodies derived from human embryonic stem cells. Endocrinology. 2004;145:1517–24.
34. Wolfgang MJ, Marshall VS, Eisele SG, Schotzko ML, Thomson JA, Golos TG. Efficient method for expressing transgenes in nonhuman primate embryos using a stable episomal vector. Mol Reprod Dev. 2002;62:69–73.
35. Wolfgang MJ, Eisele SG, Knowles L, Browne MA, Schotzko ML, Golos TG. Pregnancy and live birth from nonsurgical transfer of in vivo- and in vitro-produced blastocysts in the rhesus monkey. J Med Primatol. 2001;30:148–55.
36. Wolfgang MJ, Eisele SG, Browne MA, Schotzko ML, Garthwaite MA, Durning M, Ramezani A, Hawley RG, Thomson JA, Golos TG. Rhesus monkey placental transgene expression after lentiviral gene transfer into preimplantation embryos. Proc Natl Acad Sci U S A. 2001;98:10728–32.
37. McKiernan SH, Bavister BD, Tasca RJ. Energy substrate requirements for in-vitro development of hamster 1- and 2-cell embryos to the blastocyst stage. Hum Reprod. 1991;6:64–75.
38. McKiernan SH, Clayton MK, Bavister BD. Analysis of stimulatory and inhibitory amino acids for development of hamster one-cell embryos in vitro. Mol Reprod Dev. 1995;42:188–99.
39. McKiernan SH, Bavister BD. Gonadotrophin stimulation of donor females decreases post-implantation viability of cultured one-cell hamster embryos. Hum Reprod. 1998;13:724–9.
40. Rozner AE, Durning M, Kropp J, Wiepz GJ, Golos TG. Macrophages modulate the growth and differentiation of rhesus monkey embryonic trophoblasts. Am J Reprod Immunol. 2016;76:364–75.
41. Schramm RD, Paprocki AM, VandeVoort CA. Causes of developmental failure of in-vitro matured rhesus monkey oocytes: impairments in embryonic genome activation. Hum Reprod. 2003;18:826–33.
42. McKiernan SH, Bavister BD. Culture of one-cell hamster embryos with water soluble vitamins: pantothenate stimulates blastocyst production. Hum Reprod. 2000;15:157–64.
43. Seshagiri PB, Hearn JP. In-vitro development of in-vivo produced rhesus monkey morulae and blastocysts to hatched, attached, and post-attached blastocyst stages: morphology and early secretion of chorionic gonadotropin. Hum Reprod. 1993;8:279–87.
44. Ziegler TE, Matteri RL, Wegner FH. Detection of urinary gonadotropins in Callitrichid monkeys with a sensitive immunoassay based upon a unique monoclonal-antibody. Am J Primatol. 1993;31:181–8.
45. Munro CJ, Laughlin LS, Illera JC, Dieter J, Hendrickx AG, Lasley BL. ELISA for the measurement of serum and urinary chorionic gonadotropin concentrations in the laboratory macaque. Am J Primatol. 1997;41:307–22.
46. Bielert C, Czaja JA, Eisele S, Scheffler G, Robinson JA, Goy RW. Mating in the rhesus monkey (Macaca mulatta) after conception and its relationship to oestradiol and progesterone levels throughout pregnancy. J Reprod Fertil. 1976;46:179–87.
47. Slukvin II, Lunn DP, Watkins DI, Golos TG. Placental expression of the nonclassical MHC class I molecule Mamu-AG at implantation in the rhesus monkey. Proc Natl Acad Sci U S A. 2000;97:9104–9.
48. Bondarenko GI, Burleigh DW, Durning M, Breburda EE, Grendell RL, Golos TG. Passive immunization against the MHC class I molecule Mamu-AG disrupts rhesus placental development and endometrial responses. J Immunol. 2007;179:8042–50.
49. McConkey CA, Delorme-Axford E, Nickerson CA, Kim KS, Sadovsky Y, Boyle JP, Coyne CB. A three-dimensional culture system recapitulates placental syncytiotrophoblast development and microbial resistance. Sci Adv. 2016;2: e1501462.
50. Enders AC, Meyers S, Vandevoort CA, Douglas GC. Interactions of macaque blastocysts with epithelial cells in vitro. Hum Reprod. 2005;20:3026–32.
51. Pankov R, Cukierman E, Katz BZ, Matsumoto K, Lin DC, Lin S, Hahn C, Yamada KM. Integrin dynamics and matrix assembly: tensin-dependent translocation of alpha(5)beta(1) integrins promotes early fibronectin fibrillogenesis. J Cell Biol. 2000;148:1075–90.
52. Burrows TD, King A, Smith SK, Loke YW. Human trophoblast adhesion to matrix proteins: inhibition and signal transduction. Hum Reprod. 1995;10: 2489–500.
53. Davidson LM, Coward K. Molecular mechanisms of membrane interaction at implantation. Birth Defects Res C Embryo Today. 2016;108:19–32.
54. Fisher SJ, Cui TY, Zhang L, Hartman L, Grahl K, Zhang GY, Tarpey J, Damsky CH. Adhesive and degradative properties of human placental cytotrophoblast cells in vitro. J Cell Biol. 1989;109:891–902.
55. Aplin JD, Haigh T, Jones CJ, Church HJ, Vicovac L. Development of cytotrophoblast columns from explanted first-trimester human placental villi: role of fibronectin and integrin alpha5beta1. Biol Reprod. 1999;60: 828–38.
56. Blankenship TN, Enders AC. Trophoblast cell-mediated modifications to uterine spiral arteries during early gestation in the macaque. Acta Anat (Basel). 1997;158:227–36.
57. Kliman HJ, Nestler JE, Sermasi E, Sanger JM, Strauss JF 3rd. Purification, characterization, and in vitro differentiation of cytotrophoblasts from human term placentae. Endocrinology. 1986;118:1567–82.
58. Seshagiri PB, Terasawa E, Hearn JP. The secretion of gonadotrophin-releasing hormone by peri-implantation embryos of the rhesus monkey: comparison with the secretion of chorionic gonadotrophin. Hum Reprod. 1994;9:1300–7.
59. Blaschitz A, Weiss U, Dohr G, Desoye G. Antibody reaction patterns in first trimester placenta: implications for trophoblast isolation and purity screening. Placenta. 2000;21:733–41.
60. Haigh T, Chen C, Jones CJ, Aplin JD. Studies of mesenchymal cells from 1st trimester human placenta: expression of cytokeratin outside the trophoblast lineage. Placenta. 1999;20:615–25.
61. Muhlhauser J, Crescimanno C, Kasper M, Zaccheo D, Castellucci M. Differentiation of human trophoblast populations involves alterations in cytokeratin patterns. J Histochem Cytochem. 1995;43:579–89.
62. DaSilva-Arnold S, James JL, Al-Khan A, Zamudio S, Illsley NP. Differentiation of first trimester cytotrophoblast to extravillous trophoblast involves an epithelial-mesenchymal transition. Placenta. 2015;36:1412–8.
63. Boyson JE, Iwanaga KK, Golos TG, Watkins DI. Identification of a novel MHC class I gene, Mamu-AG, expressed in the placenta of a primate with an inactivated G locus. J Immunol. 1997;159:3311–21.

17

Construction and analysis of a lncRNA (*PWRN2*)-mediated ceRNA network reveal its potential roles in oocyte nuclear maturation of patients with PCOS

Xin Huang[*†], Jiaping Pan[†], Bi Wu and Xiaoming Teng[*]

Abstract

Background: Polycystic ovary syndrome (PCOS) is a common endocrine and metabolic disorder in women. An lncRNA, namely, Prader-Willi region nonprotein coding RNA 2 (*PWRN2*), was up-regulated in the cumulus cells of patients with PCOS. However, the molecular mechanism of *PWRN2* in PCOS remains largely unknown.

Methods: In this study, the expression levels of *PWRN2* were tested in cumulus cells through qRT-PCR analysis to confirm its potential roles in oocyte nuclear maturation of PCOS. A *PWRN2*-mediated ceRNA network was constructed based on three microarray datasets to investigate the molecular mechanism of *PWRN2* in oocyte development of patients with PCOS. The direct interactions of the candidate genes of the ceRNA network were also demonstrated by dual-luciferase reporter assay.

Results: *PWRN2* was found to be associated with oocyte nuclear maturation in patients with PCOS in contrast to that in normal patients. Based on the microarray data, 176 lncRNAs (118 up-regulated and 58 down-regulated) and 131 mRNAs (84 up-regulated and 47 down-regulated) were identified to be regulated by *PWRN2*. A *PWRN2*-miR-92b-3p-*TMEM120B* ceRNA network was constructed based on results of analysis of the combined three microarray datasets (lncRNA+mRNA microarray in KGN/shPWRN2 in this study, miRNAs microarray and lncRNA+mRNA microarray in PCOS cumulus cells reported in previous studies). The coexpression characteristics of the genes (*PWRN2*, miR-92b-3p and *TMEM120B*) were detected in the cumulus cells of cumulus-oocyte complexes at different nuclear maturity stages in PCOS. These results are in accordance with the ceRNA hypothesis. Moreover, luciferase activity assay revealed that miR-92b-3p directly binds to *PWRN2* and targets *TMEM120B*.

Conclusions: *PWNR2* plays important roles in oocyte nuclear maturation in PCOS by functioning as a ceRNA to reduce the availability of miR-92b-3p for *TMEM120B* target binding during oocyte maturation in PCOS. Our findings would provide new information and clarify abnormal oocyte development in PCOS.

Keywords: ceRNA, Oocyte maturation, Polycystic ovary syndrome, *PWRN2* , miR-92b-3p, *TMEM120B*

* Correspondence: huangxin92129@163.com; tengxiaoming@hotmail.com
[†]Xin Huang and Jiaping Pan contributed equally to this work.
Department of Assisted Reproductive Medicine, Shanghai First Maternity and Infant Hospital, Tongji University School of Medicine, 2699 Gaoke Road West, Shanghai 200001, People's Republic of China

Background

Polycystic ovary syndrome (PCOS) is a common endocrinopathy in women of reproductive age [1] and accounts for approximately 75% of anovulatory infertility disorders [2]. The phenotype of PCOS is variable and includes hyperandrogenism, menstrual irregularity and polycystic ovarian morphology [3]. Patients suffering from PCOS are often diagnosed with obesity, hirsutism, insulin resistance, increased risk of endometrial cancer, metabolic syndrome [4], type 2 diabetes (T2D) and cardiovascular diseases [5, 6]. Although the aetiology of PCOS remains unclear, most researchers regard PCOS as multifactorial and suggest that genetic factors play a pivotal role in its development and maintenance [7, 8]. Many studies have reported gene expression profiles based on tissues (i.e. theca cells [9], ovaries [10, 11], oocytes [12] and cumulus cells [13]) from controls and patients with PCOS. Genes associated with PCOS are involved in the insulin receptor signalling pathway, steroid biosynthesis and regulation of gonadotropin secretion [14]. However, the mechanism by which these genes are regulated has not been thoroughly elucidated.

Long noncoding RNAs (lncRNAs) are defined as noncoding RNAs with greater than 200 base pairs [15]. LncRNAs were previously regarded as transcriptional 'noise' without biological functions [16]; however, increasing lines of evidence indicate that lncRNAs play key roles in normal development and diseases [17]. To date, several reports have demonstrated that lncRNAs may function in PCOS-related diseases, including T2D, obesity and cardiac diseases. For instance, a β-cell-specific lncRNA (*HI-LNC25*) is dysregulated in T2D by down-regulating the mRNA expression levels of *GLIS3* (Kruppel like zinc finger transcription factor) [18].

In our previous research [19], we used microarrays [Agilent human lncRNA+mRNA Array v2.0 (4 × 180 K format)] to describe lncRNA profiles in cumulus cells isolated from 10 patients (five patients with PCOS and five normal women). A total of 623 lncRNAs were differentially expressed in PCOS and may contribute to its occurrence [19].Among these lncRNAs, Prader-Willi region nonprotein coding RNA 2 (*PWRN2*) (transcript ID: ENST00000567246.1), which is expressed in the testes and is up-regulated after meiosis during spermatogenesis [20], was found to be up-regulated (3.11-fold) in the cumulus cells of patients with PCOS. Oocyte nuclear maturation has two meiosis resumption processes at the MI (the first meiosis resumption) and MII (the second meiosis resumption) stages. Hence, *PWRN2* may be associated with oocyte nuclear maturation in PCOS. In addition, abnormal folliculogenesis is regarded as a common characteristic of PCOS although its clinical and biochemical signs are typically heterogeneous [21, 22]. Thus, studying the abnormal regulatory mechanisms in oocyte development of PCOS is important.

Increasing lines of evidence suggest that lncRNAs function as miRNA sponges or competing endogenous RNAs (ceRNAs) to reduce the availability of miRNAs for mRNA target binding [23, 24]. In the present study, we confirmed the potential roles of *PWRN2* in oocyte nuclear maturation of PCOS. We then constructed a *PWRN2*- mediated ceRNA network by analysing three microarray datasets (lncRNA+mRNA microarray in PCOS cumulus cells [19], miRNAs microarray in PCOS cumulus cells [25] and lncRNA+mRNA microarray in KGN/shPWRN2 in this study) to investigate the mechanism of *PWRN2*. Results revealed the potential roles of ceRNA in oocyte maturation in PCOS. This work highlights a novel mechanism of oocyte nuclear maturation in PCOS and provides new targets for PCOS treatment.

Methods

Patients and IVF treatment

The inclusion criteria for the recruited patients (PCOS and normal) and the methods for collecting CCs were based on our previous reports [19, 26]. This study was approved by the Institutional Ethical Review Board of Tongji University School of Medicine. Sixty participants (30 patients with PCOS and 30 normal) who were referred to our centre for IVF were included in this study after obtaining written informed consent. All patients had no history of taking drugs that affect glucose and lipid metabolism and did not have any known medical conditions or diseases, such as Cushing's syndrome, congenital adrenal hyperplasia, androgen-secreting tumours and endometriosis. Patients with PCOS were diagnosed according to the revised Rotterdam European Society of Human Reproduction and Embryology/ American Society for Reproductive Medicine Criteria [3]. The patients were required to present at least two of the following criteria: chronic oligo-ovulation or anovulation, androgen excess and polycystic ovaries. The inclusion criteria for the recruited patients in this study were as follows: age < 36 years, BMI ranging between 20 and 26 kg/m^2, basal serum LH/FSH more than 2.0, serum testosterone more than 0.5 ng/mL, antral follicle count ranging between 18 and 35 and number of obtained oocytes ranging between 12 and 28 per cycle. Control patients had regular menstrual cycles, normal ovary sonographs and normal ovulation with bilateral tube occlusion, were nondiabetic and showed no clinical signs of hyperandrogenism and anovulation. The clinical characteristics of control patients and those with PCOS are summarised in Table 1.

Patients in both groups received an agonist protocol as described previously [27]. All patients received the GnRH agonist triptorelin acetate (0.05 mg/day, Diphereline;

Table 1 Clinical characteristics of patients

	Normal (n = 30)	PCOS (n = 30)	*P*-value
Age (years)	33.6 ± 2.2	32.6 ± 3.1	NS
BMI (kg/m^2)	21.4 ± 1.6	21.6 ± 1.5	NS
FSH (mIU/ml)	6.51 ± 1.2	5.41 ± 1.3	< 0.05
LH (mIU/ml)	4.30 ± 1.4	11.91 ± 2.6	< 0.001
Basal LH/FSH	0.65 ± 0.2	2.52 ± 0.61	< 0.001
E2 (pg/ml)	38.5 ± 4.3	41.3 ± 9.5	NS
Testosterone (ng/ml)	0.12 ± 0.05	0.68 ± 0.05	< 0.001
Progesterone (ng/ml)	0.55 ± 0.22	0.70 ± 0.23	NS
Antral follicle count	10.2 ± 1.1	24.1 ± 3.7	< 0.001
Oocytes obtained	8.5 ± 3.0	17.8 ± 5.2	< 0.001
No of MII oocytes	6.3 ± 1.8	14.5 ± 4.6	< 0.001

Data are the mean ± SEM, *NS* not statistically significant
BMI body mass index, *E2* oestradiol, *FSH* follicle-stimulating hormone, *LH* luteotropic hormone, *PCOS* polycystic ovary syndrome

Ipsen Pharma Biotech, Paris, France) subcutaneously starting at the mid-luteal phase. Once adequate pituitary down-regulation was confirmed [serum LH levels < 3.0 ng/mL and serum estradiol (E_2) levels < 30 pg/mL], the patients received recombinant FSH (150–187.5 IU; Gonal-f, Follitropin Alfa, Serono) subcutaneously for COS. When two or more follicles were at least 18 mm in diameter and the serum E_2 levels were at least 300 pg/mL per dominant follicle, all patients received 250 μg of hCG (Profasi, Serono).

Retrieval of cumulus cells

Collection of CCs and assessment of oocytes were conducted as previously described [27, 28]. Cumulus-oocyte complex (COC) retrieval was performed by vaginal puncture under ultrasound echo-guidance 36 h after hCG administration. After COC retrieval, a portion of CCs surrounding a single oocyte was removed using a sharp needle. For RNA extraction, the cumulus cells were lysed in 80 μL of lysis buffer (mirVana miRNA Isolation Kit; Ambion, Austin, TX, USA) and stored at − 80 °C. For vector transfection and luciferase activity assay, the cumulus cells were firstly digested with trypsin and then cultured directly. Oocytes were further inseminated by ICSI and cultured in sequential media of SAGE (CooperSurgical, Leisegang Medical, Berlin) individually in 20 μL of droplets covered with mineral oil. The embryos were transferred or vitrified on day 3, and the other embryos were cultured to blastula stage on days 5–6.

Assessment of oocyte and division of the groups of cumulus cells

The morphological characteristics of the oocytes were individually recorded. The oocytes were denudated to assess the maturation stage before ICSI. Few of germinal vesicle (GV)-stage COCs (12 in patients with PCOS and only 3 in normal patients) were retrieved. We classified the COCs into two categories based on nuclear status: (i) MI/GV group: immature MI oocytes exhibiting no polar bodies (PB) or immature oocytes at the GV stage, and (ii) MII group: mature MII oocytes that extruded a clearly visible PB. The corresponding cumulus cells were divided into $CC_{MI/GV}$ and CC_{MII} groups. Each group had ≥ three replicates. Each subgroup, containing at least 15 cumulus cells, represented a biological replicate. Each $CC_{MI/GV}$ subgroup has one CC_{GV}.

RNA extraction

Total RNA was isolated using a Qiagen RNeasy Mini Kit (Qiagen, Hilder, Germany) according to the manufacturer's instructions. This RNA isolation kit significantly reduced contamination from genomic DNA and proteins. The purity and concentration of RNA were determined from OD260/280 readings using a spectrophotometer (NanoDrop ND-1000). RNA integrity was determined using 1% formaldehyde denaturing gel electrophoresis.

qRT-PCR

The expression levels of *PWRN2* in the $CC_{MI/GV}$ and CC_{MII} groups of normal patients and those with PCOS were tested by qRT-PCR analysis to evaluate the correlation of changes in *PWRN2* with oocyte maturation. The potential ceRNA network was constructed to investigate the action mechanism of *PWRN2*.The co-expression characteristics of the candidate genes of the ceRNA network were also tested in the CCs corresponding to oocytes at different nuclear maturity stages (MI/GV and MII) of patients with PCOS through qRT-PCR analysis.

Total RNA was reverse transcribed into cDNA by using a miScript Reverse Transcription Kit (Qiagen). qRT-PCR analysis was performed using SYBR green assay (Takara Bio, Inc., Dalian, China) according to the manufacturer's protocols. PCR was performed in a total reaction volume of 20 μL containing 10 μL of 2× QuantiTest SYBR Green PCR Master Mix, 1 μL of cDNA template, 1 μL of each primer and RNase-free water. The primers used in this study are listed in Additional file 1: Table S1. All reactions were performed using the ABI PRISM 7300 system. The amplification conditions were as follows: 10 min at 98 °C; 40 cycles of 15 s at 95 °C, 1 min at 60 °C; and a final extension for 5 min at 72 °C. Amplification efficiency was evaluated by standard curve analysis. *PWRN2* and mRNA expression data were normalised to those of *GAPDH*. The miRNA expression data were normalised to U6. Each set of qRT-PCR reactions was repeated at least three times, and fold change in the expression of each gene was analysed by the ΔΔCt method [29].

KGN cell culture

PWRN2-regulated genes were identified using RNA interference technology to inhibit the expression of *PWRN2* in KGN cell lines and eliminate differences in the genetic backgrounds of different patients with PCOS. KGN (RCB1154; RIKEN, Wako, Japan) is a steroidogenic human ovarian granulosa tumour cell line. KGN cells were cultured in 1:1 Dulbecco's modified Eagle's medium and Ham's F-12 medium (DMEM/ F12; Nissui Pharmaceutical, Tokyo, Japan) supplemented with 10% foetal bovine serum (FBS) and antibiotics (100 IU/mL penicillin and 100 μg/mL streptomycin). On the day before lentivirus transfection, KGN cells were placed into the medium without serum and incubated overnight.

Construction of lentivirus shRNA and cell transfections

Lentivirus shRNA construction and cell transfection were conducted using previously described methods [30, 31]. We selected three target sequences to construct lentiviral shRNAs (LV-*PWRN2*-homo-502, LV-*PWRN2*-homo-1574 and LV-*PWRN2*-homo-1261) and included a negative control (LV-NC) (Table 2). The target sequences were used to design two complementary oligonucleotides, which were synthesised and cloned into pGLV3/H1/GFP + Puro Vector (GenePharma, China). The positive purified lentiviral shRNA-expressing plasmids were transfected with packaging plasmids into 293 T cells for lentivirus generation (GenePharma, China). The vectors described above were used to infect KGN cells. Stable KGN cell lines were selected using 3 μg/mL bulk puromycin-resistance culture (puromycin, Sigma, St Louis, MO, USA) for 5 days. Afterwards, the cells were examined microscopically for lentiviral GFP expression. The expression levels of *PWRN2* in KGN/sh*PWRN2* cells and the corresponding negative-control KGN cells were tested by qRT-PCR to validate the effects of RNA interference.

Microarray hybridisation and data analysis

For microarray analysis, three KGN/shPWRN2 cell lines with down-regulated (FC < 0.5) *PWRN2* mRNA levels were selected as shPWRN2 groups. The corresponding three KGN cell lines with negative control vectors were used as the control groups. The methods for RNA labelling, array hybridisation and data analysis were described in our previous report [19]. The purified RNA extracted from KGN/sh*PWRN2* samples or normal KGN cells was amplified and transcribed into fluorescent cDNA for hybridisation to the Agilent human lncRNA+ mRNA Array v4.0 (4 × 180 K format) with each array containing probes interrogating approximately 41,000 human lncRNAs and approximately 34,000 human mRNAs. The lncRNA+mRNA array data were analysed to summarise, normalise and assess the quality of the data using GeneSpring software V11.5 (Agilent). To select differentially expressed genes, we used threshold values of ≥2.0- and ≤ − 2.0-fold changes and a Benjamini–Hochberg corrected *P* value of 0.05. The data were log2 transformed and median centred by genes using the Adjust Data function of the CLUSTER 3.0 software. The data were further analysed using hierarchical clustering with average linkages. Finally, we visualised the tree using Java TreeView (Stanford University School of Medicine, Stanford, CA, USA). Microarray hybridisation and data analysis were performed by CapitalBio Corporation, Beijing, P. R. China.

Table 2 Target sequences of lentiviral shRNAs for interfering *PWRN2*

LV-sh*PWRN2*	Site	Target sequences
PWRN2-homo-502	502–522	5′-GCCATTCGGTTACCATCTACT-3′
PWRN2-homo-1574	1574–1594	5′-GCAAAGGAATTACCGTTTACA-3′
PWRN2-homo-1261	1261–1281	5′-GGCAGAAAGCAATGAAGAAGA-3′
NC	Nonsense	5′-TTCTCCGAACGTGTCACGT-3′

Gene ontology (GO) and KEGG pathway analyses

GO analysis was performed to describe genes and gene product attributes in any organism (http://www.geneontology.org). This ontology covers three domains: biological processes, cellular components and molecular functions. The *P* value denotes the significance of the GO term enrichment among differentially expressed genes (P value ≤0.05 is recommended). For pathway analysis, we used the free web-based Molecular Annotation System 3.0 (MAS 3.0; http://bioinfo.capitalbio.com/mas3/), which integrates three different open-source pathway resources: KEGG, BioCarta and GenMAPP. The significantly altered pathways were selected using the threshold of the P value and FDR (corrected P value) < 0.05 derived from the hypergenomic test. GO and KEGG pathway analyses were performed by CapitalBio Corporation, Beijing, P. R. China.

Construction of the *PWRN2*-mediated ceRNA network based on microarray data

A potential *PWRN2*-mediated ceRNA network was constructed based on three microarray datasets to explain whether *PWRN2* functions as miRNA sponges or ceRNAs. The putative miRNAs and mRNAs included in the construction of the *PWRN2*-mediated ceRNA network are as follows: (i) miRNA selection: miRNAs were predicted to possess *PWRN2* binding sites by using miRanda v3.3a software and were compared with previous miRNA microarray data of PCOS; putative miRNAs with MREs in *PWRN2* and identified from previous microarray data of PCOS were selected; and (ii) mRNA selection: the target genes of the miRNAs were predicted using miRbase (http://www.mirbase.org/) and compared with the lncRNA+mRNA microarray data from KGN cells with *PWRN* interference. The selected mRNAs met two criteria: 1) differentially expressed mRNAs identified from our lncRNA+mRNA microarray data; and 2) putative target genes of miRNAs with MREs in *PWRN2*.

Luciferase reporter constructs and luciferase activity assay

The direct interaction between the candidate genes of *PWRN2*-mediated ceRNA network was evaluated by luciferase activity assay. A luciferase reporter vector (pmirGLO Dual-Luciferase miRNA Target Expression Vector; Promega) was used for luciferase constructs. *PWRN2* and the 3'UTR of *TMEM120B* were cloned by RT-PCR. *PWRN2*-WT, *PWRN2*-mutant and *TMEM120B*- 3′UTR (WT and mutant) were constructed as previously reported [26, 32]. Cumulus cells of patients with PCOS were digested with 0.25% trypsin for 5 min. The digestion was inhibited by adding 2.5 mL of DMEM: F12 containing 10% FBS and by incubating at room temperature for 5–10 min. The cumulus cells were pooled in a sterile 15 mL conical tube on ice, centrifuged at 200 g for 10 min, washed once with sterile saline, centrifuged again and resuspended in 3 mL of culture media. The number of viable cells was determined by trypan blue exclusion and ranged between 35 and 45%. The cumulus cells were plated onto 24-well plates and allowed to grow for ~ 24 h before transfection. The constructed reporter vectors (300 ng) were transfected into cells together with the miRNA and control mimics (100 nM) in Lipofectamine 2000 (2 μL). The cells were lysed after ~ 24 h of transfection. Luciferase activity was assayed using the Dual-Luciferase Reporter Assay System (Promega). Firefly luciferase activities were normalised to Renilla luciferase activities. The experiments were performed independently in triplicate.

Statistical analysis

All statistical analyses were performed using SPSS 17.0 software (SPSS Inc.) unless otherwise noted. Differences in the expression levels of the candidate genes of the *PWRN2*–mediated ceRNA network in cumulus cell samples were evaluated by two-tailed t-test. Differences were considered statistically significant at $P < 0.05$.

Results

Expression levels of *PWRN2* in cumulus cells according to oocyte nuclear maturity in normal patients and those with PCOS

The transcript levels of *PWRN2* were detected in the $CC_{MI/GV}$ and CC_{MII} groups to evaluate the involvement of *PWRN2* in the oocyte nuclear maturity in patients with PCOS ($n = 30$) and normal patients ($n = 30$). For PCOS, the mean transcript levels of *PWRN2* in the CC_{MII} group was significantly down-regulated by 4.55–fold compared with that in the $CC_{MI/GV}$ group (1.006 ± 0.028 versus 4.602 ± 0.128; Fig. 1A). In normal patients, the expression levels of *PWRN2* exhibited no significant differences between the CC_{MII} and $CC_{MI/GV}$ groups (1.02 ± 0.029 versus 0.98 ± 0.049; Fig. 1B). These results indicated that the *PWRN2* expression pattern during oocyte maturation differed between normal patients and those with PCOS.

Expression profiles of lncRNAs and mRNAs in KGN/sh*PWRN2* cell lines

To avoid the different genetic backgrounds of paitents with PCOS, we used KGN cell lines to identify *PWRN2*-regulated genes by RNA interference. Lentiviral shRNAs were constructed to inhibit *PWRN2* expression in KGN cells. The results of qRT-PCR analysis indicated that the relative expression levels of *PWRN2* mRNA were 0.23, 0.25 and 0.19 in KGN cells treated with LV-*PWRN2*-homo-502, LV-*PWRN2*-homo-1574 and LV-*PWRN2*-homo-1261, respectively, compared with those in the LV-NC group (Fig. 2A). These results indicated that the three lentiviral shRNAs effectively inhibited *PWRN2* replication in KGN cells.

The lncRNA and mRNA expression profiles of KGN/sh*PWRN2* cells infected with LV-*PWRN2*-homo-502, LV-*PWRN2*-homo-1574 or LV-*PWRN2*-homo-1261 were examined by microarrays and compared with those of the three KGN cell lines infected with control LV-NC. The raw microarray data were deposited in NCBI's Gene Expression Omnibus (GEO; http://www.ncbi.nlm.nih.-gov/geo/) and can be accessed through the GEO series accession number GSE97772. The microarray analysis revealed thousands of lncRNAs and mRNAs expressed in KGN/sh*PWRN2*.

The expression of 176 lncRNAs significantly changed in KGN/sh*PWRN2* cells relative to the control KGN cell lines. A total of 118 lncRNAs were up-regulated, whereas 58 lncRNAs were down-regulated. A total of 131 mRNAs significantly changed in the KGN/sh*PWRN2* cell lines. About 84 mRNAs were up-regulated and 47 mRNAs were down-regulated (fold change ≥2.0, $P < 0.05$). Clustering analysis of the microarrays based on the differentially expressed lncRNAs or mRNAs clustered the KGN/sh*PWRN2* groups and the control groups (Fig. 2B).

The top 20 up and down-regulated lncRNAs and mRNAs are listed in Tables 3 and 4, respectively. From the microarray data, the expression level of *PWRN2* was down-regulated (FC = – 2.526) in the KGN/sh*PWRN2* groups. The results were in concordance with the

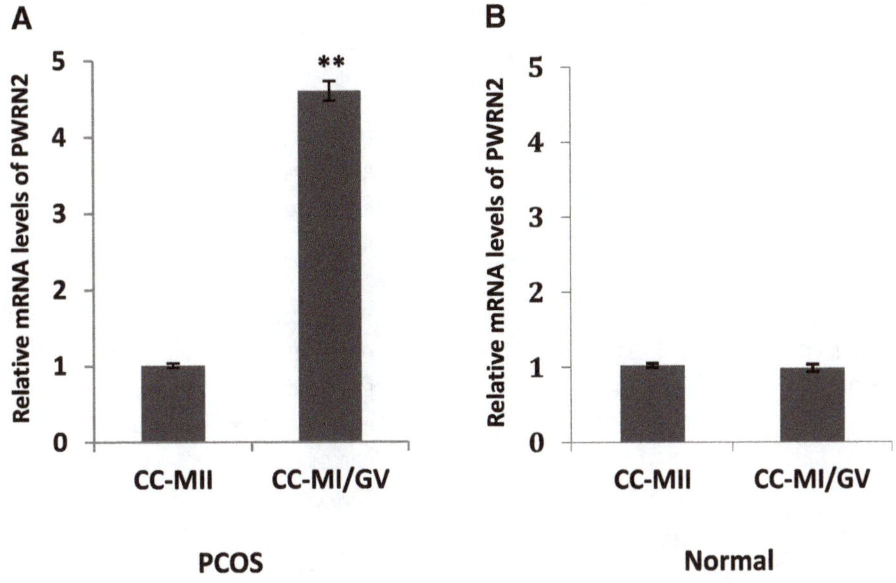

Fig. 1 Transcript levels of *PWRN2* according to oocyte nuclear maturity in PCOS ($n = 30$) and normal patients ($n = 30$). Expression levels of *PWRN2* in cumulus cells of different oocyte nuclear maturity stages (MI/GV stage and MII stage) of patients with PCOS (**a**) and normal patients (**b**). The signal intensity for *PWRN2* is shown on the y-axis in arbitrary units determined by qRT-PCR analysis with *GAPDH* as an endogenous reference. * indicates a significant difference in gene expression between CC categories (** $P < 0.01$, * $P < 0.05$). The results are presented as means ± SEM. $CC_{MI/GV}$: cumulus cells from oocytes at the MI or GV stage; CC_{MII}: cumulus cells from oocytes at the MII stage

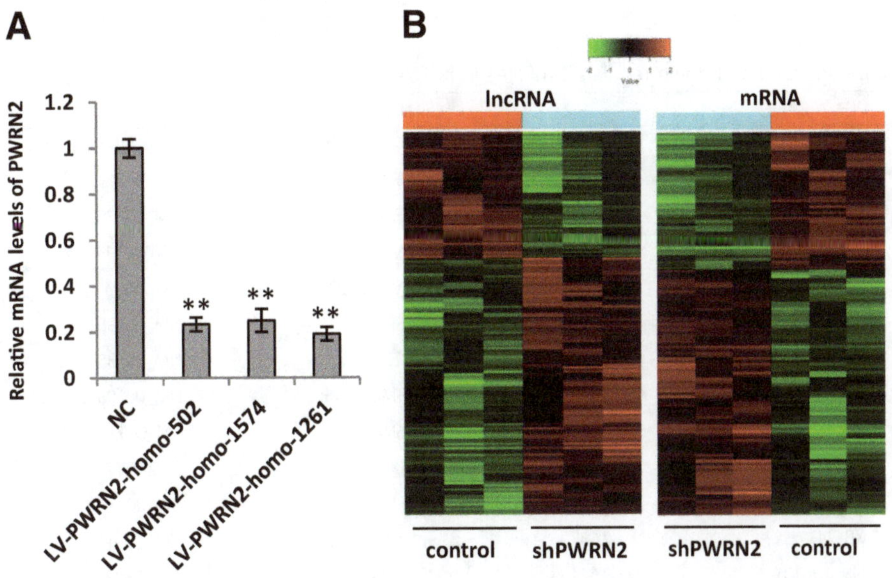

Fig. 2 Expression profiles of lncRNAs and mRNAs in KGN/shPWRN2 cell lines. **a** Relative expression of *PWRN2* mRNA was examined in KGN cells infected with different lentiviral shRNAs (LV-*PWRN2*-homo-502, LV-*PWRN2*-homo-1574, LV-*PWRN2*-homo-1261, or LV negative control) using qRT-PCR analysis with *GAPDH* as an endogenous reference. The KGN cells treated with different lentiviral shRNAs are shown on the x-axis, and the relative change of *PWRN2*/*GAPDH* is shown on the y-axis. Each set of qRT-PCR reactions was repeated at least three times. The results are presented as mean ± SEM. ** indicates $P < 0.01$. **b** Cluster of lncRNAs and mRNAs that were dyexpressed in KGN/sh*PWRN2* cells. From this lncRNA +mRNA microarray data, 176 lncRNAs changed significantly in KGN/sh*PWRN2* cells compared with those in the control cell lines. Among these lncRNAs, 118 were up-regulated, whereas 58 lncRNAs were down-regulated; and 131 mRNAs changed significantly in the KGN/sh*PWRN2* cell lines. Among these, 84 mRNAs were up-regulated, and 47 mRNAs were down-regulated. The supervised hierarchical clustering of genes overexpressed in KGN/sh*PWRN2* cells is shown. Distinct signatures were observed in the KGN/sh*PWRN2* cells. The value of each gene was adjusted with a median-centring algorithm on a log scale; the colours indicate the relative gene expression in the red-green heat map. Pure black indicates 0.00 and represents no change in the median gene expression levels in all samples. Pure green indicates − 2.00 and represents lower expression. Pure red indicates + 2.00 and relatively higher expression

Table 3 The top 20 up-regulated and down-regulated lncRNAs in KGN/shPWRN2 cells

Up-regulated lncRNAs		Down-regulated lncRNAs	
lncRNA ID (or known lncRNA name)	Fold-change	lncRNA ID (or known lncRNA name)	Fold-change
XR_110904.1	5.369	TCONS_00001136	4.033
XR_430233.1	4.498	ENST00000557828.1	3.875
ENST00000584157.1	4.485	RNA143578	3.422
RNA147334|p0438_imsncRNA843	4.185	RNA143598	3.292
uc003qmi.3	4.118	RNA146915|p0019_imsncRNA52	3.097
ENST00000543573.1	4.072	TCONS_00019731	3.092
TCONS_00012676	3.934	TCONS_00025502	3.088
ENST00000500823.2(GS1-24F4.2)	3.730	HIT000271588	3.068
ENST00000428520.2(LINC00710)	3.440	ENST00000567517.1(LINC00515)	3.029
ENST00000502766.2	3.253	RNA147684|p0788_imsncRNA576	2.963
ENST00000608299.1	3.252	HIT000468529	2.883
ENST00000607195.1	3.047	TCONS_00019573	2.882
XR_245201.2	3.035	ENST00000452741.1	2.725
uc.311-	3.034	RNA143600	2.707
TCONS_00009112	3.013	TCONS_00010743	2.638
ENST00000570809.1	2.997	TCONS_00010435	2.628
uc.211-	2.975	ENST00000489626.1	2.551
ENST00000602984.1(MIR137HG)	2.960	uc022caj.1	2.548
TCONS_00000870	2.943	ENST00000566245.1(PWNR2)	2.526
ENST00000513586.1	2.928	ENST00000439960.1	2.445

Table 4 The top 20 up-regulated and down-regulated mRNAs in KGN/shPWRN2 cells

Up-regulated mRNAs			Down-regulated mRNAs		
GeneSymbol	Genbank Accession	Fold-change	GeneSymbol	Genbank Accession	Fold-change
CACTIN	NM_021231	5.976	FTH1	NM_002032	7.358
ND3	HV963894	4.613	FAM154A	NM_153707	3.460
NUB1	NM_016118	4.417	MOP-1	AB014771	3.421
CCDC6	NM_005436	3.410	MARVELD2	AK055094	3.176
MLF1	NM_022443	3.227	RPL19	NM_000981	3.175
GPI	NM_000175	3.108	CCNG2	NM_004354	3.162
ADAM11	NM_002390	3.066	TMEM120B	NM_001080825	3.090
SYNGR4	NM_012451	2.916	SNX22	XM_005254677	3.058
TMEM234	NM_019118	2.855	RGS4	BC000737	3.051
PHIP	NM_017934	2.711	FBRSL1	NM_001142641	2.985
HIF3A	XR_243952	2.685	MB21D1	NM_138441	2.961
NIP7	NM_016101	2.644	ND4	AK097322	2.779
C11orf45	NM_145013	2.636	FMNL1	NM_005892	2.754
VWA1	NM_022834	2.565	NHS	NM_198270	2.753
ZSCAN32	NM_017810	2.562	SEMA6B	NM_032108	2.752
RPPH1	CA413366	2.553	RPL32	NM_001007074	2.729
EPHA4	NM_004438	2.551	TLE6	NM_024760	2.564
CCDC102B	NM_024781	2.403	GRIP2	NM_001080423	2.545
NOS1AP	NM_014697	2.378	LOC100287036	NM_001242885	2.454
CEP70	NM_024491	2.377	RPS2	NM_002952	2.372

qRT-PCR data of *PWRN2* expression levels in the KGN/sh*PWRN2* groups, indicating the reliability of lncRNA +mRNA microarray data.

GO and KEGG pathway analyses

The genes regulated by *PWRN2* were selected to identify the associated signalling pathways and biological functions. Regarding GO annotation, the biological processes, cellular components and molecular function associated with the target genes are presented in Additional file 2: Table S2. The GO analysis showed that the most significantly altered biological processes were nuclear-transcribed mRNA catabolic process, RNA catabolic process, SRP-dependent co-translational protein targeting to the membrane, protein targeting to the ER and others. Moreover, the KEGG pathway analysis demonstrated that the most significantly altered pathways were mRNA surveillance pathways, carbon metabolism, nitrogen metabolism and axon guidance (Additional file 3: Table S3). These results indicated that *PWRN2*-regulated genes were mostly involved in different metabolic pathways, thereby confirming that PCOS is a complex metabolic disease.

Construction of a *PWRN2*-regulated ceRNA network based on three microarray datasets

Recent studies reported that lncRNAs have been reported to function as competing endogenous RNAs [33] by mopping up miRNAs, thereby regulating their function [34]. Given that lncRNAs can interact with miRNAs through their MREs within a ceRNA network [23], we searched for putative miRNAs with MREs in *PWRN2* by using miRanda software. A total of 69 miRNAs were predicted to possess *PWRN2* binding sites. The potential target mRNAs of these 69 miRNAs were also predicted (Additional file 4: Table S4).

We further compared the 69 potential *PWRN2*-regulated miRNAs with the differentially expressed miRNAs (21 up-regulated and 38 down-regulated) in the cumulus cells of patients with PCOS [25]. Two miRNAs (miR-92b-3p and miR-365b-5p) were found. *PWRN2* was up-regulated in PCOS cumulus cells in our previous report [19], and the miRNAs (miR-92b-3p and miR-365b-5p) that possess *PWRN2* binding sites were down-regulated [25]. Hence, *PWRN2* may function as ceRNA to regulate miRNAs (miR-92b-3p and miR-365b-5p) in cumulus cells in PCOS.

By comparing the potential target genes of miR-92b-3p and miR-365b-5p with the *PWRN2*-regulated mRNAs identified by KGN/shPWRN2 microarray, we found 12 mRNAs, including *UPF2, VSIG10, CCDC144A, LRRC1, ZNF654, FHL2, NOS1AP, TMEM120B, GPI, CCDC6, RCAN3* and *AMOTL1*. Thus, a credible *PWRN2*-miRNA-mRNA ceRNA network was constructed using the combined analyses of the three microarrays (lncRNA+mRNA microarray in PCOS, miRNA microarray in PCOS and lncRNA+mRNA microarray in KGN/sh*PWRN2*; Figs. 3A, B).

According to our previous analysis of lncRNA and mRNA microarray data, *PWRN2* and *TMEM120B* were over-expressed in PCOS cumulus cells [19]. In this study, the expression level of *TMEM120B* was down-regulated in KGN/sh*PWRN2* cells. The results indicated that the expression trends of *PWRN2* and *TMEM120B* were consistent with PCOS. Moreover, miR-92b, which was predicted to process the MREs in *PWRN2* and to have a binding site in the 3′-UTR of *TMEM120B*, was down-regulated in PCOS cumulus cells (Table 5). Therefore, we regarded the *PWRN2*-miR-92b-*TMEM120B* ceRNA network as more reasonable and credible.

Co-expression characteristics of genes of the *PWRN2*-miR-92b-3p-*TMEM120B* ceRNA network in PCOS

The expression of the three candidate genes (*PWRN2*, miR-92b-3p and *TMEM120B*) in cumulus cell according to oocyte nuclear maturity ($CC_{MI/GV}$ and CC_{MII}) in patients with PCOS ($n = 30$) were detected by qRT-PCR to validate the potential ceRNA network. Based on comparison between CC_{MII} and $CC_{MI/GV}$ groups, the mean transcript level of miR-92b-3p in CC_{MII} group was significantly 4.95–fold higher than that in the $CC_{MI/GV}$ group (0.99 ± 0.14 versus 0.20 ± 0.03) (Fig. 4A); by contrast, the expression levels of the other genes (*PWRN2* and *TMEM120B*) significantly decreased in the CC_{MII} samples, with 5.23– and 2.73–fold decrease observed for *PWRN2* (0.98 ± 0.05 versus 5.13 ± 0.75) (Fig. 4B) and *TMEM120B* (1.0 ± 0.06 versus 2.73 ± 0.85) (Fig. 4C), respectively. A significant positive correlation was observed between *PWRN2* and *TMEM120B* (Fig. 4D). The co-expression characteristics observed were in accordance with the ceRNA hypothesis.

Confirmation of the direct interactions of the candidate genes of the *PWRN2*-miR-92b-3p-*TMEM120B* ceRNA network

According to the prediction results, *PWRN2* has one putative miR-92b-3p binding site. We recombined the *PWRN2* cDNA (*PWRN2*-WT) and mutational cDNA (*PWRN2*-MUT) with the presumed miR-92b-3p deleted recognition sequences downstream the luciferase reporter gene (Fig. 5A). The vectors were transfected in PCOS cumulus cells along with the corresponding miRNA mimics. After miR-92b-3p mimics transfection, luciferase activity was reduced by 60% compared with the control miRNA (Fig. 5B). Hence, miR-92b-3p directly binds to *PWRN2*.

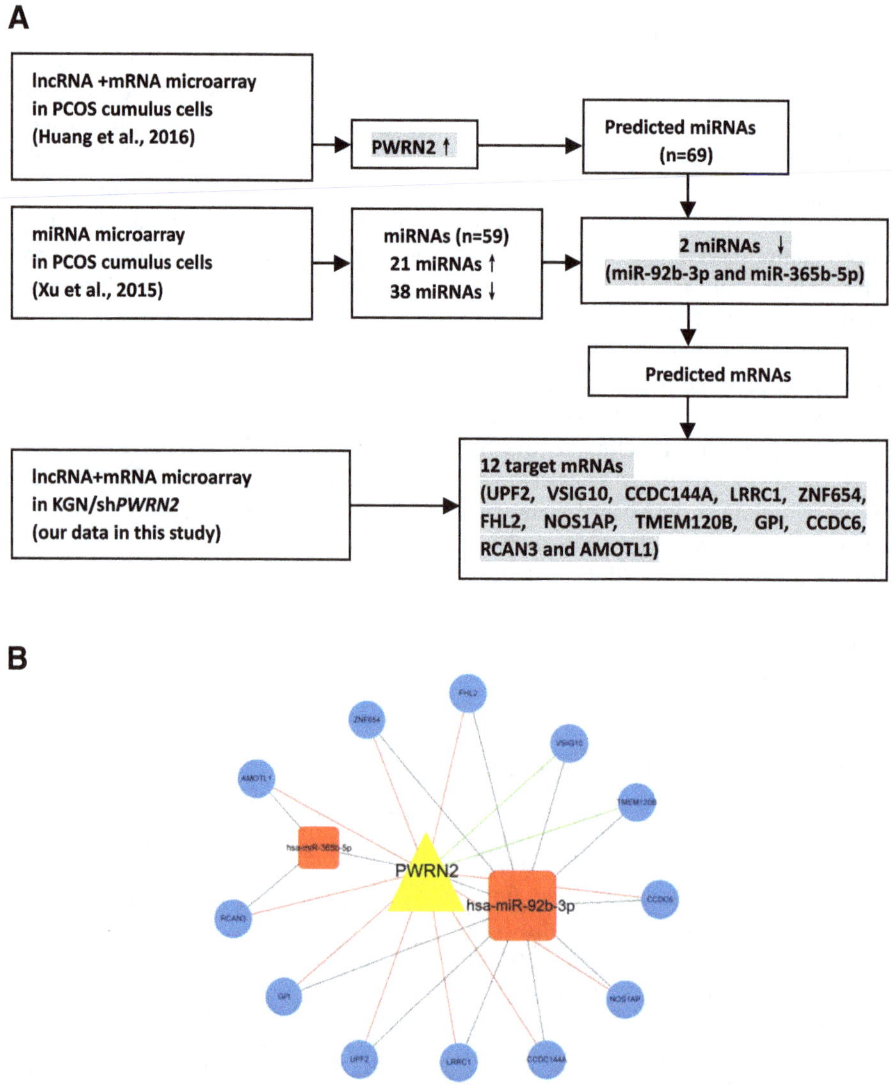

Fig. 3 Construction of a *PWRN2*-mediated ceRNA network based on microarray datasets. **a** Flow chart of building a *PWRN2*-mediated ceRNA network based on three microarray datasets: lncRNA+mRNA microarray in PCOS cumulus cells, miRNA microarray in PCOS cumulus cells and lncRNA+mRNA microarray in KGN/sh*PWRN2*. **b** *PWRN2*-mediated ceRNA network. The ceRNA network is based on lncRNA/miRNA, lncRNA/mRNA and miRNA/mRNA interactions. In this network, black edges represent sequence matching, green edges represent positive correlations and red edges represent negative correlations

To determine whether *TMEM120B* is a direct target of miR-92b-3p, we constructed luciferase reporter constructs by cloning the DNA segment-encoding part of the WT or mutant (which cannot bind miR-92b-3p) 3′ UTR of *TMEM120B* mRNA downstream of the Renilla luciferase gene (Fig. 5A) and transfected them with miR-92b-3p mimics into the PCOS cumulus cells. As shown in Fig. 5C, the relative luciferase activity significantly decreased in cumulus cells co-transfected with the *TMEM120B* WT constructs and miR-92b-3p mimics but not in cells co-transfected with the *TMEM120B* mutant constructs and miR-92b-3p mimics. Thus, miR-92b-3p suppressed the expression of *TMEM120B* in the cumulus cells by directly binding to the 3′UTR of *TMEM120B* mRNA.

Discussion

PWRN2 was up-regulated in PCOS cumulus cells and could be involved in oocyte development [19]. In the present study, we proved that *PWRN2* is associated with oocyte nuclear maturation in patients with PCOS, in contrast to that in normal patients. Hence, *PWRN2* plays important roles during the oocyte development in PCOS.

To elucidate the roles of *PWRN2* in oocyte development, we identified *PWRN2*-regulated genes in KGN

Table 5 The expression levels of *PWRN2*, miR-92b, and *TMEM120B* in three microarray data

Microarray data	*PWRN2*	miR-92b	*TMEM120B*
lncRNA+mRNA array in PCOS cumulus cells (Huang et al., 2016)	Up-regulated FC = 3.11	no	Up-regulated FC = 2.02
miRNA array in PCOS cumulus cells (Xu et al., 2015)	no	Down-regualted FC = −2.27	no
lncRNA+mRNA array in KGN/shPWRN2 array (this study)	Down-regulated FC = −2.52	no	Down-regulated FC = −3.09

cells by using RNA interference technology. A total of 176 lncRNAs and 131 mRNAs were identified and determined to be regulated by *PWRN2*.The GO and KEGG pathway analyses of these DEGs showed that the differentially expressed genes were mostly involved in various catabolic processes (e.g. nuclear-transcribed mRNA and RNA catabolic processes) and metabolism pathways (e.g. carbon and nitrogen metabolism). These results indicated that *PWRN2* may play an important role in metabolic processes. Metabolic abnormalities in cumulus cells in PCOS change the follicular microenvironment during oocyte development and subsequently affect oocyte quality [35, 36]. This deduction is consistent with PCOS because it is a metabolic disease often accompanied by poor oocyte developmental potential.

Although potential target genes of *PWRN2* were identified, the molecular mechanism of *PWRN2* remains largely unknown. Several recent reports provided support for the ceRNA hypothesis, which accounts for the function of a substantial proportion of uncharacterised lncRNAs [37–40]. To examine if *PWRN2* functions as a ceRNA, we developed a new method for elucidating specific lncRNA-mediated ceRNA networks. The most widely used methods for exploring potential lncRNA-miRNA-mRNA networks largely depend on shared MREs that are predicted by miRNA target discovery algorithms [41, 42]. We predicted miRNAs that possess *PWRN2* binding sites and potential miRNA-mRNA pairs. We then obtained *PWRN2*-mediated miRNAs by combining the analyses of predicted

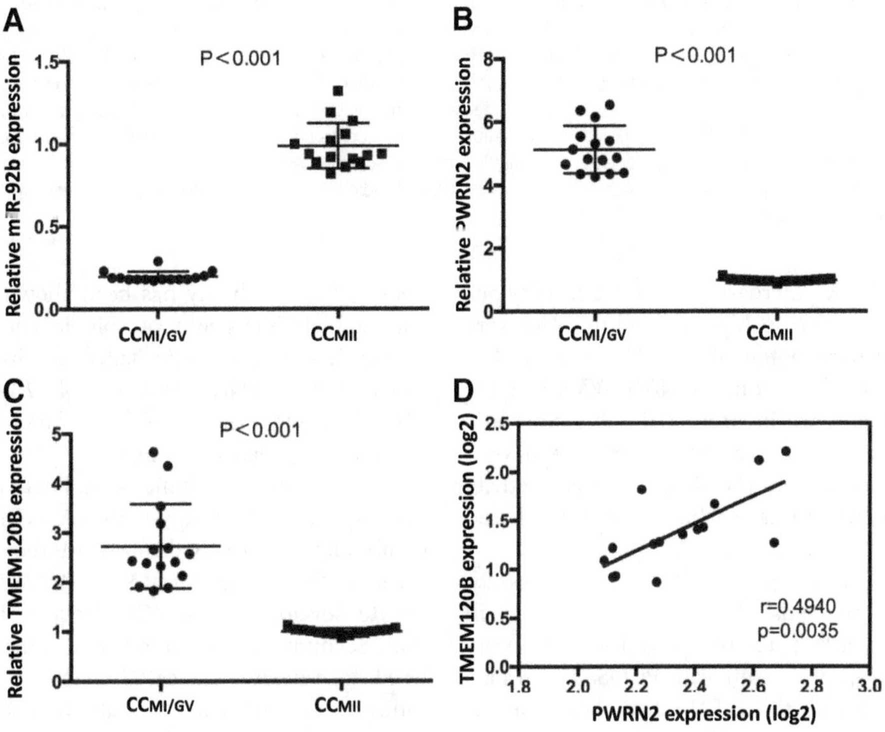

Fig. 4 Transcripts levels of the candidate genes of *PWRN2*-miR-92b-3p-*TMEM120B* ceRNA network according to oocyte nuclear maturity in patients with PCOS ($n = 30$). The transcript levels of miR-92b-3p (**a**), *PWRN2* (**b**) and *TMEM120B* (**c**) were detected by qRT-PCR. **d** Relationship between the expression levels of *PWRN2* and *TMEM120B*. The signal intensity for the genes is shown on the y-axis in arbitrary units determined by qRT-PCR analysis. *GAPDH* was used as internal control for *PWRN2* and *TMEM120B*, while U6 was used as internal control for miR-92b-3p. * indicates a significant difference in gene expression between CC categories (** $P < 0.01$, * $P < 0.05$). The results were presented as means ± SEM. $CC_{MI/GV}$: cumulus cells from oocyte at the MI or GV stage; CC_{MII}: cumulus cells from oocyte at the MII stage

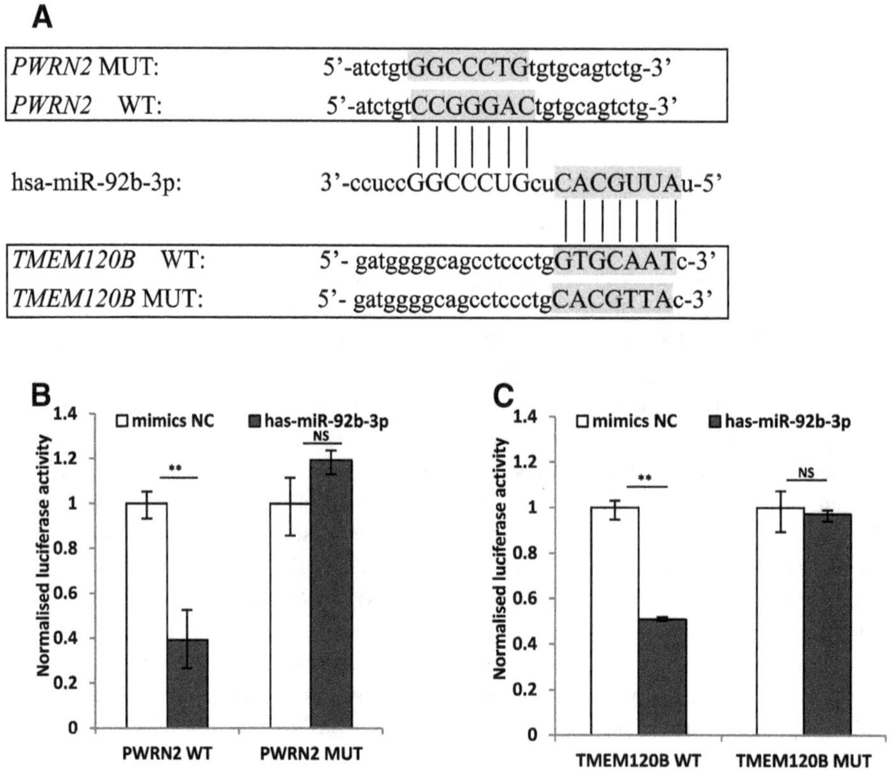

Fig. 5 Validation miR-92b-3p directly binds to *PWRN2* and the direct interaction between miR-92b-3p and its predictive target gene (*TMEM120B*) by the dual luciferase activity assay. **a** Interaction regions of *PWRN2*/miR-92b-3p and miR-92b-3p/*TMEM120B* predicted by miRanda software. MiR-92b-3p, which is predicted to process the MREs in *PWRN2*, also has a binding site in the 3'-UTR of *TMEM120B*. **b** The relative luciferase activity was assayed following co-transfection of miR-92b-3p mimics with the constructs encoding the wild-type or mutant *PWRN2* cDNA into the cumulus cells. **c** The relative luciferase activity was assayed following co-transfection of miR-92b-3p mimics with the constructs encoding the wild-type or mutant miR-92b-3p binding site of *TMEM120B* 3'-UTR into the cumulus cells. The constructed reporter vectors (WT or MUT) are shown on the x-axis, and the y-axis represents the normalised luciferase activity (firefly luciferase activities were normalised to renilla luciferase activities). The experiments were performed independently in triplicate. * indicates $P < 0.05$, ** indicates $P < 0.01$, NS indicates no significant difference. The results are presented as means ±S.E.M

miRNAs and miRNA microarray data from previous report [25]. Meanwhile, *PWRN2*-regulated mRNAs were obtained by comparing potential miRNA-target mRNA with the microarray data from KGN/sh*PWRN2* in the present study. Finally, we incorporated a bioinformatic prediction tool to construct a *PWRN2*-miRNA-mRNA ceRNA network. Based on the dual-luciferase activity assay, the ceRNA network is reliable because it is based on datasets from three microarrays.

Furthermore, we investigated *PWRN2* and miR-92b-*TMEM120B* pair and validated their expression levels in cumulus cells according to oocyte nuclear maturity ($CC_{MI/GV}$ and CC_{MII}) of patients with PCOS. The results were in accordance with the ceRNA hypothesis. In this regard, *PWRN2* functions as ceRNA to reduce the availability of miR-92b-3p for *TMEM120B* target binding. *TMEM120B* is a fat-specific nuclear envelope transmembrane protein that may play a contributory role in adipogenesis [43]. In PCOS, up-regulated *TMEM120B* will promote adipocyte differentiation/metabolism and induce obesity. Severe obesity has been shown to be associated with a high prevalence of spindle anomalies and non-aligned chromosomes in failed fertilised oocytes [44]. Thus, the ceRNA network of *PWRN2*-miR-92b-*TMEM120B* provides a basis for explaining the poor quality of oocyte in patients with PCOS.

Our study presents limitations. Firstly, we cannot identify large lncRNA-miRNA-mRNA ceRNA networks by combining microarray datasets. Moreover, the molecular roles of the *PWRN2*-miR-92b-*TMEM120B* network in oocyte development in PCOS require further investigation. Secondly, a large number of samples must be analysed to validate the ceRNA network in PCOS. Our future work will further validate the *PWRN2*-miR-92b-*TMEM120B* network and elucidate its role in the pathogenesis of PCOS, especially in oocyte development.

In conclusion, our results proved that lncRNA (*PWRN2*) is associated with oocyte nuclear maturation in PCOS. The constructed *PWRN2*-miR-92b-*TMEM120B* ceRNA network based on three microarray datasets indicated that

PWRN2 functions as ceRNA to reduce the availability of miR-92b-3p for *TMEM120B* target binding during oocyte nuclear maturation in PCOS. This ceRNA network provides new information and helps clarify the metabolic disorder that induces abnormal oocyte development in PCOS.

Abbreviations

CCs: Cumulus cells; ceRNA: competing endogenous RNAs; COC: Cumulus-oocyte complex; lncRNA: long non-coding RNAs; PCOS: Polycystic ovary syndrome; *PWRN2*: Prader-Willi region non-protein coding RNA 2

Acknowledgements

The authors gratefully acknowledge the CapitalBio Corporation for conducting the RNA extractions and microarrays.

Funding

This study was supported by the National Natural Science Foundation of China (Grant 81401172 and 81771532), Special Fund for Clinical Medicine Scientific Research of Chinese Medical Association (Grant 16020180634). Shanghai municipal medical and health discipline construction projects (Grant 2017ZZ02015).

Authors' contributions

Xin Huang conducted the experiments and generated the manuscript. Xiaoming Teng contributed to study design and data interpretation. Jiaping Pan contributed to data interpretation and manuscript editing. Bi Wu contributed to study design, data interpretation and manuscript preparation and editing. All authors read and approved the final manuscript.

Competing interests

The authors declare no conflicts of interest.

References

1. Shi Y, Zhao H, Cao Y, Yang D, Li Z, Zhang B, Liang X, Li T, Chen J, Shen J, et al. Genome-wide association study identifies eight new risk loci for polycystic ovary syndrome. Nat Genet. 2012;44:1020–5.
2. Diao FY, Xu M, Hu Y, Li J, Xu Z, Lin M, Wang L, Zhou Y, Zhou Z, Liu J, Sha J. The molecular characteristics of polycystic ovary syndrome (PCOS) ovary defined by human ovary cDNA microarray. J Mol Endocrinol. 2004;33:59–72.
3. Revised 2003 Consensus on diagnostic criteria and long-term health risks related to polycystic ovary syndrome. Fertil Steril. 2004;(81):19–25.
4. Kandaraki E, Christakou C, Diamanti-Kandarakis E. Metabolic syndrome and polycystic ovary syndrome... and vice versa. Arq Bras Endocrinol Metabol. 2009;53:227–37.
5. Carmina E. Cardiovascular risk and events in polycystic ovary syndrome. Climacteric. 2009;12(Suppl 1):22–5.
6. Wild S, Pierpoint T, Jacobs H, McKeigue P. Long-term consequences of polycystic ovary syndrome: results of a 31 year follow-up study. Hum Fertil (Camb). 2000;3:101–5.
7. Diamanti-Kandarakis E, Piperi C. Genetics of polycystic ovary syndrome: searching for the way out of the labyrinth. Hum Reprod Update. 2005;11: 631–43.
8. Vink JM, Sadrzadeh S, Lambalk CB, Boomsma DI. Heritability of polycystic ovary syndrome in a Dutch twin-family study. J Clin Endocrinol Metab. 2006;91:2100–4.
9. Wood JR, Ho CK, Nelson-Degrave VL, McAllister JM, Strauss JF 3rd. The molecular signature of polycystic ovary syndrome (PCOS) theca cells defined by gene expression profiling. J Reprod Immunol. 2004;63:51–60.
10. Jansen E, Laven JS, Dommerholt HB, Polman J, van Rijt C, van den Hurk C, Westland J, Mosselman S, Fauser BC. Abnormal gene expression profiles in human ovaries from polycystic ovary syndrome patients. Mol Endocrinol. 2004;18:3050–63.
11. Oksjoki S, Soderstrom M, Inki P, Vuorio E, Anttila L. Molecular profiling of polycystic ovaries for markers of cell invasion and matrix turnover. Fertil Steril. 2005;83:937–44.
12. Wood JR, Dumesic DA, Abbott DH, Strauss JF 3rd. Molecular abnormalities in oocytes from women with polycystic ovary syndrome revealed by microarray analysis. J Clin Endocrinol Metab. 2007;92:705–13.
13. Kenigsberg S, Bentov Y, Chalifa-Caspi V, Potashnik G, Ofir R, Birk OS. Gene expression microarray profiles of cumulus cells in lean and overweight-obese polycystic ovary syndrome patients. Mol Hum Reprod. 2009;15:89–103.
14. Mohamed-Hussein ZA, Harun S. Construction of a polycystic ovarian syndrome (PCOS) pathway based on the interactions of PCOS-related proteins retrieved from bibliomic data. Theor Biol Med Model. 2009;6:18.
15. Mattick JS. Non-coding RNAs: the architects of eukaryotic complexity. EMBO Rep. 2001;2:986–91.
16. Ponting CP, Belgard TG. Transcribed dark matter: meaning or myth? Hum Mol Genet. 2010;19:R162–8.
17. Ponting CP, Oliver PL, Reik W. Evolution and functions of long noncoding RNAs. Cell. 2009;136:629–41.
18. Moran I, Akerman I, van de Bunt M, Xie R, Benazra M, Nammo T, Arnes L, Nakic N, Garcia-Hurtado J, Rodriguez-Segui S, et al. Human beta cell transcriptome analysis uncovers lncRNAs that are tissue-specific, dynamically regulated, and abnormally expressed in type 2 diabetes. Cell Metab. 2012; 16:435–48.
19. Huang X, Hao C, Bao H, Wang M, Dai H. Aberrant expression of long noncoding RNAs in cumulus cells isolated from PCOS patients. J Assist Reprod Genet. 2016;33:111–21.
20. Wawrzik M, Spiess AN, Herrmann R, Buiting K, Horsthemke B. Expression of SNURF-SNRPN upstream transcripts and epigenetic regulatory genes during human spermatogenesis. Eur J Hum Genet. 2009;17:1463–70.
21. Christakou C, Diamanti-Kandarakis E. Polycystic ovary syndrome--phenotypes and diagnosis. Scand J Clin Lab Invest Suppl. 2014;244:18–22. discussion 21
22. Fux Otta C, Fiol de Cuneo M, Szafryk de Mereshian P. polycystic ovary syndrome: physiopathology review. Rev Fac Cien Med Univ Nac Cordoba. 2013;70:27–30.
23. Salmena L, Poliseno L, Tay Y, Kats L, Pandolfi PP. A ceRNA hypothesis: the Rosetta stone of a hidden RNA language? Cell. 2011;146:353–8.
24. Tay Y, Rinn J, Pandolfi PP. The multilayered complexity of ceRNA crosstalk and competition. Nature. 2014;505:344–52.
25. Xu B, Zhang YW, Tong XH, Liu YS. Characterization of microRNA profile in human cumulus granulosa cells: identification of microRNAs that regulate notch signaling and are associated with PCOS. Mol Cell Endocrinol. 2015; 404:26–36.
26. Huang X, Liu C, Hao C, Tang Q, Liu R, Lin S, Zhang L, Yan W. Identification of altered microRNAs and mRNAs in the cumulus cells of PCOS patients: miRNA-509-3p promotes oestradiol secretion by targeting MAP3K8. Reproduction. 2016;151:643–55.
27. Huang X, Hao C, Shen X, Liu X, Shan Y, Zhang Y, Chen L. Differences in the transcriptional profiles of human cumulus cells isolated from MI and MII oocytes of patients with polycystic ovary syndrome. Reproduction. 2013;145: 597–608.
28. Huang X, Hao C, Shen X, Zhang Y, Liu X. RUNX2, GPX3 and PTX3 gene expression profiling in cumulus cells are reflective oocyte/embryo competence and potentially reliable predictors of embryo developmental competence in PCOS patients. Reprod Biol Endocrinol. 2013;11:109.
29. Livak KJ, Schmittgen TD. Analysis of relative gene expression data using real-time quantitative PCR and the 2(−Delta Delta C(T)) method. Methods. 2001;25:402–8.
30. Shen T, Liu K, Miao D, Cao R, Zhou B, Chen P. Lentivirus-mediated RNA interference against Japanese encephalitis virus infection in vitro and in vivo. Antivir Res. 2014;108:56–64.
31. Su Z, Zhi X, Zhang Q, Yang L, Xu H, Xu Z. LncRNA H19 functions as a competing endogenous RNA to regulate AQP3 expression by sponging miR-874 in the intestinal barrier. FEBS Lett. 2016;590:1354–64.
32. Huang S, Lu W, Ge D, Meng N, Li Y, Su L, Zhang S, Zhang Y, Zhao B, Miao J. A new microRNA signal pathway regulated by long noncoding RNA TGFB2-OT1 in autophagy and inflammation of vascular endothelial cells. Autophagy. 2015;11:2172–83.
33. John-Aryankalayil M, Palayoor ST, Makinde AY, Cerna D, Simone CB 2nd, Falduto MT, Magnuson SR, Coleman CN. Fractionated radiation alters oncomir and tumor suppressor miRNAs in human prostate cancer cells. Radiat Res. 2012;178:105–17.

34. Shi X, Sun M, Liu H, Yao Y, Song Y. Long non-coding RNAs: a new frontier in the study of human diseases. Cancer Lett. 2013;339:159–66.
35. Arya BK, Haq AU, Chaudhury K. Oocyte quality reflected by follicular fluid analysis in poly cystic ovary syndrome (PCOS): a hypothesis based on intermediates of energy metabolism. Med Hypotheses. 2012;78:475–8.
36. Gluszak O, Stopinska-Gluszak U, Glinicki P, Kapuscinska R, Snochowska H, Zgliczynski W, Debski R. Phenotype and metabolic disorders in polycystic ovary syndrome. ISRN Endocrinol. 2012;2012:569862.
37. Thomson DW, Dinger ME. Endogenous microRNA sponges: evidence and controversy. Nat Rev Genet. 2016;17:272–83.
38. Tay Y, Karreth FA, Pandolfi PP. Aberrant ceRNA activity drives lung cancer. Cell Res. 2014;24:259–60.
39. Chen L, Wang W, Cao L, Li Z, Wang X. Long non-coding RNA CCAT1 acts as a competing endogenous RNA to regulate cell growth and differentiation in acute myeloid leukemia. Mol Cells. 2016;39:330–6.
40. Sun C, Li S, Zhang F, Xi Y, Wang L, Bi Y, Li D. Long non-coding RNA NEAT1 promotes non-small cell lung cancer progression through regulation of miR-377-3p-E2F3 pathway. Oncotarget. 2016;7:51784–814.
41. Song C, Zhang J, Liu Y, Pan H, Qi HP, Cao YG, Zhao JM, Li S, Guo J, Sun HL, Li CQ. Construction and analysis of cardiac hypertrophy-associated lncRNA-mRNA network based on competitive endogenous RNA reveal functional lncRNAs in cardiac hypertrophy. Oncotarget. 2016;7:10827–40.
42. Liu XH, Sun M, Nie FQ, Ge YB, Zhang EB, Yin DD, Kong R, Xia R, Lu KH, Li JH, et al. Lnc RNA HOTAIR functions as a competing endogenous RNA to regulate HER2 expression by sponging miR-331-3p in gastric cancer. Mol Cancer. 2014;13:92.
43. Batrakou DG, de Las Heras JI, Czapiewski R, Mouras R, Schirmer EC. TMEM120A and B: nuclear envelope transmembrane proteins important for adipocyte differentiation. PLoS One. 2015;10:e0127712.
44. Machtinger R, Combelles CM, Missmer SA, Correia KF, Fox JH, Racowsky C. The association between severe obesity and characteristics of failed fertilized oocytes. Hum Reprod. 2012;27:3198–207.

18

The effect of cinnamon on polycystic ovary syndrome in a mouse model

Lei Dou[1†], Yahong Zheng[1†], Lu Li[1], Xiaowei Gui[1], Yajuan Chen[2], Meng Yu[3] and Yi Guo[1*]

Abstract

Background: Polycystic ovary syndrome (PCOS) is the most prevalent cause of anovulatory infertility and hyperandrogenism. Evidence favors insulin resistance and compensatory hyperinsulinemia as the predominant, perhaps primary, defects in PCOS. The use of insulin-sensitizing drugs has been shown to improve both the reproductive and the metabolic aspects of PCOS. Cinnamon has been found to have insulin sensitizing effect and improve menstrual cyclicity in women with PCOS. The aim of this study was to determine the effect and mechanism of cinnamon on PCOS using a dehydroepiandrosterone (DHEA) induced PCOS mouse model.

Methods: Prepubertal C57BL/6 mice (age 25 days) were raised to developed into control group, DHEA group and DHEA plus cinnamon group for 20 days. The stages of the estrous cycle were determined based on vaginal cytology; metabolic characteristics were examined by intraperitoneal glucose tolerance test and insulin tolerance test, the serum levels of hormones (testosterone, insulin, LH, FSH, IGF-1, IGFBP-1) were checked using enzyme-linked immunosorbent assay (ELISA) method, the ovarian morphology was observed by stained with hematoxylin and eosin. IGF-1 and IGFBP-1 expression in ovary were detected by immunohistochemical stain.

Results: Cinnamon restores the cyclicity and ovary morphology in PCOS mice model induced by DHEA. There are significant differences of serum level of total testosterone (0.033 ± 0.009 ng/ml), among control group, DHEA and cinnamon group (0.052 ± 0.011 ng/ml), and DHEA group (0.079 ± 0.015 ng/ml); There was an increasing tendency of serum FSH level from DHEA group (5.02 ± 0.31 ng/ml), DHEA and cinnamon group (5.81 ± 0.51 ng/ml), to control group (7.13 ± 0.74 ng/ml); and there was a decreasing trend of serum LH level from DHEA group (3.75 ± 0.57 ng/ml), DHEA and cinnamon group (1.35 ± 0.61 ng/ml), or control group (0.69 ± 0.34 ng/ml); serum insulin level is significantly higher in DHEA treated mice (1.61 ± 0.31 ng/ml) than control group (0.93 ± 0.19 ng/ml), or DHEA and cinnamon effect (1.27 ± 0.23 ng/ml) ($p < 0.05$). The DHEA group also has a higher serum IGF-1 level (0.35 ± 0.06 ng/ml) than control group (0.17 ± 0.04 ng/ml) or DHEA and cinnamon group (0.21 ± 0.05 ng/ml) ($p < 0.05$). While DHEA group has a lower IGFBP-1 level (5.5 ± 1.6 ng/ml) than control group (15.8 ± 2.1 ng/ml) or DHEA and cinnamon group (10.3 ± 2.5 ng/ml) ($p < 0.05$). Cinnamon also attenuates DHEA induced a higher IGF-1 and lower IGFBP-1 expression in ovary by immunohistochemistry.

Conclusions: These preliminary data suggest that cinnamon supplementation improves insulin resistance and may be a potential therapeutic agent for the treatment of PCOS.

Keywords: Cinnamon, Polycystic ovary syndrome, DHEA, Mice

* Correspondence: guoyi12@hotmail.com
[†]Lei Dou and Yahong Zheng contributed equally to this work.
[1]Department of Obstetrics and gynecology, First Affiliated Hospital of China Medical University, Shenyang 110001, China
Full list of author information is available at the end of the article

Background

Polycystic ovary syndrome (PCOS) is one of the most common, complex and heterogeneous endocrine disorders affecting 5–10% of women of fertile age [1]. The manifestation of this syndrome includes oligomenhorrhea, amenorrhea, anovulation, numerous antral follicles, hypersecretion of circulating LH but with lower or equivalent FSH levels, hyperandrogenemia and hirsutism [2, 3]. Most of the patients also have metabolic abnormalities, such as obesity, dyslipidemia, and insulin resistance [4]. Women with PCOS are at increased risk of reproductive abnormalities, and two-thirds of them also have metabolic dysfunction and, thereby, have an increased risk of developing type 2 diabetes mellitus and cardiovascular disease [3]. The prevalence of insulin resistance and the compensatory hyperinsulinemia among women with PCOS is 50–70% [5] and may be as high as 95% in overweight women [6]. Hyperinsulinemia may promote abnormal androgen secretion and disrupt folliculogenesis and menstrual cyclicity which are the main characteristics of PCOS [7, 8].

Although the etiology of PCOS is still unclear, what we know is that genetic and environmental factors contribute to the origin and development of this disorder [9, 10]. Under such circumstances, Nutraceuticals may represent a valuable alternative or adjunct to lifestyle interventions and conventional prescription drugs. Cinnamon, which is a spice used to flavor foods, has been shown to possess anti-PCOS and anti-diabetic properties [11–13]. In a high-fructose diet induce insulin resistance rat model, cinnamon extract not only improves systemic insulin sensitivity and dyslipidemia by enhancing insulin signaling, but also effectively ameliorates circulating levels of adipokines partially mediated via regulation of the expression of multiple genes involved in insulin sensitivity and lipogenesis [14, 15]. Several in vitro and in vivo studies have shown cinnamon can reduce insulin resistance by increasing activation of the IRS/PI-3 kinase insulin signalling pathway [13].The extracts from cinnamon stimulate autophosphorylation of the insulin receptor and inhibit protein tyrosine phosphatase I [16]. Through these two mechanisms cinnamon extract make adipocytes to increase the glucose uptake and glycogen synthesis. Oral cinnamon extract reduced fasting glucose, triglycerides, low-density lipoprotein (LDL), and total cholesterol in patients with type 2 diabetes mellitus [17], as well as improved insulin sensitivity in women with PCOS [12]. Based on these findings, we put forward our hypothesis that cinnamon has an overall impact on PCOS treatment [11]. Previous studies proved dehydroepiandrosterone (DHEA) induced PCOS model represents similar characteristic seen in human patients, such as hyperandrogenism, abnormal maturation of ovarian follicles and anovulation [18, 19]. In this experiment, we tried to gain a deeper understanding of the effect and mechanism of cinnamon on PCOS using a DHEA induced PCOS like mice model.

Methods

Animals and experimental protocols

Sixty SPF grade female prepuberal C57BL/6 mice (21-day-old)were purchased from Beijing Vital River Laboratories animal co., LTD (license: SCXK(HU)2007–0003). All animals were raised in China Medical University Animal Center, 25 °C constant temperature (Humidity 50%), 12 h light:12 h dark cyclical alternates, with food and water available ad libitum. All procedures described here were reviewed and approved by the Ethical Committee of China Medical University. At Postnatal Day 25, these mice of comparable weights (12.89 ± 1.41 g)were randomly divided into three groups (control group, DHEA group, DHEA+cinnamon group) and treated for 20 consecutive days as followings (from the day 1 to the day 20). Control group ($n = 10$): The mice were injected subcutaneously daily with 0.1 ml sesame oil and 100 μL 0.5% methylcellulose given once daily using gavage needle. DHEA group ($n = 25$): The murine model of PCOS was developed by daily injecting DHEA (6 mg/100 g body weight dissolved in 0.1 ml of sesame oil) subcutaneously as described previously [20, 21] and 100 μL 0.5% methylcellulose given once daily using gavage needle. The DHEA +cinnamon group ($n = 25$): The mice were injected the same amount of DHEA while given cinnamon powder (10 mg/100 g body weight mixed in 100 μL 0.5% methylcellulose) via gavage as described [22]. After 20 days of the treatments, both reproductive and metabolic features were evaluated. The treatments were continued until the mice were killed. Throughout the whole treatment period, the animals were weighed every two days. All samples were run in triplicate.

Estrous cycle determination

The vaginal smears were taken daily at 9 AM from the 13 days after the first injection (Day 38 of life) for 7 consecutive days. The stages of the estrous cycle were determined daily based on vaginal cytology [23]: Vaginal cells were collected via saline lavage and then fixed with methanol and stained with methylene blue staining (0.1%). Predominant nucleated epithelial cells and some cornified epithelial cells indicated the proestrus stage; predominant cornified squamous epithelial cells indicated the estrus stage; both cornified squamous epithelial cells and leukocytes indicated the metaestrus stage; and predominant leukocytes indicated the diestrus stage.

Intraperitoneal glucose tolerance test

Right after 20 days of the treatment (Day 45 of life), Intraperitoneal(IP) glucose tolerance test (IPGTT) was performed [24]. The mice were fasted overnight (16 h) before the morning of the IPGTT. The mice were injected ip with glucose (2 g/kg as a 50% glucose stock solution). Glucose levels were measured by tail vein blood sampling using a blood glucose meter (Sinocare Inc., Changsha, China) immediately before the mice were injected intraperitoneally with glucose and then at 30, 60, 90, and 120 min after administration. Data were expressed as the absolute values of blood glucose concentrations. Total area under the curve of the glucose response (AUC) was calculated using GraphPad Prism 5.0 software.

Insulin tolerance test

Five days after the IPGTT experiment, an insulin tolerance test (ITT) was carried out (Day 51 of life) as previously described [25]. The mice were fasted for 6 h and then injected intraperitoneally with insulin (1 IU/kg body weight, Wanbang Biopharmaceuticals, China). Blood glucose was measured immediately before insulin administration and then at 30, 60, 90, and 120 min after injection. Data were expressed as the values of blood glucose concentrations corrected for fasting glucose. Total AUC of the corrected glucose values was calculated using GraphPad Prism 5.0 software.

Hormonal analysis of serum

After 21 days of treatment (47 days of life), the mice were anesthetized via an intraperitoneal injection of a mixture of 100 mg/ml Ketamine and 20 mg/ml Xylazine (Sigma-Aldrich Chemical, St. Louis, Missouri, USA) prepared in injectable saline (0.1 ml/10 g body weight) [26], then underwent a retrobulbar venous plexus blood draw after overnight fasting. Then the serum concentration level of testosterone, FSH, LH, IGF-1, IGFBP-1,and insulin were measured using by mouse ELISA Kit (R&D Systems. USA for testostereon testing, and Muyuan bio-tech company, Shanghai, China for the other hormones testing), as previously described [27]. All measurements were taken according to the manufacturer's instructions. The detection limit was 0.041 ng/mL for testosterone, 0.032 ng/ml for FSH, 0.048 ng/ml for LH, 2.05 ng/ml for IGF-1 and 0.35 ng/ml for IGFBP-1. The intra- and inter-assay variation was 5.2% and 8.6% for testosterone, 3.1% and 5.4% for FSH, 5.6% and 6.3% for LH, 4.1% and 3.9% for IGF-1, 4.7% and 4.3% for IGFBP-1.

Ovary collection and histology

At 47 days of life, immediately after the last blood draw, ovary samples were then rapidly removed from the animals. Ovaries from each mouse were fixed in 4% paraformaldehyde (PFA) and postfixed in 20% sucrose solution. Afterward, tissues were embedded into Tissue-Tek (O.C.T. compound; Sakura), frozen at − 80 °C overnight, and cut into sections (6-μm thickness) with a Leica Cryostat (LEICA CM1850). The ovary sections were stained with hematoxylin and eosin (H&E) according to the standard histological procedures. To examine ovarian morphology, every 12th section was mounted on a glass slide. Numbers of corpora lutea and large antral follicles were counted [28, 29]. The follicle diameter was calculated as the mean distance between opposite basal membrane portions, while the wall thickness was calculated as the sum of theca interna and granulosa cell layers. A cystic follicle is considered to be a large fluid filled cyst with an attenuated granulosa cell layer and thickened theca cell layer [30]. The count of large antral follicles was performed based on the mean diameter of the follicles greater than 300 μm. The area of the largest follicles was measured with ImageJ (National Institutes of Health) software.

Immunohistochemistry

Ovarian sections were prepared as described above and Immunohistochemistry was performed as described previously [31]. Sections (5 μm thickness) were deparaffinized and permeabilized with 0.5% triton X-100 in tris buffered saline (TBS) for 10 min followed by 2 washes with TBS. Endogenous peroxidase activity was quenched with 3% (vol/vol) H_2O_2 in methanol for 15 min. Antigen retrieval was performed by heating sections in 10 mM citrate buffer. Tissue sections were blocked with 1% bovine serum albumin for 20 min at 37 °C, followed by overnight incubation at room temperature with the goat anti mouse IGF-1 polyclonal antibody (1:40; AF-291-NA, R&D, USA), or anti-IGFBP-1 polyclonal antibody (1:40; AF871, R&D, USA). Nonimmune immunoglobulin G (IgG) was used as the negative control. Sections were then incubated with a polyperoxidase-conjugated rabbit anti-goat IgG (Zhongshan Golden Bridge) for 20 min at 37 °C. Immunostaining was revealed by using diaminobenzidine and counterstained with hematoxylin. Immunostaining intensity was evaluated by three independent observers not involved with the study who were asked to rate the intensity of the staining without knowing the identity of samples.

Statistical analysis

Data are presented as mean ± SEM. Statistical analyses were performed with statistical software package SPSS. A One-way analysis of variance and least significant difference Tukey's post hoc tests were used to evaluate the hormonal differences among the groups. A two-way analysis of variance with repeated measures for time was used to test significances of IPGTT and ITT experiment. Statistical significance was set at $P < 0.05$.

Results

Cinnamon restores estrous cyclicity and ovary morphology

As a result, all mice from DHEA group were completely acyclic and remained in constant estrus while control mice had normal cycle. The mice from DHEA plus cinnamon group have cycle but less than controls. Representative cyclicities of mice in three groups are showed in Fig. 1a. All of the mice (10 of 10,100%)in the control group showed normal estrous cyclity, while (20 of 25, 80%) the mice treated with DHEA displayed abnormal estrous cycles. Cinnamon treatment recover the disrupted estrous cycle induced by DHEA with a longer period (17 of 25, 68%). We did not find the difference of the weight of mice body among the three groups of mice as showed in Fig. 1b. Typical micrographs of ovarian sections of the three groups are shown in Fig. 1c. Comparing with DHEA plus Cinnamon or control group, DHEA treated mice exhibited a significant decrease of morphologically healthy large antral follicles, their identifying characteristic is a fluid-filled cavity and the oocyte lies at the edge in a mound made of granulosa epithelial cells [17]. The number of corpora lutea and oocyte in DHEA group was significantly lower than the DHEA plus Cinnamon or control group ($P < 0.05$). The thickness of the granulosa cell layer of large antral in DHEA group is less and the cells appear degenerated.

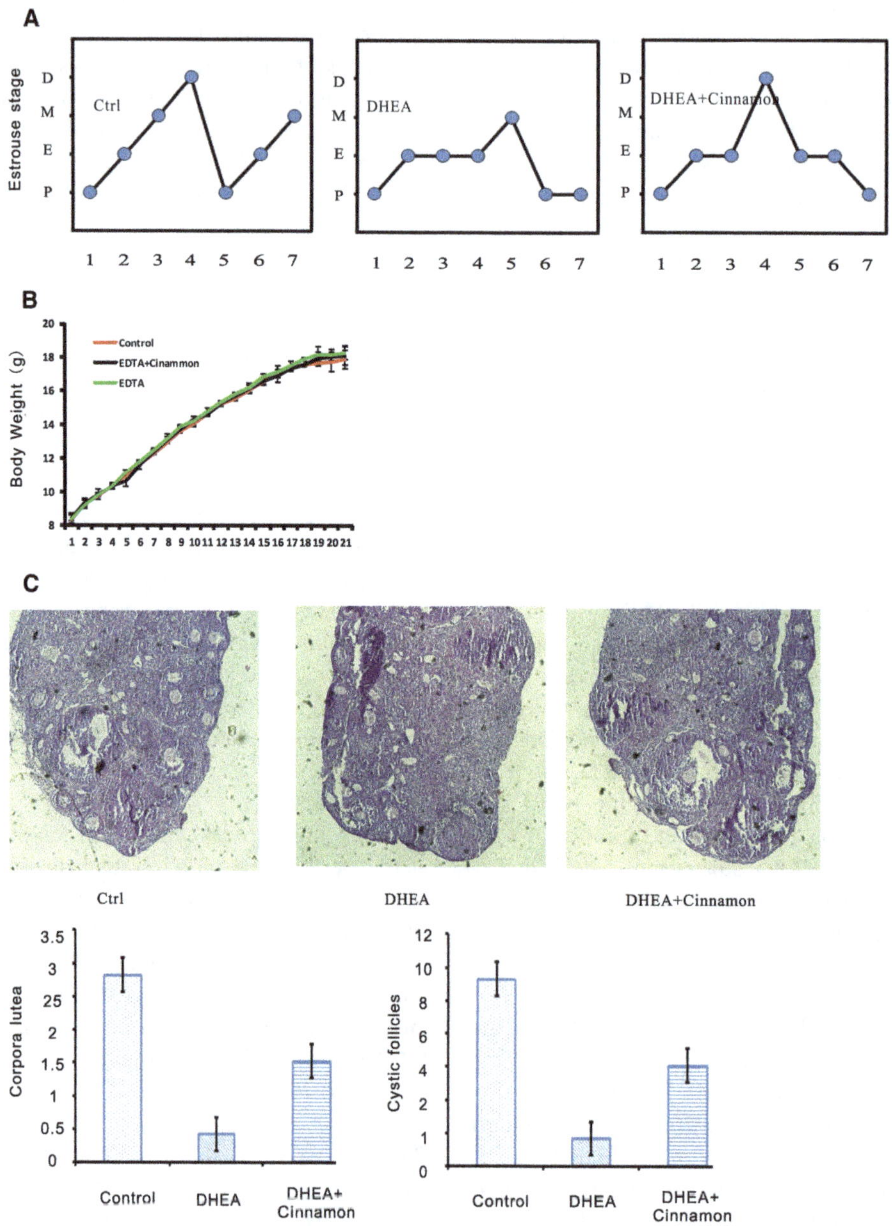

Fig. 1 Estrous cycle, body weight, and ovarian morphology in the mice. **a** Representative estrous cycle of one mouse from each group. D,diestrus; M, metestrus; E, estrus; P, proestrus. **b** Body weight. **c** Representative H&E staining of ovarian sections of one mouse from each group. Micrographs were taken at magnifications× 200

Cinnamon effect on hormone level

Total testosterone is increasing from control group (0.033 ± 0.009 ng/ml), to DHEA and cinnamon group (0.052 ± 0.011 ng/ml), to DHEA group (0.079 ± 0.015 ng/ml), the differences among them were significant ($p < 0.05$). There was an increasing tendency of serum FSH level from DHEA group (5.02 ± 0.31 ng/ml), DHEA and cinnamon group (5.81 ± 0.51 ng/ml), to control group (7.13 ± 0.74 ng/ml); and there was a decreasing trend of serum LH level from DHEA group (3.75 ± 0.57 ng/ml), DHEA and cinnamon group (1.35 ± 0.61 ng/ml), or control group (0.69 ± 0.34 ng/ml); The differences of the ration of LH to FSH among control group, DHEA group and DHEA plus cinnamon group were significant ($p < 0.05$). Serum insulin level was significant higher in DHEA treated mice (1.61 ± 0.31 ng/ml) than control group (0.93 ± 0.19 ng/ml), add cinnamon can attenuated DHEA effect on insulin in the mice model (1.27 ± 0.23 ng/ml) ($p < 0.05$). The DHEA group also have a higher serum IGF-1 level (0.35 ± 0.06 ng/ml) than control group (0.17 ± 0.04 ng/ml) or DHEA and cinnamon group (0.21 ± 0.05 ng/ml) ($p < 0.05$). While DHEA group have a lower IGFBP-1 level (5.5 ± 1.6 ng/ml) than control group (15.8 ± 2.1 ng/ml) or DHEA and cinnamon group (10.3 ± 2.5 ng/ml) ($p < 0.05$); (Fig. 2).

IPGTT and ITT experiments

We performed IPGTT to investigate cinnamon effect on glucose tolerance of DHEA induced PCOS model. There were no differences of fasting glucose level among the three groups (Fig. 3a). Neither differences in 0- to 120-min AUC value existed among the tree groups (Fig. 3b). We also performed Insulin tolerance test. Blood glucose levels were corrected for fasting glucose. There were significant differences of corrected serum glucose levels among the three groups of mice after injection ($P < 0.05$). Correspondingly, the differences of AUC were also significant among the three groups ($P < 0.05$; Fig. 3c). In addition, these data suggested the impaired glucose tolerance in DHEA induced PCOS mice was likely be mitigated by cinnamon treatment.

Cinnamon effects on IGF-1 and IGFBP-1 expression in ovary

In the normal ovary of control group, there was weak IGF-1 staining was seen in oocyte and granulosa cell of small antral follicles. Atretic follicle and the surrounding stroma in DHEA treated group showed a strong IGF-1 staining. There was a moderate IGF-1 staining in DHEA and cinnamon group (Fig. 4a). While large follicles in the ovary of control mice showed a strong IGFBP-1 staining. Atretic follicles in the ovary of DHEA treated mice have no IGFBP-1 staining. Follicles in the ovary of DHEA and cinnamon treated mice have a moderate IGFBP-1 staining (Fig. 4b).

Discussion

As a complex disorder consisting multiple phenotypic parameters, PCOS patients have neuroendocrine and ovarian impairments, as well as a high prevalence of metabolic perturbation, such as obesity and glucose intolerance [32, 33]. There is clear evidence that insulin stimulates ovarian thecal and stromal androgen secretion in vitro [34]. In women with PCOS, insulin resistance with compensatory hyperinsulinemia induces overproduction of ovarian androgens, leading to hyperandrogenism. The action of insulin on the production of androgens in the ovary is believed to be through IGF-1 receptors on theca and stroma cells [35, 36]. IGF-1 stimulates estrogen production by granulosa cell [37] and acts synergistically with FSH and LH in controlling granulosa cell aromatase concentration [38]. IGF-1 also acts synergistically with LH to stimulate androgen production on thecal cell [39]. High level of insulin and IGF-1 amplifies the effect of LH on granulosa cell, inducing terminal differentiation and leading to anovulation. IGF-1 and IGFBP-1affect follicular maturation by autocrine and/or paracrine mechanisms [40, 41]. It looks like that IGF-1 has negative impact on normal folliculogenesis and ovulation [39, 42]. Though total plasma IGF-1 level was not reported significantly higher in PCOS patients [43], there is a decreased plasma IGFBP-1 level in PCOS patients compared with normal women [44]. The reduction of IGFBP-1 concentration may raise IGF-1 bioavailability, in fact, the free plasma IGF-1 concentration is higher in PCOS patients [45].

Insulin resistance likely contributes to the hallmark symptoms of PCOS such as androgen excess and menstrual irregularity, as well as increases the risk of developing diabetes mellitus, hyperlipidemia and cardiovascular diseases [46]. Hence, reducing insulin resistance not only provides potential reproductive health benefits but more importantly is the key to improving the overall long-term health of patients with PCOS.

Cinnamon, a commonly used spice and flavoring material, has a long history as a medicine as well. The cinnamon has been recognized as insulin potentiating factor almost 20 years ago [47]. Cinnamon extracts act as enhancer of enhancer of insulin-receptor function and inhibitor of the enzyme that blocks insulin-receptor attachment, respectively. Procyanidin polyphenol type-A polymers extracted from cinnamon and has the ability to stimulate autophosphorylation of the insulin receptor and inhibit protein tyrosine phosphatase I. Insulin receptor kinase autophosphorylation and subsequent phosphorylation of its principal substrate are markedly decreased in insulin-responsive tissues of subjects with severe obesity or non-insulin-dependent diabetes mellitus (NIDDM) [48]. The inhibition of tyrosine phosphatase by cinnamon would prove that insulin resistance

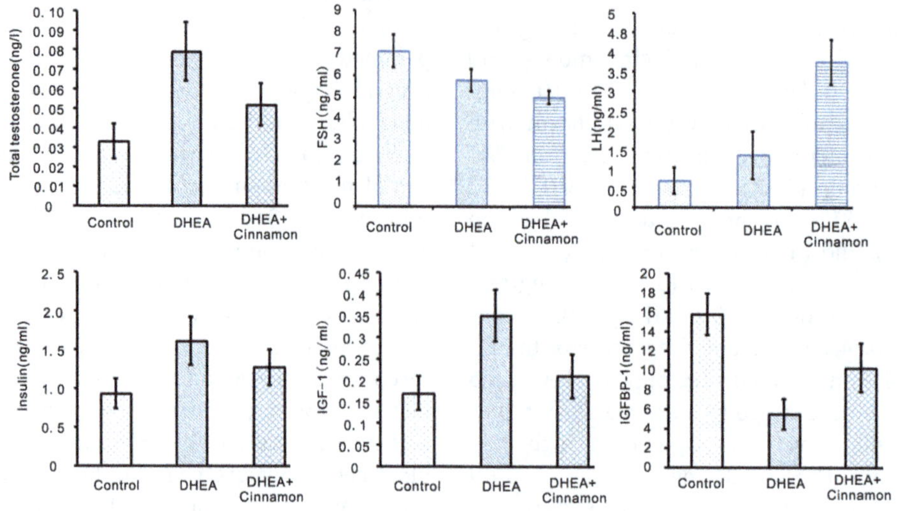

Fig. 2 Serum levels of testosterone, insulin, FSH, LH, IGF-1 and IGFBP-1in the mice. Data are presented as mean ± SEM. $n = 8$ per group

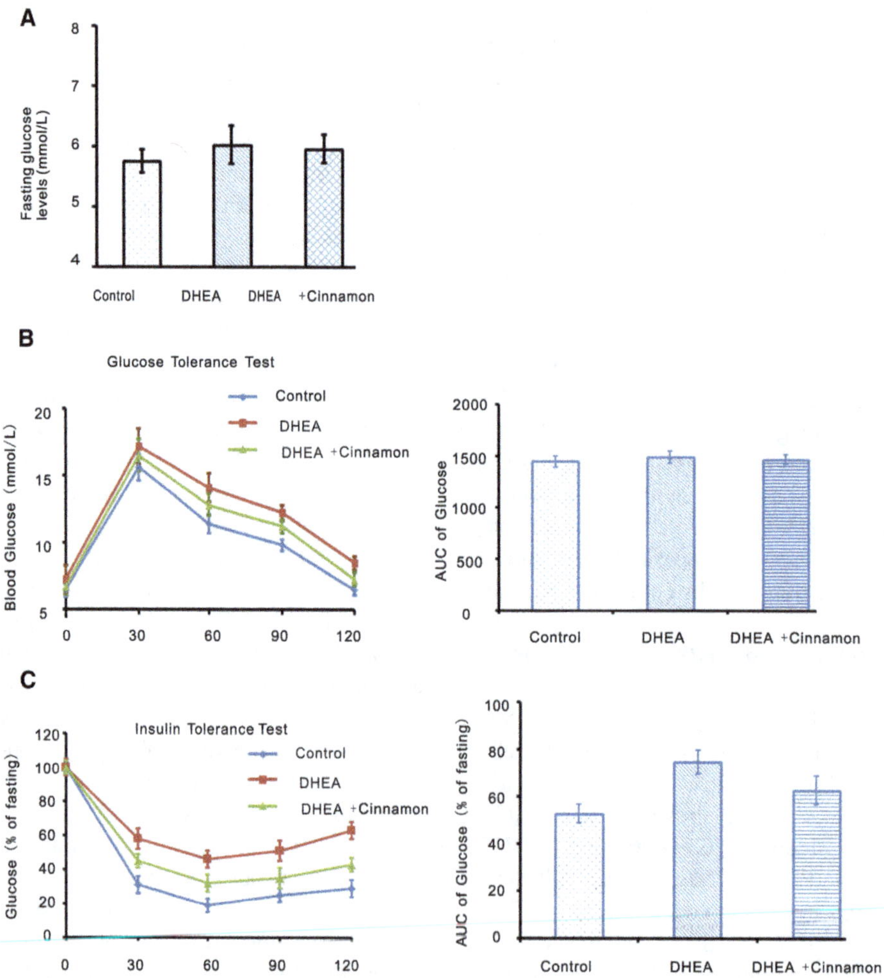

Fig. 3 Fasting glucose, IPGTT and ITT Experiments in the mice. **a** Fasting glucose. **b** IPGTT experiment, IPGTT curve and IPGTT AUC. **c** ITT experiment, Serum glucose levels corrected for fasting glucose and the AUC of the corrected glucose levels. Data are presented as mean ± SEM. $N = 8$ per group

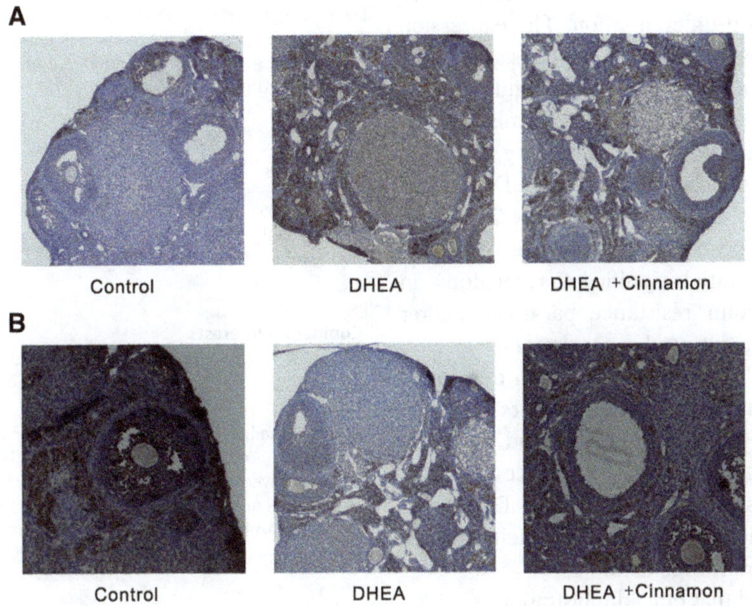

Fig. 4 a Weak staining of IGF-1 in ovary of control mice group, strong staining of DHEA mice group, moderate staining of DHEA and cinnamon group. **b** Strong staining of IGFBP-1 in ovary of control mice group, weak staining of DHEA mice group, moderate staining of DHEA and cinnamon group

may be due to elevated tyrosine phosphatase activity [49]. Cinnamon has been showed to have anti-diabetes and anti-obese properties. Cinnamon extract has been found to mitigate insulin resistance induced by high fructose diets [14] and benefit glucose utilization by enhancing insulin signaling pathway [15]. Cinnamon extract increases glycogen synthesis by activating glycogen synthase and inhibiting glycogen synthase kinase 3β [50], and reduces glucose absorption in the small intestine through increasing in glucosidase enzymes and inhibition of intestinal ATPase [51, 52]. Cinnamon also contains other polyphenolic compounds like rutin, catechin, quercetin and kaempferol which have insulin like activity [53]. In a study to explore the mechanism of cinnamon on glucose regulating, cinnamic acid with 5 and 10 mg/kg doses administered orally to diabetic rats improved glucose tolerance in a dose-dependent manner; as well as in vitro studies showed that cinnamic acid significantly enhanced glucose-stimulated insulin secretion in isolated islets [54]. So cinnamic acid exerts the function of improving glucose tolerance in vivo and stimulating insulin secretion in vitro. Cinnamaldehyde, one of the active components of cinnamon, has been tested for its antiobesity by investigating the antidifferentiation effect on 3 T3-L1 preadipocytes, and high-fat-diet-induced obese ICR mice. It was found that cinnamaldehyde significantly reduced lipid accumulation and down-regulated the expression of peroxisome proliferator-activated receptor-γ (PPAR-γ), CCAAT/enhancer-binding proteins α (C/EBPα), and sterol regulatory element-binding protein 1 (SREBP1) in concentration-dependent manners. Moreover, cinnamaldehyde markedly up-regulated AMP-activated protein kinase (AMPK) and acetyl-CoA carboxylase (ACC), and these effects were blunted in the presence of AMPK inhibitor, compound C [55, 56]. In the animal study, weight gains, insulin resistance index, plasma triglyceride (TG), nonesterified fatty acid (NEFA), and cholesterol levels in the 40 mg/kg of cinnamaldehyde-administered group were significantly decreased by 67.3, 55, 39, 31, and 23%, respectively, when compared to the high-fat diet control group [55]. Cinnamon can also modulate the insulin and IGF1 signaling pathways such as mTOR, Cyclic-AMP signaling and autophagy [57].

As a folk medicine, cinnamon shows hepatoprotective [58], anti-oxidant [59], anti-obesity [60], antihyperlipidemic [61], and antidiabetic activities [62]. A randomized controlled clinical trial has provided evidence that cinnamon supplementation improves menstrual cyclicity and may be an effective treatment option for some women with PCOS [11]. The underlying mechanism for cinnamon effects on PCOS may contribute to its improvement in insulin sensitivity. Insulin receptor is the entry of insulin signaling pathway that mediates the pleiotropic actions of insulin. Insulin receptor substrate (IRS) proteins act as docking molecules to connect tyrosine kinase receptor activation to essential downstream kinase cascades, including activation of the PI-3 kinase or MAPK cascade [63]. Phosphorylation of IRS proteins leads to the activation of these two main signaling pathways. The PI-3 kinase pathway is responsible for most of the metabolic actions of insulin, and the MAPK pathway regulates expression of some genes and cooperates with the PI-3 kinase pathway to control cell growth and differentiation. The expression level of IRS protein has been found to be significantly downregulated in the model animals and upregulated after cinnamon treatment [64]. In the first randomized, controlled trial, cinnamon at different dosages (1 g, 3 g, 6 g) decreased mean fasting glucose, triglycerides, LDL cholesterol, and total cholesterol in patients with type 2 diabetes [17]. A prospective placebo-controlled pilot study showed that cinnamon demonstrated significant reductions in fasting glucose and insulin resistance parameters after 8 weeks of oral cinnamon extract 1 g per day [12].

Different kinds of Rodent models have been developed to study the mechanisms and treatment effects of PCOS [65, 66]. DHEA, as the most abundant steroid hormone in the circulation, has been used to induce a PCOS mouse model for almost a decade [20]. The DHEA induced PCOS mice model has disturbed cyclicity, multicystic ovaries, and hyperandrogenism.

In this study, we showed that oral administration of cinnamon extract would restore cyclicity, down-regulate testosterone and improve insulin sensitivity in DHEA-induced PCOS mice with the C57BL/6 background.

The results of this study confirmed the effects that cinnamon had on the reduction of insulin resistance. Although the effects of cinnamon on diabetes and its related blood parameters and lipid profile have been studied in several trials, to our knowledge, this is the first study indicating the therapeutic effects of cinnamon on PCOS characteristics with animal model. In this study, we confirmed cinnamon effect in treating PCOS by reducing the level of IGF-I and increase the level of IGFBP-1 in plasma as well as in ovary tissue.

Conclusions

In summary, our study demonstrated that cinnamon had the ability to restore the estrous cyclicity and ovary morphology, down-regulate serum levels of testosterone and insulin, decrease IGF-1 level while increase IGFBP-1 level in plasma as well as in the ovary in DHEA induce PCOS mice model. Cinnamon may be a potential therapeutic agent for the treatment of PCOS.

Abbreviations

AUC: Area under the curve; DHEA: Dehydroepiandrosterone; ELISA: Enzyme-linked immunosorbent assay; FSH: Follicle-stimulating hormone; HE: Hematoxylin-eosin; IGF-1: Insulin-like growth factor I; IGFBP-1: Insulin like growth factor binding protein-1; IHC: Immunohistochemical; IPGTT: Intraperitoneal Glucose Tolerance Test; IRS: Insulin receptor substrate; IRS/PI: Insulin receptor substrate/Phosphoinositide; ITT: Insulin tolerance test; LDL: Low-density lipoprotein; LH: Luteinizing hormone; MAPK: Mitogen-activated protein kinase; MC: Methylcellulose; NIDDM: Non-insulin-dependent diabetes mellitus; PCOS: Polycystic ovary syndrome; SPF: Specific pathogen Free; TBS: Tris buffered saline

Acknowledgements

We are grateful to all the participants involved in this study. We thank two anonymous reviewers for constructive comments on the manuscript.

Authors'contributions

LD, YZ, MY, and YG designed the study and prepared the manuscript. YZ and LL produced the DHEA induced PCOS mice model. XG and YC performed the hormone test and immunohistochemistry. All authors read and approved the final manuscript.

Funding

This study was funded by the National Natural Science Foundation of China (No. 81572054 and No. 81171649) to Yi Guo. The funding bodies had no role in study design, collection, analysis, and interpretation of data or in manuscript preparation.

Competing interests

The authors declare that they have no competing interests.

Author details

[1]Department of Obstetrics and gynecology, First Affiliated Hospital of China Medical University, Shenyang 110001, China. [2]Department of Obstetrics and gynecology, Anshan Branch of First Affiliated Hospital of China Medical University, Anshan, China. [3]Department of Reproductive Biology and Transgenic Animals, China Medical University, Shenyang, China.

References

1. Fauser BC, Tarlatzis BC, Rebar RW, Legro RS, Balen AH, Lobo R, Carmina E, Chang J, Yildiz BO, Laven JS, et al. Consensus on women's health aspects of polycystic ovary syndrome (PCOS): the Amsterdam ESHRE/ASRM-sponsored 3rd PCOS consensus workshop group. Fertil Steril. 2012;97:28–38 e25.
2. Abbott DH, Dumesic DA, Franks S. Developmental origin of polycystic ovary syndrome - a hypothesis. J Endocrinol. 2002;174:1–5.
3. Goodarzi MO, Dumesic DA, Chazenbalk G, Azziz R. Polycystic ovary syndrome: etiology, pathogenesis and diagnosis. Nat Rev Endocrinol. 2011;7:219–31.
4. Diamanti-Kandarakis E, Dunaif A. Insulin resistance and the polycystic ovary syndrome revisited: an update on mechanisms and implications. Endocr Rev. 2012;33:981–1030.
5. Dunaif A. Insulin resistance and the polycystic ovary syndrome: mechanism and implications for pathogenesis. Endocr Rev. 1997;18:774–800.
6. Carmina E, Lobo RA. Use of fasting blood to assess the prevalence of insulin resistance in women with polycystic ovary syndrome. Fertil Steril. 2004;82:661–5.
7. Nestler JE, Jakubowicz DJ, de Vargas AF, Brik C, Quintero N, Medina F. Insulin stimulates testosterone biosynthesis by human thecal cells from women with polycystic ovary syndrome by activating its own receptor and using inositolglycan mediators as the signal transduction system. J Clin Endocrinol Metab. 1998;83:2001–5.
8. Azziz R. Androgen excess is the key element in polycystic ovary syndrome. Fertil Steril. 2003;80:252–4.
9. Franks S, Gharani N, Waterworth D, Batty S, White D, Williamson R, McCarthy M. The genetic basis of polycystic ovary syndrome. Hum Reprod. 1997;12: 2641–8.
10. Kahsar-Miller M, Azziz R. The development of the polycystic ovary syndrome: family history as a risk factor. Trends Endocrinol Metab. 1998; 9:55–8.
11. Kort DH, Lobo RA. Preliminary evidence that cinnamon improves menstrual cyclicity in women with polycystic ovary syndrome: a randomized controlled trial. Am J Obstet Gynecol. 2014;211:487 e481–6.
12. Wang JG, Anderson RA, Graham GM 3rd, Chu MC, Sauer MV, Guarnaccia MM, Lobo RA. The effect of cinnamon extract on insulin resistance parameters in polycystic ovary syndrome: a pilot study. Fertil Steril. 2007;88:240–3.
13. Qin B, Nagasaki M, Ren M, Bajotto G, Oshida Y, Sato Y. Cinnamon extract (traditional herb) potentiates in vivo insulin-regulated glucose utilization via enhancing insulin signaling in rats. Diabetes Res Clin Pract. 2003;62:139–48.
14. Qin B, Nagasaki M, Ren M, Bajotto G, Oshida Y, Sato Y. Cinnamon extract prevents the insulin resistance induced by a high-fructose diet. Horm Metab Res. 2004;36:119–25.

15. Mang B, Wolters M, Schmitt B, Kelb K, Lichtinghagen R, Stichtenoth DO, Hahn A. Effects of a cinnamon extract on plasma glucose, HbA, and serum lipids in diabetes mellitus type 2. Eur J Clin Investig. 2006;36:340–4.
16. Imparl-Radosevich J, Deas S, Polansky MM, Baedke DA, Ingebritsen TS, Anderson RA, Graves DJ. Regulation of PTP-1 and insulin receptor kinase by fractions from cinnamon: implications for cinnamon regulation of insulin signalling. Horm Res. 1998;50:177–82.
17. Khan A, Safdar M, Ali Khan MM, Khattak KN, Anderson RA. Cinnamon improves glucose and lipids of people with type 2 diabetes. Diabetes Care. 2003;26:3215–8.
18. Knudsen JF, Costoff A, Mahesh VB. Dehydroepiandrosterone-induced polycystic ovaries and acyclicity in the rat. Fertil Steril. 1975;26:807–17.
19. Knudsen JF, Mahesh VB. Initiation of precocious sexual maturation in the immature rat treated with dehydroepiandrosterone. Endocrinology. 1975;97:458–68.
20. Luchetti CG, Solano ME, Sander V, Arcos ML, Gonzalez C, Di Girolamo G, Chiocchio S, Cremaschi G, Motta AB. Effects of dehydroepiandrosterone on ovarian cystogenesis and immune function. J Reprod Immunol. 2004;64:59–74.
21. Elia E, Sander V, Luchetti CG, Solano ME, Di Girolamo G, Gonzalez C, Motta AB. The mechanisms involved in the action of metformin in regulating ovarian function in hyperandrogenized mice. Mol Hum Reprod. 2006;12: 475–81.
22. Khasnavis S, Pahan K. Cinnamon treatment upregulates neuroprotective proteins Parkin and DJ-1 and protects dopaminergic neurons in a mouse model of Parkinson's disease. J NeuroImmune Pharmacol. 2014;9:569–81.
23. Walters KA, Middleton LJ, Joseph SR, Hazra R, Jimenez M, Simanainen U, Allan CM, Handelsman DJ. Targeted loss of androgen receptor signaling in murine granulosa cells of preantral and antral follicles causes female subfertility. Biol Reprod. 2012;87:151.
24. Kaku K, Fiedorek FT Jr, Province M, Permutt MA. Genetic analysis of glucose tolerance in inbred mouse strains. Evidence for polygenic control. Diabetes. 1988;37:707–13.
25. Brennan-Speranza TC, Henneicke H, Gasparini SJ, Blankenstein KI, Heinevetter U, Cogger VC, Svistounov D, Zhang Y, Cooney GJ, Buttgereit F, et al. Osteoblasts mediate the adverse effects of glucocorticoids on fuel metabolism. J Clin Invest. 2012;122:4172–89.
26. Mulder KJ, Mulder JB. Ketamine and xylazine anesthesia in the mouse. Vet Med Small Anim Clin. 1979;74:569–70.
27. van Casteren JI, Schoonen WG, Kloosterboer HJ. Development of time-resolved immunofluorometric assays for rat follicle-stimulating hormone and luteinizing hormone and application on sera of cycling rats. Biol Reprod. 2000;62:886–94.
28. Maurya VK, Sangappa C, Kumar V, Mahfooz S, Singh A, Rajender S, Jha RK. Expression and activity of Rac1 is negatively affected in the dehydroepiandrosterone induced polycystic ovary of mouse. J Ovarian Res. 2014;7:32.
29. Kauffman AS, Thackray VG, Ryan GE, Tolson KP, Glidewell-Kenney CA, Semaan SJ, Poling MC, Iwata N, Breen KM, Duleba AJ, et al. A novel Letrozole model recapitulates both the reproductive and metabolic phenotypes of polycystic ovary syndrome in female mice. Biol Reprod. 2015;93:69.
30. Caldwell AS, Middleton LJ, Jimenez M, Desai R, McMahon AC, Allan CM, Handelsman DJ, Walters KA. Characterization of reproductive, metabolic, and endocrine features of polycystic ovary syndrome in female hyperandrogenic mouse models. Endocrinology. 2014;155:3146–59.
31. Kang J, Chapdelaine P, Parent J, Madore E, Laberge PY, Fortier MA. Expression of human prostaglandin transporter in the human endometrium across the menstrual cycle. J Clin Endocrinol Metab. 2005;90:2308–13.
32. Blank SK, McCartney CR, Marshall JC. The origins and sequelae of abnormal neuroendocrine function in polycystic ovary syndrome. Hum Reprod Update. 2006;12:351–61.
33. Moran LJ, Misso ML, Wild RA, Norman RJ. Impaired glucose tolerance, type 2 diabetes and metabolic syndrome in polycystic ovary syndrome: a systematic review and meta-analysis. Hum Reprod Update. 2010;16:347–63.
34. Barbieri RL. Hyperandrogenism, insulin resistance and acanthosis nigricans. 10 years of progress. J Reprod Med. 1994;39:327–36.
35. Nagamani M, Stuart CA. Specific binding sites for insulin-like growth factor I in the ovarian stroma of women with polycystic ovarian disease and stromal hyperthecosis. Am J Obstet Gynecol. 1990;163:1992–7.
36. Bergh C, Carlsson B, Olsson JH, Selleskog U, Hillensjo T. Regulation of androgen production in cultured human thecal cells by insulin-like growth factor I and insulin. Fertil Steril. 1993;59:323–31.
37. Erickson GF, Magoffin DA, Cragun JR, Chang RJ. The effects of insulin and insulin-like growth factors-I and -II on estradiol production by granulosa cells of polycystic ovaries. J Clin Endocrinol Metab. 1990;70:894–902.
38. Erickson GF, Garzo VG, Magoffin DA. Insulin-like growth factor-I regulates aromatase activity in human granulosa and granulosa luteal cells. J Clin Endocrinol Metab. 1989;69:716–24.
39. Cara JF, Rosenfield RL. Insulin-like growth factor I and insulin potentiate luteinizing hormone-induced androgen synthesis by rat ovarian thecal-interstitial cells. Endocrinology. 1988;123:733–9.
40. Suikkari AM, Tiitinen A, Stenman UH, Seppala M, Laatikainen T. Oral contraceptives increase insulin-like growth factor binding protein-1 concentration in women with polycystic ovarian disease. Fertil Steril. 1991; 55:895–9.
41. Katz E, Ricciarelli E, Adashi EY. The potential relevance of growth hormone to female reproductive physiology and pathophysiology. Fertil Steril. 1993;59:8–34.
42. Barbieri RL, Makris A, Randall RW, Daniels G, Kistner RW, Ryan KJ. Insulin stimulates androgen accumulation in incubations of ovarian stroma obtained from women with hyperandrogenism. J Clin Endocrinol Metab. 1986;62:904–10.
43. Homburg R, Pariente C, Lunenfeld B, Jacobs HS. The role of insulin-like growth factor-1 (IGF-1) and IGF binding protein-1 (IGFBP-1) in the pathogenesis of polycystic ovary syndrome. Hum Reprod. 1992;7:1379–83.
44. Suikkari AM, Ruutiainen K, Erkkola R, Seppala M. Low levels of low molecular weight insulin-like growth factor-binding protein in patients with polycystic ovarian disease. Hum Reprod. 1989;4:136–9.
45. Thierry van Dessel HJ, Lee PD, Faessen G, Fauser BC, Giudice LC. Elevated serum levels of free insulin-like growth factor I in polycystic ovary syndrome. J Clin Endocrinol Metab. 1999;84:3030–5.
46. Lobo RA, Carmina E. The importance of diagnosing the polycystic ovary syndrome. Ann Intern Med. 2000;132:989–93.
47. Khan A, Bryden NA, Polansky MM, Anderson RA. Insulin potentiating factor and chromium content of selected foods and spices. Biol Trace Elem Res. 1990;24:183–8.
48. Goodyear LJ, Giorgino F, Sherman LA, Carey J, Smith RJ, Dohm GL. Insulin receptor phosphorylation, insulin receptor substrate-1 phosphorylation, and phosphatidylinositol 3-kinase activity are decreased in intact skeletal muscle strips from obese subjects. J Clin Invest. 1995;95:2195–204.
49. Nadiv O, Shinitzky M, Manu H, Hecht D, Roberts CT Jr, LeRoith D, Zick Y. Elevated protein tyrosine phosphatase activity and increased membrane viscosity are associated with impaired activation of the insulin receptor kinase in old rats. Biochem J. 1994;298(Pt 2):443–50.
50. Couturier K, Qin B, Batandier C, Awada M, Hininger-Favier I, Canini F, Leverve X, Roussel AM, Anderson RA. Cinnamon increases liver glycogen in an animal model of insulin resistance. Metabolism. 2011;60:1590–7.
51. Adisakwattana S, Lerdsuwankij O, Poputtachai U, Minipun A, Suparpprom C. Inhibitory activity of cinnamon bark species and their combination effect with acarbose against intestinal alpha-glucosidase and pancreatic alpha-amylase. Plant Foods Hum Nutr. 2011;66:143–8.
52. Kreydiyyeh SI, Usta J, Copti R. Effect of cinnamon, clove and some of their constituents on the Na(+)-K(+)-ATPase activity and alanine absorption in the rat jejunum. Food Chem Toxicol. 2000;38:755–62.
53. Anderson RA, Broadhurst CL, Polansky MM, Schmidt WF, Khan A, Flanagan VP, Schoene NW, Graves DJ. Isolation and characterization of polyphenol type-a polymers from cinnamon with insulin-like biological activity. J Agric Food Chem. 2004;52:65–70.
54. Hafizur RM, Hameed A, Shukrana M, Raza SA, Chishti S, Kabir N, Siddiqui RA. Cinnamic acid exerts anti-diabetic activity by improving glucose tolerance in vivo and by stimulating insulin secretion in vitro. Phytomedicine. 2015;22: 297–300.
55. Huang B, Yuan HD, Kim DY, Quan HY, Chung SH. Cinnamaldehyde prevents adipocyte differentiation and adipogenesis via regulation of peroxisome proliferator-activated receptor-gamma (PPARgamma) and AMP-activated protein kinase (AMPK) pathways. J Agric Food Chem. 2011;59:3666–73.
56. Sheng X, Zhang Y, Gong Z, Huang C, Zang YQ. Improved insulin resistance and lipid metabolism by cinnamon extract through activation of peroxisome proliferator-activated receptors. PPAR Res. 2008;2008:581348.
57. Schriner SE, Kuramada S, Lopez TE, Truong S, Pham A, Jafari M. Extension of Drosophila lifespan by cinnamon through a sex-specific dependence on the insulin receptor substrate Chico. Exp Gerontol. 2014;60:220–30.

58. Moselhy SS, Ali HK. Hepatoprotective effect of cinnamon extracts against carbon tetrachloride induced oxidative stress and liver injury in rats. Biol Res. 2009;42:93–8.
59. Azab K, Mostafa AH, Ali EM, Abdel-Aziz MA. Cinnamon extract ameliorates ionizing radiation-induced cellular injury in rats. Ecotoxicol Environ Saf. 2011; 74:2324–9.
60. Vafa M, Mohammadi F, Shidfar F, Sormaghi MS, Heidari I, Golestan B, Amiri F. Effects of cinnamon consumption on glycemic status, lipid profile and body composition in type 2 diabetic patients. Int J Prev Med. 2012;3:531–6.
61. Shatwan IA, Ahmed LA, Badkook MM. Effect of barley flour, crude cinnamon, and their combination on glycemia, dyslipidemia, and adipose tissue hormones in type 2 diabetic rats. J Med Food. 2013;16:656–62.
62. Lee SC, Xu WX, Lin LY, Yang JJ, Liu CT. Chemical composition and hypoglycemic and pancreas-protective effect of leaf essential oil from indigenous cinnamon (Cinnamomum osmophloeum Kanehira). J Agric Food Chem. 2013;61:4905–13.
63. Fritsche L, Weigert C, Haring HU, Lehmann R. How insulin receptor substrate proteins regulate the metabolic capacity of the liver--implications for health and disease. Curr Med Chem. 2008;15:1316–29.
64. Liu Y, Li X, Xie C, Luo X, Bao Y, Wu B, Hu Y, Zhong Z, Liu C, Li M. Prevention effects and possible molecular mechanism of mulberry leaf extract and its formulation on rats with insulin-insensitivity. PLoS One. 2016;11:e0152728.
65. Moore AM, Prescott M, Marshall CJ, Yip SH, Campbell RE. Enhancement of a robust arcuate GABAergic input to gonadotropin-releasing hormone neurons in a model of polycystic ovarian syndrome. Proc Natl Acad Sci U S A. 2015;112:596–601.
66. Moore AM, Prescott M, Campbell RE. Estradiol negative and positive feedback in a prenatal androgen-induced mouse model of polycystic ovarian syndrome. Endocrinology. 2013;154:796–806.

Peroxiredoxin I maintains luteal function by regulating unfolded protein response

Hyo-Jin Park[1], Dong Gil Lee[2], Jung Bae Seong[2], Hyun-Shik Lee[2], Oh-Shin Kwon[2], Beom Sik Kang[2], Jeen-woo Park[2], Sang-Rae Lee[3] and Dong-Seok Lee[2,4*]

Abstract

Background: Mounting evidence shows that ROS regulation by various antioxidants is essential for the expression of enzymes involved in steroidogenesis and maintenance of progesterone production by the corpus luteum (CL). However, the underlying mechanisms of peroxiredoxin 1 (PRDX1), an antioxidant enzyme, in luteal function for progesterone production in mice have not been reported. The aim of this study was to evaluate the functional link between PRDX1 and progesterone production in the CL of *Prdx1* knockout (K/O) mice in the functional stage of CL.

Methods: The expression pattern of the unfolded protein response (UPR) signaling pathways, endoplasmic reticulum (ER) stress-induced apoptosis related genes and peroxiredoxins 1 (PRDX1) were investigated by western blotting analysis in CL tissue of 10 weeks mice during functional stage of CL. The protein levels of these genes after ER-stress inducer tunicamycin (Tm), ER-stress inhibitor tauroursodeoxycholic acid (TUDCA) and ROS scavenger, N-acetylcysteine (NAC) stimulation by intraperitoneal (i.p) injection were also investigated in CL tissue of wild type (WT) mice. Finally, we examined progesterone production and UPR signaling related gene expression in CL tissue of *Prdx1* K/O mice.

Results: We demonstrated that PRDX1 deficiency in the functional stage activates the UPR signaling pathways in response to ER stress-induced apoptosis. Interestingly, CL number, serum progesterone levels, and steroidogenic enzyme expression in *Prdx1* K/O mice decreased significantly, compared to those in wild type mice. Levels of UPR signaling pathway markers (GRP78/BIP, P50ATF6, and phosphorylated (p)-eIF2) and ER-stress associated apoptotic factors (CHOP, p-JNK, and cleaved caspase-3) were dramatically increased in the CL tissue of *Prdx1* K/O mice. In addition, administration of the NAC, reduced progesterone production and activated ER-stress-induced UPR signaling in the CL tissue obtained from the ovary of *Prdx1* K/O mice. Taken together, these results indicated that reduction in serum progesterone levels and activation of ER-stress-induced UPR signaling are restored by NAC injection in the CL of *Prdx1* K/O mice.

Conclusion: These observations provide the first evidence regarding the basic mechanisms connecting PRDX1 and progesterone production in the functional stage of CL.

Keywords: Corpus luteum, Peroxiredoxin 1, Unfolded protein response, Apoptosis

* Correspondence: lee1@knu.ac.kr
[2]School of Life Sciences, BK21 Plus KNU Creative BioResearch Group, Kyungpook National University, Daegu, South Korea
[4]College of Natural Sciences, Kyungpook National University, Daegu 702-701, Republic of Korea
Full list of author information is available at the end of the article

Background

Regulation of antioxidant enzymes and reactive oxygen species (ROS) production has been proposed as a major mediator of granulosa/cumulus cell communication, oocyte maturation [1], and luteal phase development in mice [2]. Previous studies showed that abnormal expression of antioxidant enzymes is associated with ROS production in female reproductive system such as those affecting adverse pregnancy outcomes [3], resumption of meiosis, ovarian functions, and reducing fertility [4, 5]. In particular, excess ROS production, especially in the corpus luteum (CL), induces hormone imbalance and luteal phase defect in female mice [5]. To protect cells against the damaging and toxic effects of ROS, antioxidant enzymes, including catalase (CAT), glutathione peroxidase (GPX), superoxide dismutase (SOD), and peroxiredoxins (PRDXs) are activated in mammalian cells [6, 7]. The peroxiredoxin family consists of six proteins (PRDX1–6), which can reduce hydrogen peroxide (H_2O_2), lipid hydroperoxides, and peroxynitrite. PRDX 1–6 are categorized as typical 2-Cys peroxiredoxins, which are distinct from the atypical 2-Cys (PRDX5) and 1-Cys peroxiredoxins (PRDX 6) [8]. Among these PRDXs, PRDX1 is localized in the cytosol, where it interacts with various signaling molecules [9, 10]. In addition, a relationship between granulosa cell stimulation and PRDX1 expression has been previously detected in the rat ovary [10].

The CL is a transient ovarian endocrine gland, which secretes progesterone, a hormone essential for regulation of the luteal phase [11]. Steroidogenic enzymes such as steroidogenic acute regulatory (StAR) protein, p450 cholesterol side-chain cleavage enzyme (P450scc), and 3β-hydroxysteroid dehydrogenase (3β-HSD) are required [12, 13] for progesterone production by the luteal cells of the CL. Loss of progesterone production, followed by loss of luteal cell function, leads to CL regression [11]. Recent studies showed that H_2O_2 production from the CL tissue is important for luteal function, such as for steroidogenic enzyme activation and regression of CL during the luteal phase [14]. Therefore, regulation of ROS production can play an important role in progesterone production and maintenance of luteal functions during the CL life span. However, the mechanisms via which PRDX1 acts as a ROS regulator and enables progesterone production in mice CL have not been reported.

ROS production is induced by endoplasmic reticulum (ER) stress and activation of unfolded protein response (UPR) [15]. The UPR alleviates ER stress, rescues ER homeostasis, and prevents cell death via the induction of ER chaperone expression, reduction of protein synthesis, and degradation of unfolded and/or misfolded proteins using three ER-localized transmembrane proteins, namely, inositol-requiring enzyme 1 (IRE1 or ERN1), protein kinase RNA (PKR)-like ER kinase (PERK), and activating transcription factor-6 (ATF6) [16]. Therefore, all three UPR pathways contribute to the induction of cell apoptosis or ER stress-associated cell death, under conditions of excessive ER stress. In addition, it is well known that C/EBP homologous protein (CHOP), cJUN NH2-terminal kinase (JNK) and caspase-12 have been implicated in apoptotic signaling in response to ER stress [17]. Previously, we demonstrated that ER stress affects progesterone production during the functional stage of CL in mice and bovine CL tissue of estrous cycle [18, 19]. Additionally, reports show that PRDX4 protects against ER-stress mediated cell death by removing H_2O_2 [20]. However, the roles of PRDX1 in regulation of ER stress and UPR signaling pathways during progesterone production in the functional stage of CL has not yet been investigated.

Therefore, the aims of present study were: i) to investigate whether PRDX1 acts as an antioxidant and ROS-regulator during progesterone production, ii) to confirm the association of PRDX1 with oxidative stress-derived ER stress response and UPR activation using an ER stress inducer and inhibitor during the functional stage of CL in mice, and iii) to evaluate the changes in progesterone production, UPR signaling, and ER stress-mediated apoptosis in the CL tissue of *Prdx1* knockout (K/O) mice compared to those in wild type (WT) mice. Finally, we investigated whether injection of the ROS scavenger, N-acetylcysteine (NAC), in *Prdx1* K/O mice effectively controls progesterone production by altering the levels of enzymes involved in steroidogenesis and regulating ER stress in mice CL.

Methods

Chemicals

Unless otherwise stated, all chemicals and reagents used in this study were purchased from Sigma Aldrich (St. Louis, MO, USA).

Animals

Female C57/B6J mice (8–10-week-old) of wild type were purchased from Hyochang Bio-Science (Daegu, Korea) and *Prdx1*-deficient (*Prdx1 −/−*) female mice (8–10-weeks old) maintained in accordance with the institutional guidelines of the Institutional Animal Care and Use Committee of the Korea Research Institute of Bioscience and Biotechnology (KRIBB, Daejeon, South Korea). Animals were maintained under standard environmental conditions (temperature at 20–22 °C, humidity at 50–60%, and 12-h-dark/light cycles) with free access to food and water.

Determination of estrous cycle

The short reproductive cycle length observed in rodents is called the estrous cycle. The normal estrous cycle in rodents follows a 4–5-day pattern, the characteristics of which vary with the day [21]. We classified mice on the basis of the predicted time of hormone induced-superovulation as described previously [18]. In all mice, superovulation was achieved by intraperitoneal (i.p) injection of 5 IU pregnant mare's serum gonadotropin/mouse (n = 5–6 in each group, 8-week-old) (PMSG; Sigma Aldrich), followed 48 h later by injection of 5 IU human chorionic gonadotropin/mouse (hCG; Sigma Aldrich). Ovulation occurred 12 h after the hCG injection, and therefore, 16 h post-hCG injection was considered as the beginning of CL formation. CL tissues were collected from the ovaries of treated mice 16, 24, 48, 72 and 96 h after hCG administration (Fig. 1a). The luteal phase was divided into two groups, namely, the functional stage (16, 24 and 48 h) and the regressing stage (72, 96 h) on the basis of serum progesterone concentration and changes in steroidogenic enzyme expression during progesterone production. Mice were killed, blood was collected, and the ovaries were removed at the indicated time intervals. CL tissues were collected from the ovaries under a dissecting microscope and immediately frozen at − 70 °C until further use. All experiments were performed in triplicate, and each experiment was independently analyzed.

Administration of tm, TUDCA, and NAC in female mice

C57BL/6 female mice (8-week-old) were administered tunicamycin (Tm; 0.5 μg/g body weight; Calbiochem, CA, USA) as an ER stress inducer, and tauroursodeoxycholic acid (TUDCA;0.5 μg/g body weight; Calbiochem) or NAC (1.0 μg/g, Sigma) as ER stress inhibitors by i.p. injection at the indicated times (16 h). Saline was injected intraperitoneally in the control animals. After

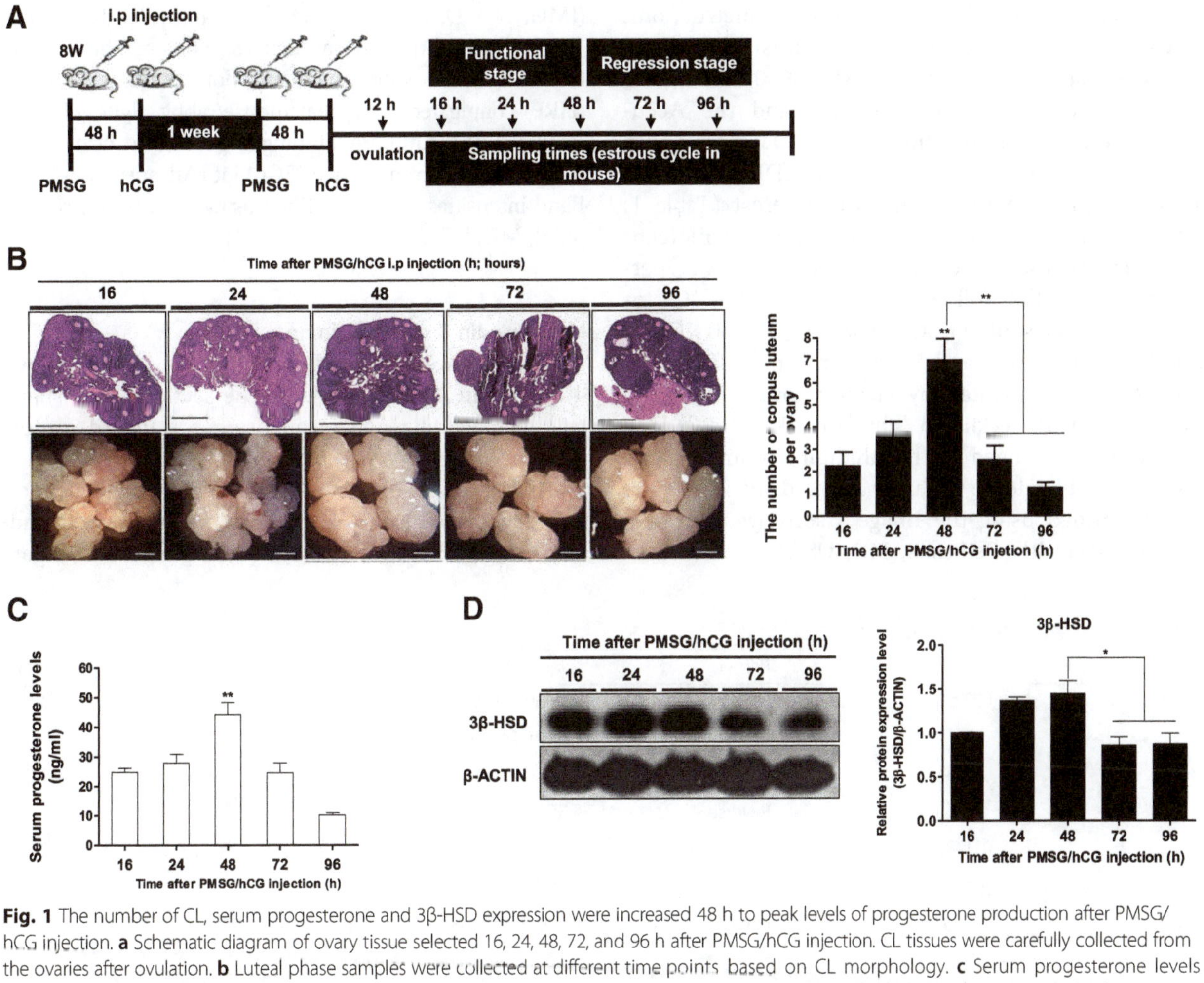

Fig. 1 The number of CL, serum progesterone and 3β-HSD expression were increased 48 h to peak levels of progesterone production after PMSG/hCG injection. **a** Schematic diagram of ovary tissue selected 16, 24, 48, 72, and 96 h after PMSG/hCG injection. CL tissues were carefully collected from the ovaries after ovulation. **b** Luteal phase samples were collected at different time points based on CL morphology. **c** Serum progesterone levels were determined by progesterone ELISA kit (ALPCO) for 4–5 animals at each time point of the luteal phase during the estrous cycle. **d** Western blotting analysis of 3β-HSD, a marker of progesterone synthesis in the CL. The 3β-HSD level was normalized to that of the β-actin control. The histogram represents values of densitometry analysis obtained using the Image J software (NIH). The data are representative of at least three independent experiments conducted in triplicate. Values represent means ± SEM (4–5 mice/group) * $P < 0.05$, ** $P < 0.01$, and *** $P < 0.001$

administration, the mice were sacrificed at the indicated times, and blood and CL tissues were collected.

Progesterone estimation by enzyme immunoassay (EIA)

For estimating serum progesterone concentration, blood was collected from female mice after each injection (16, 24, 48, 72 and 96 h after PMSG/hCG treatment). Serum was separated from blood and stored at − 20 °C until it was assayed for progesterone. Progesterone concentration was assessed using a progesterone EIA kit (ALPCO, Windham, NH, USA) according to the manufacturer's instructions.

RNA extraction and reverse transcription polymerase chain reaction (RT-PCR)

Total RNA was isolated from each individual CL tissue using the Trizol reagent (Invitrogen, Inc., CA, USA) according to the manufacturer's instructions. RNA concentration and purity were measured using a NanoDrop spectrophotometer (ASP-2680; ACTgene, NJ, USA). Next, 1 μg/μl total RNA and the AccuPower® RT-PCR premix (Bioneer Inc., Daejeon, South Korea) were used to synthesize the cDNA. Primers specific for the mouse sequences of interest (Table 1) were designed using the National Center for Biotechnology Information (NCBI) database. PCR was performed using the following condition: 95 °C for 5 min, 30 cycles of 95 °C for 30 s, 55~ 60 °C for 30 s, 72 °C for 30 s, and 72 °C for 5 min. The PCR products were separated by electrophoresis on a 2% agarose gel with a known standard (100 bp ladder, Bioneer Inc.), stained with ethidium bromide, and photographed under UV illumination. Band intensities were quantified using the Image J software (National Institute of Health, Bethesda, MD, USA).

Protein extraction and western blotting

Lysates of CL tissue from each stage were prepared in PRO-PREP protein lysis buffer (iNtRON, Daejeon, Korea). The protein concentration for each sample was estimated using a Bradford dye-binding assay with bovine serum albumin (BSA) as a standard (Bradford, 1976). Aliquots of the proteins (30 μg) were separated by sodium dodecyl sulfate-polyacrylamide gel electrophoresis (SDS-PAGE) on 12% gels. After electrophoresis, the separated proteins were transferred onto nitrocellulose (NC) membranes (Pall Corporation, Port Washington, NY, USA). After blocking with 5% non-fat milk in Tris-buffered saline (TBS) with 0.1% Tween 20 at 4 °C under mild agitation, the membranes were incubated with 1:2000 diluted anti-CHOP, anti-p90ATF6, anti-CREB-2, anti-3β-HSD (Santa Cruz, Biotechnology, CA, USA), anti-GRP78/BIP, anti-p-eIF2α, anti-IRE1, anti-eIF2a, anti-JNK, anti-p-SAPK/JNK, anti-caspase-3, anti-β-tubulin (Cell Signaling, Beverly, MA, USA), anti-p50ATF6 (IMG, San Diego, CA, USA), and anti-p-IRE1α (Abcam, Cambridge, MA, USA) antibodies. The membranes were then incubated with secondary horse radish peroxidase (HRP)-conjugated anti-goat/mouse/rabbit IgG (Thermo, Rockford, IL). Antibody binding was detected using an enhanced chemiluminescence (ECL) kit (Advansta, CA, USA). Band intensities were quantified using the Image J software (NIH, MD, USA).

Hematoxylin & eosin staining

The ovaries were isolated from the body and fixed with 4% formalin (Sigma Aldrich). The sections were stained with hematoxylin and eosin using a standard protocol described previously (Park, et al. 2013b, Park, et al. 2014) [18, 22]. Thin sections were cut with a diamond knife and mounted. The sections were observed under an Olympus BX51 microscope (Olympus, Tokyo, Japan).

Table 1 Primer sequence for reverse transcription PCR

Target	Accession numbers	Primer	Sequence reported 5′-3′	Tm°C	length (bp)
3β-hsd	NM_008293.3	Forward:5′	ACTGCAGGAGGTCAGAGCT	55	401
		Reverse:3′	GCCAGTAACACACAGAATACC		
Prdx1	NM_011034.4	Forward:5′	CACCCAAGAAACAAGGAGGA	53.5	343
		Reverse:3′	TGGTCCAGTGCTCACTTCTG		
Star	NM_011485.4	Forward:5′	GAAAAGACACGGTCATCACT	56	262
		Reverse:3′	CCGTGTCTTTTCCAATCCTC		
P450scc (Cyp11a1)	AF195119.1	Forward:5′	GCTGGAAGGTGTAGCTCAGG	57	224
		Reverse:3′	CACTGGTGTGGAACATCTGG		
Gapdh	BC145810.1	Forward:5′	ACCACAGTCCATGCCATCAC	55	452
		Reverse:3′	TCCACCACCCTGTTGCTGTA		

3β-hsd: 3β-hydroxysteroid dehydrogenase, *Prdx1*: peroxiredoxin 1, *Star*: steroidogenesis acute regulatory, *P450scc*: cytochrome P450 side-chain cleavage, Tm: melting temperature

Immunohistochemistry

The ovaries were fixed in formalin, embedded in paraffin, and cut into 3-μm-thick sections. The sections were deparaffinized and briefly heated. The sections were then treated with a protein blocking solution (Dako, CA, USA) and incubated with anti-phospho eIF2a (Cell Signaling). After washing with 0.1 M TBS containing 0.01% Tween-20 (TBST), the sections were incubated with anti-rabbit polymer (Dako). Peroxidases bound to the antibody complex were visualized after treatment with a 3, 3′-diaminobenzidine (DAB) chromogen substrate solution (Dako). The DAB reaction was monitored under a microscope to determine the optimal incubation time and stopped with several washes of 0.1 M TBS. The immunolabeled sections were dehydrated in a graded ethanol series, defatted in xylene, and mounted. The sections were examined under a bright field Olympus BX51 microscope and images were acquired using an Olympus DP 70 camera (Olympus, Japan).

Statistical analysis

All experiments were repeated at least three times, and percentage data obtained in this study are presented as the mean ± standard error of the mean (SEM). These data were subjected to one-way analysis of variance (ANOVA), followed by Dunnett's multiple comparison test. Statistical analysis was performed using paired Student's t-test. Data obtained from WT and *Prdx1* K/O mice CL tissues were compared using the unpaired Student's t-test. All calculations were performed using the GraphPad Prism 5.0 software package (GraphPad Software, San Diego, CA, USA). $P < 0.05$ was considered to be statistically significant.

Results

Measurement of progesterone production in CL tissue of mouse

For delineating the timing of the luteal phase during the estrous cycle post-PMSG/hCG injection, we used a methods of hormone injection for synchronization of estrous cycle as previously described by Park et al., [18].

We observed the morphology and determined the number of collected CL tissues microscopically at 16, 24, 48, 72 and 96 h after PMSG/hCG injection (Fig. 1a and b). Next, we determined the serum progesterone level and the expression of 3β-HSD, a classical steroidogenic enzyme involved in progesterone biosynthesis, using the progesterone ELISA kit (ALPCO) and western blot analysis during mice estrous cycle, respectively. Serum progesterone level was significantly increased ($P < 0.01$) 48 h after the PMSG/hCG injection (Fig. 1c). Protein levels of 3β-HSD showed the same pattern as that of serum progesterone till the CL functional stage, but rapidly decreased after 48 h (Fig. 1d). Based on these results, we concluded that the time point (48 h) corresponding to peak progesterone levels in CL tissues during the entire luteal phase after PMSG/hCG injection should be used for subsequent experiments.

ER-stress-induced reduction in progesterone production at the functional stage of CL is recovered by the ROS scavenger NAC

In our previous study, we demonstrated that ER stress affects progesterone production during the functional stage of CL. In addition, ER stress-mediated apoptosis induced CL regression in the mouse luteal phase [18]. Recent studies indicate that ROS production can be induced by ER stress [23]. Therefore, we investigated whether progesterone production is regulated by the ROS scavenger under ER stress in the functional stage of CL. To analyze the relationship between ROS and ER stress during progesterone production in the CL tissue at the peak of progesterone synthesis (48 h after PMSG/hCG injection), we performed the experiment as shown in Fig. 2a. We used Tm as an ER stress inducer, TUDCA as an ER stress inhibitor, or NAC as a ROS scavenger. Mice injected with Tm (0.5 μg/g) showed dynamic deficiency of luteal function with low serum progesterone and reduction in 3β-HSD and P450scc protein levels in the CL. Compared to the Tm-treated group, serum progesterone level recovered significantly ($P < 0.05$) in the group where NAC (1.0 μg/g) was added after Tm (0.5 μg/g) pre-treatment (Fig. 2b). Addition of NAC as a recovery effect like a TUDCA also significantly increased the protein levels of 3β-HSD and P450scc in CL (Fig. 2c). On the contrary, NAC or TUDCA administration in mice pre-treated with Tm decreased the expression level of CHOP as an ER stress-mediated apoptotic factors during the functional stage of CL ($P < 0.001$) (Fig. 2c). These results demonstrate that the regulation of ER stress-induced ROS production is required for maintaining progesterone production during the functional stage of CL in mice.

Prdx1 knockout reduced CL number, and levels of serum progesterone, 3β-HSD, and P450ssc

The above results underline the necessity of regulating ROS synthesis for maintaining progesterone production during the functional stage of CL (Fig. 2). We investigated whether PRDXs can act as antioxidants for maintaining progesterone production.

The expression of the PRDXs at 16, 24, 48, 72 and 96 h after PMSG/hCG injection were analyzed (Fig. 3a). Interestingly, PRDX1 was continuously expressed in CL during the entire luteal phase (Fig. 3b), irrespective of the changes in 3β-HSD expression. In contrast, western blotting showed that the other PRDX proteins (2–6) were not expressed continuously during the entire luteal

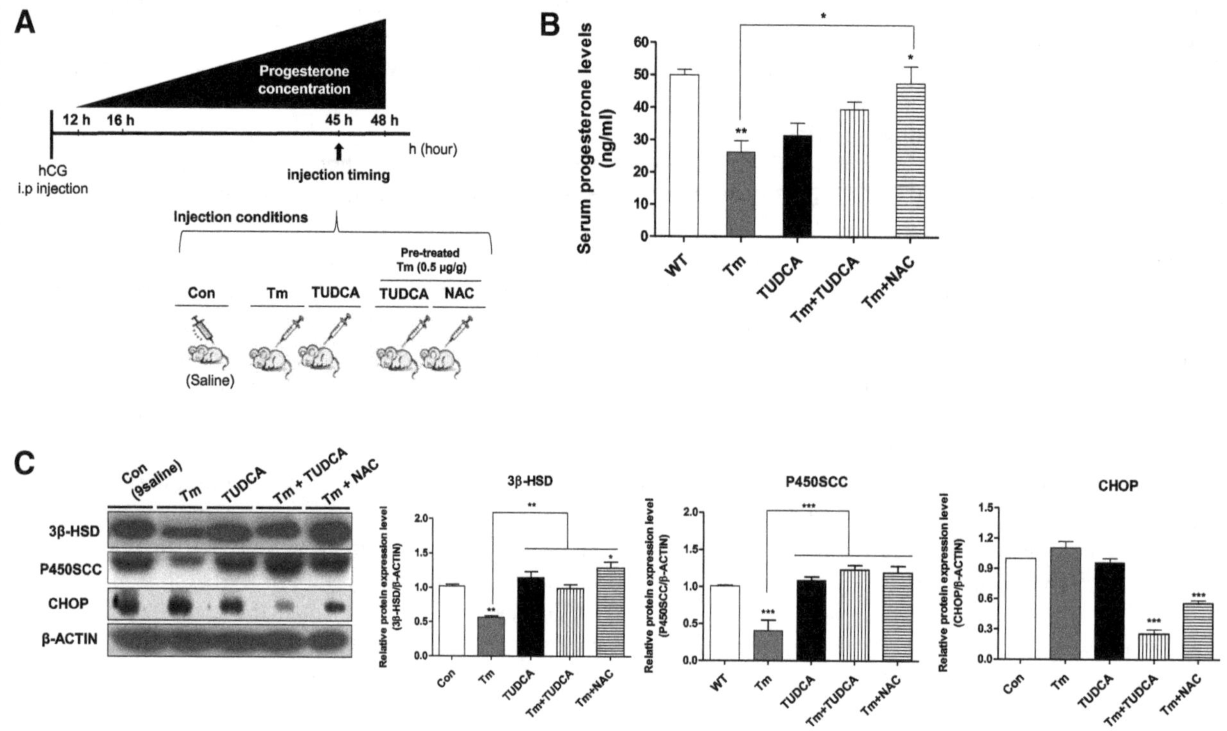

Fig. 2 ER-stress-induced reduction in progesterone production at the functional stage of CL is recovered by ROS scavenger NAC. **a** Schematic diagram showing the injection and collection times of the ER stress-regulator and ROS scavenger injection. Tm (an ER stress inducer; 0.5 μg/g body weight), TUDCA, (an ER stress inhibitor; 0.5 μg/g body weight), or NAC (a ROS scavenger; 1.0 μg/g body weight) were injected into mice 45 h after the PMSG/hCG injection. **b** Peak production of serum progesterone was measured (48 h after the PMSG/hCG injection) in the luteal phase. **c** Protein level of the UPR signaling activation marker CHOP in selected CL tissues was measured by western blot analysis after ER stress regulator and ROS scavenger stimulation. The levels of 3β-HSD, P450scc, and CHOP were normalized to that of β-actin. The histogram represents values of densitometry analysis obtained using the Image J software (NIH). The bar graphs represent the least-squares means ± SEM (4–5 mice/group) of three independent experiments. * $P < 0.05$, ** $P < 0.01$, and *** $P < 0.001$; Dunnett's multiple comparison test compared to 48 h after PMSG/hCG injection

phase (Additional file 1: Figure S1). The PRDX1 level was increased by Tm treatment and recovered by TUDCA at the peak time point of progesterone production (Fig. 3c and d). TUDCA or NAC injection after Tm also decreased PRDX1 level compared to Tm only treatment (Fig. 3c and d). These results indicated that continuously expressed PRDX1 in CL during the entire luteal phase may be involved in ROS regulation for maintaining progesterone production in the functional stage of CL. Therefore, to investigate whether PRDX1 acts as an antioxidant and ROS-regulator during progesterone production in the functional luteal stage after PMSG/hCG injection, we evaluated the changes in progesterone production and expression of ER stress marker genes in the CL tissue of *Prdx1* K/O mice and compared them with those of WT mice. First, to determine the CL number, the ovary from *Prdx1* K/O and WT mice were subjected to genotyping and H & E staining, respectively (Fig. 4a). The number of formed CL and ovary size in *Prdx1* K/O mice dramatically decreased ($P < 0.01$; fold 2.8, Fig. 4b) 48 h after the PMSG/hCG injection. Similarly, the serum progesterone concentration and protein levels of 3β-HSD and P450ssc were significantly reduced compared to those in the CL of WT mice (Fig. 4c and d). Furthermore, to determine the effect of PRDX1 on progesterone production in CL tissue, we observed the ovary morphology in wild type, and *Prdx1* heterozygous and homozygous K/O mice. Although the ovary size in *Prdx1* heterozygous mouse was slightly reduced, the levels of serum progesterone and steroidogenic enzymes in the CL tissue of *Prdx1* heterozygous mice showed the same pattern as that of WT mice 48 h after PMSG/hCG injection (Additional file 2: Figure S2). These results demonstrate that absence of PRDX1 in the functional luteal stage after PMSG/hCG injection decreased CL number and ovary size compared to those of WT mice, which reduces serum progesterone and protein levels of the steroidogenesis enzymes 3β-HSD and P450ssc.

PRDX1 deficiency induced UPR signal activation and ER stress-mediated apoptosis in CL functional stage

We investigated whether PRDX1 deficiency is involved in UPR signaling (GRP78/BIP, p-EIF2α, p50ATF6, and

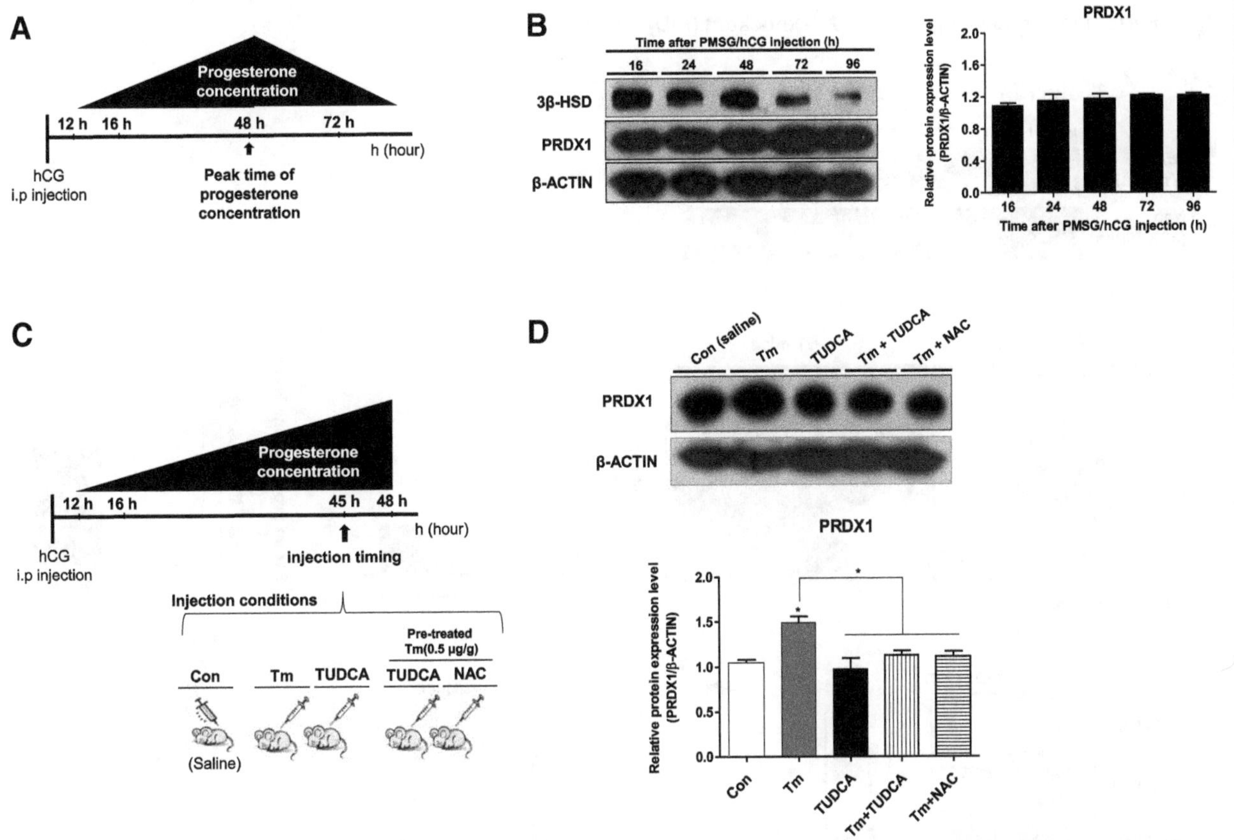

Fig. 3 Increased PRDX1 expression by injection of ER-stress inducer (Tm) in the CL tissue was recovered by ER-stress inhibitor (TUDCA) or ROS scavenger (NAC). **a** Schematic diagram showing the time taken to reach peak progesterone levels in CL 48 h after PMSG/hCG injection. **b** Protein levels of PRDX1 and 3β-HSD were measured by western blot analysis in different sampling times of the luteal phase. **c** Schematic diagram showing the timing of ER stress-regulator and ROS scavenger injection and sample collection. **d** PRDX1 levels in selected CL tissues were measured using western blot analysis in the presence of the ER stress inducer (Tm) (0.5 µg/g body weight) or ER stress inhibitor (TUDCA) (0.5 µg/g body weight). And ER stress inhibitor (TUDCA) (0.5 µg/g body weight) or ROS scavenger (NAC) (1.0 µg/g body weight) after pre-treatment with the ER stress inducer (0.5 µg/g Tm), respectively. 3β HSD and PRDX1 levels were normalized to that of β-actin. The histogram represents values densitometry analysis was performed using the Image J software (NIH). The bar graphs represent the least-squares means ± SEM (4–5 mice/group) of three independent experiments. * $P < 0.05$, ** $P < 0.01$, and *** $P < 0.001$

p-IRE1) or ER stress-mediated apoptosis (CHOP, p-JNK, and cleaved caspase-3) in the functional luteal stage using western blotting analysis and the CL tissue of WT and *Prdx1* K/O mice. As shown in Fig. 5a, the levels of GRP78/BIP, p50ATF6, and p-EIF2α were dramatically increased ($P < 0.01$) in the CL tissue of *Prdx1* K/O mice, but, the levels of total EIF2α and p-IRE1 showed no change compared to those of WT mice. The levels of CHOP, p-JNK, and cleaved caspase-3 were also significantly increased (CHOP; $P < 0.05$, p-JNK, and cleaved caspase-3; $P < 0.01$) in the CL of *Prdx1* K/O mice (Fig. 5b). In addition, immunohistochemistry (IHC) showed that the levels of p-EIF2α, ATF6, and cleaved caspase-3 were higher in the ovary of *Prdx1* K/O mice than in the ovary of WT mice (Fig. 5c). Therefore, these results demonstrated that PRDX1 deficiency during functional luteal stage activates the UPR signaling pathways in response to ER stress-mediated apoptosis.

Restoration of impaired progesterone production and UPR signaling activation in response to ER stress by NAC injection in Prdx1 knockout mice

As shown in Fig. 2, the NAC-mediated decrease in ER stress-induced ROS levels is required for maintaining progesterone production during the luteal functional stage. Thus, we investigated whether NAC injection in *Prdx1* K/O mice restores the reduced serum progesterone concentration and protein levels of steroidogenesis enzymes in the ovaries of *Prdx1* K/O mice. First, we injected NAC 45 h after the PMSG/hCG injection, and collected CL tissue from the ovary 3 h after the NAC injection. As shown in the Fig. 6a, serum progesterone production, which was rapidly reduced ($P < 0.01$; compared to WT mice) in the CL tissue of *Prdx1* K/O mice, recovered significantly ($P < 0.05$; compared to *Prdx1* K/O mice) after the NAC injection. We also investigated whether NAC treatment of *Prdx1* K/O mice recovered steroidogenic enzyme expression and

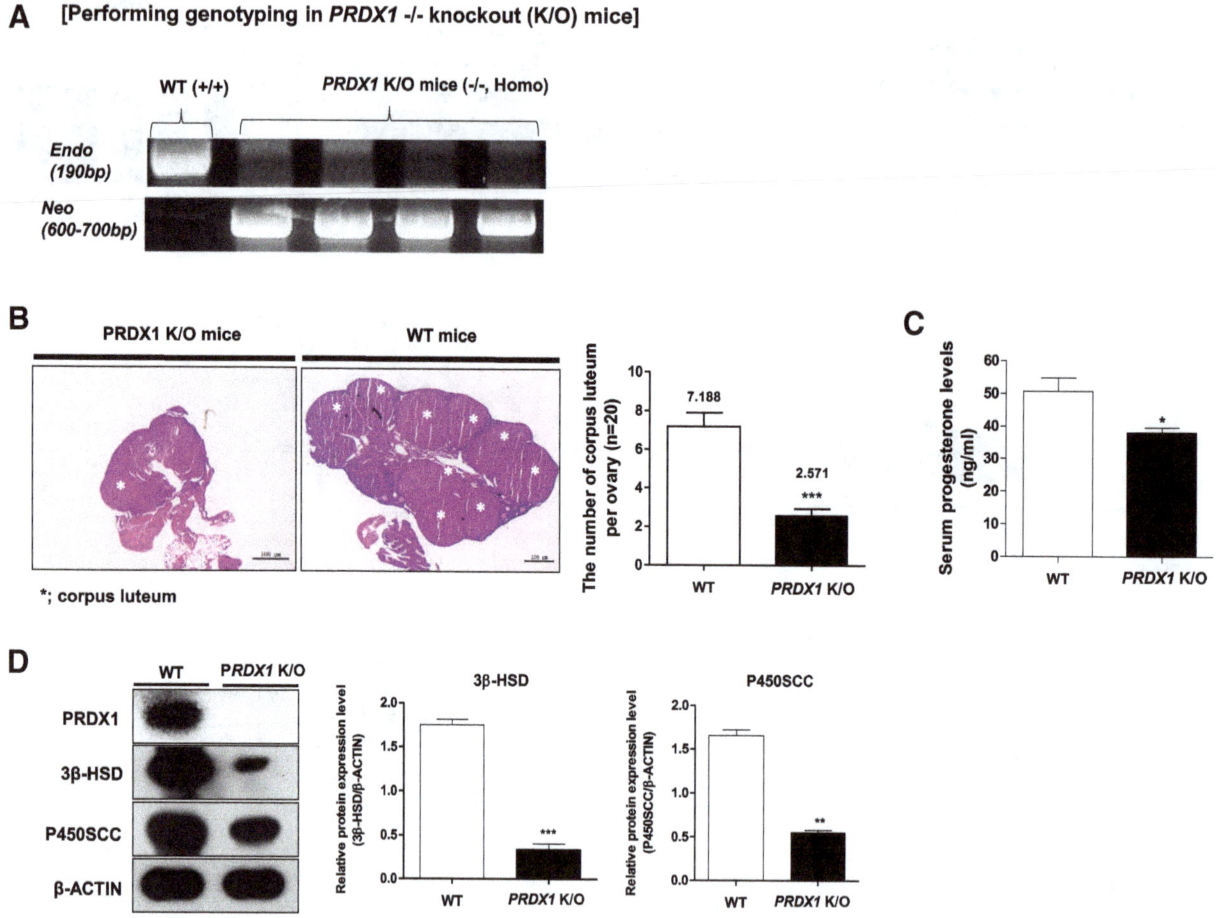

Fig. 4 The CL number, serum progesterone, 3β-HSD, and P450ssc expression were decreased in *Prdx1* K/O mice. **a** We performed genotyping of PRDX1 by PCR in the tail of *Prdx1* K/O mice. **b** CL number in the ovary of *Prdx1* K/O mice was observed by hematoxylin and eosin (H & E) staining. **c** Serum progesterone levels were measured using a progesterone kit in *Prdx1* K/O mice. **d** The levels of the steroidogenic enzymes 3β-HSD and P450SCC were determined in CL tissue by western blot analysis. The relative levels of these proteins were obtained after normalization with β-actin levels. The histogram values of densitometry analysis were obtained using the Image J software. The bars represent the mean of two independent experiments means ± SEM (4–5 mice/group) * $P < 0.05$, ** $P < 0.01$, and *** $P < 0.001$; two-tailed Student's *t*-test compared to WT mice

decreased activation of UPR signaling in response to ER stress during the functional luteal stage. We observed that the mRNA levels of the steroidogenic enzymes 3β-HSD, StAR ($P < 0.001$; compared to *Prdx1* K/O mice), and P450scc ($P < 0.01$; compared to *Prdx1* K/O mice) were recovered by NAC treatment (Fig. 6b). In contrast, the mRNA levels of CHOP ($P < 0.001$ compared to *Prdx1* K/O mice), GRP78/BIP, and p50ATF6 ($P < 0.05$ compared to *Prdx1* K/O mice) in the CL tissue of NAC-treated *Prdx1* K/O mice were significantly reduced (Fig. 6c). These results suggested that decrease in serum progesterone production and activation of UPR signaling in response to ER stress are restored by injecting NAC, a ROS scavenger, during the luteal stage of PRDX I KO mice.

Discussion

In this study, we demonstrated that the antioxidant activity of PRDX1 is required for maintaining progesterone production and the protein levels of enzymes involved in steroidogenesis via regulation of the UPR signaling pathway and ER stress response in the functional stage of mice CL. In addition, injection of the ROS scavenger NAC restored the reduction in progesterone production and activation of the UPR signaling pathway in response to ER stress in the CL tissue of *Prdx1* K/O mice. Therefore, PRDX1 may act as a regulator for progesterone production by reducing ER stress during the luteal functional stage.

It is well known that regulation of ROS production by various antioxidant enzymes is essential for the expression of enzymes related to steroidogenesis, and maintenance of progesterone production and hormone secretion by the CL [24]. During the secretory phase of the CL, H_2O_2 is produced from the CL tissue by monooxygenation, which is catalyzed by the P450scc steroidogenic enzyme [14, 25]. The differential expression of antioxidant

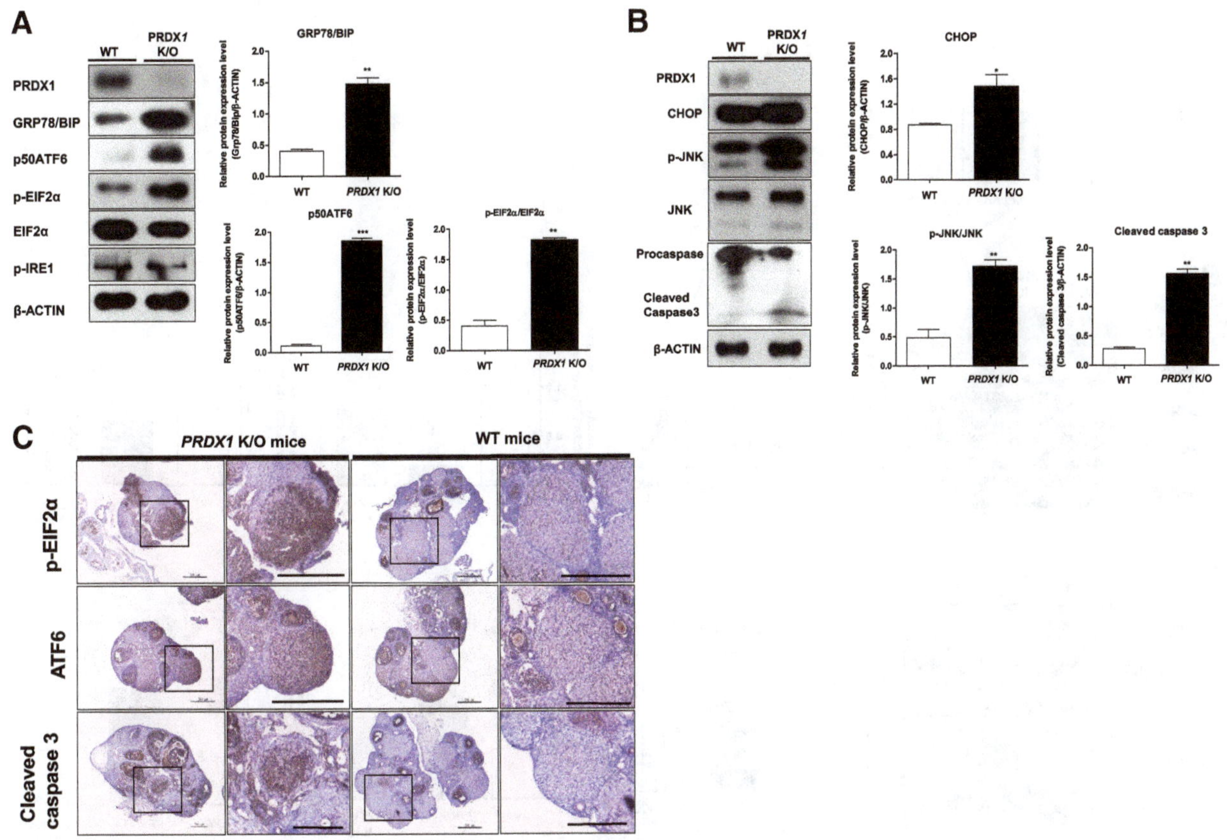

Fig. 5 Protein levels of UPR signal activation and ER stress-mediated apoptosis in CL functional stage were induced in the CL tissue of *Prdx1* K/O mice. **a** Western blot analysis to evaluate the levels of PRDX1 and UPR signaling-related proteins (GRP78/BIP, p-EIF2α, EIF2α, p50ATF5, and p-IRE1) and (**b**) ER stress-mediated apoptotic factors (CHOP, p-JNK, JNK, and caspase-3) in the CL. The relative levels of these proteins were obtained after normalization with β-actin levels. The histogram values of densitometry analysis were obtained using the Image J software. The bars represent the means of two independent experiments ± SEM (4–5 mice/per group) * $P < 0.05$, ** $P < 0.01$, and *** $P < 0.001$; two-tailed Student's t-test compared to WT mice. **c** IHC staining for UPR markers (p-EIF2α and ATF6) and ER stress apoptosis marker (cleaved caspase-3) in CL tissue from ovary of *Prdx1* K/O mice. Scale bar = 200 μm

enzymes such as superoxide dismutase (SOD), catalase, and peroxiredoxins (PRDXs) suggest that oxidative stress affects ROS-related cellular mechanisms and the steroidogenic status of rat CL [26] and the bovine estrous cycle [27]. In this respect, although the roles of various antioxidant enzymes have been reported for female reproduction [5, 28], no direct information is available regarding the PRDX1 antioxidant system and its effect on progesterone production during the luteal phase.

Among these PRDXs, the protein levels of PRDX1 were continuously and highly expressed in the CL during the entire luteal phase (Fig. 3b). The levels of PRDX1, which protects against ER stress-mediated cell death by removing H_2O_2, was increased in the CL regression stage (Additional file 1: Figure S1). Protein level patterns of PRDX2, 3, 5, and 6 were irregularly expressed unrelated to CL formation, maintenance and regression progression in the CL during the entire luteal phase. The continuous high production of PRDX1 may stimulate ROS production from the CL tissue due to active metabolism and steroidogenesis during entire luteal phase (16–96 h PMSG/hCG injection). In addition, in *Prdx1* K/O mice, the number of CL tissues in the ovary, serum progesterone levels, and expression of the main steroidogenesis enzymes were dramatically reduced compared to those in WT mice (Fig. 4). The luteal phase requires adequate secretions of progesterone by the CL [29]. In luteal phase deficiency or CL insufficiency is widely accepted to be female reproductive function defects, perhaps due to poor follicular development and an abnormality of ovarian function [30, 31]. Also, luteal phase defect is induced an ovulatory disorder of considerable clinical importance that is implicated in infertility and recurrent spontaneous abortion [32]. As a results of Fig. 4, depending on the decrease in the size of the ovaries in Prdx1 K/O mice, we speculated that the CL formation number and progesterone production level at CL functional stage (48 h) can reduced. Also, we analogized that it would appear that impaired follicular growth and ovulation can occur by decreased in CL formation

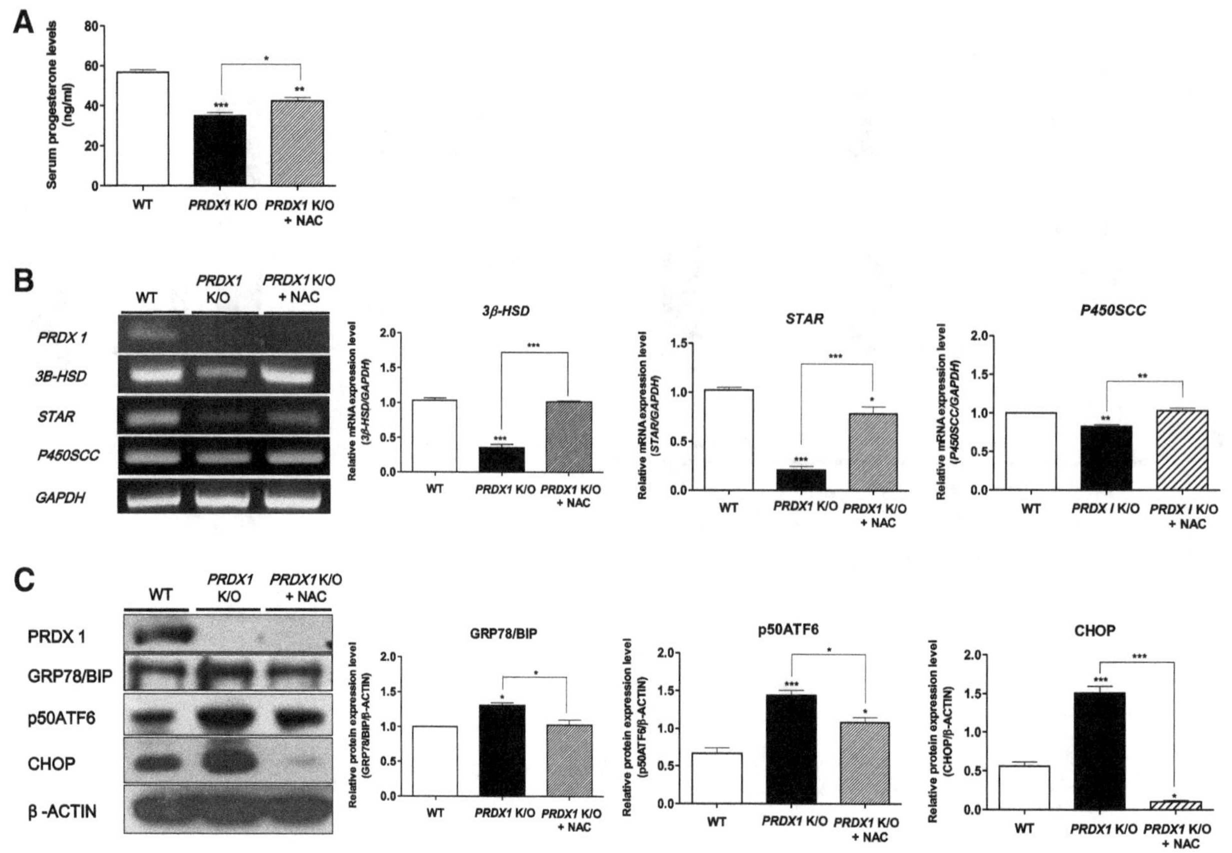

Fig. 6 Deceased serum progesterone, steroidogenesis enzymes, and increased activation of UPR signaling in response to ER stress in *Prdx1* K/O mice are restored by injecting NAC, a ROS scavenger. **a** Serum progesterone levels of PRDX1 were measured using a progesterone kit after NAC (1.0 μg/g) i.p injection. **b** RT-PCR analysis of *Prdx1* and three major genes encoding steroidogenesis enzymes (3β-HSD, StAR, and P450scc). **c** The levels of PRDX1, UPR signaling-related proteins (GRP78/BIP and p50ATF5), and ER stress-mediated apoptotic factors (CHOP) were determined in the CL tissue of *Prdx1* K/O mice by western blot analysis after NAC (1.0 μg/g) i.p injection. The relative mRNA/protein levels were normalized to those of GAPDH/β-actin controls. The histogram values of densitometry analysis were obtained using Image J software. The data are representative of at least three independent experiments conducted in triplicate and shown as means ± SEM (3–5 mice/group). * $P < 0.05$, ** $P < 0.01$, and *** $P < 0.001$; Dunnett's multiple comparison test, compared to 48 h after PMSG/hCG injection

number in Prdx1 K/O mice. Therefore, our results demonstrate a link between the antioxidant enzyme PRDX1 and progesterone production in the CL of *Prdx1* K/O mice, which may be critical in regulating ROS production by the anti-oxidative effects of PRDX1 during the functional stage of mouse CL.

The ER stress-associated oxidative environment may also be correlated with ER stress-associated ROS production [33]. ROS is generated during protein unfolding due to the depletion of antioxidant enzymes [33]. Thus, secreted proteins such as steroid hormones involved in ER-regulated protein folding may be more susceptible to higher levels of oxidative stress. ER stress and oxidative stress are closely linked events [33]. Reports show that prolonged ER stress leads to ROS production and oxidative stress via ER stress-mediated pro-apoptotic signaling [34, 35]. We believe that the ER of luteal cells plays an important role as the site for steroidogenic enzyme synthesis and progesterone production during the CL functional stage. Previously, we observed that the progesterone production capacity of the CL tissue reduced after ER-stress inducer treatment [18].

We investigated whether N-acetyl-L-cysteine (NAC), which is widely used as a thiol-containing antioxidant [36], could protect progesterone production in WT mice after Tm administration. We also verified whether reduced progesterone production of *Prdx1* K/O mice could be rescued by NAC administration. As shown in Fig. 2, serum progesterone level was recovered by NAC treatment in Tm pre-treated WT mice. In addition, the levels of 3β-HSD and P450scc steroidogenic enzymes were recovered and that of CHOP (ER stress-mediated apoptotic factor) was reduced by NAC or TUDCA treatment. Based on these results, we concluded that the regulation of ER stress-induced ROS is required for maintaining progesterone production during the mouse luteal phase. In *Prdx1* K/O mice, NAC administration also recovered progesterone production and the levels of steroidogenic enzymes and CHOP (Fig. 6). In addition, the levels of serum progesterone and steroidogenic enzymes in *Prdx1* heterozygous mice showed the same pattern as in WT mice (Additional file 2: Figure S2). PRDX1 expression is upregulated following exposure to oxidative stress [10]. In agreement with this observation, we observed that Tm treatment increased PRDX1 expression, which was significantly recovered by NAC or TUDCA (Fig. 3c and d). We believe that the antioxidant enzyme PRDX1 is upregulated by the ER stress-associated oxidative environment of the mouse luteal phase. In the present study, NAC administration rescued luteal function by restoring progesterone production and reducing ER stress in the CL of *Prdx1* K/O mice (Fig. 6). Therefore, these results demonstrate that PRDX1 is a regulator of ER stress-induced ROS production that is required for maintaining progesterone production during the functional stage in mouse CL.

Several studies have demonstrated a crosstalk between the production of ROS and UPR signal-induced ER stress response [15, 37, 38]. Previously, we showed that UPR is involved in steroidogenic enzyme expression in hCG-stimulated Leydig cells [22] and regulation of CL function in mice luteal phase [18]. The UPR signaling pathways were activated in response to ER stress, which plays important roles in the regulation of CL function, and ER stress-mediated apoptosis occurs via three activated UPR pathways (PERK, ATF6, and IRE1) in the CL regression stage. To determine whether the loss in progesterone production depends on PRDX1, we attempted to identify a functional link between PRDX1 and UPR signaling (GRP78/BIP, p-eIF2α, p50ATF6, and p-IRE1) and ER-stress mediated apoptotic factors (p-JNK, CHOP, and cleaved caspase-3) in the functional stage using WT and *Prdx1* K/O mice. As shown in Fig. 5a and b, GRP78/BIP, p-eIF2α, p50ATF6, p-JNK, CHOP, and cleaved caspase-3 were upregulated in the CL functional stage in the *Prdx1* K/O mice. In addition, p50ATF6, p-eIF2α and cleaved caspase-3 were detected in the CL tissue of *Prdx1* K/O mice by immunohistochemical staining (Fig. 5c). Interestingly, although the exact molecular mechanism has not been fully elucidated, phosphorylation of the UPR marker IRE1 was not affected in the *Prdx1* K/O mice. Activation of GRP78/BIP and p50ATF6 were also significantly reduced by NAC administration in *Prdx1* K/O mice (Fig. 6c.). Therefore, the present study demonstrates a link between the antioxidant enzyme PRDX1 and progesterone production via regulation of UPR signaling and ER stress response. Consequently, PRDX1 deficiency activated the UPR signaling pathways and ER stress-mediated apoptosis in the CL functional stage. These novel observations suggest that PRDX1 may be component of a regulatory network for luteal functions that specifically reduce ROS.

Conclusion

In conclusion, our findings demonstrate that PRDX1 is an antioxidant enzyme, which is essential for preserving progesterone production against ER stress-associated oxidative stress in the CL functional stage (Fig. 7). PRDX1 deficiency decreased progesterone production via ER-stress induced ROS generation in CL tissue. Therefore, PRDX1 is required for the maintenance of luteal function via regulation of UPR signaling pathways in response to ER stress in mice. These findings highlight the basic mechanisms underlying PRDX1 antioxidant activity, which will enhance our understanding of the relationship between antioxidant enzymes and progesterone production in CL functional stage.

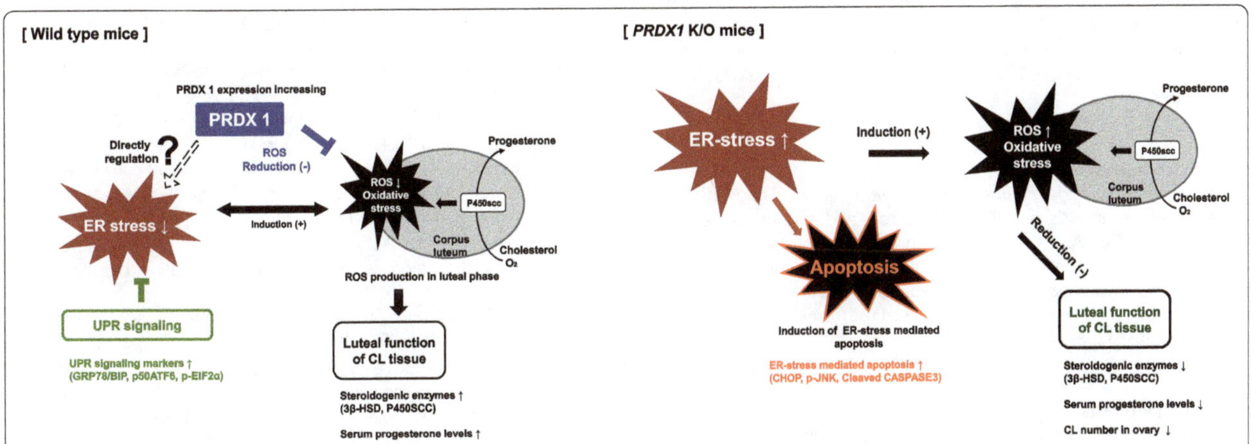

Fig. 7 Roles of PRDX1 on progesterone production, and UPR signaling activation in CL tissue of mice. Graphical summary. *Right panel*; ROS reduction by PRDX1 during the luteal functional stage (48 h after PMSG/hCG injection) in WT mice decreased activated UPR signaling in response ER stress and increased steroidogenesis enzymes expression in the CL to promote progesterone production. *Left panel*; Increasing ROS by PRDX1 deficiency during the luteal functional stage of *Prdx1* K/O mice increased activated UPR signaling in response ER stress mediated apoptosis and decreased progesterone production related steroidogenesis enzymes expression in CL tissue and serum progesterone levels

Additional files

Additional file 1: Figure S1. Changes in PRDX family (2–6) protein levels in luteal phase of WT mice. Protein levels of PRDX 2–6 were confirmed in CL tissue by western blot analysis (A). The relative levels of PRDX proteins were obtained after normalization to β-actin levels. The histogram values of densitometry analysis were obtained using the Image J software. The bar graph data represent the least-squares means ± SEM of three independent experiments. $*P < 0.05$, $**P < 0.01$, and $***P < 0.001$; Dunnett's multiple comparison test compared to 16 h after PMSG/hCG injection. (DOCX 281 kb)

Additional file 2: Figure S2. Effects of PRDX1 on progesterone production in CL tissue using *Prdx1* heterozygous and K/O mice. We observed ovary morphology in wild type, *Prdx1* K/O and heterozygous mice (A). Serum progesterone levels were measured using a progesterone kit in *Prdx1* K/O and heterozygous mice (B). The levels of steroidogenic enzymes 3β-HSD and P450SSC were determined in the CL tissue using western blot analysis. The relative levels of the steroidogenic enzymes were normalized to β-actin levels (C). Western blotting analysis of the ER stress marker CHOP in CL tissue of *Prdx1* heterozygous and K/O mice. The relative levels of CHOP were normalized to β-tubulin levels (control). (D) The histogram values of densitometry analysis were obtained using the Image J software. The bar graphs represent the least-squares means ± SEM of three independent experiments. $*P < 0.05$, $**P < 0.01$, and $***P < 0.001$; Dunnett's multiple comparison test compared to 48 h after PMSG/hCG injection. (DOCX 331 kb)

Abbreviations

3β-HSD: 3β-hydroxysteroid dehydrogenase; ANOVA: One-way analysis of variance; ATF6: Activating transcription factor-6; BSA: Bovine serum albumin; CAT: Catalase; CHOP: C/EBP homologous protein; CL: Corpus luteum; DAB: 3'-diaminobenzidine; ECL: Enhanced chemiluminescence; ER: Endoplasmic reticulum; GPX: Glutathione peroxidase; H_2O_2: Hydrogen peroxide; hCG: Human chorionic gonadotropin/mouse; HRP: Horse radish peroxidase; IHC: immunohistochemistry; IRE1 or ERN1: Inositol-requiring enzyme 1; JNK: cJUN NH2-terminal kinase; K/O: Knockout; NAC: N-acetylcysteine; NC: Nitrocellulose; P450scc: P450 cholesterol side-chain cleavage enzyme; PERK: Protein kinase RNA (PKR)-like ER kinase; PMSG: Pregnant mare's serum gonadotropin; PRDX1: Peroxiredoxin 1; PRDXs: Peroxiredoxins; ROS: Reactive oxygen species; SDS-PAGE: Sodium dodecyl sulfate-polyacrylamide gel electrophoresis; SEM: Standard error of the mean; SOD: Superoxide dismutase; StAR: Steroidogenic acute regulatory; TBS: Tris-buffered saline; Tm: Tunicamycin; UPR: Unfolded protein response; WT: Wild type

Funding

This research was supported by grants from the National Research Foundation of Korea Government (NRF-2017R1A5A2015391, NRF- 2017R1A2B4008176 and NRF-2015R1A4A1042271), and by grants from the Korea Research Institute of Bioscience & Biotechnology (KRIBB) Research Initiative Program (KGM4611821), Republic of Korea.

Author's contributions

HJP conceived the study, performed the in vitro culture of pig oocytes, western blotting analysis, and RT-PCR, and collected and interpreted the data. DGL, JBS, SRL, SL: data collection, analysis, and interpretation. HSL, OSK, JWP, BSK: study design and financial support. DSL conceived and designed the study, analyzed and interpreted data, wrote the manuscript, arranged for financial support, and finally approved the manuscript. All authors read and approved the final manuscript.

Competing interests

The authors declare that they have no competing interests.

Author details

[1]College of Engineering, Daegu University, Biotechnology, Gyeongsan, South Korea. [2]School of Life Sciences, BK21 Plus KNU Creative BioResearch Group, Kyungpook National University, Daegu, South Korea. [3]Korea Research Institute of Bioscience and Biotechnology (KRIBB), National Primate Research Center (NPRC), Daejeon, South Korea. [4]College of Natural Sciences, Kyungpook National University, Daegu 702-701, Republic of Korea.

References

1. Tanghe S, Van Soom A, Nauwynck H, Coryn M, de Kruif A. Minireview: functions of the cumulus oophorus during oocyte maturation, ovulation, and fertilization. Mol Reprod Dev. 2002;61:414–24.
2. Al-Gubory KH, Garrel C, Faure P, Sugino N. Roles of antioxidant enzymes in corpus luteum rescue from reactive oxygen species-induced oxidative stress. Reprod BioMed Online. 2012;25:551–60.
3. Al-Gubory KH, Fowler PA, Garrel C. The roles of cellular reactive oxygen species, oxidative stress and antioxidants in pregnancy outcomes. Int J Biochem Cell Biol. 2010;42:1634–50.
4. Behrman HR, Kodaman PH, Preston SL, Gao S. Oxidative stress and the ovary. J Soc Gynecol Investig. 2001;8:S40–2.
5. Agarwal A, Aponte-Mellado A, Premkumar BJ, Shaman A, Gupta S. The effects of oxidative stress on female reproduction: a review. Reprod Biol Endocrinol. 2012;10:49.
6. Pham-Huy LA, He H, Pham-Huy C. Free radicals, antioxidants in disease and health. Int J Biomed Sci. 2008;4:89–96.
7. Agarwal A, Gupta S, Sharma RK. Role of oxidative stress in female reproduction. Reprod Biol Endocrinol. 2005;3:28.
8. Nicolussi A, D'Inzeo S, Capalbo C, Giannini G, Coppa A. The role of peroxiredoxins in cancer. Mol Clin Oncol. 2017;6:139–53.
9. Immenschuh S, Baumgart-Vogt E. Peroxiredoxins, oxidative stress, and cell proliferation. Antioxid Redox Signal. 2005;7:768–77.
10. Lee YI, Kang WD, Kim MY, Cho MK, Chun SY. Expression of peroxiredoxin I regulated by gonadotropins in the rat ovary. Clin Exp Reprod Med. 2011;38: 18–23.
11. Niswender GD, Juengel JL, Silva PJ, Rollyson MK, McIntush EW. Mechanisms controlling the function and life span of the corpus luteum. Physiol Rev. 2000;80:1–29.
12. Black VH, Sanjay A, van Leyen K, Lauring B, Kreibich G. Cholesterol and steroid synthesizing smooth endoplasmic reticulum of adrenocortical cells contains high levels of proteins associated with the translocation channel. Endocrinology. 2005;146:4234–49.
13. Christenson LK, Devoto L. Cholesterol transport and steroidogenesis by the corpus luteum. Reprod Biol Endocrinol. 2003;1:90.
14. Fujii J, Iuchi Y, Okada F. Fundamental roles of reactive oxygen species and protective mechanisms in the female reproductive system. Reprod Biol Endocrinol. 2005;3:43.
15. Zeeshan HM, Lee GH, Kim HR, Chae HJ. Endoplasmic reticulum stress and associated ROS. Int J Mol Sci. 2016;17:327.
16. Schroder M, Kaufman RJ. ER stress and the unfolded protein response. Mutat Res. 2005;569:29–63.
17. Oyadomari S, Mori M. Roles of CHOP/GADD153 in endoplasmic reticulum stress. Cell Death Differ. 2004;11:381–9.
18. Park HJ, Park SJ, Koo DB, Lee SR, Kong IK, Ryoo JW, Park YI, Chang KT, Lee DS. Progesterone production is affected by unfolded protein response (UPR) signaling during the luteal phase in mice. Life Sci. 2014;113:60–7.
19. Park HJ, Park SJ, Koo DB, Kong IK, Kim MK, Kim JM, Choi MS, Park YH, Kim SU, Chang KT, et al. Unfolding protein response signaling is involved in development, maintenance, and regression of the corpus luteum during the bovine estrous cycle. Biochem Biophys Res Commun. 2013;441:344–50.
20. Tavender TJ, Bulleid NJ. Peroxiredoxin IV protects cells from oxidative stress by removing H2O2 produced during disulphide formation. J Cell Sci. 2010; 123:2672–9.
21. Byers SL, Wiles MV, Dunn SL, Taft RA. Mouse estrous cycle identification tool and images. PLoS One. 2012;7:e35538.
22. Park SJ, Kim TS, Park CK, Lee SH, Kim JM, Lee KS, Lee IK, Park JW, Lawson MA, Lee DS. hCG-induced endoplasmic reticulum stress triggers apoptosis and reduces steroidogenic enzyme expression through activating transcription factor 6 in Leydig cells of the testis. J Mol Endocrinol. 2013;50:151–66.
23. Burrill JS, Long EK, Reilly B, Deng Y, Armitage IM, Scherer PE, Bernlohr DA. Inflammation and ER stress regulate branched-chain amino acid uptake and metabolism in adipocytes. Mol Endocrinol. 2015;29:411–20.
24. Foyouzi N, Cai Z, Sugimoto Y, Stocco C. Changes in the expression of steroidogenic and antioxidant genes in the mouse corpus luteum during luteolysis. Biol Reprod. 2005;72:1134–41.

25. Riley JC, Behrman HR. In vivo generation of hydrogen peroxide in the rat corpus luteum during luteolysis. Endocrinology. 1991;128:1749–53.
26. Lee SY, Lee JY, Oh SJ, Kim HC, Kim SK. Expression of hepatic and ovarian antioxidant enzymes during estrous cycle in rats. Toxicol Lett. 2012;212:329–36.
27. Rapoport R, Sklan D, Wolfenson D, Shaham-Albalancy A, Hanukoglu I. Antioxidant capacity is correlated with steroidogenic status of the corpus luteum during the bovine estrous cycle. Biochim Biophys Acta. 1998;1380:133–40.
28. Banmeyer I, Marchand C, Verhaeghe C, Vucic B, Rees JF, Knoops B. Overexpression of human peroxiredoxin 5 in subcellular compartments of Chinese hamster ovary cells: effects on cytotoxicity and DNA damage caused by peroxides. Free Radic Biol Med. 2004;36:65–77.
29. Mesen TB, Young SL. Progesterone and the luteal phase: a requisite to reproduction. Obstet Gynecol Clin N Am. 2015;42:135–51.
30. Ayabe T, Tsutsumi O, Momoeda M, Yano T, Mitsuhashi N, Taketani Y. Impaired follicular growth and abnormal luteinizing hormone surge in luteal phase defect. Fertil Steril. 1994;61:652–6.
31. Hinney B, Henze C, Kuhn W, Wuttke W. The corpus luteum insufficiency: a multifactorial disease. J Clin Endocrinol Metab. 1996;81:565–70.
32. Ginsburg KA. Luteal phase defect. Etiology, diagnosis, and management. Endocrinol Metab Clin N Am. 1992;21:85–104.
33. Bhandary B, Marahatta A, Kim HR, Chae HJ. An involvement of oxidative stress in endoplasmic reticulum stress and its associated diseases. Int J Mol Sci. 2012;14:434–56.
34. Malhotra JD, Kaufman RJ. Endoplasmic reticulum stress and oxidative stress: a vicious cycle or a double-edged sword? Antioxid Redox Signal. 2007;9: 2277–93.
35. Malhotra JD, Miao H, Zhang K, Wolfson A, Pennathur S, Pipe SW, Kaufman RJ. Antioxidants reduce endoplasmic reticulum stress and improve protein secretion. Proc Natl Acad Sci U S A. 2008;105:18525–30.
36. Halasi M, Wang M, Chavan TS, Gaponenko V, Hay N, Gartel AL. ROS inhibitor N-acetyl-L-cysteine antagonizes the activity of proteasome inhibitors. Biochem J. 2013;454:201–8.
37. Cao SS, Kaufman RJ. Endoplasmic reticulum stress and oxidative stress in cell fate decision and human disease. Antioxid Redox Signal. 2014;21:396–413.
38. Eletto D, Chevet E, Argon Y, Appenzeller-Herzog C. Redox controls UPR to control redox. J Cell Sci. 2014;127:3649–58.

Associations between the maternal circulating lipid profile in pregnancy and fetal imprinted gene alleles

Clive J. Petry[1*], Albert Koulman[2,3], Liangjian Lu[1,4], Benjamin Jenkins[2], Samuel Furse[3], Philippa Prentice[1], Lee Matthews[2], Ieuan A. Hughes[1], Carlo L. Acerini[1], Ken K. Ong[1,3,5] and David B. Dunger[1,3]

Abstract

Background: Imprinted genes, which are expressed in a parent of origin-specific manner, are thought to mediate the genetic priorities of each parent in pregnancy. Recently we reported that some fetal imprinted gene variants are associated with maternal glucose concentrations and blood pressures in pregnancy. We suggest that the conflict between the effects of paternal and maternal transmitted genes starts at conception and may already be evident in measures of maternal metabolism in early pregnancy, before gestational diabetes is manifest.

Methods: Lipid fractions in maternal non-fasting serum collected around week 15 of pregnancy were profiled using direct infusion mass spectrometry in a subset Discovery Cohort ($n = 200$) of women from the Cambridge Baby Growth Study using direct infusion mass spectrometry. Associations between 151 haplotype-tag fetal polymorphisms in 16 imprinted genes and lipids were determined using partial least squares discriminant analysis. Variable importance in projection scores were used to identify those lipid species that contribute most to the underlying variation in the lipid profile and the concentrations of these species tested for associations with fetal imprinted gene alleles using linear regression. In an internal Validation Cohort ($n = 567$ women from the same cohort) the lipid fraction was profiled using liquid chromatography-mass spectrometry and tested for associations with the same fetal imprinted gene variants as above, followed by meta-analysis of associations from the Discovery and Validation Cohorts.

Results: The most significant associations were between a monounsaturated triglyceride (44:1) and both paternally-transmitted fetal *H19* rs7950932 ($R = 0.14$, $p = 2.9 \times 10^{-3}$, $n = 386$) and maternally-transmitted fetal *FAM99A* rs7131362 ($R = 0.18$, $p = 6.2 \times 10^{-3}$, $n = 351$; association with maternal-untransmitted allele $R = 0.08$, $p = 0.07$, $n = 328$). This same triglyceride isoform was also associated with subsequent week 28 fasting glucose concentrations ($R = 0.09$, $p = 9.9 \times 10^{-3}$, $n = 673$) and homeostasis model assessment of insulin resistance ($R = 0.09$, $p = 0.01$, $n = 664$).

Conclusions: Fetal imprinted genes may influence maternal circulating clinically relevant triglyceride concentrations early in pregnancy.

Keywords: Lipidomics, Lipid profiling, Triglycerides, Gestational diabetes, Development, Parent-of-origin

* Correspondence: cjp1002@cam.ac.uk
[1]Department of Paediatrics, University of Cambridge, Box 116, Cambridge Biomedical Campus, Hills Road, Cambridge CB2 0QQ, UK
Full list of author information is available at the end of the article

Background

The Kinship (or Conflict) Hypothesis [1, 2] suggests that paternally-expressed fetal imprinted genes will tend to increase fetal growth whereas maternally-expressed genes will tend to restrain it. It has been suggested that this is achieved through modifying fetal and placental nutritional demand and supply [3]. This is supported by evidence that polymorphic variation in the fetal genome, particularly in fetal growth genes, could lead to alterations in maternal metabolism in pregnancy [4]. This long-standing hypothesis suggests that imprinted genes mediate the separate reproductive genetic priorities of the mother and the father in pregnancies [1, 2], through their parent-of-origin-mediated expression. Which parentally-transmitted copy of the gene is expressed, and which is repressed, is governed by the particular gene and the tissue in question, as well as the stage of development. We suggested that in altering both maternal metabolism and physiology, variation in the fetal genome could lead to an alteration in maternal glucose concentrations and blood pressures, leading to a change in the risk of individuals developing adverse conditions of pregnancy such as gestational diabetes (GDM) and gestational hypertension [5, 6]. Following up the equivalent results that we found in an *H19* knockout mouse model [7], in humans we observed that paternally-transmitted fetal alleles in the *IGF2* gene were associated with maternal glucose concentrations in late pregnancy [8] and GDM when contributing towards fetal imprinted gene allele scores [9]. We have also found other fetal imprinted gene variants that are associated with maternal blood pressure in pregnancy [10]. None of the other maternal circulating nutrient groups that could contribute to fetal growth and development appear to have been tested for associations with polymorphic variation in the fetal genome thus far. This includes lipids such as triglycerides.

In addition to the influence of the mother's dietary intake, concentrations of triglycerides in the maternal circulation during pregnancy appear to be able to be influenced by polymorphic variation in the maternal genome (e.g. [11]). As well as with maternal circulating lipid concentrations, associations with fatty acids in cord blood have been reported for both maternal and fetal polymorphisms (e.g. [12]). Triglycerides in the maternal circulation appear to have a number of positive effects on the pregnancy including being: (a) a mobile energy source, (b) a reservoir of fatty acids in the mother and (c) an important contributor to fetal growth and potentially newborn development (via the de novo biosynthesis of lipids and triglycerides in mammary glands) [13]. However they have also been linked to negative effects of the high abundance of triglycerides in the maternal circulation, e.g. pre-eclampsia, pre-term birth, macrosomia and maternal cardiovascular disease later in life. Triglycerides are strongly associated with fetal growth in women with GDM [14], and changes in their abundance in their circulating concentrations and isoform profile can precede the development of adverse conditions of pregnancy [15]. Whilst acknowledging that there are many factors in pregnancy that may affect the abundance of lipids in the maternal circulation, including variation in the maternal genome, given the potential influence of these triglyceride species on fetal growth and development it seems reasonable to suggest that polymorphic variation in the fetal genome may have its own influence on maternal circulating lipid levels in pregnancy. This could contribute to the regulation of fetal growth and development.

Previously we have found associations between paternally-transmitted fetal *IGF2* and late pregnancy maternal glucose concentrations [8, 9]. This led us to the hypothesis that the interaction between the fetal genotype and maternal metabolism occurs early in pregnancy, when GDM is less well defined. We therefore used mass spectrometry-based lipid profiling to identify metabolic signals and test the hypothesis that fetal variants in imprinted genes are associated with the profile of maternal serum lipids during the first half of pregnancy.

Methods

Cohort and sample selection

The prospective and longitudinal Cambridge Baby Growth Study recruited mothers (and their partners and offspring) attending ultrasound clinics during early pregnancy at the Rosie Maternity Hospital, Cambridge, U.K. between 2001 and 2009 [8–10, 16]. Where possible venous blood (non-fasting) was collected from mothers at recruitment (at the pregnancy booking clinic, around 15 weeks of gestation). After allowing time for clotting, these samples were centrifuged at 3000 g for 10 min. and the serum separated and stored at – 80 °C until they were used. In total, 845 DNA triads were collected from the families of 1074 mothers recruited to the study for whom week 28 75 g oral glucose tolerance test (OGTT) data were collected for GDM studies [8, 9]. Blood and/or mouth swab samples for DNA extraction were collected from the father and the offspring *post-partum*. In this cohort 96.9% of the offspring were Caucasian, 0.8% were mixed race, 0.6% were Black (African or Caribbean), 0.8% were Oriental and 0.9% were Indo-Asian.

The current analysis was restricted to 767 women for whom we had both DNA family triad samples available and serum samples from around week 15 of pregnancy. To be of use in a range of studies, 200 of these samples ("the Discovery Cohort") were specifically chosen to have broadly equal: (1) numbers drawn from tertiles of the venous glucose concentration 60 min. post glucose load at the week 28 OGTT, (2) proportions of pregnancies where the baby exhibited "normal", "catch-up" or "catch-down" growth (defined as > − 0.67 and < + 0.67, > + 0.67, and < − 0.67 respectively, change in weight z-scores over the first year of life) and (3) numbers of the various combinations of compound fetal alleles formed from the paternally-transmitted *IGF2* rs1077025 allele [8, 9] and the maternally-transmitted *H19* rs2071094 allele [16]. The remaining participants in this analysis (n = 567), were used as an internal Validation Cohort. Clinical characteristics of participants in the Discovery and Validation Cohorts are shown in Table 1. The only detectable difference between the two groups was a slightly shorter mean gestational age at delivery in the Validation Cohort of around 2 days.

Gene selection and genetics

Genomic DNA was extracted from blood samples or mouth swabs using an Autopure LS Machine (Qiagen Ltd., Crawley, U.K.). The 16 genes that were studied (*DLK1, FAM99A, GNAS, GRB10, H19, IGF2, INS, KCNQ1OT1, MEST, NNAT, PEG3, PEG10, PLAGL1, SGCE, SNRPN, ZIM2*) were chosen because they were all imprinted at some stage of development in certain tissues. They were also all placentally-expressed [17], although by the time in pregnancy that the placenta was fully functional some of them may have been biallelically expressed. The variants that were genotyped were haplotype tag SNPs covering the gene and 20 kb either side of it, identified by Tagger (r^2 > 0.8 and minor allele frequency > 0.2) from the Centre d'Etude du Polymorphisme Human population (Utah residents with ancestry from Northern and Western Europe) of HapMap Project Build 36 using Haploview [18]. The one exception to this was *IGF2* where 11 of the tagging SNPs were identified by Rodríguez et al. [19]. The SNPs that were genotyped are listed in Table 2. The DNA samples were genotyped using KASPar assays, which are competitive allele-specific PCR SNP genotyping assays using FRET quencher cassette oligonucleotides (designed and performed by LGC Genomics, Hoddesdon, U.K.). The SNP genotypes that were used in this study were consistent with Hardy Weinberg equilibrium (p > 0.05 using the χ^2 test) and had a repeat genotyping discordancy rate of < 1.0%. For each of the 151 SNPs that were successfully designated, genotypes from both parents and their child were used to infer parental allelic transmission to the fetus according to Table 3.

Lipid profiling: Sample extraction and mass spectrometry

The lipid profiles of maternal serum from the Discovery Cohort were analysed using the direct infusion mass spectrometry method that we developed for use with dried blood spots [20, 21], which was originally based on a method for plasma [22]. All solvents were of at least liquid chromatography–mass spectrometry (LC–MS) grade and were purchased from Sigma Aldrich (Gillingham, Dorset, U.K.). All internal standards were obtained from Avanti Polar lipids (through Instruchem, Delfzijn, The Netherlands) except for undecanoic acid and trilaurin (Sigma Aldrich).

Samples were subjected to a balanced randomisation to achieve an approximately equal number of genotypes in each batch (2 × 68 samples and 1 × 64 samples). A serum pool was created by using 5 μL of a random subset of samples, to create the first quality control (QC1). Part of the pooled sample was diluted with phosphate buffered saline (PBS), either mixing the pooled sample 1:1 with PBS (to create QC2) or 1:4 with PBS (to create QC3). From the QC material 15 μL was aliquoted into 1.2 mL Cryovials and stored at − 80 °C prior to use. Quality assurance (QA) samples used were based on commercially available human plasma. Each batch had 6 x blanks, 6 x QAs, 4 x QC1, 4 x QC2, 4 xQC3. The

Table 1 Characteristics of the study participants drawn from the Cambridge Baby Growth Study

Characteristic	Discovery Cohort (n = 200)	Validation Cohort (n = 567)	p-value
Age at delivery (years)	33.4 (32.8, 34.0)	33.2 (32.8, 33.6)	0.6
Gestational age at delivery (weeks)	40.1 (39.9, 40.3)	39.8 (39.7, 40.0)	0.02
Parity (n)	1.7 (1.6, 1.8)	1.7 (1.6, 1.8)	0.6
Pre-pregnancy BMI (kg/m^2)	23.9 (23.2, 24.6)	24.2 (23.8, 24.6)	0.5
Weight gain during pregnancy (kg)	9.2 (8.0, 10.4)	9.0 (8.2, 9.7)	0.8
Week 28 OGTT fasting glucose concentration (mmol/L)	4.3 (4.2, 4.4)	4.3 (4.3, 4.3)	0.9
Week 28 OGTT 60 min. glucose concentration (mmol/L)	6.4 (6.2, 6.7)	6.6 (6.5, 6.8)	0.1
Week 28 fasting insulin concentration (pmol/L)	44.9 (41.7, 48.4)	45.6 (43.7, 47.6)	0.7
Week 28 fasting insulin resistance (HOMA IR)	0.915 (0.850, 0.985)	0.925 (0.886, 0.965)	0.8
Carrying a male fetus (%)	49.2	52.6	0.4
Smoking during pregnancy (%)	2.6	4.9	0.2

Data are mean (95% confidence interval) or counts (%) for those study participants where the information was available. Categorical data was assessed using the χ^2 test, all other testing was performed using linear regression

Table 2 The SNPs that were genotyped for this study

Gene	No. of SNPs	Single nucleotide polymorphisms
DLK1	5	rs12147008, rs7155375, rs10139403, rs1802710, rs7147586
*FAM99A**	7	rs4752779, rs4752781, rs11600502, rs10839220, rs11607954, rs1489945, rs7131362
GNAS	20	rs6123832, rs965808, rs6128441, rs6026561, rs6026560, rs12625436, rs4810148, rs7271854, rs6100260, rs6026576, rs6128461, rs6123837, rs13831, rs234630, rs919196, rs3730168, rs919197, rs7121, rs234623, rs234621
GRB10	17	rs4245555, rs12669770, rs7802879, rs7777754, rs2715129, rs3807549, rs2299150, rs11769934, rs2237441, rs1468450, rs6948959, rs980716, rs2715116, rs737292, rs7794604, rs17133917, rs2237450
H19	13	rs2071094, rs2735466, rs7950932, rs217222, rs217727, rs2251375, rs217228, rs3741216, rs1706879, rs2735971, rs7950715, rs7950787, rs12417375
*IGF2**	17	rs6578987, *rs734351, *rs4341514, rs680, *rs3741212, *rs11603378, *rs3213216, *rs10770125, *rs3741205, *rs3741206, rs1004446, *rs4320932, *rs3842752, *rs7924316, *rs7483056, *rs6356, *rs10743152
*INS**	16	*rs734351, *rs4341514, rs2585, *rs3741212, *rs11603378, *rs3213216, *rs10770125, *rs3741205, *rs3741206, *rs4320932, rs3741211, *rs3842752, *rs7924316, *rs7483056, *rs6356, *rs10743152
*KCNQ1OT1**	14	rs231352, rs463924, rs4930005, rs231841, rs10832514, rs756852, rs7128926, rs10832430, rs231361, rs760419, rs9666537, rs7929804, rs10766218, rs6578283
MEST	6	rs12706933, rs13234660, rs765205, rs13225903, rs1047456, rs10954272
NNAT	3	rs6066671, rs12481150, rs6019103
*PEG3**	8	rs17207579, rs11084466, *rs2079877, *rs7256072, *rs382592, rs758752, rs7248098, *rs1860565
PEG10	5	rs1568214, rs13073, rs1533831, rs6948099, rs6465422
PLAGL1	20	rs12528289, rs9484833, rs1884087, rs10499846, rs2268440, rs6930726, rs7770529, rs2268443, rs2876578, rs9373409, rs2268445, rs17073273, rs9403542, rs9484836, rs6570599, rs2328537, rs9321957, rs6937128, rs9767615, rs2207851
SGCE	2	rs1879854, rs7778237
SNRPN	12	rs7164801, rs17114774, rs7171320, rs1453556, rs4028398, rs1982981, rs736008, rs9806682, rs7164989, rs8042562, rs12592279, rs8029318
*ZIM2**	8	*rs2079877, rs12981689, rs1476830, *rs7256072, *rs382592, *rs1860565, rs2286751, rs10401139

Genes are named according to their HUGO (Human Genome Organisation) abbreviation
*indicates that some of the SNPs are shared with another gene (*IGF2* with *INS*, *PEG3* with *ZIM2*, *PLAGL1* with *HYMAI*, *KCNQ1OT1* with *KCNQ1*, and *FAM99A* with *FAM99B and KRTAP5-6*). A total of 155 SNPs were genotyped. The following SNP genotypes failed as either the assay was unsuitable or the genotypes did not pass the quality control procedures: (*GNAS*) rs6123837, (*GRB10*) rs2237450, (*PLAGL1*) rs12528289, (*ZIM2*) rs2286751

Table 3 Imputation table of parentally transmitted fetal alleles based on family triad genotypes

Paternal Genotype	Maternal Genotype	Fetal Genotype	Paternally-transmitted Allele	Maternally-transmitted Allele
A/A	A/A	A/A	A	A
A/A	A/a	A/A	A	A
A/A	A/a	A/a	A	a
A/A	a/a	A/a	A	a
A/a	A/A	A/A	A	A
A/a	A/A	A/a	a	A
A/a	A/a	A/A	A	A
A/a	A/a	A/a	Uninformative	Uninformative
A/a	A/a	a/a	a	a
A/a	a/a	A/a	A	a
A/a	a/a	a/a	a	a
a/a	A/A	A/a	a	A
a/a	A/a	A/a	a	A
a/a	A/a	a/a	a	a
a/a	a/a	a/a	a	a

"A" represents the major allele of a SNP and "a" the minor allele based on frequency

extraction method for the lipids used a Flexus automated liquid handler (Anachem, Milton Keynes, UK) for pipetting. 15 μL serum samples were extracted using *tert*-butyl methyl ether (MTBE), containing the following internal standards: 1,2-di-*O*-octadecyl-glycero-*sn*-3-phosphatidylcholine, 1,2-di-*O*-phytanyl-glycero-*sn*-3-phophatidylethanolamine, C8-ceramide, N-heptadecanoyl-D-erythro-sphingosylphosporylcholine, undecanoic acid and trilaurin on glass coated 2.4 mL deep well plates (Plate+TM, Esslab, Hadleigh, UK) as described [20]. A 96 head micro-dispenser (Hydra Matrix, Thermo Fisher Ltd., Hemel Hampstead, U.K.) was used to transfer 25 μL of the lipid extract to a glass coated low well plate (Plate +TM, Esslab, Hadleigh, U.K.) and with 90 μL of MS-mix (7.5 mM NH_4Ac IPA:MeOH (2:1)) using a Hydra Matrix, after which the plate was sealed using Corning aluminium microplate sealing tape (Sigma-Aldrich Company, U.K.) and stored at − 20 °C until analysis.

At 15 °C throughout, 5 μL of sample was dispensed into the mass spectrometer (Thermo Fisher Exactive benchtop orbitrap; Hemel Hempstead, U.K.) using an Advion Triversa Nanomate (Ithaca, New York, U.S.A.) electrospray ioniser under 0.2 psi nitrogen pressure. Ionisation was achieved with a potential of 1.2 kV. Data acquisition started 20 s. after sample aspiration began. After 72 s. of acquisition in positive mode, negative mode was adopted by changing the potential to − 1.5 kV. The spray was maintained for another 66 s.

Liquid chromatography–mass spectrometry

Lipids were identified using a selected subset of samples analysed using a LTQ Orbitrap Velos Elite coupled to a Surveyor (both Thermo Fisher, Hemel Hampstead, U.K.) LC system as described [21]. The Orbitrap was set-up using the data-dependent precursor selection. Generally the selected masses were isolated with a 1.5 m/z width in the linear ion trap and then fragmented using either linear ion trap with 35% relative collision energy or in the higher-energy collision-induced dissociation collision cell, with a range from 5 to 75% relative collision energy. All spectra were recorded in the Orbitrap set at 100,000 resolution. All species recorded were identified based on accurate mass and subsequently based on accurate mass MS2 spectra and retention time from the LC–MS experiment.

The maternal serum lipid profiles of the Validation Cohort were subsequently analysed by LC–MS rather than by the direct infusion mass spectrometry that was used for the Discovery Cohort [23], using the method described previously [24].

The raw mass spectrometry data were converted to .mzXML format using MS Convert, parsed to R and 50 spectra averaged per mode using XCMS (http://bioconductor.org/packages/release/bioc/html/xcms.html). Additional processing was then conducted using an in-house R script (Peakpicker version 2.0) to select peaks, deisotope and annotate direct-infusion mass spectrometry data sets. Only those lipid species where more than 70% (140) of the samples contained detectable concentrations and showed a linear correlations with diluted QC range were used. Accordingly 173 lipid/triglyceride species were considered for statistical analysis.

Other assays and calculations

Blood glucose concentrations were measured using a routine glucose oxidase-based method. Maternal plasma insulin concentrations were measured using a DSL ELISA (London, U.K.) run according to the manufacturer's instructions. Homeostatic model assessment of insulin resistance (HOMA IR) was estimated using the HOMA calculator [25]. Body mass index (BMI) was calculated as the body weight (kg) divided by the height (m) squared.

Statistical power

In the Discovery Cohort there was 80% statistical power to detect a difference of 1.37 standard deviations in lipid species concentrations for a variant with a minor allele frequency of 0.4 ($\alpha = 0.05$). The equivalent value for the Validation Cohort was 1.21. There was 80% statistical power in the random-effects meta-analysis with moderate heterogeneity for a small effect size (Cohen's d) of 0.29 ($\alpha = 0.05$).

Statistical analyses

Lipid profiles in the Discovery Cohort were analysed by Partial Least Squares – Discriminant Analysis (PLS-DA), a multivariate dimensionality-reduction tool with awareness of class labels, using Metaboanalyst 3.0 [26]. The peak intensity table from the mass spectrometry was loaded into the software and the default data integrity check accepted. Without data filtering, the log-transformed data was normalised using the median and scaled using mean centring. Fitted models were considered significant if the value of Q^2 (representing the predictive capability of the model, as estimated by cross-validation) was positive [23]. The importance of individual lipid species was quantified via the variable importance in projection (VIP) score, a weighted sum of squares of the PLS-DA loadings that takes into account the amount of explained lipid profile variance for each component, and used to identify individual candidate lipid species (with a threshold VIP score of greater than 2.0 in this study) that may be significantly associated with fetal imprinted gene alleles. These associations (and those with maternal genotypes) were then tested using linear regression models in both the Discovery and Validation Cohorts. Analysis of the associations in the full cohort was by meta-analysis rather than combining results from both sub-Cohorts into one because of the different laboratory methods used to assess the lipid profiles. The meta-analysis was analysed using the Der Simonian-Laird approach [27] for random effects models implemented into the R Metacor package, version 1.0–2 (https://cran.r-project.org/packages/metacor/index.html). Additional analyses were then performed to assess potential imprinting effects on the associations, by testing associations between the lipid species and the maternal genotypes, the maternal untransmitted allele and the fetal imprinted allele transmitted from the parent whose allele did not produce significant fitted models in Metaboanalyst.

Categorical and ordinal data were analysed using the χ^2 or Fisher's exact tests, or logistic regression. Associations with $p < 0.05$ were considered significant throughout. Apart from the use of Metaboanalyst, and the meta-analyses which were performed in R (version 3.2.2; https://cran.r-project.org/bin/windows/base/), all other statistical analyses were performed in Stata (version 13.1; StataCorp LP, College Station, TX, U.S.A.).

Results

Associations between fetal imprinted gene alleles and the maternal lipid profile around week 15 of pregnancy

The associations between the peak intensities of individual lipid species (that produced significant fitted models in the PLS-DA analysis of the Discovery Cohort) and fetal imprinted gene alleles are shown in Table 4. The most significant fetal imprinted gene allele associations

Table 4 Associations between fetal genotypes and candidate lipid species' peak intensity

SNP	Gene	Parental Transmission	Lipid	VIP Score of lipid species*	Discovery Cohort			Validation Cohort			Meta-Analysis	
					R	*p*-value	n	R	*p*-value	n	R	*p*-value
rs10839220	*KRTAP5–6*	Maternal	TG(44:1)	3.4	0.175	0.03	163	0	0.96	197	0.09 (− 0.09, 0.25)	0.17
rs10839220	*KRTAP5–6*	Maternal	LysoPCP(18:0)	2.8	0.243	1.8×10^{-3}	163	0.092	0.16	233	0.16 (0.01, 0.31)	0.02
rs10839220	*KRTAP5–6*	Maternal	PE(34:0)	2.2	0.279	3.2×10^{-4}	163	0.014	0.85	233	0.15 (−0.12, 0.39)	0.14
rs10839220	*KRTAP5–6*	Maternal	DG(36:3)	2.1	0.271	4.6×10^{-4}	163	0.118	0.09	209	0.19 (0.04, 0.34)	7.4×10^{-3}
rs4752779	*FAM99B*	Maternal	TG(44:1)	3.2	0.161	0.03	173	0.030	0.67	201	0.09 (−0.04, 0.22)	0.08
rs7131362	*FAM99A*	Maternal	TG(44:1)	4.7	0.257	9.7×10^{-4}	161	0.114	0.12	190	0.18 (0.04, 0.32)	6.2×10^{-3}
rs7131362	*FAM99A*	Maternal	TG(48:0)	2.1	0.197	0.01	161	0	0.95	217	0.10 (−0.10, 0.28)	0.17
rs17073273	*PLAGL1*	Maternal	TG(44:1)	3.5	0.181	0.02	175	0.014	0.83	206	0.09 (−0.07, 0.25)	0.13
rs17073273	*PLAGL1*	Maternal	TG(55:9)	2.7	0.234	1.8×10^{-3}	175	0.079	0.23	235	0.15 (0.00, 0.30)	0.03
rs17073273	*PLAGL1*	Maternal	TG(48:0)	2.5	0.226	2.6×10^{-3}	175	0.035	0.59	235	0.13 (−0.06, 0.31)	0.09
rs2268445	*PLAGL1*	Maternal	TG(44:1)	3.6	0.189	0.01	176	0.035	0.62	212	0.11 (−0.04, 0.26)	0.08
rs7950932	*H19*	Paternal	TG(44:1)	2.6	0.167	0.02	183	0.117	0.10	203	0.14 (0.04, 0.24)	2.3×10^{-3}

Only those lipid species that tagged components with significant fitted models in Metaboanalyst are shown
*in the PLSDA component with a significant Q^2 in the Discovery Cohort dataset

both related to TG(44:1), namely paternally-transmitted *H19* rs7950932 and maternally-transmitted *FAM99A* rs7131362. Of the associations in this list, not all of which reached statistical significance, there was a predominance of associations of species with maternally-expressed fetal alleles in the Discovery Cohort analyses ($p = 0.01$). Due to this we also tested associations between the same species and both the maternal genotype (Table 5) and the untransmitted maternal allele (Table 6) to investigate whether the associations were most likely fetally- or maternally-mediated. All other associations were considered non-significant (data not shown). To assess whether the associations highlighted in Table 4 were parent-of-origin effects we also tested associations between the same species and fetal alleles transmitted from the parent whose allele did not produce significant fitted models in the PLS-DA analysis of the Discovery Cohort (Table 7). Fetal *H19* rs7950932 alleles transmitted from both parents showed significant associations with maternal TG(44:1) peak intensity (Tables 4 and 7), and we also found significant associations with the fetal rs7950932 genotype (Discovery Cohort $R = 0.17$, $p = 0.01$, $n = 191$; Validation cohort $R = 0.10$, $p = 0.08$, $n = 220$; meta-analysis $R = 0.13$ (0.04–0.23), $p = 3.6 \times 10^{-3}$).

Associations between the abundance of TG(44:1) at around week 15 of pregnancy and clinically significant parameters

The species most heavily represented in the list of associations with fetal imprinted gene variant alleles by the VIP scores was TG(44:1), a monounsaturated triglyceride. It is also the triglyceride involved in the two most

Table 5 Associations between maternal imprinted gene SNP genotypes and candidate lipid species' peak intensity

SNP	Gene	Lipid	Discovery Cohort			Validation Cohort			Meta-Analysis	
			R	*p*-value	n	R	*p*-value	n	R	*p*-value
rs10839220	*KRTAP5–6*	TG(44:1)	0.157	0.04	179	0.017	0.78	225	0.08 (−0.05, 0.22)	0.12
rs10839220	*KRTAP5–6*	LysoPCP(18:0)	0.205	5.8×10^{-3}	179	0	0.92	267	0.10 (−0.10, 0.29)	0.17
rs10839220	*KRTAP5–6*	PE(34:0)	0.194	9.2×10^{-3}	179	0.051	0.41	267	0.12 (− 0.02, 0.25)	0.05
rs10839220	*KRTAP5–6*	DG(36:3)	0.224	2.6×10^{-3}	179	0.062	0.34	240	0.14 (−0.02, 0.29)	0.04
rs4752779	*FAM99B*	TG(44:1)	0.102	0.17	180	0.045	0.51	227	0.07 (−0.03, 0.17)	0.08
rs7131362	*FAM99A*	TG(44:1)	0.222	2.9×10^{-3}	178	0.041	0.54	221	0.13 (−0.05, 0.30)	0.08
rs7131362	*FAM99A*	TG(48:0)	0.150	0.05	178	0.030	0.64	251	0.08 (−0.03, 0.20)	0.08
rs17073273	*PLAGL1*	TG(44:1)	0.042	0.56	188	0.033	0.61	234	0.04 (−0.06, 0.13)	0.23
rs17073273	*PLAGL1*	TG(55:9)	0.125	0.09	188	0.117	0.06	267	0.12 (0.03, 0.21)	5.2×10^{-3}
rs17073273	*PLAGL1*	TG(48:0)	0.084	0.25	188	0.057	0.35	267	0.07 (− 0.02, 0.16)	0.07
rs2268445	*PLAGL1*	TG(44:1)	0.046	0.54	187	0.071	0.28	231	0.06 (−0.04, 0.16)	0.11

Only those lipid species that tagged components with significant fitted models in Metaboanalyst using maternally-transmitted fetal variants are shown

Table 6 Associations between maternal untransmitted alleles and candidate lipid species' peak intensity

SNP	Gene	Lipid	Discovery Cohort			Validation Cohort			Meta-Analysis	
			R	*p*-value	n	R	*p*-value	n	R	*p*-value
rs10839220	*KRTAP5–6*	TG(44:1)	0.113	0.16	154	0.067	0.38	179	0.09 (−0.02, 0.19)	0.05
rs10839220	*KRTAP5–6*	LysoPCP(18:0)	0.095	0.24	154	0.114	0.10	213	0.11 (0, 0.21)	0.02
rs10839220	*KRTAP5–6*	PE(34:0)	0.068	0.54	154	0.042	0.40	213	0.05 (−0.05, 0.15)	0.16
rs10839220	*KRTAP5–6*	DG(36:3)	0.122	0.13	154	0	0.98	190	0.06 (−0.06, 0.17)	0.18
rs4752779	*FAM99B*	TG(44:1)	0.020	0.81	161	0.054	0.47	185	0.04 (−0.07, 0.14)	0.24
rs7131362	*FAM99A*	TG(44:1)	0.119	0.14	153	0.050	0.51	175	0.08 (−0.03, 0.19)	0.07
rs7131362	*FAM99A*	TG(48:0)	0.080	0.43	153	0.065	0.26	198	0.07 (−0.03, 0.18)	0.09
rs17073273	*PLAGL1*	TG(44:1)	0.131	0.09	170	0.024	0.74	201	0.07 (−0.03, 0.18)	0.09
rs17073273	*PLAGL1*	TG(55:9)	0	0.98	170	0.123	0.06	228	0.07 (−0.05, 0.19)	0.13
rs17073273	*PLAGL1*	TG(48:0)	0.094	0.22	170	0.067	0.31	228	0.08 (−0.02, 0.18)	0.06
rs2268445	*PLAGL1*	TG(44:1)	0.092	0.23	172	0.022	0.76	201	0.05 (−0.05, 0.16)	0.15

Only those lipid species that tagged components with significant fitted models in Metaboanalyst using maternally-transmitted fetal variants are shown

significant associations between fetal imprinted gene alleles and triglycerides in analyses of lipid species where PLS-DA analysis of the Discovery Cohort data led to significant fitted models (Table 4). To investigate whether this isoform was clinically relevant in our population we tested associations between its peak intensities, maternal pre-pregnancy BMI and indices derived from the OGTT (Table 8). Of these in the two sub-cohorts the strongest associations were with fasting glucose concentrations and HOMA IR, both of which were positively related to the abundance of TG(44:1). In turn week 28 fasting glucose concentrations (odds ratio (OR) 4.8×10^{10} (8.5×10^{8}, 2.7×10^{12}), $p = 5.7 \times 10^{-33}$, $n = 1083$) and HOMA IR (OR 7.7 (4.8, 12.1), $p = 2.7 \times 10^{-18}$, $n = 1059$) were also both positively associated with GDM in the Cambridge Baby Growth Study as a whole. In addition they were both positively associated with baby's birth weight (fasting glucose concentrations: standardised $\beta = 0.116$, $p = 3.7 \times 10^{-6}$, $n = 813$; HOMA IR: standardised $\beta = 0.065$, $p = 0.048$, n = 813; both adjusted for gestational age at birth, sex, parity and maternal BMI).

Discussion

In this detailed investigation of the associations between fetal imprinted gene alleles and the circulating maternal lipid profile around week 15 of pregnancy, we found several significant associations with particular triglyceride isoform peak intensities in the maternal circulation. There was an overrepresentation of maternally-transmitted fetal alleles in the list of associations with fitted models in the PLS-DA analysis. Whilst unexpected this may relate to an influence of triglycerides on fetal growth [13] and the

Table 7 Associations between candidate lipid species' peak intensity and alleles transmitted from the other parent than those with significant fitted models

SNP	Gene	Parental Transmission	Lipid	Discovery Cohort			Validation Cohort			Meta-Analysis	
				R	*p*-value	n	R	*p*-value	n	R	*p*-value
rs10839220	*KRTAP5–6*	Paternal	TG(44:1)	0.12	0.14	161	0.08	0.26	200	0.10 (−0.01, 0.20)	0.03
rs10839220	*KRTAP5–6*	Paternal	LysoPCP(18:0)	0.07	0.40	161	0.12	0.07	235	0.07 (−0.03, 0.17)	0.08
rs10839220	*KRTAP5–6*	Paternal	PE(34:0)	0.10	0.20	161	0.11	0.10	235	0.11 (0.01, 0.20)	0.02
rs10839220	*KRTAP5–6*	Paternal	DG(36:3)	0.05	0.53	161	0.18	8.4×10^{-3}	213	0.12 (−0.01, 0.25)	0.03
rs4752779	*FAM99B*	Paternal	TG(44:1)	0.03	0.66	174	0.04	0.61	205	0.04 (−0.07, 0.14)	0.25
rs7131362	*FAM99A*	Paternal	TG(44:1)	0.05	0.57	159	0.01	0.86	204	0.03 (−0.08, 0.13)	0.30
rs7131362	*FAM99A*	Paternal	TG(48:0)	0.03	0.68	159	0.03	0.64	232	0.03 (−0.07, 0.13)	0.26
rs17073273	*PLAGL1*	Paternal	TG(44:1)	0.14	0.07	174	0.08	0.26	216	0.11 (0.01, 0.20)	0.02
rs17073273	*PLAGL1*	Paternal	TG(55:9)	0.13	0.08	174	0.03	0.66	248	0.07 (−0.03, 0.17)	0.08
rs17073273	*PLAGL1*	Paternal	TG(48:0)	0.19	0.01	174	0.10	0.10	248	0.14 (0.04, 0.23)	2.4×10^{-3}
rs2268445	*PLAGL1*	Paternal	TG(44:1)	0.14	0.06	177	0.14	0.04	218	0.14 (0.04, 0.24)	2.7×10^{-3}
rs7950932	*H19*	Maternal	TG(44:1)	0.09	0.21	183	0.09	0.22	209	0.09 (−0.01, 0.19)	0.04

Table 8 Associations between week 15 TG (44:1) peak intensities and biomarkers derived from the week 28 OGTT

Biomarker	Discovery Cohort			Validation Cohort			Meta-Analysis	
	R	*p*-value	n	R	*p*-value	n	R	*p*-value
Pre-pregnancy BMI	−0.10	0.21	170	−0.06	0.31	356	−0.07 (− 0.16, 0.01)	0.05
Fasting glucose concentration	0.04	0.54	195	0.11	0.02	478	0.09 (0.01, 0.16)	9.9×10^{-3}
Glucose concentration 60 min. post 75 g load	0.16	0.03	195	0.05	0.26	478	0.09 (−0.01, 0.19)	0.04
Fasting insulin concentration	0.03	0.65	189	0.10	0.03	476	0.08 (0, 0.16)	0.02
HOMA IR	0.03	0.65	189	0.12	8.8×10^{-3}	475	0.09 (0.01, 0.17)	0.01
HOMA B	0.03	0.72	189	0.05	0.26	475	0.04 (−0.03, 0.12)	0.13

extra influence that maternal genes may have on the resulting offspring birth weight in particular in comparison to paternal genes [28]. In previous studies we observed an influence of fetal imprinted genes on maternal glucose concentrations in pregnancy, although these were much later in pregnancy around week 28 [8, 9]. Results from the current study provide the first evidence for a potential role for fetal imprinted genes in modifying maternal metabolism, in particular circulating levels of certain lipid species, relatively early in pregnancy.

The strongest association was detected with the abundance of maternal circulating TG(44:1), which may include configurations 15:0/15:0/14:1 and/or 15:1/14:0/15:0 [29]. This lipid species was linked to the development of insulin resistance and type 2 diabetes in the Framingham Offspring Study [30]. Importantly, in the current study this isoform was associated with paternally-transmitted fetal rs7950932 (Table 4). This variant is one of the single nucleotide polymorphisms (SNPs) that was used to tag *H19*, which is generally expressed only from the maternally-transmitted allele [31]. However there was also an association between the maternally-transmitted rs7950932 allele and TG(44:1) (Table 7), possibly resulting from biallelic expression in some tissues at this stage of development (which would be consistent with there also being a significant association with the fetal rs7950932 genotype). In other tissues, however, the alleles may have been expressed only from the paternally-transmitted allele: this interpretation being consistent with the association with the paternally-transmitted allele having a higher regression coefficient (and being more statistically significant) than that with the maternally-transmitted allele. Although when expressed in an imprinted fashion *H19* is expressed only from the maternal allele, the rs7950932 locus is located in the proximity of *H19*'s differentially methylated region [32] which helps regulate paternally-expressed *IGF2* as well as *H19* expression [33], making the association with the paternally-transmitted allele plausible. Interestingly the abundance of TG(44:1) in maternal serum around week 15 of pregnancy correlated with subsequent (week 28) fasting glucose concentrations and HOMA IR in our population, which in turn were associated with both GDM and offspring birth weight. We have previously found several paternally-transmitted fetal *IGF2* variants that were associated with late pregnancy glucose concentrations [8, 9]. Together all these results suggest that the associations between fetal rs7950932 alleles and week 15 maternal TG(44:1) levels may be related to both *IGF2* and *H19* expression.

The second strongest association in our population was between fetal rs7131362, a downstream variant of the *FAM99A* gene, and the abundance of maternal week 15 TG(44:1) again. The association was with the maternally-transmitted fetal allele, and with the associations having larger regression coefficients (and greater statistical significance) than those of the equivalent associations with the maternal genotype and the untransmitted maternal alleles, it appears to be directly related to the transmitted fetal allele itself rather than the maternal gene per se. The lack of association with the paternally-transmitted allele is consistent with the fetal effect being modified by imprinting. This variant is in a chromosomal region populated by reciprocally imprinted genes a number of which are maternally-expressed [34]. Although a parent-of-origin effect of this variant on maternal circulating lipid levels has not been evident before, other published studies suggest why such an association may be plausible. Data from the 1000 Genomes project [35] shows a degree of linkage disequilibrium between rs7131362 and rs2334499 (D' = 0.86), whose maternally-transmitted allele has been associated with risk of type 2 diabetes [36] (with the protective allele in [36] being in linkage disequilibrium with the allele associated with the lower TG(44:1) peak intensity in the present study). In recent years it has become apparent that there is a strong correlation between genetic risk variants for type 2 diabetes and those for GDM [37]. As described above, in our population the abundance of the triglyceride isoform TG(44:1) was associated with factors themselves associated with risk of GDM.

Even the most significant associations found in this study should be considered preliminary in nature. The main limitation of the study is that it was only powered to detect associations with large effect sizes. Nevertheless the main associations in our population appear biologically plausible based on current knowledge in the published literature. The associations need external validation in other cohorts, rather than the internal validation that was used in this study, but they will be useful for meta-analyses once studies in other populations have been completed. Our results suggest that associations with TG(44:1) in pregnancy may be particularly important.

Conclusion

The results of this study suggest that the interaction between the fetal imprinted genotype and maternal metabolism may be detected early in pregnancy through alterations in serum levels of clinically relevant triglycerides in the maternal circulation. This result is remarkable because it suggests that triglycerides, traditionally regarded as merely energy storage molecules, may be involved in the metabolic signalling that controls fetal development. However further validation in more highly powered studies is required to establish this.

Abbreviations

BMI: Body mass index; GDM: Gestational diabetes mellitus; HOMA B: Homeostasis model assessment of β-cell function; HOMA IR: Homeostasis model assessment of insulin resistance; LC-MS: Liquid chromatography–mass spectrometry; MTBE: Methyl *tert*-butyl ether; OGTT: Oral glucose tolerance test; OR: Odds ratio; PBS: Phosphate-buffered saline; PLS-DA: Partial least squares discriminant analysis; QA: Quality assurance; QC: Quality control; SNP: Single nucleotide polymorphism; TG(44:1): Triglyceride with 44 carbon atoms and 1 double bond; VIP: Variable importance in projection
Individual lipid species are abbreviated according to LIPID MAPS (http://www.lipidmaps.org/data/classification/lipid_cns.html)

Acknowledgements

The authors acknowledge the excellent technical assistance in the laboratory for this project that was provided by Dianne Wingate, Rachel Seear, Katrin Mooslehner and Radka Platte. The authors would like to thank all the families that took part in the Cambridge Baby Growth Study, and acknowledge the crucial role played by the research nurses especially Suzanne Smith, Ann-Marie Wardell and Karen Forbes, staff at the Addenbrooke's Wellcome Trust Clinical Research Facility, and midwives at the Rosie Maternity Hospital in collecting data for this study.

Funding

The genotyping part of the Cambridge Baby Growth Study was funded by the Evelyn Trust (EW9035322), Diabetes U.K. (11/0004241) and the Wellbeing of Women (the Royal College of Obstetricians and Gynaecologists, U.K.) (RG1644). The lipidomics assays were supported by the Medical Research Council (UD99999906) and Cambridge Lipidomics Biomarker Research Initiative (G0800783). Other core funding has come from the Medical Research Council (G1001995); European Union Framework 5 (QLK4-1999-01422); the Mothercare Charitable Foundation (RG54608); Newlife Foundation for Disabled Children (07/20) and the World Cancer Research Fund International (2004/03). In addition there has been support from National Institute for Health Research Cambridge Biomedical Research Centre. KO is supported by the Medical Research Council (Unit Programme number: MC_UU_12015/2). The various funding bodies took no part in the design of the study, the collection, analysis, and interpretation of the data, or in the writing of the manuscript.

Authors' contributions

CP, AK and DD designed the experiment. CP and AK performed the statistical analysis. CP also oversaw the genotyping. AK, BJ, SF, and LM performed the lipidomics experiments, with PP contributing towards the laboratory methodology. IH, CA, KO and DD devised and oversee the Cambridge Baby Growth Study. CP, RS and AK drafted the initial version of the manuscript. All authors commented on initial drafts of the manuscript and approved the submitted version of it.

Competing interests

The authors declare that they have no competing interests.

Author details

[1]Department of Paediatrics, University of Cambridge, Box 116, Cambridge Biomedical Campus, Hills Road, Cambridge CB2 0QQ, UK. [2]Medical Research Council Human Nutrition Research, Cambridge, UK. [3]The Institute of Metabolic Science, University of Cambridge, Cambridge, UK. [4]Khoo Teck Puat-National University Children's Medical Institute, National University Hospital, National University Health System, Singapore, Singapore. [5]Medical Research Council Epidemiology Unit, University of Cambridge, Cambridge, UK.

References

1. Haig D, Westoby M. Parent-specific gene expression and the triploid endosperm. Am Nat. 1989;134:147–55.
2. Haig D. Genetic conflicts in human pregnancy. Q Rev Biol. 1993;68:495–532.
3. Reik W, Constância M, Fowden A, Anderson N, Dean W, Ferguson-Smith A, et al. Regulation of supply and demand for maternal nutrients in mammals by imprinted genes. J Physiol. 2003;547:35–44.
4. Haig D. Placental hormones, genomic imprinting, and maternal–foetal communication. J Evol Biol. 1996;9:357–80.
5. Petry CJ, Ong KK, Dunger DB. Does the foetal genotype affect maternal physiology during pregnancy? Trends Mol Med. 2007;13:414–21.
6. Petry CJ, Beardsall K, Dunger DB. The potential impact of the foetal genotype on maternal blood pressure during pregnancy. J Hypertens. 2014; 32:1553–61.
7. Petry CJ, Evans ML, Wingate DL, Ong KK, Reik W, Constância M, et al. Raised late pregnancy glucose concentrations in mice carrying pups with targeted disruption of H19delta13. Diabetes. 2010;59:282–6.
8. Petry CJ, Seear RV, Wingate DL, Manico L, Acerini CL, Ong KK, et al. Associations between paternally transmitted fetal IGF2 variants and maternal circulating glucose concentrations in pregnancy. Diabetes. 2011; 60:3090–6.
9. Petry CJ, Mooslehner K, Prentice P, Hayes MG, Nodzenski M, Scholtens DM, Hughes IA, Acerini CL, Ong KK, Lowe WL Jr, Dunger DB. Associations between a fetal imprinted gene allele score and late pregnancy maternal glucose concentrations. Diabetes Metab. 2017;43:323–31.
10. Petry CJ, Sanz Marcos N, Pimentel G, Hayes MG, Nodzenski M, Scholtens DM, et al. Associations between fetal imprinted genes and maternal blood pressure in pregnancy. Hypertension. 2016;68:1459–66.
11. Simopoulos AP. Genetic variants in the metabolism of omega-6 and omega-3 fatty acids: their role in the determination of nutritional requirements and chronic disease risk. Exp Biol Med (Maywood). 2010;235:785–95.
12. Lattka E, Koletzko B, Zeilinger S, Hibbeln JR, Klopp N, Ring SM, et al. Umbilical cord PUFA are determined by maternal and child fatty acid desaturase (FADS) genetic variants in the Avon longitudinal study of parents and children (ALSPAC). Br J Nutr. 2013;109:1196–210.
13. Ghio A, Bertolotto A, Resi V, Volpe L, Di Cianni G. Triglyceride metabolism in pregnancy. Adv Clin Chem. 2011;55:133–53.
14. Schaefer-Graf UM, Graf K, Kulbacka I, Kjos SL, Dudenhausen J, Vetter K, et al. Maternal lipids as strong determinants of foetal environment and growth in pregnancies with gestational diabetes mellitus. Diabetes Care. 2008;31: 1858–63.
15. Vrijkotte TG, Krukziener N, Hutten BA, Vollebregt KC, van Eijsden M, Twickler MB. Maternal lipid profile during early pregnancy and pregnancy complications and outcomes: the ABCD study. J Clin Endocrinol Metab. 2012;97:3917–25.

16. Petry CJ, Seear RV, Wingate DL, Acerini CL, Ong KK, Hughes IA, et al. Maternally transmitted foetal H19 variants and associations with birth weight. Hum Genet. 2011;130:663–70.
17. Frost JM, Moore GE. The importance of imprinting in the human placenta. PLoS Genet. 2010;6:e1001015.
18. Barrett JC, Fry B, Maller J, Daly MJ. Haploview: analysis and visualization of LD and haplotype maps. Bioinformatics. 2005;21:263–5.
19. Rodríguez S, Gaunt TR, O'Dell SD, Chen XH, Gu D, Hawe E, et al. Haplotypic analyses of the IGF2-INS-TH gene cluster in relation to cardiovascular risk traits. Hum Mol Genet. 2004;13:715–25.
20. Koulman A, Prentice P, Wong MC, Matthews L, Bond NJ, Eiden M, et al. The development and validation of a fast and robust dried blood spot based lipid profiling method to study infant metabolism. Metabolomics. 2014;10: 1018–25.
21. Prentice P, Koulman A, Matthews L, Acerini CL, Ong KK, Dunger DB. Lipidomic analyses, breast- and formula-feeding, and growth in infants. J Pediatr. 2015;166:276–81.
22. Graessler J, Schwudke D, Schwarz PE, Herzog R, Shevchenko A, Bornstein SR. Top-down lipidomics reveals ether lipid deficiency in blood plasma of hypertensive patients. PLoS One. 2009;4:e6261.
23. Lu L, Koulman A, Petry CJ, Jenkins B, Matthews L, Hughes IA, et al. An unbiased lipidomics approach identifies early second trimester lipids predictive of maternal glycemic traits and gestational diabetes mellitus. Diabetes Care. 2016;39:2232–9.
24. Koulman A, Woffendin G, Narayana VK, Welchman H, Crone C, Volmer DA. High-resolution extracted ion chromatography, a new tool for metabolomics and lipidomics using a second-generation orbitrap mass spectrometer. Rapid Commun Mass Spectrom. 2009;23:1411–8.
25. Levy JC, Matthews DR, Hermans MP. Correct homeostasis model assessment (HOMA) evaluation uses the computer program. Diabetes Care. 1998;21: 2191–2.
26. Xia J, Sinelnikov IV, Han B, Wishart DS. MetaboAnalyst 3.0 - making metabolomics more meaningful. Nucleic Acids Res. 2015;43:W251–7.
27. Schulze R. Meta-analysis: a comparison of approaches. Cambridge, MA: Hogrefe & Huber Pub; 2004.
28. Rice F, Thapar A. Estimating the relative contributions of maternal genetic, paternal genetic and intrauterine factors to offspring birth weight and head circumference. Early Hum Dev. 2010;86:425–32.
29. Roberts LD, Murray AJ, Menassa D, Ashmore T, Nicholls AW, Griffin JL. The contrasting roles of PPARδ and PPARγ in regulating the metabolic switch between oxidation and storage of fats in white adipose tissue. Genome Biol. 2011;12:R75.
30. Rhee EP, Cheng S, Larson MG, Walford GA, Lewis GD, McCabe E, et al. Lipid profiling identifies a triacylglycerol signature of insulin resistance and improves diabetes prediction in humans. J Clin Invest. 2011;121:1402–11.
31. Lustig O, Ariel I, Ilan J, Lev-Lehman E, De-Groot N, Hochberg A. Expression of the imprinted gene H19 in the human fetus. Mol Reprod Dev. 1994;38: 239–46.
32. Sandovici I, Kassovska-Bratinova S, Vaughan JE, Stewart R, Leppert M, Sapienza C. Human imprinted chromosomal regions are historical hot-spots of recombination. PLoS Genet. 2006;2:e101.
33. Vu TH, Li T, Nguyen D, Nguyen BT, Yao XM, Hu JF, Hoffman AR. Symmetric and asymmetric DNA methylation in the human IGF2-H19 imprinted region. Genomics. 2000;64:132–43.
34. Smith AC, Choufani S, Ferreira JC, Weksberg R. Growth regulation, imprinted genes, and chromosome 11p15.5. Pediatr Res. 2007;61:43R–7R.
35. 1000 Genomes Project Consortium, Auton A, Brooks LD, Durbin RM, Garrison EP, Kang HM, et al. A global reference for human genetic variation. Nature. 2015;526:68–74.
36. Kong A, Steinthorsdottir V, Masson G, Thorleifsson G, Sulem P, Besenbacher S, et al. Parental origin of sequence variants associated with complex diseases. Nature. 2009;462:868–74.
37. Petry CJ. Genetic risk factors for gestational diabetes. In: Petry CJ, editor. Gestational diabetes: origins, complications and treatment. Boca Raton, Florida, U.S.A.: CRC Press; 2014. p. 69–94.

21

Escherichia coli recombinant sperm immobilizing factor RecX as a potential vaginal contraceptive

Monika Answal and Vijay Prabha*

Abstract

Background: To control the overpopulation and unintended pregnancies, vaginal contraceptives have gained recent surge of interest because of its topical application with possible avoidance of systemic effects. However non-specific cytotoxicity associated with detergent-based synthetic vaginal contraceptive agents limits their use and generates considerable interest in the development of vaginal contraceptives of biological origin for controlling reproduction and ultimately growing population. In this study, we have cloned, over-expressed an *Escherichia coli* gene encoding a sperm immobilizing factor (SIF) that inhibits sperm motility for the development of vaginal contraceptive from a biological source i.e. *E. coli*. The contraceptive efficacy of the *Escherichia coli* recombinant sperm immobilizing factor (r-SIF) was also determined.

Methods: Genomic DNA library of an *E. coli* strain isolated from semen sample of an infertile male was constructed for the identification and cloning of *E. coli* SIF coding gene. This gene was sub-cloned in pBADmycHisB for over-expression and the r-SIF was purified using Ni-NTA affinity chromatography. Effect of r-SIF on mouse sperm motility, viability and on morphology was evaluated. Binding of r-SIF to mouse sperm was demonstrated by fluorescent labeling. Contraceptive efficacy of r-SIF was checked in murine model.

Results: Genomic library resulted in five hundred transformants; five clones were found positive for sperm immobilizing activity. The protein product of the insert DNA sequence in one of the transformants showed maximum sperm immobilizing activity. Sequence analysis of ORFs in the insert revealed homology to *recX* on both nucleotide and protein level. 40 μg of the purified r-SIF showed immediate spermicidal activity in vitro for mouse sperm. Scanning electron micrograph of the r-SIF treated sperm showed intense morphological damage to sperm. FITC labeled r-SIF showed highest fluorescence at the head region of the sperm. 5 μg of purified r-SIF exhibited a complete contraceptive effect in mouse model.

Conclusion: r-SIF could be seen as potential target to be developed as potent and safe vaginal contraceptive in future.

Keywords: Vaginal contraceptives, Reproduction, Sperm, Cloning, Sperm immobilizing factor, Contraceptive agents, Spermicidal, Fertility control

* Correspondence: satishvijay11@yahoo.com
Department of Microbiology, Panjab University, Chandigarh 160014, India

Background

During the twentieth century alone, the population in the world has grown from 1.65 billion to 6 billion and is projected to touch 9.4 billion by 2050. Population explosion and a higher rate of unintended pregnancies are affecting the resources worldwide [1]. Contraception is an essential component of preventive measures that allows women to have planned pregnancies that ultimately lead optimal health, social and economic outcomes for women, families and society. However available contraceptive methods still have associated side effects, failure rate or irreversibility [2]. Oral contraceptive pills have highest contraceptive efficacy and reversibility, but these sex-steroid based pills are not without risks [3]. Intrauterine devices carry the possibility of expulsion and upper genital tract infections [4]. Contraceptive efficacy of condoms is compromised by their improper and inconsistent use [5]. Their use is coitus-related and depends on the co-operation of a male partner. Men being reluctant to use condoms and women being unable to negotiate with a partner; limits the use of this simple option of fertility control. Cultural biases and improper use or breakage during intercourse are some other compromising issues related to the efficacy of condoms [6]. Other approaches such as emergency contraception are not popular due to high cost and requirement of clinical supervision to certain extent [7]. Natural family planning is not sure and safe as many couples find them difficult to calculate safe period for the copulation, especially in women with irregular menstrual cycles. Reliance on surgical sterilization increases with age and can be used by women who are certain about their desired childbearing. The whole playscript reflects that only 5% of unwanted births are due to contraceptive failure and remaining 95% above burden is from women who do not use any contraception, experience gaps in the use of contraception, or use contraception incorrectly or inconsistently [8]. To turn this enormity corner, scientific predilections should be inclined on new targets that might be exploited for the development of safe, effective and inexpensive contraceptive agents.

Vaginal contraceptives being topical agents avoid systemic consequences and can address many of the issues and fit in women agreement hence may give them the power to safeguard themselves. However, available vaginal contraceptive formulations such as nonoxynol-9 (N-9), sodium dodecyl sulfate (SDS) and benzalkonium chloride exhibit detergent-type cytotoxic effect on cervicovaginal epithelium and normal vaginal flora. Their repeated use renders the user to discomfort, vaginal irritation and more susceptible to sexually transmitted diseases, including HIV [9, 10]. These limitations encourage researchers to develop vaginal contraceptives from biological sources, e.g., Immotilin [11], Magainin [12] and Nisin [13] are being examined as spermicidal agents. Microorganisms are also known to block sperm motility either by agglutination or by secreting extracellular substances. Reports are also available for microbial spermicidal factors [14–17]. Likewise, we observed, our laboratory *Escherichia coli* strain was producing a sperm motility inhibiting factor i.e. sperm immobilizing factor (SIF). Potential of SIF to inhibit sperm motility in vitro strengthened its utilization for the development of new vaginal contraceptive of biological origin. However, further progress with SIF in its crude form was not possible. Therefore, to obtain SIF in pure form it was necessary to characterize it at molecular level. In the present study the gene encoding for SIF was cloned, over expressed and pure recombinant factor was obtained. The r-SIF was evaluated both in vitro and in vivo for its spermicidal activity and contraceptive efficacy respectively.

Methods

Bacterial strains, plasmids, and enzymes

Sperm immobilizing factor producing *Escherichia coli* was previously isolated in our laboratory from semen sample of an infertile male, from the Department of Urology, PGIMER, Chandigarh [18]. *E. coli* DH5α and *E. coli* BL21 cells used as cloning host and expression host respectively, were cultured in Luria-Bertani (LB) broth (Himedia Labs, India) containing ampicillin (100 μg/ml). Plasmid pSMART-LCAmp (Lucigen, USA) was used for the preparation of genomic library and pBADmycHisB (Invitrogen, India) used for expression of SIF. Restriction enzymes and T4 ligase were purchased from Thermo Scientific, India. Ni-NTA resin was purchased from Qiagen (India). The primers used were synthesized from Eurofins genomics, India (Table 1).

Animals

Sexually mature, 5–6 weeks old male (26 ± 2 g) and 4–5 weeks old female (23 ± 2 g) Balb/c mice (Mus musculus) were used in the present study. The animals were housed in polypropylene cages and kept in the animal house of the Department of Microbiology, Panjab University Chandigarh. The animals were maintained in laboratory conditions (12:12, dark: light cycle), fed with standard pellet diet (Hindustan Lever products, India) and water ad libitum. All the experimental protocols were approved by Institutional Animal Ethics

Table 1 Primers used in the study

Primer	5′-3′ sequence	Restriction site
recX F	5′-GTTGTAAGGATATGCCATGGCAGAATC-3′	NcoI
recX R	5′-GTATGCGGTCGACCGGCAAAATTTC-3′	SalI
SL1	5′-CAGTCCAGTTACGCTGGAGTC-3′	–
SR2	5′-GGTCAGGTATGATTTAAATGGTCAGT-3′	–

Committee of the Panjab University, Chandigarh, India, vide letter number PU/IAEC/S/15/71 dated 15.09.2015 and were performed in accordance with the guidelines of the Committee for the Purpose of Control and Supervision of Experiments on Animals, India.

Construction of genomic library

Genomic DNA of *Escherichia coli* producing sperm immobilizing factor (Qiagen DNA extraction kit) was partially digested with HaeIII and the DNA fragments were separated by gel electrophoresis to obtain 2–6 kb DNA fragments which were purified from agarose gel (Qiagen gel purification kit). Genomic DNA fragments were cloned at the blunt ends of pSMART-LCAmp plasmid and transformed into *E. coli* DH5α cells using heat shock technique [19]. The transformants were obtained on LB agar containing 100 μg/ml of ampicillin and transferred to fresh LB-ampicillin plates.

Screening of genomic library

Transformants were screened for sperm immobilizing activity. In brief, each of the transformants was grown separately in 50 ml LB broth supplemented with ampicillin and incubated at 37 °C/200 rpm for 14–16 h. Cell pellet obtained after centrifugation at 10,000 rpm for 10 min was re-suspended in 10 ml of phosphate buffer saline (PBS) pH 7.4 and sonicated (30% amplitude, 10 s on, 20 s off; total time 2 min). Cell debris was removed after centrifugation at 10,000 rpm for one hr. The motile population of sperm was obtained from vas deferens of mouse excised after the autopsy. Sperm were collected in physiological saline and motile sperm count was adjusted to a concentration of 40×10^6/ ml. The cell lysate was mixed with mouse sperm in equal proportions and incubated for different time intervals, i.e., 5 min, 15 min, 30 min and 1 h and analyzed under a light microscope at 400X (Olympus India Pvt. Ltd) for sperm immobilizing activity. Cell lysate obtained from the culture of *E. coli* DH5α containing pSMART-LCAmp was also checked for sperm immobilizing activity. Plasmid from transformants that displayed maximum sperm immobilizing activity was isolated (QIAprep Spin Miniprep Kit) and DNA sequencing was performed for the determination of the insert sequence (Chromous Biotech India Ltd.).

Sequencing of insert DNA fragment and bioinformatics analyses

Insert DNA fragment was analyzed for the presence of ORFs in all reading frames using 'ORF Finder' program (https://www.ncbi.nlm.nih.gov/orffinder/). Database homology searches of nucleotide and deduced amino acid sequences obtained were carried out using BlastX and BlastP (https://blast.ncbi.nlm.nih.gov/Blast.cgi) on the NCBI website. The primers to amplify the target gene were designed using 'Gene runner' software.

Construction of an over-expression system

To over-express SIF encoding gene, the identified ORF region was amplified by PCR using primers RecX F1 (5′-GTTGTAAGGATATG**CCATGG**CAGAATC-3′) and RecX R1 (5′-GTATGCG**GTCGAC**CGGCAAAATTTC-3′) containing NcoI and SalI sites, respectively. For amplification, the PCR conditions were as follows: a hot start at 95 ° C for 5 min, 30 cycles of 95 °C for 1 min, 56 °C for 1 min and 72 °C for 45 s, followed by one cycle of 72 °C for 10 min. The amplified PCR product was purified and digested by the restriction enzymes mentioned above and cloned into pBADmycHisB between NcoI and SalI sites. Cloning at SalI site ensured the presence of 6X histidine residues at C-terminal of the expressed protein. The cloned gene was transformed and expressed in *E. coli* BL21.

Production and purification of recombinant *E. coli* sperm immobilizing factor (r-SIF)

E. coli BL21 transformant cells were cultured in 500 ml LB broth at 37 °C/200 rpm till absorbance at 600 nm (OD_{600}) reached 0.5–0.6. The production of sperm immobilizing factor was induced by addition of 0.4% of L-arabinose (Sigma Aldrich, India) and subsequent growth for 4 h. Cells were harvested by centrifugation (7000 rpm, 20 min), re-suspended in lysis buffer [50 mM phosphate buffer, 0.3 M NaCl, 1 mM PMSF, 2 mM β-mercaptoethanol (pH 7.4)] and sonicated. Soluble proteins were separated from cell debris by centrifugation at 10,000 rpm for 1 h. Clarified cell supernatant was applied to 2 ml of Ni-NTA affinity column (Qiagen), preequilibrated with 15 ml of equilibration buffer (50 mM phosphate buffer, 0.3 M NaCl), followed by the column washing with 25 ml of Buffer A [50 mM phosphate buffer, 0.3 M NaCl, 10 mM imidazole (pH 7.4)] to remove loosely bound proteins. Recombinant protein containing histidine-tag was eluted from the column with Buffer A containing different concentration of imidazole (10–100 mM). Fractions containing tagged protein identified by SDS-PAGE were pooled and dialyzed overnight against sodium phosphate buffer (pH 7.4) at 4 °C and subsequently concentrated using Amicon concentrator (< 10 kDa) (Millipore). The protein concentration was measured by BCA protein estimation assay kit (Thermo Scientific, India) according to manufacturer's recommendations. Molecular weight and purity of r-SIF were determined using 15% SDS-polyacrylamide gel with MiniProtean III system (Bio-Rad, India). The gel was stained with Coomassie Brilliant Blue R-250 and molecular weight was estimated with reference to the broad range molecular weight protein marker (Thermo Scientific, India).

In vitro effect of r-SIF on mouse sperm parameters

(a) Sperm motility: Mouse sperm were mixed with different concentration of r-SIF (10–100 μg), after 20 s a drop of the mixture was observed on a microscopic slide under a light microscope at 400X. A control containing PBS mixed with mouse sperm was set up simultaneously. Complete immobilization of motile sperm within 20 s was recorded as a positive result and the corresponding highest dilution was taken as the minimum effective concentration (MEC).

(b) Viability: Mouse sperm viability was checked with Eosin staining method. Mouse sperm were mixed with PBS and MEC of r-SIF which served as negative and positive controls, respectively. After 20 s two drops of 1% Eosin were added to each and mixed well. A smear prepared from the mixture on a clean glass slide was observed under light microscopy at 400X to ascertain pink stained headed dead sperm from unstained headed live sperm.

(c) Sperm morphology: Scanning electron microscopy (SEM) was done to study the effect of r-SIF on the morphology of mouse sperm using Jeol scanning microscope (JSM-6100, SM Jeol 20 kV, Japan) by standard method [20] with slight modifications. Briefly, mouse sperm suspension was centrifuged at 500 rpm for 10 min, mixed with PBS as control and MEC of purified r-SIF as test; both incubated at 37 °C for 1 h. To each tube, 4 ml of 2.5% phosphate-buffered glutaraldehyde was added and mixed gently. After 30 min, samples were centrifuged for 5 min at 500 rpm and washed twice with PBS. One drop of fixed and washed sperm was placed on a silver painted adhesive tape mounted on brass stubs and air dried. 100 Å gold coating was done on Jeol fine coat ion sputter (Jeol, Japan) and the specimens were observed at different magnifications under the scanning electron microscope at sophisticated analytical instrumentation facility, Panjab University, Chandigarh, India.

Binding of FITC labeled r-SIF to mouse sperm

r-SIF was conjugated with Fluorescein isothiocyanate (FITC) using FITC protein labeling kit (Bangalore Genei, India) according to manufacturer's instructions. Mouse sperm washed twice with PBS, resuspended in 500 μL of PBS and were incubated with FITC labeled r-SIF. After incubation at 37 °C for 40 min, the sperm were fixed with 3% formaldehyde, washed twice with PBS and observed under fluorescent microscope (Nikon, Japan) at 400X. Sperm incubated with unconjugated FITC dye; unlabeled r-SIF with sperm and sperm suspended in PBS were set as negative control.

Contraceptive efficacy of r-SIF in mice

Animals were divided into two groups i.e. control and test; six female and three male animals were used for each group. Control mice received 20 μL of PBS whereas different concentration of r-SIF (2.5, 5, 10, 25, 40 and 50 μg; 20 μL of each) was administered in the vagina of test groups. The mice were held in a supine position during the application. All females were immediately mated with proven breeder males in the ratio of 2:1. Mating was confirmed by the presence of a vaginal plug and females were kept under observation for pregnancy outcome. The contraceptive effect of r-SIF was determined based on prevention of pregnancy in test group as compared to controls and the consistency of this response.

Results

Construction and screening of genomic library

The genomic library containing 2–6 kb partially digested *E. coli* genomic DNA fragments resulted in five hundred transformants. Screening for SIF positive clones resulted in five positive transformants which exhibited sperm immobilizing activity while *E. coli* DH5α harboring plasmid pSMART did not show sperm immobilizing activity. Recombinant plasmids were recovered from transformed *E. coli* DH5α cells and confirmed for the presence of insert by the digestion (Fig. 1). Plasmid from one transformant

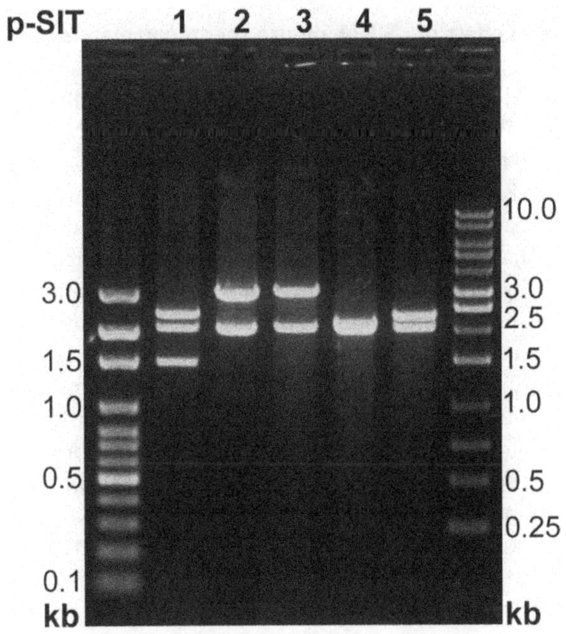

Fig. 1 EcoRI-digested pSMART-LCAmp plasmids isolated from transformants carrying *E.coli* DNA fragments (p-SIT) and expressed sperm immobilizing activity. Lanes 1, 2, 3, 4 and 5 correspond to digested plasmid from different transformants, the size of the DNA fragments generated by the digestion correspond to the DNA size ladder.

designated as sperm immobilizing transformant (SIT-5), showing maximum sperm immobilizing activity in minimum time (5 min) was sequenced.

Nucleotide sequence analysis of gene encoding the SIF

Recombinant pSMART from transformant SIT-5 subjected to DNA sequencing showed an insert DNA fragment of ~ 2.2 kb. The gene sequence has been submitted to GenBank under accession number MG269998. One ORF of 501 nucleotides was found which showed 100% identity with the regulatory protein RecX of *Enterobacteriaceae* (Fig. 2). The deduced amino acid sequence is 99% identical to RecX protein. The putative RecX consists of 167 amino acids with a theoretical molecular weight of 19.4 kDa. Conclusively, based on NCBI conserved domain database and amino acid sequence similarity, the identified gene belonged to the RecX superfamily [21].

Expression and purification of recombinant sperm immobilizing factor(r-SIF)

E. coli BL21 cells harboring recombinant plasmid with His-tagged RecX were induced with 0.4% of L-arabinose for protein expression. The recombinant protein was purified by Ni-NTA chromatography and a single protein band between 15 kDa and 25 kDa on comparison to broad range protein marker was obtained in fractions eluted with buffer containing 40–50 mM imidazole (Fig. 3).

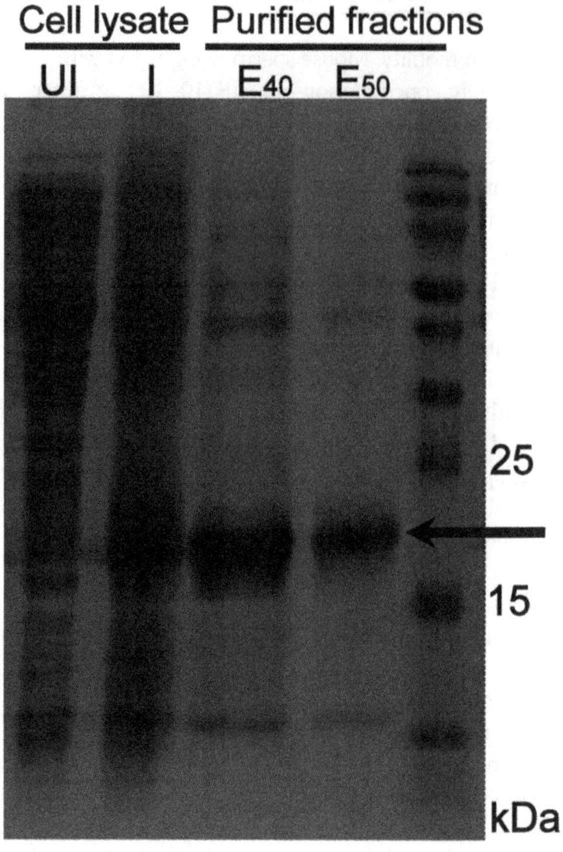

Fig. 3 SDS-PAGE analysis of purified RecX: Lane 'UI', lysate of un-induced cells from *E. coli* BL21; lane 'I', cell lysate of induced cells from *E. coli* BL21; lane 'E_{40}', fractions containing expressed RecX obtained at 40 mM; lane 'E_{50}', fractions containing expressed RecX obtained at 50 mM of imidazole.

In vitro effect of r-SIF on mouse sperm parameters

(a) Motility & viability: Complete sperm motility inhibition was observed immediately (within 20 s) with a minimum concentration of 40 μg of r-SIF (Fig. 4). At this concentration, r-SIF not only caused immobilization of spermatozoa but also had a spermicidal effect which was investigated by eosin staining. Pink stained head of dead sperm were distinguished from the unstained head of live spermatozoa (Fig. 5a and b).

(b) Sperm morphology: The scanning electron micrographs of mouse sperm treated with PBS showed normal morphology, sperm membrane remained smooth and intact all over the whole sperm viz. head, midpiece, and tail (Fig. 6a). In contrast, r-SIF treated mouse sperm resulted in

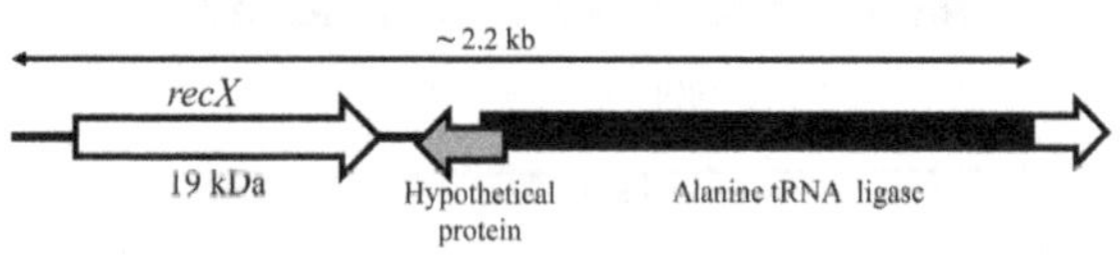

Fig. 2 Organization of genes in insert DNA fragment cloned in pSMART-LCAmp.

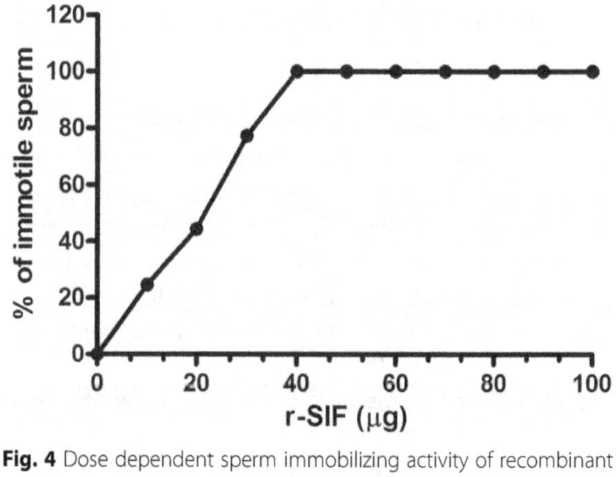

Fig. 4 Dose dependent sperm immobilizing activity of recombinant sperm immobilizing factor (r-SIF).

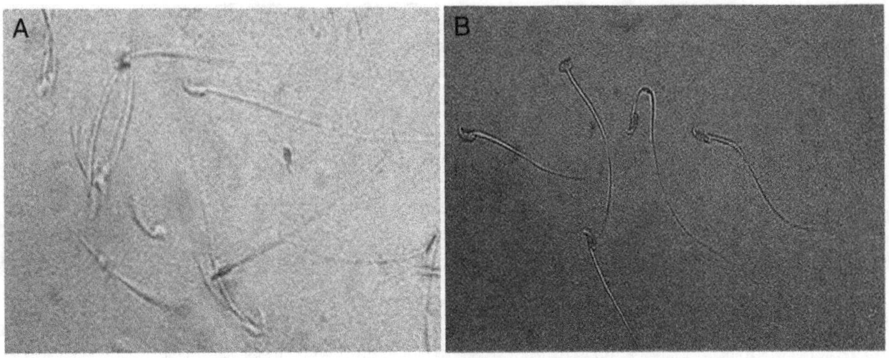

Fig. 5 Eosin staining of mouse spermatozoa after 20 s of incubation with (**a**) PBS, unstained head (live) spermatozoa. (**b** Recombinant sperm immobilizing factor, pink stained head (dead) spermatozoa. Magnification for both **a** and **b**: 400X.

prominent morphological defects, disruption of the head surface membrane (Fig. 6b) and detachment of head region from midpiece (Fig. 6c).

Binding of FITC labeled r-SIF to mouse sperm

Binding of r-SIF to mouse sperm was evaluated by fluorescence microscopy. Incubation of sperm with FITC-r-SIF resulted in staining of the whole sperm viz. head, neck, midpiece, and tail. Head and neck region showed more fluorescence as compared to whole sperm pointing major binding of FITC at these regions (Fig. 7b). In control samples, mouse spermatozoa incubated with FITC dye did not give any fluorescence from head and neck region of mouse spermatozoa as compared to spermatozoa incubated with FITC labeled r-SIF (Fig. 7a). In unlabeled r-SIF mixed with sperm and sperm in PBS there was no fluorescence (Fig. 7c and d).

Contraceptive effect of r-SIF

Pregnancy-related changes, i.e., abdominal distension, protrusion of mammary glands, a string of pearls were observed by 12–14 days of gestation period in control group and group received 2.5 μg of r-SIF (Fig. 8a, b, c) whereas these changes were absent in groups treated with ≥5 μg of r-SIF. On the parturition after 21 days, 6–8 pups were delivered by pregnant animals (Fig. 8d), but animals received r-SIF(dose ≥5 μg) did not delivered pups. Hence, a minimum concentration of 5 μg of r-SIF resulted in the complete inhibition of conception. The effect of different doses of r-SIF on fertility outcome is presented in Table 2.

Discussion

The present-day scenario of increasing population and number of unintended pregnancies looks alarming. Over the years considerable efforts and resources are being spent in controlling the population by available contraceptive methods. Although some progress has been made using these in bringing down the birth rate in urban areas but it has not made much impact on the decrease in overall population. However problems associated with these methods limit their use. Vaginal contraceptives; the topical agents emerge as a replacement to current chemical and physical method of fertility control. However, their mode of action lacks in any cellular specificity and repeated use render the user to discomfort, vaginal irritation and more susceptible to STDs. Several European nations have banned the use of N-9 related compounds due to health risks and potential environmental toxicity [22]. Due to these problems, various products of biological origin which may be either from plant source like CONSAP,

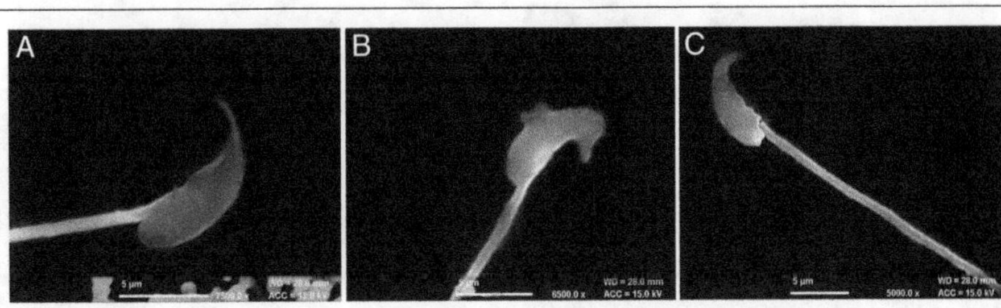

Fig. 6 Scanning electron micrograph of mouse sperm upon (**a**) treatment with PBS showed normal morphology at 7500X magnification; (**b**) treatment with recombinant sperm immobilizing factor indicated morphological changes in sperm head membrane at 6500X, and (**c**) detachment of sperm head from mid piece after treatment at 5000X.

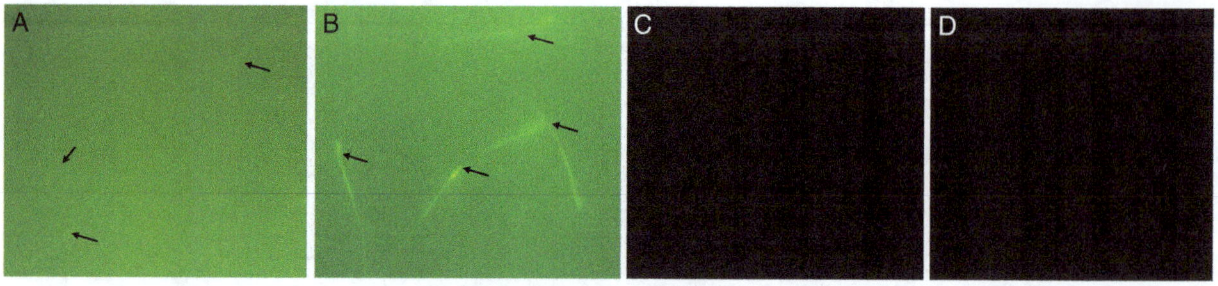

Fig. 7 Binding of Fluorescein isothiocyanate labeled recombinant sperm immobilizing factor to mouse sperm. (**a**) Mouse sperm with FITC dye alone showed no florescence from head and neck region of sperm (**b**) Fluorescence was observed on whole sperm. Intensity of fluorescence was more in head and neck regions. Magnification: 400X. (**c**) & (**d**) Mouse sperm incubated with un-labelled r-SIF and sperm suspended in PBS did not show any fluorescence.

NIM-76 or of the microbial source, e.g., Nisin are being developed as vaginal contraceptives.

With an aim to develop safe and effective vaginal contraceptives which not only instantly arrest sperm movement but also overcome the genital epithelial toxicity of available vaginal contraceptives, the present study assessed a recombinant sperm immobilizing factor, produced by *Escherichia coli* for its sperm immobilizing property and contraceptive efficacy in a series of in vitro and in vivo experiments respectively in murine model.

To the best of our knowledge and extensive literature survey, there are no reports about SIF encoding genes. Hence, lack of gene sequence hampered the production of SIF in pure form. In this respect, our approach was to identify SIF encoding gene by the construction of genomic library from *E. coli* genome. Out of approximately five hundred *E. coli* transformants obtained, five transformants expressed the sperm immobilizing activity. SIT-5 showed maximum sperm immobilizing activity indicated by exhibiting its effect on sperm motility in the least time, i.e., 5 min. The nucleotide sequence of the SIT-5 insert showed the presence of a complete ORF, which displayed 100% homology with regulatory protein RecX of *Enterobacteriaceae*, as well as two incomplete ORFs lacking stop codon (Fig.2). The amino acid sequence of the protein product of ORF1 exhibited high sequence identity (99%) with recombination regulator RecX *Escherichia coli*. Further, *recX was* over-expressed in a heterologous host which is a good substitute to overcome the problem of low protein production [23]· *recX* with 6X-his-tag was sub-cloned in pBADmycHisB plasmid downstream of arabinose promoter and transformed in *E. coli* BL21 cells. The optimal expression of tagged RecX was observed with L-arabinose which was purified by Ni-NTA affinity chromatography. The purified factor was homogeneous on SDS-PAGE and its molecular weight was estimated 19 kDa which is close to the expected value of the monomeric form.

In vitro r-SIF showed complete mouse sperm immobilizing activity (within 20 s) at a concentration of 40 μg. In our work, sperm immobilizing activity of *recX* can be related to the antagonistic effect of RecX on RecA

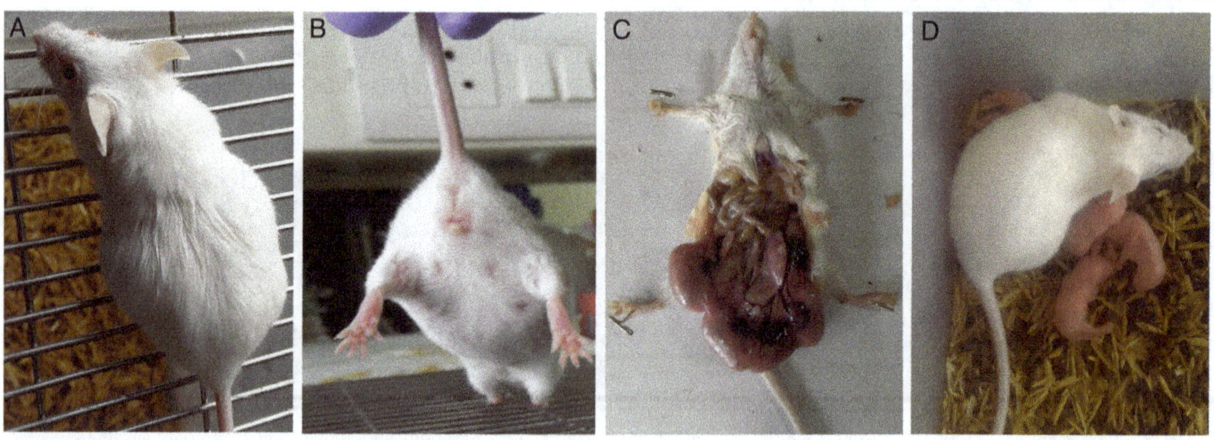

Fig. 8 Representative photomicrograph of pregnancy related changes in pregnant mice (**a**) abdominal distension (**b**) protrusion of mammary glands (**c**) string of pearls on day 14 (**d**) pups delivered after 21 days of gestation.

Table 2 Effect of r-SIF on fertility outcome in female mice

Dose instilled (20 μl each)	Number of female mice (per group)	Fertility outcome
Placebo (PBS)	6	6/6 (100%)
2.5 μg of r-SIF	6	6/6 (100%)
5 μg of r-SIF	6	0/6 (0%)
10 μg of r-SIF	6	0/6 (0%)
25 μg of r-SIF	6	0/6 (0%)
40 μg of r-SIF	6	0/6 (0%)
50 μg of r-SIF	6	0/6 (0%)

activity. *recX* is found just downstream of *recA* gene and act as a repressor of *recA* mediated DNA-dependent ATP hydrolysis, DNA recombinase and co-protease function both in vitro and in vivo in *Escherichia coli* [24]. *recA* reported in *E. coli* has a homolog *rad51* which shares structural similarities and exhibits same comparable molecular functions including DNA dependent ATP-hydrolysis and ATP-dependent recombinase [25–27]. Literature supported that *rad51* has been identified in various higher eukaryotes, including human, mouse, hamster and other higher eukaryotes [28]. For sperm immobilizing activity we hypothesize that as RecX suppresses RecA mediated ATP hydrolysis, most likely it may also inhibit the ATP hydrolysis activity of Rad51. It has been reported that flagellar/sperm movement is driven by dynein motor proteins, which use the energy of ATP hydrolysis to slide the microtubules [29] and absence of ATP hydrolysis inhibits sperm motility. So, the sperm motility inhibition by RecX may be a result of suppression of ATP hydrolysis.

Further experimentation showed that r-SIF exerts spermicidal action confirmed by eosin staining. Pink-headed mouse sperm in test sample confirmed their death as compared to unstained headed live mouse sperm in control. Viability test indicated the rapid sperm damage by r-SIF, which was further validated by scanning electron microscopy. Plasma membrane (PM) plays a vital role in the process of sperm migration and fertilization therefore several spermicidal agents act via structural and functional modulation of the PM, like, disruption of the membrane was observed after exposure of sperm to spermicide [30]. This statement supports the similar obseravtion of our study wherein profound disruption in head membrane and detachment of head were observed during scanning electron microscopy of r-SIF treated sperm. These changes are may be due to loosening of PM, stretching and breakdown of the head membrane. SEM results illustrate that r-SIF exerts spermicidal action by damaging membrane integrity of sperm. Since sperm motility and viability are most essential features for successful fertilization, the spermicidal action of r-SIF makes it a highly desirable candidate for vaginal contraceptive for the future.

Above findings were also suggestive of some interaction between mouse sperm and r-SIF, which were further assessed by fluorescent microscopy. Although fluorescence was observed over the entire surface of the FITC labeled r-SIF sperm, but the intensity of fluorescence was more at head and neck regions indicating the presence of receptors on mouse sperm for r-SIF that might play a role in their interaction. In one of the negative control; sperm and FITC dye, head and neck region of sperm did not show any fluorescence. There was no fluorescence observed with the other two negative controls i.e. sperm incubated with unlabeled r-SIF and sperm suspended in PBS. This indicated that r-SIF specifically binds to mouse spermatozoa at head and neck region.

The contraceptive agents that impair sperm motility in vitro are not necessarily effective in vivo [31]. Therefore, in vivo spermicidal efficacy of r-SIF was assessed using murine model. Fertility outcome experiments showed that animals from groups treated with dose ≥5 μg of r-SIF did not conceive whereas control group animals and group received dose of 2.5 μg delivered the pups. Our studies suggest, r-SIF effectively blocks sperm motility and prevents the establishment of pregnancy in mice. These results are in agreement with studies done by Reddy *et al.* where they reported contraceptive potential of a microbial compound Nisin [13] and with earlier studies of our laboratory which demonstrated the contraceptive potential of a microbial factor [32].

Conclusion

Our study concludes that RecX is an efficient spermicidal agent which effectively prevents pregnancy in mice and could be developed as a potential vaginal contraceptive for future use in women. Further studies in this direction are under way to evaluate the safety of r-SIF in mouse model.

Abbreviations

FITC: Fluorescein isothiocyanate; MEC: Minimum effective concentration; r-SIF: Recombinant sperm immobilizing factor; SEM: Scanning electron microscopy; SIF: Sperm immobilizing factor; SIT: Sperm immobilizing transformant

Acknowledgments

We would like to thank Dr. Ravinder Kumar, Institute of Microbial Technology Chandigarh for his guidance during cloning and overexpression experiments.

Funding

The authors acknowledge funding from Indian council of Research, New Delhi vide letter No. 3/1/3/JRF-2012/HRD dated 31.08.2012.

Authors' contributions

VP conceived the idea of study. MA performed all experiments and wrote the main manuscript text. Both authors analyzed and interpreted the experimental results. Both authors read and approved the final manuscript.

Competing interests

The authors declare that they have no competing interests.

References

1. Naz RK. Can curcumin provide an ideal contraceptive. Mol Reprod Dev. 2011;78:116–23.
2. Singh KK, Parmar S, Tatke PA. Contraceptive efficacy and safety of HerbOshieldTM vaginal gel in rats. Contraception. 2012;85:122–7.
3. Spevack E. The long-term health implications of depo-provera. Int Med. 2013;12:27–34.
4. Naz RK. Contraceptive vaccines. Drugs. 2005;65:593–603.
5. Macaluso M, Blackwell R, Jamieson DJ, et al. Efficacy of the male latex condom and of the female polyurethane condom as barriers to semen during intercourse: a randomized clinical trial. Am J Epidemiol. 2007;166:88–96.
6. Shoupe D, Mishell DR. In: Goldman MB, Troisi R, Rexrode KM, editors. Contraception. Women and health. 2nd ed. London: Academic Press; 2013.
7. LaValleur J. Emergency contraception. Obstet Gynecol Clin N Am. 2000;27: 817–39.
8. Sitruk-Ware R, Nath A, Mishell DR. Contraception technology: past, present and future. Contraception. 2013;87:319–30.
9. Fichorova RN, Tuker LD, Anderson DJ. The molecular basis of nonoxynol-9-induced vaginal inflammation and its possible relevance to human immunodeficiency virus type 1 transmission. J Infect Dis. 2001;84:418–28.
10. Van Damme L, Ramjee LG, Alary M, et al. Effectiveness of COL-1492, a nonoxynol-9 vaginal gel, on HIV-1 transmission in female sex workers: a randomised controlled trial. Lancet. 2002;360:971–7.
11. Mukherjee M, Datta M, Biswas S, et al. Immotilin, a novel sperm immobilizing protein. Fertil Steril. 2003;79:673–5.
12. Reddy KVR, Manjramkar DD. Evaluation of antifertility effect of magainin-a in rabbits: in vitro and in vivo studies. Fertil Steril. 2000;73:353–8.
13. Reddy KVR, Aranha C, Gupta SM, Yedery RD. Evaluation of antimicrobial peptide Nisin as a safe vaginal contraceptive agent in rats: in vitro and in vivo studies. Reproduction. 2004;128:117–26.
14. Tian YH, Xiong JW, Hu L, Huang DH, Xiong CL. *Candida albicans* and filtrates interfere with human spermatozoal motility and alter the ultrastructure of spermatozoa: an in vitro study. Int J Androl. 2007;30:421–9.
15. Schulz M, Sanchez R, Soto L, Risopatron J, Villegas J. Effect of *Escherichia coli* and its soluble factors on mitochondrial membrane potential, phosphatidylserine translocation, viability, and motility of human spermatozoa. Fertil Steril. 2010;94:619–23.
16. Barbonetti A, Vassallo MRC, Cinque B, et al. Soluble products of *Escherichia coli* induce mitochondrial dysfunction-related sperm membrane lipid peroxidation which is prevented by lactobacilli. PLoS One. 2013;8:e83136.
17. Cano-Chaves A, Galarzo-Pardo S, Puerta-Suarez J, Giraldo M, Cadavid P, Cardona-Maya WD. Effect of uropathogenic bacteria and soluble factors of their metabolism on sperm quality: *Escherichia coli* and *Enterococcus faecalis*. Clin Res Gynecol Obstet. 2017;44:106–12.
18. Prabha V, Sandhu R, Kaur S, et al. Mechanism of sperm immobilization by *Escherichia coli*. Adv Urol. 2010;2010:240268.
19. Sambrook J, Russell DW. Molecular cloning: a laboratory manual. 3rd ed. New York: Cold Spring Harbor Laboratory Press; 2001.
20. Hafez ESE, Kanagawa H. Scanning electron microscopy of human, monkey and rabbit spermatozoa. Fertil Steril. 1973;24:776–8.
21. Marchler-Bauer A, Derbyshire MK, Gonzales NR, et al. CDD/SPARCLE: functional classification of proteins via subfamily domain architectures. Nucleic Acids Res. 2017;45:200–3.
22. Renner R. European bans on surfactant trigger transatlantic debate. Environ Sci Technol. 1997;31:316–20.
23. Zou G, Shi S, Jiang Y, et al. Construction of a cellulase hyper-expression system in *Trichoderma reesei* by promoter and enzyme engineering. Microb Cell Factories. 2012;11:21.
24. Stohl EA, Brockman JP, Burkle KL, Morimatsu K, Kowalczykowski SC, Seifert HS. *Escherichia coli* RecX inhibits RecA recombinase and coprotease activities in vitro and in vivo. J Biol Chem. 2003;278:2278–85.
25. Story RM, Weber I, Steitz TA. The structure of the *E. coli* recA protein monomer and polymer. Nature. 1992;355:318–25.
26. Conway AB, Lynch TW, Zhang Y, et al. Crystal structure of a Rad51 filament. Nat Struct Mol Biol. 2004;11:791–6.
27. Chen Z, Yang H, Pavletich NP. Mechanism of homologous recombination from the RecA-ssDNA/dsDNA structures. Nature. 2007;453:489–94.
28. Arnaudeau C, Helleday T, Jenssen D. The RAD51 protein supports homologous recombination by an exchange mechanism in mammalian cell. J Mol Biol. 1999;289:1231–8.
29. Pereira R, Rosália SA, Barros A, Sousa M. Major regulatory mechanisms involved in sperm motility. Asian J Androl. 2017;19:5–14.
30. Debanjana C, Arindam M, Tarun J, Nirup BM. Spermicidal and contraceptive potential of desgalactotigonin: a prospective alternative of nonoxynol-9. PLoS One. 2014;9:1–9.
31. UDCP Update. US HIV and AIDS cases reported through December 1996. HIV/AIDS Surveill Rep. 1997;8:1–33.
32. Aggarwal J, Prabha V. Contraceptive effect of sperm-agglutinating factor isolated from *Staphylococcus aureus* in mouse. BJOG. 2006;113:1039–43.

22

Structure of preantral follicles, oxidative status and developmental competence of in vitro matured oocytes after ovary storage at 4 °C in the domestic cat model

Anna Rita Piras, Giovanni Pietro Burrai, Federica Ariu, Laura Falchi, Maria Teresa Zedda, Salvatore Pau, Sergio Domenico Gadau, Elisabetta Antuofermo, Daniela Bebbere, Sergio Ledda and Luisa Bogliolo*

Abstract

Background: Storage conditions during transportation of explanted ovaries are a critical step in setting up fertility preservation protocols in both animal and human fields. Here, we evaluated the effects of ovary storage at 4 °C on the preservation of preantral follicles and oocytes retrieved from antral follicles using the domestic cat as model.

Methods: Ovaries were harvested from fifty-five healthy domestic queens during ovariectomy and stored at 4 °C for 0 (control), 24, 48, 72 and 96 h. In Experiment 1, the effects of the storage period at 4 °C on the morphology, cytoskeleton (α/β tubulin) and DNA integrity (phosphorylation of histone H2AX) of preantral follicles were investigated. In Experiment 2, oocytes recovered from antral follicles were matured and fertilized in vitro to evaluate their meiotic and developmental competence. Reactive oxygen species (ROS), glutathione (GSH) and lipid peroxidation were measured in matured oocytes.

Results: The results showed that: a) storage up to 24 h did not affect the morphology and the DNA integrity of preantral follicles; b) extended storage times caused progressive morphological abnormalities, disassembling of microtubules and DNA damage; c) storage up to 48 h did not influence in vitro meiotic maturation of oocytes nor cleavage after in vitro fertilization. However, only oocytes stored within the ovary for 24 h produced blastocysts in a percentage similar to control oocytes; d) GSH levels of in vitro matured oocytes did not change at any time during ovary storage; a progressive increase in ROS levels was detected from 48 h associated with elevated lipid peroxidation at 72 and 96 h of storage.

Conclusions: Storage of cat ovaries for up to 24 h caused minimal alteration of preantral follicles and oocytes. The extension of the storage period beyond 24 h progressively impaired the structure of follicles, and modified the oxidative status of in vitro matured oocytes and their developmental competence after in vitro fertilization. This information may help when setting up programs for fertility conservation, especially for wild feline species which die in geographic areas located far away from ARTs centers.

* Correspondence: luis@uniss.it
Department of Veterinary Medicine, University of Sassari, Via Vienna 2, 07100 Sassari, Italy

Background

Most of the 36 living species of wild cats are formally listed as threatened by extinction mainly due to poaching, habitat destruction and infectious diseases [1]. Assisted Reproductive Technologies (ARTs) contribute to the preservation of endangered feline species. In domestic felids considerable progress has been made in the development of modern methodologies of ARTs including in vitro embryo production and banking of genetic resources. Some of these techniques have been included in programs for the conservation of feline wildlife species [2, 3].

The possibility of rescuing germplasm from feline females after sudden death in their natural habitat or zoos or after medical ovariohysterectomy may at times require the shipment of ovaries for long distances, from the retrieval site to the ART centres. Therefore, storage conditions (temperature, duration, medium) during transportation of explanted ovaries are a critical step in setting up of fertility preservation protocols.

In this context, studies conducted to establish the appropriate transportation temperature for ovaries provided evidence that feline oocytes, in contrast to other species, have a unique tolerance to cold storage at 4 °C [4–6]. A pivotal study by Johnston et al. [7] found that oocytes from rare wild species could be matured and fertilized in vitro following ovary storage for as long as 36 h in cold (4 °C) phosphate buffer saline (PBS). Histological evaluation of cold stored ovaries of domestic cats further supported the concept that immature oocytes have some degree of cold tolerance [8]. Other studies reported unaffected in vitro maturation (IVM) rates when domestic cat ovaries were stored at 4 °C up to 72 h. However, only oocytes stored within the ovary for 24 h could produce blastocysts after in vitro fertilization [9] and retained competence to develop into live offspring after transfer into recipients [10]. More recently, findings by Luu et al. [11] indicated that the addition of relaxin to the IVM medium improved the rate of blastocyst development of cat oocytes from ovaries stored for 24 h at 4 °C. Furthermore, superoxide dismutase (SOD) supplementation to ovary transportation medium enhanced in vitro embryo production from oocytes of domestic cat ovaries preserved at 4 °C for up to 72 h [12].

Most studies on the cold storage of feline ovaries have focused on the preservation of oocytes from antral follicles. This is a limitation as an ovary contains a large amount of preantral follicles, which represents the female's ovarian reserve and includes more than 90% of the follicular population [13]. Therefore, the pool of preantral follicles constitutes a potentially rich source of genetic material which could be used in fertility preservation programs for genetically valuable animals, including females of endangered species that die before reaching sexual maturity [14]. In fact, the ovarian cortex can be cryopreserved and utilized for xenotrasplantation or, alternatively, preantral follicles can be isolated and cultured in vitro until maturity. Slow freezing of cat ovarian cortex in conjunction with xenotransplantation was first reported by Bosch et al. [15]. Moreover, mature oocytes have been obtained after long-term transplantation of ovarian cortex from female lions into immunodeficient mice [16]. In several animal species, including cats, attempts have been made to develop in vitro culture systems for the growth of preantral follicles with variable results [17–20]. Full term culture of primordial follicles to a mature stage and birth of viable offspring after in vitro fertilization and embryo transfer have only been achieved in mice and were first described by Eppig and O'Brien [21].

Nowadays, to the best of our knowledge, there is little information about the impact of cold storage on the health status of preantral follicles of feline ovaries and on the maximal tolerable storage duration [22]. Evidence from other animal models indicates that cold temperature favors the preservation of preantral follicles [23–27].

The storage of ovarian tissue during transportation has great importance not only for rare and endangered species, but also for humans. Indeed, transportation of human ovarian tissue from cancer patients to a single central national center is conducted in several countries [28]. In Denmark [29, 30] Germany, Switzerland, Austria [31, 32] and in the United States [33–36] ovarian tissue is cryostored only in specific centers and finding the optimal transportation conditions will probably also be a benefit to such centers.

In the present study, the domestic cat was used as an experimental model to evaluate the preservation of preantral follicles and of oocytes retrieved from antral follicles in ovaries stored at 4 °C for different time periods. Therefore, we analyzed: a) morphology, microtubular cytoskeleton and DNA damage in preantral follicles and, b) developmental competence of oocytes after in vitro maturation and fertilization as well as oxidative status in matured oocytes.

Methods

Chemicals

All chemicals, in this study, were purchased from Sigma Chemical CO. (St. Louis, MO, USA) unless stated otherwise.

Ovary collection and storage

Ovaries were harvested from fifty five healthy, domestic queens (*Felis catus*, 8 months-2 years of age) at random stages of their oestrus cycles during routine ovariectomy at the Veterinary Teaching Hospital of the University of Sassari (Italy). The ovaries were placed in sterile 15-ml tubes containing Phosphate Buffered Saline (PBS, cat n°

18,912–014, Gibco, Life Technologies, Carlsbad, California, USA) with penicillin (100 mg/L), streptomycin (100 mg/L) [8, 12]., Calcium Dichloride Hydrate ($CaCl_2H_2O$, 133 mg/L) and Magnesium Chloride Hexahydrate ($MgCl_2{\bullet}6H_2O$, 100 mg/L). The divalent cations, calcium and magnesium, were added to the PBS solution in order to preserve cellular adhesion and tissue integrity in the ovary during storage at 4 °C [37, 38]. The ovaries were immediately transported to the laboratory at room temperature (22–25 °C) and randomly divided in two groups: fresh ovaries (0 h, control group) and ovaries to be stored at 4 °C (stored group). The ovaries from each storage group were transferred under sterile conditions to a 15-ml tube containing 4 ml of fresh pre-cooled PBS and held at 4 °C in a refrigerator for different lengths of times (24, 48, 72, 96 h). Control and stored ovaries were processed according to the following experimental design.

Experimental design

The experimental design includes two experiments. Experiment 1 was performed to evaluate the effect of different storage times (0, 24, 48, 72 and 96 h) at 4 °C on the morphology, organization of microtubular cytoskeleton and DNA integrity of preantral follicles.

In Experiment 2, the in vitro meiotic and developmental competence of oocytes collected from antral follicles of control and stored ovaries were evaluated. Moreover, the oxidative status of in vitro matured oocytes from each experimental group was analyzed by quantifying the intracellular levels of Reactive Oxygen Species (ROS), Glutathione (GSH) and lipid peroxidation.

Experiment 1

Morphological evaluation of preantral follicles

Both control and stored ovaries were fixed in Bouin's solution for 12 h, embedded in paraffin, serially sectioned (5 μm), and mounted onto microscope slides. The sections were either stained with Hematoxylin and Eosin (HE) or used for immunohistochemistry, as described below. In order to evaluate follicular morphology, three sections from each sample were examined. Preantral follicles were classified according to their developmental status as: i) primordial with one layer of flattened cells; ii) primary with one layer of cuboidal cells; iii) secondary with two or more layers of cuboidal cells and a theca cell layer [39]. Moreover, they were graded according to their morphology: structurally normal follicles presented a spherical oocyte with a non-pyknotic nucleus surrounded by well-arranged granulosa cells, while abnormal follicles were characterized by contraction and clumping of oocyte chromatin surrounded by disorganized granulosa cells. To avoid double counting in adjacent sections, the follicles were only analyzed when an oocyte nucleus was present.

Fluorescent immunoistochemistry

The histological sections were immersed for 20 min in a 98 °C preheated solution (WCAP, citrate pH 6, BiOptica, Milan, Italy) which simultaneously allows dewaxing, rehydration and antigen unmasking. Slides were mounted in a sequenza chamber (Shandon, Runcorn, UK) before performing immunostaining.

Assessment of microtubular cytoskeleton organization

Microtubules are ubiquitous cytoskeletal structures that are formed by the polymerization of α and β tubulin heterodimers [40]. Accordingly, we used monoclonal anti α and β tubulin antibodies to detect the effect of cold storage on the microtubular cytoskeleton organization of ovarian tissue.

Ovarian sections were incubated overnight at 4 °C with a mixture of mouse monoclonal anti α-tubulin (1:1000, Sigma Chemical CO, St. Louis, MO, USA; Cat n° T5168) and mouse monoclonal anti β-tubulin (1:100; Sigma Chemical CO, Cat n° T-7941) antibodies then labeled with donkey anti-mouse Alexa Fluor 488 (1:100, Cat n° A21202, Life Technologies, Invitrogen, Carlsbad, California, USA) for 1 h at room temperature. These specific primary antibodies were chosen for immunofluorescence due to their high affinity to α and β tubulin as indicated by the manufacturer and other Authors [41–44].

The nuclei were counter-stained with Hoechst 33,342 (10 μg/ml; Cat n° B2261) in 1:1 (*v*/*v*) glycerol/PBS solution. The sections were covered with coverslips, sealed with nail polish, and kept at 4 °C in the dark until observation. Images were acquired by a laser-scanning confocal fluorescence microscope (Leica TCS SP5), equipped with 543 nm HeNe, 488 nm Argon and 405 nm 405-diode laser using an oil immersion 40x objective (NA = 1,25). The parameters related to fluorescence intensity (laser energy, gain, offset and pinhole size) were maintained at constant values during all image acquisitions.

Detection of histone H_2AX phosphorylation

We investigated whether cold storage induced DNA damage in preantral follicles, examining histone H_2AX phosphorylation (γH_2AX), a marker of DNA double-strand breaks (DSBs) [45]. The ovary sections were incubated overnight at 4 °C with mouse monoclonal anti-γH_2AX (phospho S139) antibody (Cat n° ab26350, Abcam, Cambridge; UK) and labeled with donkey anti-mouse Alexa Fluor 488 (1:100) for 1 h at room temperature. The nuclei were counter-stained with propidium iodide (1 μg/ml, Cat n°4170) in 1:1 (*v*/*v*) glycerol/PBS solution. Images were acquired as described above.

Experiment 2

Oocyte recovery and in vitro maturation

Ovaries from control and stored groups were sliced with a scalpel blade to release the cumulus-oocyte complexes

(COCs). The COCs were collected in sterile Petri dishes in dissection medium (DM; 25 mM Hepes-buffered TCM 199) supplemented with 0.1% (*w/v*) polyvinyl alcohol (PVA) and antibiotics (100 µg/ml penicillin and streptomycin). Only the oocytes with darkly pigmented ooplasm and completely surrounded by at least one layer of cumulus cells were selected for in vitro maturation (IVM). The COCs were matured in groups of 25–35 in 650 µl of TCM 199 supplemented 0.36 mM pyruvate, 2 mM glutamine, 2.2 mM calcium lactate, 1.2 mM cysteine, 4 mg/ml BSA fatty acid free and FSH 1 IU / ml and LH 1 IU / ml (Pluset; Bio98, Milan, Italy) under mineral oil, in 4-well dishes (Nunc Cell Culture, Thermo Fisher Scientific, Waltham, Massachusetts, USA) in a humidified atmosphere of 5% CO_2, at 38.5 °C for 24 h [46].

Assessment of oocyte nuclear maturation

After IVM, groups of oocytes were completely denuded of granulosa cells via gentle pipetting with a fine bore glass pipette in DM, stained with Hoechst 33,342 (10 µg/ml) in 1:1 (*v*/v) glycerol/PBS solution, placed on a slide and overlaid with a coverslip supported by four droplets of vaseline. The nuclear configuration was classified under an epifluorescent microscope (Olympus IX 70, Italy) as germinal vesicle (GV), germinal vesicle breakdown (GVBD), metaphase I (MI), or metaphase II (MII). The oocytes with the diffusely stained cytoplasm typical of nonviable cells and those with unidentifiable or invisible chromatin were classified as degenerated (Deg).

Measurement of intracellular ROS and GSH levels

Groups of matured oocytes (MII) from all experimental groups were selected on the basis of the presence of the first polar body and sampled for intracellular Reactive Oxygen Species (ROS) and Glutathione (GSH) level measurement [47].

Briefly, 2′7′-dichlorodihydrofluorescein diacetate (H2DCFDA, Cat n° D 6883) and 4-chloromethyl-6,8-difluoro-7-hydroxycoumarin (CMF2HC, Cell Tracker Blue, Cat n° C12881, Molecular Probes, Oregon, USA) were used to detect intracellular ROS as green fluorescence and GSH level as blue fluorescence. A total of 30–35 oocytes from each treatment group were incubated in the dark for 30 min at 38.5 °C in 5% CO_2 in air in PBS-PVA containing 10 µM H_2DCFDA or 10 µM CellTracker Blue. After incubation, the oocytes were washed with PBS-PVA, placed in 50 µL droplets, and observed using an epifluorescence microscope (Olympus IX 70, Italy) with UV filters (460 nm for ROS and 370 nm for GSH). The oocytes were positioned in the plane of focus, and the area of measurement was adapted to the size of the oocyte. Microscope adjustments and photomultiplier settings were kept constant for all experiments. The data of emission intensity/oocyte were reduced by compensation for the background fluorescence. The fluorescent images were saved as graphic files in. TIFF format. Fluorescence intensitiy was analyzed with Image J software (version 1.40; National Institute of health, Bethesda, MD). Results were normalized to control values for each experiment. The experiments were performed in triplicate.

Lipid peroxidation assay

Lipid peroxidation assay was performed with 4, 4-difluoro-5- (4- phenyl-1, 3-buttadienyl)-4-bora 3a, 4a-diaza-s-indacene-3-undecanoic acid 581/591C11 (BODIPY D3861, Life Technologies, Invitrogen, Carlsbad, California, USA) [48]. Briefly, a total of 30–35 MII oocytes recovered from the different groups were incubated with 10 mM BODIPY stain for 30 min at 38.5 °C in 5% CO_2 in air. The dye loaded oocytes were then washed twice in DM and mounted on slides. Green and red fluorescence of BODIPY were determined using a confocal laser scanning microscope equipped with Argon and Helium/Neon lasers at excitation wavelengths of 488 and 543 nm and emission spectra of 500–530 nm (green) and greater than 560 nm (red). Levels of lipid peroxidation were measured by the ratio of green to red fluorescence. Results were normalized to control values for each experiment. The experiments were performed in triplicate.

In vitro fertilization and embryo culture

Spermatozoa were collected from epididymides of cats following routine orchiectomy [49, 50] and frozen according to the procedure described by Tsutsui et al. [51]. Before IVF, straws of semen were thawed by immersion in a 37 °C water bath for 30s and centrifuged at 620 x g for 5 min. The supernatant was discarded and the pellet was re-suspended in synthetic oviductal fluid (SOF) containing 6 mg/ml BSA, 50 µg/ml gentamicin (IVF medium). After maturation, the COCs were co-incubated with 1×10^6 motile spermatozoa/mL in IVF medium at 38.5 C in 5% CO_2 in air with maximum humidity [52].

After 22 h, the presumptive zygotes were washed and cultured in SOF containing 4 mg/ml BSA, 100 IU/ml penicillin and 1% MEM non-Essential amino acids. On day 3 after IVF (day = 0) the embryos were transferred to SOF supplemented with 10% fetal calf serum and 2% MEM essential amino acids [52]. On day 2 and day 7 of IVC, respectively, the number of embryos cleaved and developing to blastocyst stage was determined. Blastocysts were stained with Hoechst 33,342 (10 µg/mL), mounted on a glass slide and examined under epifluorescent microscope (Olympus IX70, Italy). A digital image of each embryo was taken, and the number of nuclei was counted.

Statistical analysis

All statistical analyses were performed using Stata/IC 11.2 (StataCorp LP, USA). In continuous data, normal distribution was checked by Shapiro-Wilk test. When the assumption of normality was met (follicles expressing > 3 γH2AX foci, ROS and GSH, blastocyst cell number) the data were analysed by one way ANOVA using Bonferroni as post-hoc test. When the data were not normally distributed (normal preantral follicles) a non-parametric Kruskal-Wallis test was used. Categorical data of meiotic progression, cleavage and development to blastocyst stage were analyzed by chi-square test. The level of statistical significance was set at $P < 0.05$.

Results

Experiment 1

Morphology of preantral follicles after ovary storage at 4°

A total of 998 preantral follicles were examined (mean ± SD for each group: 199.6 ± 24.3). The distribution of preantral follicles at each developmental stage was similar among storage groups. Most of the preantral follicles were at primordial stage (77.2 ± 1.2%), while primary (15.7 ± 1.1%) and secondary follicles (6.8 ± 1.2%) were represented in lower percentages.

The percentage of morphologically normal follicles at different storage times is shown in Fig. 1. Storage for 24 h maintained the proportion of follicles with normal morphology (86.3 ± 2.8%) similar to control values (87.7 ± 2.5%). A progressive decrease ($P < 0.05$) in the percentage of normal follicles was observed following 48 h (65.0 ± 6.1%), 72 h (39.7 ± 2.8%) and 96 h (20.0 ± 3.2%) of storage compared to 0 and 24 h groups.

Effect of ovary storage at 4 °C on the organization of the microtubular cytoskeleton

A storage time-dependent change of the tubulin organization was evident in cellular components of ovarian tissue (Fig. 2). In control sections, large amounts of tubulin were visible in the granulosa cell layers and a

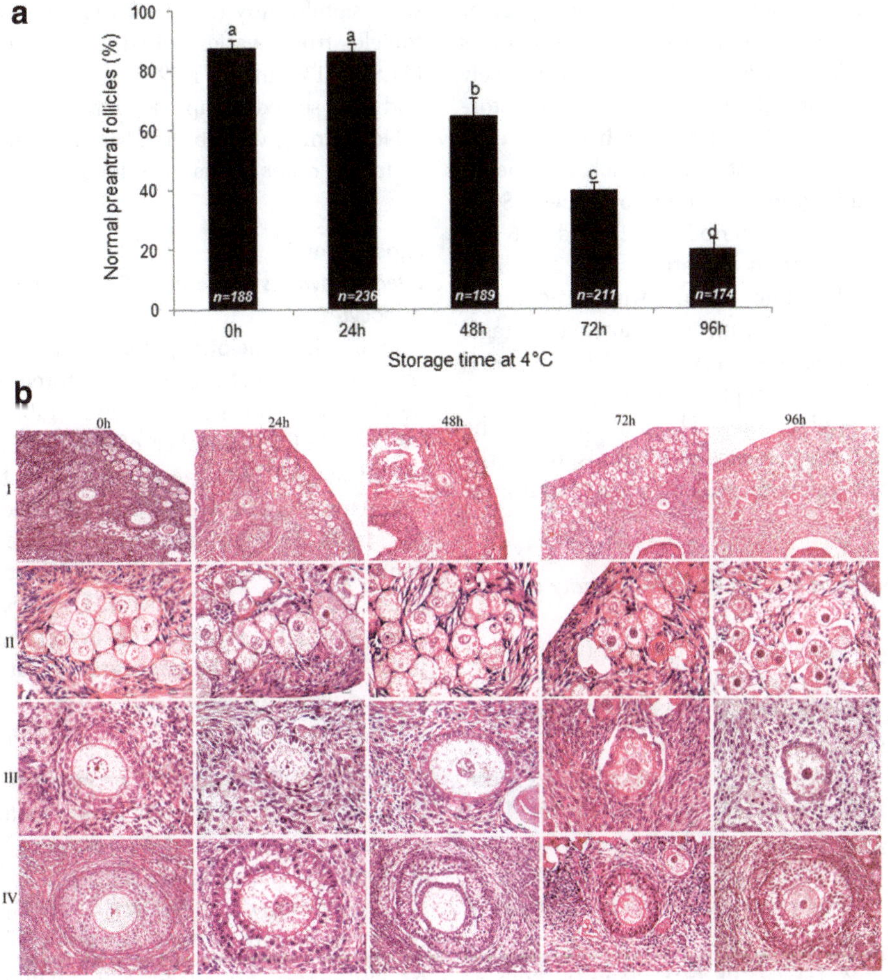

Fig. 1 **a** Percentage (mean ± S.E.M) of morphologically normal preantral follicles after different time of ovary storage at 4 °C. **b** Representative images of sections of ovarian tissue (I) and different classes of preantral follicles (II-IV) stained by hematoxylin and eosin. Different superscripts (a, b, c, d) among storage times indicate $P < 0.05$. n = number of preantral follicles analyzed

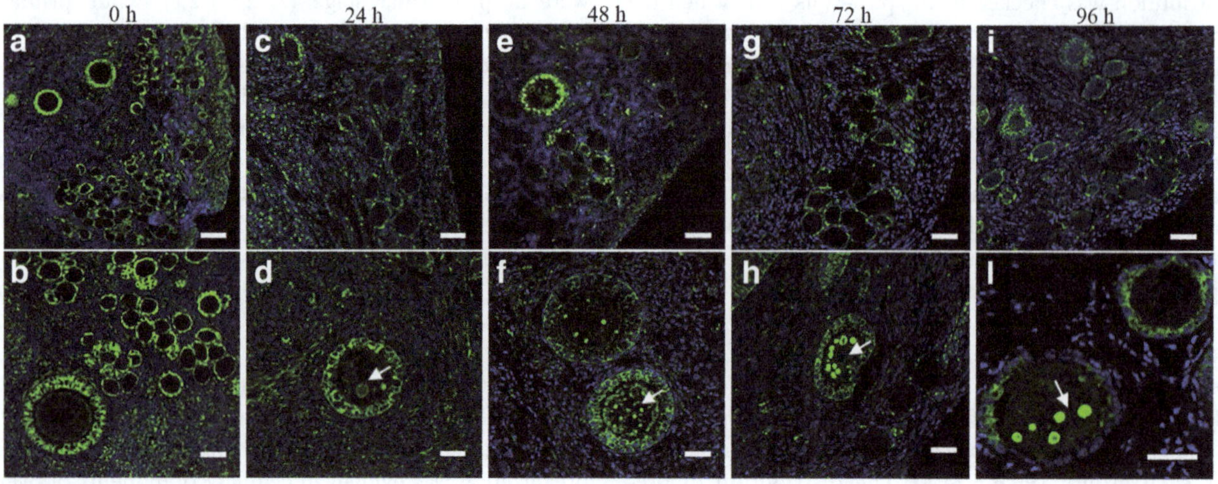

Fig. 2 Representative images of tubulin organization of preantral follicles after different times of ovary storage at 4 °C. Tubulin staining of granulosa and stromal cells is progressively reduced with increasing storage time (**a**-**i**) and bright spots of tubulin appear in the cytoplasm of follicle enclosed oocyte (**d**-**l**, white arrow). Nuclei were stained with Hoechst 33,342 (blue). Scale bar = 20 μm (**a**, **c**, **e**, **g**, **i**); 10 μm (**b**, **d**, **f**, **h**, **l**)

well detectable microtubular network was present throughout the cytoplasm of follicle-enclosed oocytes (Fig. 2 a, b). The tubulin distribution was progressively disrupted when increasing the storage time. Ovary storage at 4 °C for 24 h (Fig. 2 c,d) and 48 h (Fig. 2 e, f) caused a decrease in tubulin staining, which became irregularly distributed in granulosa and stromal cells. Storage for more extended periods (72 and 96 h) progressively induced tubulin alterations (Fig. 2 g,h,i, l). Similarly, the network of microtubules within the oocyte became irregular and disorganized following storage; spots of tubulin staining (see arrow in Fig. 2 f, h, and l) were observed inside the cytoplasm of the primary/secondary follicle-enclosed oocytes. The alterations in the tubulin network and the presence of tubulin spots in the oocyte cytoplasm were more evident when the storage time was prolonged.

Effect of ovary storage at 4 °C on the DNA integrity of preantral follicles

The presence of characteristic bright points (foci) within oocyte nuclei after immunostaining for γH2AX was considered to represent the induction of DNA DSBs. The percentage of follicles expressing distinct γH2AX foci and the number of foci they presented were assessed in preantral follicles after different times of ovary storage at 4 °C (Fig. 3). Since the control samples had very few oocytes with more than three foci (Fig. 3a, A, C), detection of three or more foci\nucleus was considered an indicator of DNA damage induced by ovary storage (Fig. 3a, B, D).

Low percentages of γH2AX-positive preantral follicles with > 3 foci/oocyte were observed in the 24 h stored group (6.2 ± 2.3) and did not differ from the control group (0.3 ± 0.3%). In contrast, γH2AX-positive foci were significantly ($P < 0.05$) more abundant in preantral follicles from ovaries stored for 48 h (16.6 ± 2.6%), 72 h (21.8 ± 2.1%) and 96 h (23.7 ± 3.1%) compared to control and 24 h stored groups (Fig. 3b).

No staining was observed in individual granulosa cells or in any other ovarian cell types.

Experiment 2

Effect of ovary storage at 4 °C on the meiotic competence of oocytes

The in vitro meiotic progression of oocytes retrieved from antral follicles of ovaries stored at 4 °C for 0, 24, 48, 72 and 96 h is summarized in Table 1. A significantly higher ($P < 0.05$) number of oocytes in the 96 h group stayed at the GV stage compared to the other groups. The percentage of oocytes that resumed meiosis (GVBD/MI stage) did not differ among the five groups. The percentages of oocytes reaching MII stage were similar among 0, 24 and 48 h stored groups. A significantly lower ($P < 0.05$) MII rate was detected following storage for 72 and 96 h. The degeneration rate significantly increased with storage time ($P < 0.05$).

Effect of ovary storage at 4 °C on intracellular levels of GSH, ROS, and lipid peroxidation of in vitro matured oocytes

The intracellular level of GSH was not statistically different among groups (Fig. 4a, a').

A significantly higher level ($P < 0.05$) of ROS was recorded in in vitro matured oocytes recovered from ovaries stored for 48, 72 and 96 h compared to oocytes obtained from ovaries stored for 0 and 24 h (Fig. 4b, b').

The levels of lipid peroxidation of in in vitro matured oocytes retrieved from ovaries stored for 72 and 96 h

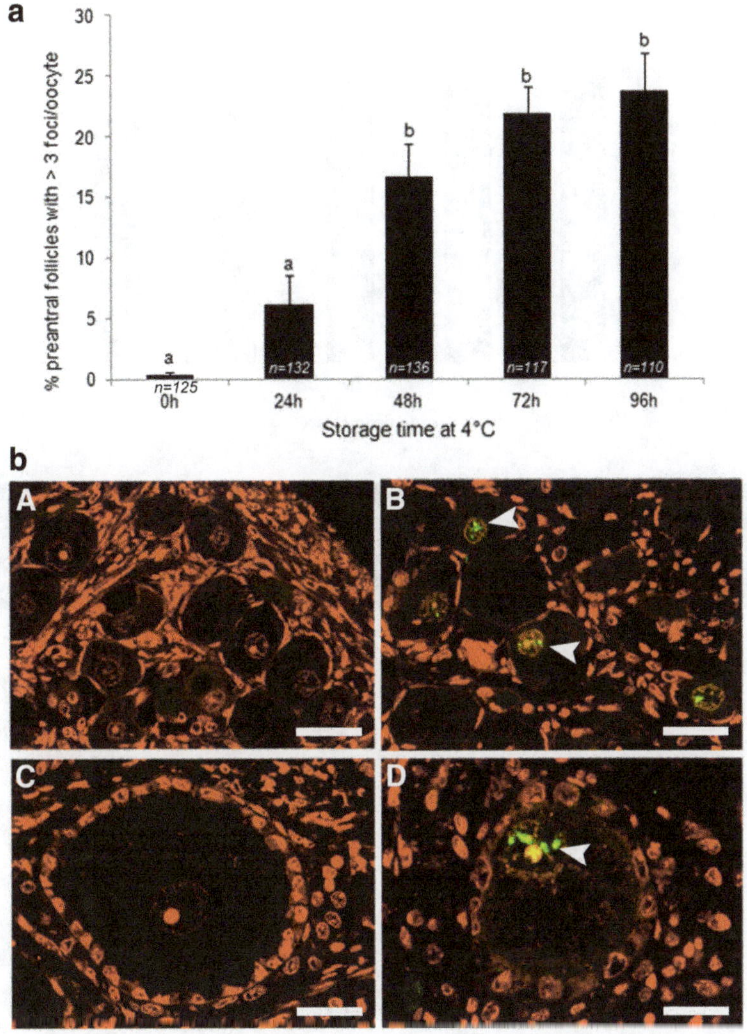

Fig. 3 a. Representative images of fluorescent immunodetection of γH2AX phosphorylation: follicle-enclosed oocytes with nuclei without bright foci (A, C) or expressing green fluorescent foci (B, D, white arrows). **b** Percentage (mean ± S.E.M) of preantral follicles with 3 or more foci/oocyte after different time of ovary storage at 4 °C. Nuclei were stained with propidium iodide (red). Scale bar =10 μm. Different superscripts (a, b) among storage times indicate $P < 0.05$. n = number of preantral follicles analyzed per storage time

Table 1 In vitro maturation of cat oocytes retrieved from ovaries stored for different times at 4 °C

Nuclear configuration after IVM					
Storage time (h)	n° oocytes	GV (%)	GVBD/MI (%)	MII (%)	Deg (%)
0	109	25 (22.9%)[a]	14 (12.8%)	67 (61.5%)[a]	3 (2.8%)[a]
24	114	24 (21.1%)[a]	8 (7.0%)	70 (61.4%)[a]	12 (10.5%)[b]
48	83	11 (13.2%)[a]	4 (4.8%)	58 (69.9%)[a]	10 (12.1%)[b]
72	58	16 (27.6%)[a]	2 (3.5%)	19 (32.7%)[b]	21 (36.2%)[c]
96	62	28 (45.2%)[b]	4 (6.5%)	11 (17.7%)[b]	19 (30.6%)[c]

GV germinal vesicle, *GVBD* germinal vesicle breakdown, *MI* metaphase I, *MII* metaphase II, *Deg* degenerated
Different superscripts (a, b, c) $P < 0.05$

were higher than those in oocytes from 0, 24 and 48 h groups (Fig. 5a, b).

Effect of ovary storage at 4 °C on oocyte developmental competence

The proportion of oocytes that progressed to the first cleavage stage after in vitro fertilization was similar among 0, 24 and 48 h stored groups. A significantly ($P < 0.05$) decrease of cleavage rate was observed following 72 and 96 h of ovary storage (Table 2). The percentages of blastocysts relative to the number of cleaved embryos (developmental competence) and to the total number of oocytes (blastocyst yield) were lower in 48, 72 and 96 h stored groups compared to those in 0 and 24 h groups (Table 2, Fig. 6). Cell numbers in blastocysts from 0 and 24 h

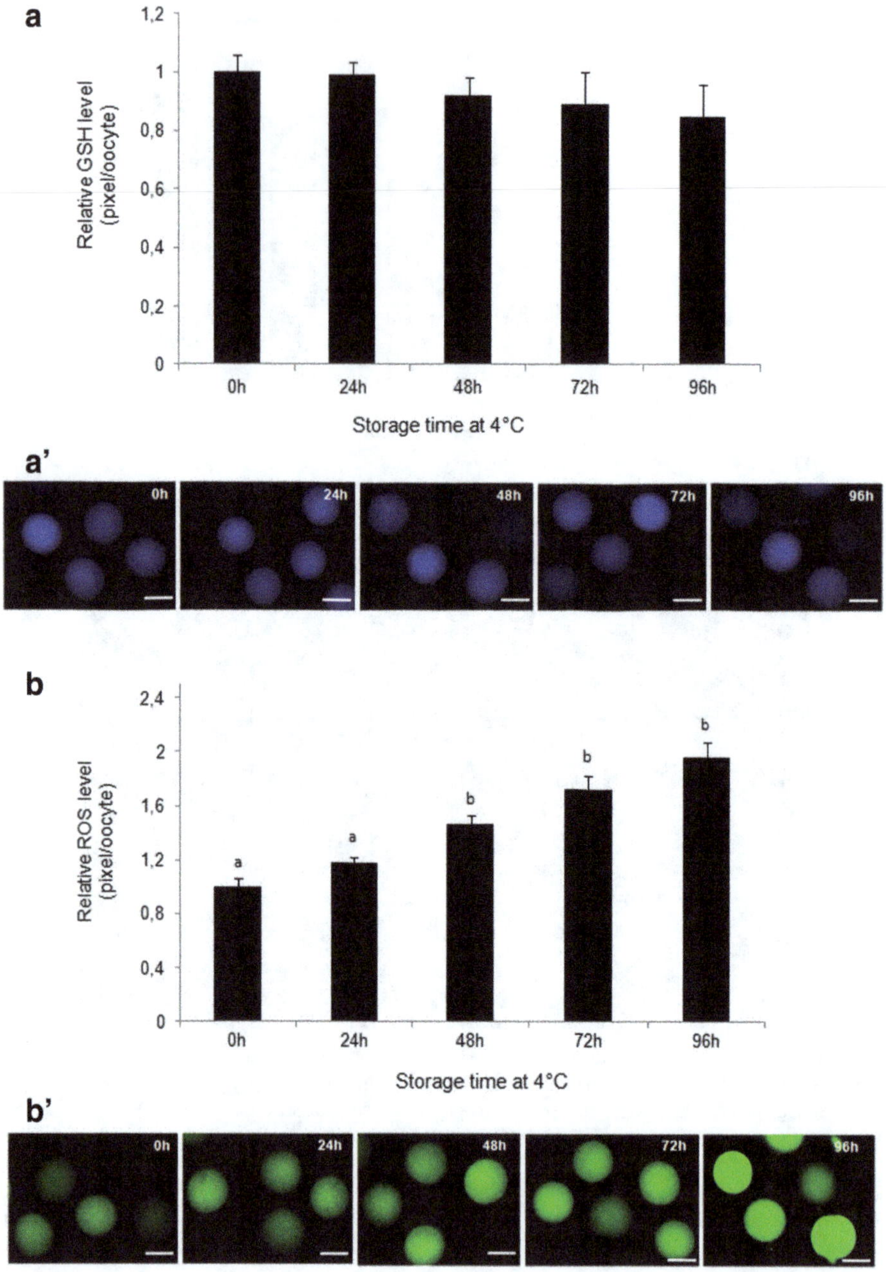

Fig. 4 Effect of ovary storage time at 4 °C on intracellular GSH (**a**) and ROS levels (**b**) of in vitro matured oocytes. Epifluorescence photomicrographs of MII oocytes that were stained with CellTracker Blue to determine the level of GSH (**a'**) and with 2'7'-dichlorodihydrofluorescein diacetate (H2DCFDA) to detect ROS (**b'**). Different superscripts (a, b, c, d) among storage times indicate $P < 0.05$. Scale bar =50 µm

groups were similar. Only one blastocyst with 98 cells developed after 48 h of ovary storage.

Discussion

This study is the first to examine the effect of cat ovary storage at 4 °C for an extended period of time (up to 96 h) on the morphology, microtubular cytoskeleton and DNA damage in preantral follicles. We also investigated the in vitro meiotic and developmental competence of oocytes recovered from antral follicles and parameters of oxidative stress as indicators of the quality of matured oocytes. The main findings of the research were: a) storage up to 24 h did not affect the morphology and DNA integrity of preantral follicles, whereas the organization of the microtubular cytoskeleton was moderately altered; b) extended storage times (48, 72, 96 h) caused progressive structural changes of preantral follicles as showed by morphological abnormality, disassembling of

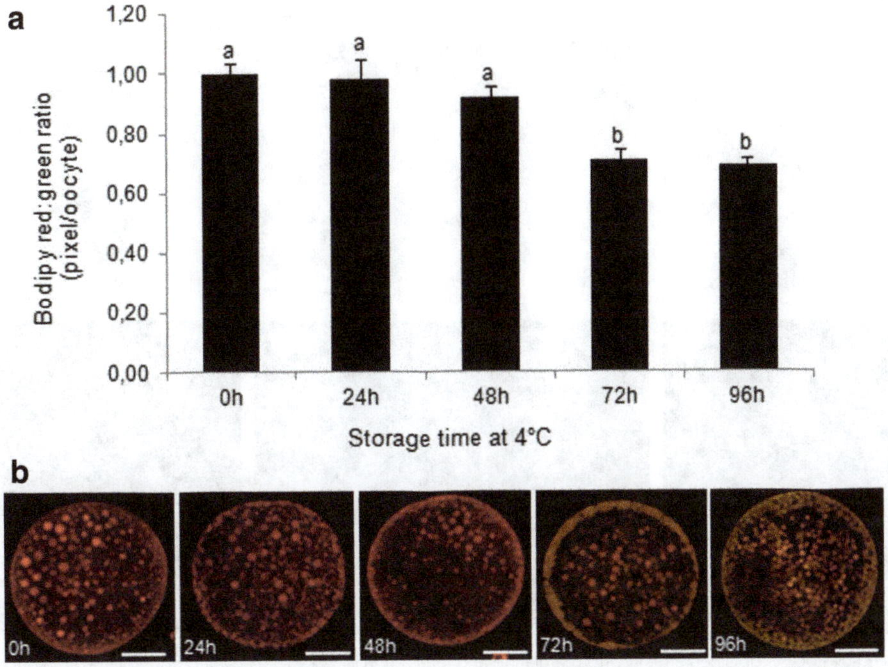

Fig. 5 a Levels of lipid peroxidation as measured by the ratio of red: green fluorescence of in vitro matured oocytes recovered from ovaries stored at 4 °C for different times. **b** Epifluorescence photomicrographs of matured oocytes that were stained with BODIPY. Scale bar =100 μm. Different superscripts (a, b) among storage times indicate $P < 0.05$.

microtubules and DNA damage; c) ovary storage up to 48 h did not influence the in vitro meiotic maturation ability of the oocytes retrieved from antral follicles but only the oocytes stored within the ovary for 24 h developed to blastocyst stage in percentage similar to control oocytes; d) the duration of storage did not affect the GSH levels, whereas increased levels of ROS were detected starting from 48 h and lipid peroxidation at 72 and 96 h of storage.

Hypothermic storage (0–7 °C) of organs is normally used to minimize tissue metabolism and prevent ischemic injury, and the maximum storage time depends on the specific organs. Several studies described transportation at cold temperature of mammalian, including human, ovarian tissue for fertility preservation. Indeed, the transportation of human ovarian tissue at low temperature and within a period of 4 to 26 h didn't affect human ovarian tissue morphology, viability, and follicle development in vitro and in vivo [53–57]. On the other hand, a study by Klocke et al. [58] investigating the effects that storage at 4 °C for 24 or 48 h before vitrification has on the human ovarian cortex highlighted significant negative consequences within 24 h.

Some investigators [55, 56, 59] recommended cooling human ovarian tissue to low positive temperatures before cryopreservation independently of transportation purposes. The Storage of human ovarian cortex for 24 h at 5 °C before cryopreservation increased the viability of the follicles after thawing and in vitro culture in the chorioallantoic membrane system [56]. Moreover, the same group also showed, after in vitro culture, a significant increase of neo-vascularisation in human ovarian tissue pre-cooled at 5 °C for 24 h compared to non-cooled control tissue [55] and a reduced translocation of

Table 2 In vitro embryo development after in vitro fertilization of cat oocytes retrieved from ovaries stored for different times at 4 °C

Storage time (h)	n°oocytes fertilized	n°cleaved embryos	n°blastocysts/ cleaved/embryos	n°blastocysts/ total oocytes	Blastocyst cell number (mean ± SD)
0	56	25 (44.6%)^{a}	15 (60%) ^{a}	15 (26.8%) ^{a}	178.5 ± 40.5 ^{a}
24	48	19 (39.6%) ^{a}	11 (57.9%) ^{a}	11 (22.9%) ^{a}	171.9 ± 44.6 ^{a}
48	43	16 (37.2%) ^{a}	1 (6.2%) ^{b}	1 (2.3%) ^{b}	98 ^{h}
72	41	2 (4.9%)^{b}	0 (0%) ^{b}	0 (0%) ^{b}	–
96	39	0 (0%) ^{b}	0 (0%) ^{b}	0 (0%) ^{b}	–

Different superscripts (a, b) $P < 0.05$

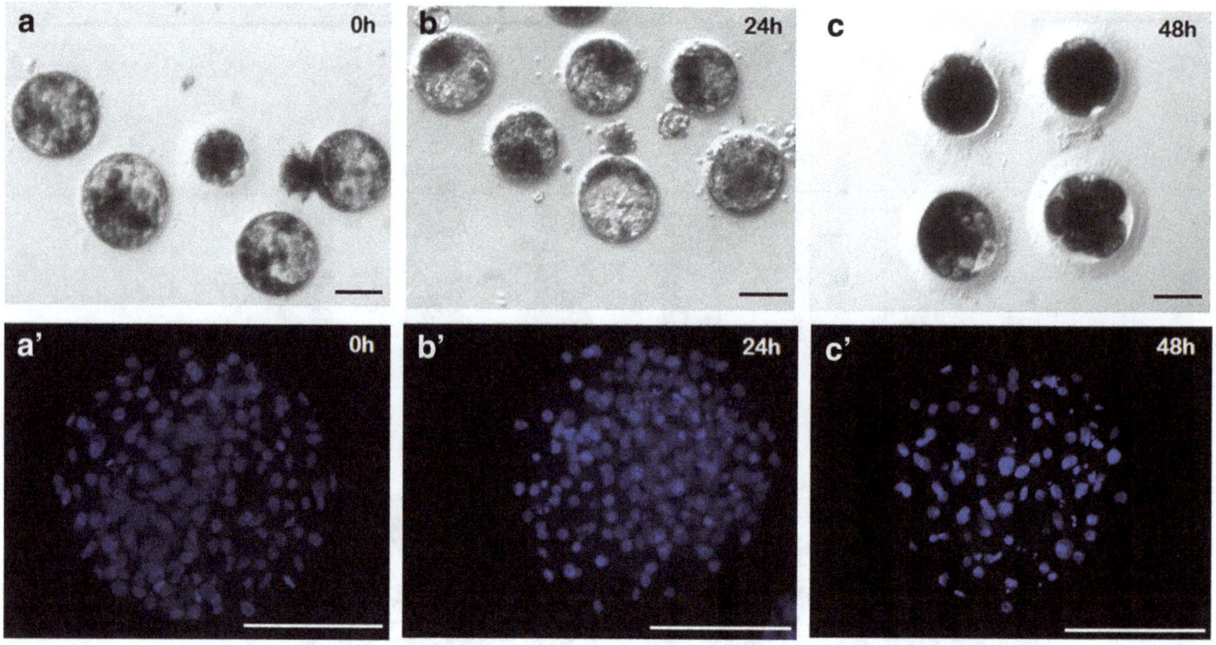

Fig. 6 In vitro produced blastocysts obtained after in vitro maturation and fertilization of oocytes recovered from ovaries stored for 0, 24 and 48 h at 4 °C under phase contrast microscopy (**a**, **b**, **c**) and under epifluorescent microscopy after staining with Hoechst 33,342 (**a'**, **b'**,**c'**). Scale bar =100 μm

phosphatidylserine, a membrane component with a key role in the mechanisms of necrosis and apoptosis [59].

Certainly the proof of the efficiency of ovarian tissue storage at cold temperatures during transportation are the successful births reported in European countries where ovarian transportation for long distance is conducted [29, 60–63].

Evidence from animal studies has shown that chilling ovarian tissue at 4 °C during transportation provides optimal conditions to preserve follicular morphology and viability for longer times than at higher temperatures. In the mouse, storage at 4 °C for up to 24 h has no deleterious effect on histological morphology of ovarian tissue or on mature gametes [27]. Similarly, ovarian follicles from sheep and goat [23, 64] were successfully preserved for up to 24 h and ovarian follicles from zebu cows for up to 18 h [65]. In the canine [24] and equine models [25], the morphology of preantral follicles was best maintained when ovaries were stored at 4 °C for shorter periods (12 and 4 h respectively).

Our study clearly demonstrated that morphological changes in the preantral follicle population of cat ovaries stored at 4 °C was modest for at least 24 h, maintaining about 86.3% of morphologically normal follicles. Longer storage times caused a progressive damage to preantral follicles as shown by the percentages of normal follicles following 48 h (65%), 72 h (39.7%) and 96 h (20%) of storage.

Vitrification is an ideal option for preserving ovarian tissue especially for wildlife species because it doesn't require specialized equipment and can be performed in the field. To date, there are only few studies on vitrification of feline ovarian tissue [66–71] and, despite recent progress, this procedure still requires modification and optimization. The percentage of vitrified-warmed morphologically normal follicles, immediately after warming, ranged from 5.9% [66] to a maximum 58.8% [69] under the optimal conditions. The storage at 4 °C can be a useful method for short-term preservation of ovarian tissue because the normal morphology of preantral follicles remains high even after 48 h storage, allowing xenotrasplantation into recipient animals or in vitro culture of follicles.

Information regarding the influence of cold storage on preantral follicles of cat ovaries is scarce. A study by Cocchia et al. [12] explored cell viability in cat ovaries stored at 4 °C up to 72 h and reported a storage time-dependent increase in the percentage of apoptotic areas in the ovarian tissue. Recently, the impact of holding of cat ovaries at 4 °C for 24 and 72 h followed by vitrification has been investigated by monitoring the survival and morphology of preantral follicles with neutral red staining, histology and ultrastructural analysis by transmission electron microscopy [22]. Results indicated a reduction in the number of intact and viable follicles after 24 and 72 h storage without significant differences between groups and time points. As reported by the Authors, the large variation in the number of follicles evaluated and the high standard deviations probably masked differences between groups and time points. The variability of sample numbers as well as differences in experimental design and methodology make it difficult to compare these data with our results. Indeed, cortical slices of ovaries stored for 24 and 72 h were incubated for 16 h with neutral red before viability and morphology assessment. The small number of follicles utilized for transmission electron microscopy affected the accuracy of the ultrastructural evaluation, although it revealed the preservation of subcellular structures after cooling for 24 h. Authors finally concluded that the ovarian tissue can be maintained for a maximum of 24 h at 4 °C before cryopreservation.

A further goal of our study was to investigate the response of the microtubular cytoskeleton of preantral follicles to chilling at 4 °C. The presence of an intact cytoskeleton and its dynamic organization are crucial during folliculogenesis and oogenesis [72]. The effect of cold temperature is known to induce depolimerization of microtubules [73] in mammalian cells. Chilling injuries on meiotic spindles of fully grown oocytes have been extensively reported in several species [74–76]. A previous study on mice [42] investigated the effect of chilling at 0 °C on the cytoskeleton organization of isolated early preantral follicles. The results showed that chilling for only 1 min was sufficient to cause depolymerization of microtubules in the oocytes and the surrounding granulosa cell layer. In the present study, an alteration of microtubular network in preantral follicles of ovaries stored at 4 °C for different times has been detected. Observed changes included tubulin depolimerization and disassembling in the granulosa cell layer and the appearance of tubulin spots in the oocytes of preantral follicles. The extent of microtubule modifications depended on the time of ovary storage: these started from 24 h of storage and became more evident following 48, 72 and 96 h. Further studies are needed to understand the reversibility of the cooling effect on the microtubular cytoskeleton. Preliminary evaluations (data not shown) indicated that the microtubule modification was fully reversible when ovaries stored at 4 °C for 24 and 48 h were re-warmed at 38.5 °C for 2 h.

Beside the morphological and structural analysis of ovarian tissue, the preservation of DNA integrity is fundamental in order to understand the effect of low temperature on preantral follicles. DNA double-strand breaks in oocytes enclosed in preantral follicles have never been investigated after storing of cat ovaries at 4 °C. Cocchia et al. [12] previously evaluated apoptosis by TUNEL assay in the cat ovarian tissue stored at 4 °C up to 72 h and indicated that the addition of the antioxidant enzyme superoxide dismutase (SOD) to transportation medium reduced cellular apoptosis, albeit these differences were not statistically relevant. Double-strand breaks of DNA (DSBs) are a marker of severe DNA damage, which can activate apoptosis [45] if not repaired. We have demonstrated that ovary storage at 4 °C for over 24 h induces DSBs in oocytes enclosed in preantral follicles and that DNA damage increases as storage is prolonged. Additional analysis is needed to assess the DNA repair capability of oocytes to ultimately confirm the exact extent of the DNA damage.

Our explorative study focuses mainly on the evaluation of morphological and structural modifications in preantral follicles in feline ovarian tissue after storage at 4 °C for a prolonged period. The next step should be to validate the quality and survival of stored ovarian tissue by assessing the developmental competence of the preantral follicles following xenotrasplantation of ovarian cortex into immunodeficient recipients or after in vitro culture.

The second part of our study was aimed to determine the adverse effects of cold storage on the oocytes harvested from antral follicles by analyzing their meiotic and developmental competence after in vitro fertilization.

Our findings indicated that when ovaries were stored at 4 °C for 24 and 48 h, oocytes retained the ability to progress to metaphase II at a rate similar to control oocytes, while a significant reduction of nuclear maturation was registered after 72 and 96 h of storage. The storage of ovarian tissue at 4 °C (at least for 48 h) may offer the possibility to preserve viability and meiotic competence of oocytes retrieved from antral follicles otherwise compromised by vitrification of ovarian tissue. Indeeed, Luvoni et al... [66] reported that oocytes recovered from vitrified ovarian tissue showed higher degeneration rate and lower rate of meiosis resumption compared to those collected from fresh tissue.

Our data corroborate the results previously reported by other Authors [4, 6, 9], showing that ovary storage at 4 °C for 24 and 48 h has no effect on the in vitro meiotic competence of cat oocytes. Conversely, Evecen et al. [77] documented that, while storing ovaries for 24 h at 4 °C did not affect the meiotic competence of oocytes in vitro, 48 h of storage decreased it dramatically. Unaffected IVM rates were reported when cat ovaries were stored at 4 °C up to 72 h; however, only oocytes stored within the ovary for 24 h could produce blastocysts after in vitro fertilization [9, 10]. These developed into live kittens after transfer to recipients [10]. Similarly, our results showed that cleavage frequency, in vitro development to blastocyst stage and blastocyst cell number did not were not different after recovery of oocytes from fresh and 24 h stored ovaries. Moreover, we observed that the developmental competence of oocytes declined markedly after 24 h of storage. Recently, Cocchia et al [12] showed that SOD supplementation in the transportation medium of domestic cat ovaries enhances embryo production after 48 and 72 h of storage.

Our rates of blastocyst formation in the 24 h stored group (22.9%) are higher than those obtained after in vitro maturation of cat oocytes in presence of relaxin [11] or with the addition of SOD during ovary storage [12].

One of the main factors contributing to the poor quality of in vitro matured oocytes may be oxidative stress (OS). Under physiological conditions the antioxidant defense mechanism of oocytes and ovaries, consisting of enzymatic antioxidants such as superoxide dismutase (SOD), catalase (CAT) and glutathione peroxidase (GPx) and non-enzymatic antioxidants (GSH), detoxifies excess ROS maintaining the oxidant/antioxidant balance. However, increased levels of ROS beyond the physiological range may lead to OS and cause a wide range of molecular damages, including lipid peroxidation and protein and DNA damage resulting in deterioration of oocyte quality [78, 79]. The ROS scavenging ability of oocytes decreases under pathological conditions, different types environmental stress, and aging or elevated oxygen tension during in vitro manipulation [80, 81]. Glutathione is the major non-protein sulphydryl compound in mammalian cells and protects them from oxidative damage [82]. The level of GSH in oocytes increases as the oocyte resumes meiosis, and higher concentrations are found in mature oocytes than in immature ones [83–85].

Several studies underlined that the GSH content in oocytes at the end of IVM appears to reflect the degree of cytoplasmic maturation and quality of oocytes [86–89].

Our results showed that when ovaries were stored for different times at 4 °C the content of intracellular GSH of in vitro matured oocytes was slightly lower than that in control oocytes, but without statistical difference among groups. We speculate that, given the availability of cysteine in the maturation medium, GSH may be properly synthesized as long as the oocytes retain the ability to complete maturation. A previous study provided evidence that the availability of constitutive amino acids, in particular cysteine, is the limiting factor for GSH synthesis in mammalian oocytes [87].

Beside constant levels of GSH, the analysis of the selected oxidative stress markers in matured oocytes showed a progressive increase in ROS levels from 48 h of ovary storage associated with elevated lipid peroxidation at 72 and 96 h of storage. Lipids are highly susceptible to the attack of ROS [90] and their peroxidation may damage the oocyte membrane, modifying its structure and function.

Long-term storage of ovaries at 4 °C (72 and 96 h) may have altered the activity of other enzymes which are involved in modulating the antioxidant defense system in oocytes during in vitro maturation. Further evaluation is necessary to improve knowledge on the redox state of oocytes recovered from cold stored ovaries.

In light of these results, we suggest that oxidative stress is one of the factors hindering the developmental capacity of in vitro matured oocytes following ovary storage for more than 24 h. Strategies aimed at reducing oxidative stress, including the addition of antioxidants in the oocyte maturation medium or in the transportation medium of the ovaries, may improve oocyte quality.

Collectively, the results provide additional information on the effect of cold storage on preantral follicles and on oocytes from antral follicles and may help in setting up programs for fertility conservation, especially for wild feline species which die in geographic areas located far from ARTs centers.

Conclusions

In summary, the results of our study revealed that morphological and structural changes of preantral follicles are minimal after storage for up to 24 h. These alterations progressively increase from 48 h onwards and become more severe at 72 and 96 h of storage. The extension of the storage period beyond 24 h negatively influences the oxidative status of oocytes after in vitro maturation and their developmental competence.

Authors' contributions

AP, LB designed the study, analyzed data and wrote the paper. AP, GPB, FA, SG, DB, LF, EA, LS conducted experimental procedures of the study and collaborated in analyzing data and drafting the paper. SP and MT Z performed ovariectomies. LB supervised experiments and performed critical data analysis. All authors read and approved the paper.

Competing interests

The authors declare that they have no competing interests.

References

1. IUCN 2018.The IUCN Red List of Threatened Species.Version 2018-1. http://www.iucnredlist.org
2. Pope CE, Gomez MC, Dresser BL. In vitro embryo production and embryo transfer in domestic and non-domestic cats. Theriogenology. 2006;66:1518–4.
3. Amstislavsky S, Lindeberg H, Luvoni G. Reproductive technologies relevant to the genome resource bank in Carnivora. Reprod Domest Anim. 2012;47:164–75.
4. Luu VV, Namula Z, Do LT, Sato Y, Taniguchi M, Karja NW, Otoi T. Nuclear status and DNA fragmentation of oocytes from porcine, bovine and feline ovaries stored at 4 degrees C for 5 days. Cryo Letters. 2014;35:48–53.
5. Naoi H, Otoi T, Shimamura T, Karja NW, Agung B, Shimizu R, Taniguchi M, Nagai T. Developmental competence of cat oocytes from ovaries stored at various temperature for 24 h. J Reprod Dev. 2007;53:271–7.
6. Otoi T, Murakami M, Ooka A, Karja NW, Suzuki T. Effects of size and storage temperature on meiotic competence of domestic cat oocytes. Vet Rec. 2001;148:116–8.
7. Johnston LA, Donoghue AM, O'Brien SJ, Wildt DE. Rescue and maturation in vitro of follicular oocytes collected from nondomestic felid species. Biol Reprod. 1991;45:898–906.
8. Wood TC, Montali RJ, Wildt DE. Follicle-oocyte atresia and temporal taphonomy in cold-stored domestic cat ovaries. Mol Reprod Dev. 1997;46:190–200.
9. Wolfe BA, Wildt DE. Development to blastocysts of domestic cat oocytes matured and fertilized *in vitro* after prolonged cold storage. J Reprod Fertil. 1996;106:135–41.
10. Pope CE, Gomez MC, King AL, Harris RF, Dresser BL. Embryos produced in vitro after recovery of oocytes from cat ovaries stored at 4 °C for 24–28 h retain the competence to develop into live kittens after transfer to recipients. Theriogenology. 2003;59:308.
11. Luu VV, Hanatate K, Tanihara F, Sato Y, Do LT, Taniguchi M, Otoi T. The effect of relaxin supplementation of *in vitro* maturation medium on the development of cat oocytes obtained from ovaries stored at 4 degrees C. Reprod Biol. 2013;13:122–6.

12. Cocchia N, Corteggio A, Altamura G, Tafuri S, Rea S, Rosapane I, Sica A, Landolfi F, Ciani F. The effects of superoxide dismutase addition to the transport medium on cumulus-oocyte complex apoptosis and IVF outcome in cats (Felis catus). Reprod Biol. 2015;15:56–64.
13. Jewgenow K, Paris MC. Preservation of female germ cells from ovaries of cat species. Theriogenology. 2006;66:93–100.
14. Comizzoli P, Holt WV. Recent advances and prospects in germplasm preservation of rare and endangered species. Adv Exp Med Biol. 2014;753:331–56.
15. Bosch P, Hernandez-Fonseca HJ, Miller DM, Wininger JD, Massey JB, Lamb SV, Brackett BG. Development of antral follicles in cryopreserved cat ovarian tissue transplanted to immunodeficient mice. Theriogenology. 2004;61:581–94.
16. Wiedemann C, Hribal R, Ringleb J, Bertelsen MF, Rasmusen K, Andersen CY, Kristensen SG, Jewgenow K. Preservation of primordial follicles from lions by slow freezing and xenotransplantation of ovarian cortex into an immunodeficient mouse. Reprod Domest Anim. 2012;47(Suppl 6):300–4.
17. Fujihara M, Comizzoli P, Keefer CL, Wildt DE, Songsasen N. Epidermal growth factor (EGF) sustains in vitro primordial follicle viability by enhancing stromal cell proliferation via MAPK and PI3K pathways in the prepubertal, but not adult, cat ovary. Biol Reprod. 2014;90:86.
18. Alves AE, Padilha-Nakaghi LC, Pires-Butler EA, Apparicio M, Silva N, Motheo TF, Vicente W, Luvoni GC. Viability and growth of feline preantral follicles in vitro cultured with insulin growth factor and epidermal growth factor supplemented medium. Reprod Domest Anim. 2016;52(Suppl 2):93–7.
19. Green LJ, Shikanov A. *In vitro* culture methods of preantral follicles. Theriogenology. 2016;86:229–38.
20. Vilela JM, Leonel EC, D'Oliveira L, Paiva RE, Miranda-Vilela AL, Amorim CA, Pic-Taylor A, Lucci CM. Culture of domestic cat ovarian tissue *in vitro* and in the chick embryo chorioallantoic membrane. Theriogenology. 2016;86:1774–81.
21. Eppig JJ, O'Brien MJ. Development in vitro of mouse oocytes from primordial follicles. Biol Reprod. 1996;54:197–207.
22. Martins JLA, Lopes MD, de Souza FF, Possebon FS, Wibbelt G, Jewgenow K. Cat preantral follicle survival after prolonged cooled storage followed by vitrification. Cryobiology. 2018;81:94–100.
23. Silva JR, Lucci CM, Carvalho FC, Bao SN, Costa SH, Santos RR, Figueiredo JR. Effect of coconut water and Braun-Collins solutions at different temperatures and incubation times on the morphology of goat preantral follicles preserved in vitro. Theriogenology. 2000;54:809–22.
24. Lopes CA, dos Santos RR, Celestino JJ, Melo MA, Chaves RN, Campello CC, Silva JR, Bao SN, Jewgenow K, de Figueiredo JR. Short-term preservation of canine preantral follicles: effects of temperature, medium and time. Anim Reprod Sci. 2009;115:201–14.
25. Gomes RG, Andrade ER, Lisboa LA, Ciquini A, Barreiros TR, Fonseca NA, Seneda MM. Effect of holding medium, temperature and time on structural integrity of equine ovarian follicles during the non-breeding season. Theriogenology. 2012;78:731–6.
26. Henry L, Fransolet M, Labied S, Blacher S, Masereel MC, Foidart JM, Noel A, Nisolle M, Munaut C. Supplementation of transport and freezing media with anti-apoptotic drugs improves ovarian cortex survival. J Ovarian Res. 2016;9:4.
27. Kamoshita K, Okamoto N, Nakajima M, Haino T, Sugimoto K, Okamoto A, Sugishita Y, Suzuki N. Investigation of *in vitro* parameters and fertility of mouse ovary after storage at an optimal temperature and duration for transportation. Hum Reprod. 2016;31:774–81.
28. Fisch B, Abir R. Female fertility preservation: past, present and future. Reproduction. 2018; 156(1):F11-F27.
29. Jensen AK, Kristensen SG, Macklon KT, Jeppesen JV, Fedder J, Ernst E, Andersen CY. Outcomes of transplantations of cryopreserved ovarian tissue to 41 women in Denmark. Hum Reprod. 2015;30:2838–45.
30. Rosendahl M, Schmidt KT, Ernst E, Rasmussen PE, Loft A, Byskov AG, Andersen AN, Andersen CY. Cryopreservation of ovarian tissue for a decade in Denmark: a view of the technique. Reprod BioMed Online. 2011;22:162–71.
31. Von Wolff M, Montag M, Dittrich R, Denschlag D, Nawroth F, Lawrenz B. Fertility preservation in women-a practical guide to preservation techniques and therapeutic strategies in breast cancer, Hodgkin's lymphoma and borderline ovarian tumours by the fertility preservation network. FertiPROTEKT. Arch Gynecol Obstet. 2011;284(2):427–35.
32. Bastings L, Liebenthron J, Westphal JR, Beerendonk CCM, Van der Ven H, Meinecke B, Montag M, Braat DDM, Peek R. Efficacy of ovarian tissue cryopreservation in a major European center. J Assist Reprod Genet. 2014;31(8):1003–12.
33. Woodruff TK. The Oncofertility consortium--addressing fertility in young people with cancer. Nat Rev Clin Oncol. 2010;7:466–675.

29. Jensen AK, Kristensen SG, Macklon KT, Jeppesen JV, Fedder J, Ernst E, Andersen CY. Outcomes of transplantations of cryopreserved ovarian tissue to 41 women in Denmark. Hum Reprod. 2015;30:2838–45.
30. Rosendahl M, Schmidt KT, Ernst E, Rasmussen PE, Loft A, Byskov AG, Andersen AN, Andersen CY. Cryopreservation of ovarian tissue for a decade in Denmark: a view of the technique. Reprod BioMed Online. 2011;22:162–71.
31. Von Wolff M, Montag M, Dittrich R, Denschlag D, Nawroth F, Lawrenz B. Fertility preservation in women-a practical guide to preservation techniques and therapeutic strategies in breast cancer, Hodgkin's lymphoma and borderline ovarian tumours by the fertility preservation network. FertiPROTEKT. Arch Gynecol Obstet. 2011;284(2):427–35.
32. Bastings L, Liebenthron J, Westphal JR, Beerendonk CCM, Van der Ven H, Meinecke B, Montag M, Braat DDM, Peek R. Efficacy of ovarian tissue cryopreservation in a major European center. J Assist Reprod Genet. 2014;31(8):1003–12.
33. Woodruff TK. The Oncofertility consortium--addressing fertility in young people with cancer. Nat Rev Clin Oncol. 2010;7:466–675.

34. Gracia CR, Chang J, Kondapalli L, Prewitt M, Carlson CA, Mattei P, Jeffers S, Ginsberg JP. Ovarian tissue cryopreservation for fertility preservation in cancer patients: successful establishment and feasibility of a multidisciplinary collaboration. J Assist Reprod Genet. 2012;29:495–502.
35. Duncan FE, Zelinski M, Gunn AH, Pahnke JE, O'Neill CL, Songsasen N, Woodruff DR, Woodruff TK. Ovarian tissue transport to expand access to fertility preservation: from animals to clinical practice. Reproduction. 2016;152(6):201–10.
36. Armstrong AG, Kimler BF, Smith BM, Woodruff TK, Pavone ME, Duncan FE. Ovarian tissue cryopreservation in young females through the Oncofertility Consortium's National Physicians Cooperative. Future Oncol. 2018;14(4):363–78.
37. Irving Zeidman MD. Chemical factors in the mutual adhesiveness of epithelial cells. AACR Journals. 1947;7:386–9.
38. Ueda MJ, Takeichi M. Two mechanisms in cell adhesion revealed by effects of divalent cations. Cell structure and function. 1976;1:377–88.
39. Bristol-Gould S, Woodruff TK. Folliculogenesis in the domestic cat (Felis catus). Theriogenology. 2006;66:5–13.
40. Dowing KH, Nogales E. Tubulin and microtubule structure. Cell Biology. 1998;10:16–22.
41. Comizzoli P, Wildt DE, Pukazhenthi BS. Effect of 1,2-propanediol versus 1,2-ethanediol on subsequent oocytes maturation, spindle integrity, fertilization, and embryo development in vitro in the domestic cat. Biol Reprod. 2004;71:598–604.
42. Vanhoutte L, Cortvrindt R, Nogueira D, Smitz J. Effects of chilling on structural aspects of early preantral mouse follicles. Biol Reprod. 2004;70:1041–8.
43. Yin XJ, Lee YH, Jin JY, Kim NH, Kong IK. Nuclear and microtubule remodeling and in vitro development of nuclear transferred cat oocytes with skin fibroblasts of the domestic cat (Felis silvestris catus) and leopard cat (Prionailurus bengalensis). Anim Reprod Sci. 2006;95:307–15.
44. Jin YX, Cui XS, Yu XF, Han JY, Kong IK, Kim NH. Alterations of spindle and microfilament assembly in aged cat oocytes. Reprod Dom Anim. 2010;45:865–71.
45. Petrillo SK, Desmeules P, Truong TQ, Devine PJ. Detection of DNA damage in oocytes of small ovarian follicles following phosphoramide mustard exposures of cultured rodent ovaries *in vitro*. Toxicol Appl Pharmacol. 2011;253:94–102.
46. Bogliolo L, Leoni G, Ledda S, Zedda MT, Bonelli P, Madau L, Santucciu C, Naitana S, Pau S. M-phase promoting factor (MPF) and mitogen activated protein kinases (MAPK) activities of domestic cat oocytes matured *in vitro* and *in vivo*. Cloning Stem Cells. 2004;6(1):15–23.
47. Sovernigo TC, Adona PR, Monzani PS, Guemra S, Barros F, Lopes FG, Leal C. Effects of supplementation of medium with different antioxidants during in vitro maturation of bovine oocytes on subsequent embryo production. Reprod Domest Anim. 2017;52(4):561–9.
48. Sobinoff AP, Beckett EL, Jarnicki AG, Sutherland JM, McCluskey A, Hansbro PM, McLaughlin EA. Scrambled and fried: cigarette smoke exposure causes antral follicle destruction and oocyte dysfunction through oxidative stress. Toxicol Appl Pharmacol. 2013;271(2):156–67.
49. Bogliolo L, Leoni G, Ledda S, Naitana S, Zedda M, Carluccio A. Pau S: intracytoplasmic sperm injection of in vitro matured oocytes of domestic cats with frozen-thawed epididymal spermatozoa. Theriogenology. 2001;56(5):955–67.
50. Niżanski W, Dejneka GJ, Klimowicz M, Dubiel A. Evaluating some properties of domestic cat epididymal spermatozoa and their cryopreservation. Med Weter. 2005;61:173–8.
51. Tsutsui T, Wada M, Anzai M, Hori T. Artificial insemination with frozen epididymal sperm in cats. J Vet Med Sci. 2003;3:397–9.
52. Sananmuang T, Tharasanit T, Nguyen C, Phutikanit N, Techakumphu M. Culture medium and embryo density influence on developmental competence and gene expression of cat embryos. Theriogenology. 2011;75:1708–19.

53. Schmidt KL, Ernst E, Byskov AG, Andersen AN, Andersen CY. Survival of primordial follicles following prolonged transportation of ovarian tissue prior to cryopreservation. Hum Reprod. 2003;18:2654–9.
54. Isachenko E, Isachenko V, Nawroth F, Rahimi G, Weiss JM. Effect of long-term exposure at suprazero temperatures on activity and viability of human ovarian cortex. Fertil Steril. 2009;91:1556–9.
55. Isachenko V, Isachenko E, Mallmann P, Rahimi G. Long-time cooling of human ovarian tissue before cryopreservation as obvious procedure: stimulation of follicular development and neo-vascularisation. Clin Lab. 2012;58:1293–300.
56. Isachenko V, Isachenko E, Mallmann P, Rahimi G. Increasing follicular and stromal cell proliferation in cryopreserved human ovarian tissue after long-term precooling prior to freezing: in vitro versus chorioallantoic membrane (CAM) xenotransplantation. Cell Transplant. 2013;22:2053–61.
57. Laronda MM, Duncan FE, Hornick JE, Xu M, Pahnke JE, Whelan KA, Shea LD, Woodruff TK. Alginate encapsulation supports the growth and differentiation of human primordial follicles within ovarian cortical tissue. J Assist Reprod Genet. 2014;31(8):1013–28.
58. Klocke S, Tappehorn C, Griesinger G. Effects of supra-zero storage on human ovarian cortex prior to vitrification-warming. Reprod BioMed Online. 2014;29(2):251–8.
59. Isachenko V, Todorov P, Isachenko E, Rahimi G, Tchorbanov A, Mihaylova N, Manoylov I, Mallmann P, Merzenich M. Long-time cooling before cryopreservation decreased translocation of phosphatidylserine (Ptd-L-Ser) in human ovarian tissue. PLoS One. 2015;10(6):e0129108.
60. Andersen CY, Rosendahl M, Byskov AG, Loft A, Ottosen C, Dueholm M, Schmidt KL, Andersen AN, Ernst E. Two successful pregnancies following autotransplantation of frozen/thawed ovarian tissue. Hum Reprod. 2008;23:2266–72.
61. Ernst E, Bergholdt S, Jorgensen JS, Andersen CY. The first woman to give birth to two children following transplantation of frozen/thawed ovarian tissue. Hum Reprod. 2010;25:1280–1.
62. Dittrich R, Lotz L, Keck G, Hoffmann I, Mueller A, Beckmann MW, van der Ven H, Montag M. Live birth after ovarian tissue autotransplantation following overnight transportation before cryopreservation. Fertil Steril. 2012;97:387–90.
63. Muller A, Keller K, Wacker J, Dittrich R, Keck G, Montag M, Van der Ven H, Wachter D, Beckmann MW, Distler W. Retransplantation of cryopreserved ovarian tissue: the first live birth in Germany. Dtsch Arztebl Int. 2012;109:8–13.
64. Andrade ER, Rodrigues AP, Amorim CA, Carvalho FC, Dode MA, Figueiredo JR. Short term maintenance of sheep preantral follicles in situ in 0.9% saline and Braun-Collins solution. Small Rumin Res. 2001;41:141–9.
65. Lucci CM, Kacinskis MA, Rumpf R, Bao SN. Effects of lowered temperatures and media on short-term preservation of zebu (Bos indicus) preantral ovarian follicles. Theriogenology. 2004;61:461–72.
66. Luvoni GC, Tessaro I, Apparício M, Ruggeri E, Luciano AM, Modina SC. Effect of vitrification of feline ovarian cortex on follicular and oocyte quality and competence. Reprod Domest Anim. 2012;47(3):385–91.
67. Tanpradit N, Comizzoli P, Srisuwatanasagul S, Chatdarong K. Positive impact of sucrose supplementation during slow freezing of cat ovarian tissues on cellular viability, follicle morphology, and DNA integrity. Theriogenology. 2015;83:1553–61.
68. Brito DCC, Domingues SFS, Silva JK, Wu X, Santos RR, Pieczarka JC. Detrimental effect of phenol red on the vitrification of cat (Felis catus) ovarian tissue. Biopreserv Biobank. 2016;14:17–22.
69. Mouttham L, Comizzoli P. The preservation of vital functions in cat ovarian tissues during vitrification depends more on the temperature of the cryoprotectant exposure than on the sucrose supplementation. Cryobiology. 2016;73(2):187–95.
70. Brito DCC, Domingues SFS, Rodrigues APR, Maside C, Lunardi FO, Wu X, Figueiredo JR, Pieczarka JC, Santos RR. Cryopreservation of domestic cat (Felis catus) ovarian tissue: comparison of two vitrification methods. Theriogenology. 2018;111:69–77.
71. Demirel MA, Acar DB, Ekim B, Çelikkan FT, Alkan KK, Salar S, Erdemli EA, Özkavukçu S, Yar SS, Kanca H, Baştan A. The evaluation of xenotransplantation of feline ovarian tissue vitrified by needle immersed vitrification technique into male immunodeficient mice. Cell Tissue Bank. 2018;19(1):133–47.
72. Albertini DF. Cytoplasmic microtubular dynamics and chromatin organization during mammalian oogenesis and oocyte maturation. Mutat Res. 1992;296:57–68.
73. Brinkley BR, Cartwright J Jr. Cold-labile and cold-stable microtubules in the mitotic spindle of mammalian cells. Ann N Y Acad Sci. 1975;253:428–39.
74. Pickering SJ, Johnson MH. The influence of cooling on the organization of the meiotic spindle of the mouse oocyte. Hum Reprod. 1987;2:207–16.
75. Vincent C, Johnson MH. Cooling, cryoprotectants, and the cytoskeleton of the mammalian oocyte. Oxf Rev Reprod Biol. 1992;14:73–100.
76. Liu RH, Sun QY, Li YH, Jiao LH, Wang WH. Effects of cooling on meiotic spindle structure and chromosome alignment within in vitro matured porcine oocytes. Mol Reprod Dev. 2003;65:212–8.
77. Evecen M, Cirit U, Demir K, Karaman E, Hamzaoglu AI, Bakirer G. Developmental competence of domestic cat oocytes from ovaries stored at various durations at 4 degrees C temperature. Anim Reprod Sci. 2009;116:169–72.
78. Devine PJ, Perreault SD, Luderer U. Roles of reactive oxygen species and antioxidants in ovarian toxicity. Biol Reprod. 2012;86:27.
79. Prasad S, Tiwari M, Pandey AN, Shrivastav TG, Chaube SK. Impact of stress on oocyte quality and reproductive outcome. J Biomed Sci. 2016;23:36.
80. Combelles CM, Gupta S, Agarwal A. Could oxidative stress influence the in-vitro maturation of oocytes? Reprod BioMed Online. 2009;18:864–80.
81. Lord T, Aitken RJ. Oxidative stress and ageing of the post-ovulatory oocyte. Reproduction. 2013;146:217–27.
82. Pastore A, Federici G, Bertini E, Piemonte F. Analysis of glutathione: implication in redox and detoxification. Clin Chim Acta. 2003;333:19–39.
83. Perreault SD, Barbee RR, Slott VL. Importance of glutathione in the acquisition and maintenance of sperm nuclear decondensing activity in maturing hamster oocytes. Dev Biol. 1988;125:181–6.
84. Yoshida M, Ishigaki K, Nagai T, Chikyu M, Pursel VG. Glutathione concentration during maturation and after fertilization in pig oocytes: relevance to the ability of oocytes to form male pronucleus. Biol Reprod. 1993;49:89–94.
85. Miyamura M, Yoshida M, Hamano S, Kuwayama M. Glutathione concentration during maturation and fertilization in bovine oocytes. Theriogenology. 1995;43:282.
86. Funahashi H, Day BN. Effect of cumulus cells on glutathione content of porcine oocytes during in vitro maturation. J Anim Sci. 1995;73:90.
87. Furnus CC, de Matos DG, Picco S, Garcia PP, Inda AM, Mattioli G, Errecalde AL. Metabolic requirements associated with GSH synthesis during *in vitro* maturation of cattle oocytes. Anim Reprod Sci. 2008;109:88–99.
88. Jiao GZ, Cao XY, Cui W, Lian HY, Miao YL, Wu XF, Han D, Tan JH. Developmental potential of prepubertal mouse oocytes is compromised due mainly to their impaired synthesis of glutathione. PLoS One. 2013;8:e58018.
89. Abazari-Kia AH, Mohammadi-Sangcheshmeh A, Dehghani-Mohammadabadi M, Jamshidi-Adegani F, Veshkini A, Zhandi M, Cinar MU, Salehi M. Intracellular glutathione content, developmental competence and expression of apoptosis-related genes associated with G6PDH-activity in goat oocyte. J Assist Reprod Genet. 2014;31:313–21.
90. Repetto M, Semprine J, Boveris A. Lipid peroxidation: chemical mechanism, biological implications and analytical determination. In: InTech, editor. Lipid Peroxidation; 2012. p. 4–29.

Permissions

All chapters in this book were first published in RBE, by BioMed Central; hereby published with permission under the Creative Commons Attribution License or equivalent. Every chapter published in this book has been scrutinized by our experts. Their significance has been extensively debated. The topics covered herein carry significant findings which will fuel the growth of the discipline. They may even be implemented as practical applications or may be referred to as a beginning point for another development.

The contributors of this book come from diverse backgrounds, making this book a truly international effort. This book will bring forth new frontiers with its revolutionizing research information and detailed analysis of the nascent developments around the world.

We would like to thank all the contributing authors for lending their expertise to make the book truly unique. They have played a crucial role in the development of this book. Without their invaluable contributions this book wouldn't have been possible. They have made vital efforts to compile up to date information on the varied aspects of this subject to make this book a valuable addition to the collection of many professionals and students.

This book was conceptualized with the vision of imparting up-to-date information and advanced data in this field. To ensure the same, a matchless editorial board was set up. Every individual on the board went through rigorous rounds of assessment to prove their worth. After which they invested a large part of their time researching and compiling the most relevant data for our readers.

The editorial board has been involved in producing this book since its inception. They have spent rigorous hours researching and exploring the diverse topics which have resulted in the successful publishing of this book. They have passed on their knowledge of decades through this book. To expedite this challenging task, the publisher supported the team at every step. A small team of assistant editors was also appointed to further simplify the editing procedure and attain best results for the readers.

Apart from the editorial board, the designing team has also invested a significant amount of their time in understanding the subject and creating the most relevant covers. They scrutinized every image to scout for the most suitable representation of the subject and create an appropriate cover for the book.

The publishing team has been an ardent support to the editorial, designing and production team. Their endless efforts to recruit the best for this project, has resulted in the accomplishment of this book. They are a veteran in the field of academics and their pool of knowledge is as vast as their experience in printing. Their expertise and guidance has proved useful at every step. Their uncompromising quality standards have made this book an exceptional effort. Their encouragement from time to time has been an inspiration for everyone.

The publisher and the editorial board hope that this book will prove to be a valuable piece of knowledge for researchers, students, practitioners and scholars across the globe.

List of Contributors

Michal Elbaz and Eran Gershon
Department of Ruminant Science, Agricultural Research Organization, 50250 Rishon LeZion, Israel

Ron Hadas
Department of Biological Regulation, Weizmann Institute of Science, 76100 Rehovot, Israel

Louise M. Bilezikjian
Clayton Foundation Laboratories for Peptide Biology and Laboratory of Neuronal Structure and Function, Salk Institute for Biological Studies, La Jolla, San Diego, CA 92037, USA

Basmah Al Omrani and Nadia Al Eisa
Zoology Department, King Saud University, Riyadh, Saudi Arabia

Murid Javed and Hamad Al Sufyan
Assisted Reproductive Technology Laboratories, Thuriah Medical Center, Riyadh, Saudi Arabia

Maher Al Ghedan
Genetics Laboratory, Thuriah Medical Center, Riyadh, Saudi Arabia

Hamoud AlMatrafi
Urology and Andrology Unit, Thuriah Medical Center, Riyadh, Saudi Arabia

Kristian Leisegangs
School of Natural Medicine, University of the Western Cape, Private Bag X17, Bellville 7535, South Africa

Ralf Henkel
Department of Medical Biosciences, University of the Western Cape, Private Bag X17, Bellville 7535, South Africa

Yanwen Jiang, Yun Zhao, Shuxiong Chen, Lu Chen, Chunjin Li and Xu Zhou
College of Animal Science, Jilin University, 5333 Xian Road, Changchun, Jilin 130062, China

Shaoquan Zhan, Shanbo Cao, Hongzi Du, Yuan Sun, Li Li, Haiyan Zheng and Junjiu Huang
Center for Reproductive Medicine, Key Laboratory for Reproductive Medicine of Guangdong Province, Key Laboratory for Major Obstetric Diseases of Guangdong Province, and Key Laboratory for Reproduction and Genetics of Guangdong Higher Education Institutes, the Third Affiliated Hospital of Guangzhou Medical University, Guangzhou 510150, China

Shanbo Cao
Beijing Acorndx Biotechnology Co. Ltd, Beijing 100176, China

Chenhui Ding and Junjiu Huang
Key Laboratory of Reproductive Medicine of Guangdong Province, School of Life Sciences and the First Affiliated Hospital, Sun Yat-sen University, Guangzhou 510275, China

Angela Köninger, Annette Mathan, Pawel Mach, Rainer Kimmig and Alexandra Gellhaus
Department of Gynecology and Obstetrics, University of Duisburg-Essen, Hufelandstrasse 55, 45122 Essen, Germany

Annette Mathan
Department of Gynecology and Obstetrics, Klinikum Würzburg Mitte, Salvatorstrasse 7, 97074 Würzburg, Germany

Mirjam Frank and Boerge Schmidt
Institute for Medical Informatics, Biometry and Epidemiology (IMIBE), University of Duisburg-Essen, Hufelandstrasse 55, 45122 Essen Germany

Ekkehard Schleussner
Department of Obstetrics, Jena University Hospital, Am Klinikum 1, 07747 Jena, Germany

Hans Dieplinger
Division of Genetic Epidemiology, Department of Medical Genetics, Molecular and Clinical Pharmacology, Medical University of Innsbruck, Schöpfstrasse 41, 6020 Innsbruck, Austria Vitateq Biotechnology GmbH, 6020 Innsbruck, Austria

Hongjuan Ye, Hui Tian and Lihua Sun
Centre of assisted reproduction, Shanghai East Hospital, Tongji University, Shanghai, People's Republic of China

Wen He, Qifeng Lyu, Yanping Kuang and Qiuju Chen
Department of Assisted Reproduction, Shanghai Ninth People's Hospital, Shanghai Jiaotong University School of Medicine, Shanghai, People's Republic of China

Irma Virant-Klun and Andrej Vogler
Reproductive Unit, Department of Obstetrics and Gynecology, University Medical Centre Ljubljana, Zaloska cesta 002, 1000 Ljubljana, SI, Slovenia

Viola Maria Schmidt, Vladimir Isachenko, Gohar Rahimi, Bettina Hanstein, Bernd Morgenstern, Peter Mallmann and Evgenia Isachenko
Research Group for Reproductive Medicine and IVF-Laboratory, Department of Obstetrics and Gynaecology, University Maternal Hospital, Cologne University, Kerpener Str. 34, 50931 Cologne, Germany

Gunter Rappl
Cell Sort Service Department, Center for Molecular Medicine Cologne University (CMMC), Robert Koch Str. 21, 50931 Cologne, Germany

Menglu Ji, Xingling Wang, Wenbin Wu, Yichun Guan, Jing Liu, Jingyan Wang, Wenxia Liu and Chunyan Shen
Department of Reproductive Medical Center, Third Affiliated Hospital of Zhengzhou University, 7 Kangfuqian Road, Zhengzhou 450052, Henan, People's Republic of China

Chen-Yu Huang, Guan-Yeu Chen, Miawh-Lirng Shieh and Hsin-Yang Li
Division of Reproductive Endocrinology and Infertility, Department of Obstetrics and Gynecology, Taipei Veterans General Hospital, 201, Shih-Pai Road Section 2, Taipei 112, Taiwan, Republic of China

Hsin-Yang Li
Division of Obstetrics and Gynecology, Faculty of Medicine, School of Medicine, National Yang-Ming University, Taipei, Taiwan, Republic of China

Chen-Yu Huang
Institute of Clinical Medicine, National Yang-Ming University, Taipei, Taiwan, Republic of China

Semra Kahraman, Caroline Pirkevi Çetinkaya, Murat Çetinkaya, Mehmet Ali Tüfekçi and Cumhur Gökhan Ekmekçi
Istanbul Memorial Hospital, Assisted Reproductive Technologies and Reproductive Genetics Centre, Piyale Pasa Bulvari 34385 Okmeydani Sisli, Istanbul, Turkey

Markus Montag
ilabcomm GmbH, Eisenachstr. 34, 53757 Sankt Augustin, Germany

Bo Liang, Ling Wu, Hui Xu, Chun Wai Cheung, Wen Ying Fung, Sze Wai Wong and Chi Chiu Wang
Department of Obstetrics and Gynaecology, The Chinese University of Hong Kong, c/o 1st Floor, Special Block E, Prince of Wales Hospital, Shatin, Hong Kong

Chi Chiu Wang
Reproduction and Development Laboratory, Li Ka Shing Institute of Health Sciences, The Chinese University of Hong Kong, Shatin, Hong Kong
School of Biomedical Sciences, The Chinese University of Hong Kong, Shatin, Hong Kong

Laura Falchi, Gian Mario Dore, Maria Teresa Zedda, Salvatore Pau, Luisa Bogliolo, Federica Ariu, Stefano Nieddu and Sergio Ledda
Dipartimento di Medicina Veterinaria, Università degli Studi di Sassari, Sassari, Italy

Grazia Galleri
Dipartimento di Medicina Clinica e Sperimentale, Università degli Studi di Sassari, Sassari, Italy

Alessandra Pinna
Department of Materials, Imperial College London, South Kensington Campus, London, UK

Plinio Innocenzi
Dipartimento di Chimica e Farmacia, Università degli Studi di Sassari, Sassari, Italy

Jean Damascene Niringiyumukiza, Hongcai Cai and Wenpei Xiang
Family Planning Research Institute/Center of Reproductive Medicine, Tongji Medical College, Huazhong University of Science and Technology, Wuhan 430030, Hubei, China

T. Arthur Chang, Gennadiy I. Bondarenko, Behzad Gerami-Naini, Jessica G. Drenzek, Maureen Durning, Mark A. Garthwaite, Jenna Kropp Schmidt and Thaddeus G. Golos
Wisconsin National Primate Research Center, University of Wisconsin-Madison, 1223 Capitol Court, Madison, Wisconsin 53715-1299, USA

Thaddeus G. Golos
Department of Comparative Biosciences, School of Veterinary Medicine, University of Wisconsin-Madison, Madison, WI, USA
Department of Obstetrics and Gynecology, School of Medicine and Public Health, University of Wisconsin-Madison, Madison, WI, USA

T. Arthur Chang
Department of Obstetrics and Gynecology, University of Texas Health Science Center, San Antonio, TX, USA

Gennadiy I. Bondarenko
Covance Laboratories, Madison, WI, USA

Behzad Gerami-Naini
School of Dental Medicine, Tufts University, Boston, MA, USA

Jessica G. Drenzek
Illumina-Madison, Madison, WI, USA

Xin Huang, Jiaping Pan, Bi Wu and Xiaoming Teng
Department of Assisted Reproductive Medicine, Shanghai First Maternity and Infant Hospital, Tongji University School of Medicine, 2699 Gaoke Road West, Shanghai 200001, People's Republic of China

Lei Dou, Yahong Zheng, Lu Li, Xiaowei Gui and Yi Guo
Department of Obstetrics and gynecology, First Affiliated Hospital of China Medical University, Shenyang 110001, China

Yajuan Chen
Department of Obstetrics and gynecology, Anshan Branch of First Affiliated Hospital of China Medical University, Anshan, China

Meng Yu
Department of Reproductive Biology and Transgenic Animals, China Medical University, Shenyang, China

Hyo-Jin Park
College of Engineering, Daegu University, Biotechnology, Gyeongsan, South Korea

Dong Gil Lee, Jung Bae Seong, Hyun-Shik Lee, Oh-Shin Kwon, Beom Sik Kang, Jeen-woo Park, and Dong-Seok Lee
School of Life Sciences, BK21 Plus KNU Creative BioResearch Group, Kyungpook National University, Daegu, South Korea

Sang-Rae Lee
Korea Research Institute of Bioscience and Biotechnology (KRIBB), National Primate Research Center (NPRC), Daejeon, South Korea

Dong-Seok Lee
College of Natural Sciences, Kyungpook National University, Daegu 702-701, Republic of Korea

Clive J. Petry, Liangjian Lu, Philippa Prentice, Ieuan A. Hughes, Carlo L. Acerini Ken K. Ong and David B. Dun
Department of Paediatrics, University of Cambridge, Cambridge Biomedical Campus, Hills Road, Cambridge CB2 0QQ, UK

Albert Koulman, Benjamin Jenkins and Lee Matthews
Medical Research Council Human Nutrition Research, Cambridge, UK

Albert Koulman, Samuel Furse, Ken K. Ong and David B. Dun
The Institute of Metabolic Science, University of Cambridge, Cambridge, UK

Liangjian Lu
Khoo Teck Puat-National University Children's Medical Institute, National University Hospital, National University Health System, Singapore, Singapore

Ken K. Ong
Medical Research Council Epidemiology Unit, University of Cambridge, Cambridge, UK

Monika Answal and Vijay Prabha
Department of Microbiology, Panjab University, Chandigarh 160014, India

Anna Rita Piras, Giovanni Pietro Burrai, Federica Ariu, Laura Falchi, Maria Teresa Zedda, Salvatore Pau, Sergio Domenico Gadau, Elisabetta Antuofermo, Daniela Bebbere, Sergio Ledda and Luisa Bogliolo
Department of Veterinary Medicine, University of Sassari, Via Vienna 2, 07100 Sassari, Italy

Index

www.ingramcontent.com/pod-product-compliance
Lightning Source LLC
LaVergne TN
LVHW080735210926
848485LV00003B/564